Handbook of Neurosurgery, Neurology, and Spinal Medicine for Nurses and Advanced Practice Health Professionals

This practical handbook allows nurses, physician assistants, and allied health professionals practicing in the fields of neurosurgery, neurology, and spinal care to quickly review essentials while in the work environment. It emphasizes procedural steps and critical elements in patient management, including intensive care, the neurological examination, differential diagnoses, and pain management. Written by a multidisciplinary team of experts, this handbook is expected to become a well-worn companion and essential aid to the busy practitioner.

Handbook of Neurosurgery, Neurology, and Spinal Medicine for Nurses and Advanced Practice Health Professionals

Edited by
Michael Y. Wang, Andrea L. Strayer, Odette A. Harris,
Cathy M. Rosenberg, Praveen V. Mummaneni

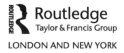

Routledge
Taylor & Francis Group

LONDON AND NEW YORK

Thank you to Roberto Suazo, Graphic Design Project Manager for the Department of Neurological Surgery, University of Miami Miller School of Medicine, who drew the majority of the figures.

First published 2018
by Routledge
711 Third Avenue, New York, NY 10017
and by Routledge
2 Park Square, Milton Park, Abingdon, Oxon, OX14 4RN

Routledge is an imprint of the Taylor & Francis Group, an informa business
© 2018 Taylor & Francis

International Standard Book Number-13: 978-1-1385-5695-9 (Hardback)

The right of Michael Y. Wang, Andrea L. Strayer, Odette A. Harris, Cathy M. Rosenberg and Praveen V. Mummaneni to be identified as the author of the editorial material, and of the authors for their individual chapters, has been asserted in accordance with sections 77 and 78 of the Copyright, Designs and Patents Act 1988.

Library of Congress Cataloging-in-Publication Data

Names: Wang, Michael Y., 1971- editor. | Strayer, Andrea, editor. | Harris,
Odette A., editor. | Rosenberg, Cathy, 1963- editor. | Mummaneni, Praveen V., editor.
Title: Handbook of neurosurgery, neurology, and spinal medicine for nurses
and advanced practice health professionals / edited by Michael Wang,
Andrea Strayer, Odette Harris, Cathy Rosenberg, Praveen Mummaneni.
Description: Abingdon, Oxon ; New York, NY : Routledge, 2018. | Includes
bibliographical references and index.
Identifiers: LCCN 2017028274| ISBN 9781138556959 (hardback) | ISBN
9781498719421 (pbk.) | ISBN 9781315382760 (ebook)
Subjects: | MESH: Nervous System Diseases | Neurosurgical Procedures--nursing
| Neurologic Examination--nursing | Perioperative Care--nursing
Classification: LCC RC350.5 | NLM WL 140 | DDC 616.8/04231–dc23
LC record available at https://lccn.loc.gov/2017028274

Visit the Taylor & Francis Web site at
http://www.taylorandfrancis.com

and the CRC Press Web site at
http://www.crcpress.com

CONTENTS

Contents

CONTRIBUTORS

Aminul I. Ahmed, MD, PhD
Miami Project to Cure Paralysis
Miller School of Medicine
University of Miami
Coral Gables, Florida

Junyoung Ahn, BS
Department of Orthopedic Surgery
Rush University Medical Center
Chicago, Illinois

Vincent J. Alentado, BS
Department of Neurological Surgery
Cleveland Clinic Center for Spine Health
    and
Case Western Reserve University School of
    Medicine
Cleveland, Ohio

Khalid Al-Rayess, MD
Department of Neurosurgery
University of California San Francisco
San Francisco, California

Arun Paul Amar, MD
Department of Neurosurgery
Keck School of Medicine
University of Southern California
    and
LAC+USC Medical Center
Los Angeles, California

Jimmi Amick, RN, BSN
Children's of Alabama Section of Pediatric
    Neurosurgery
University of Alabama School of Medicine
Birmingham, Alabama

Jaclyn Baloga, MPAS, PA-C
University of Miami Hospital and Clinics
Miami, Florida

Gregory Basil, MD
Department of Neurological Surgery
Miller School of Medicine
University of Miami
Miami, Florida

Mustafa Baskaya, MD
Department of Neurological Surgery
University of Wisconsin Medical School
Madison, Wisconsin

**J.J. Baumann, MS, RN, CNS-BC, CNRN,
    SCRN**
Department of Neurosurgery
Stanford Stroke Center
Stanford University School of Medicine
Stanford, California

Marianne J. Beare, RN, MSN, ANP-BC
Department of Neurosciences
Inova Medical Group—Neurosurgery
Fairfax, Virginia

Bianca Belcher, MPH, PA-C
Department of Neurosurgery
Brigham and Women's Hospital
Boston, Massachusetts

Teresa Bell-Stephens, RN, BSN, CNRN
Department of Neurosurgery
Stanford Stroke Center
Stanford University School of Medicine
Stanford, California

David Benglis, MD
Atlanta Brain and Spine Care
Atlanta, Georgia

Nicole Bennett, MS, RN, ACNS-BC, APNP, CNRN, SCRN
Comprehensive Stroke Program
University of Wisconsin Hospital and Clinics
Madison, Wisconsin

Karen Bond, PA-C
Center for Spine Health
Cleveland Clinic
Cleveland, Ohio

Christine Boone, BS, MD, PhD
Department of Neurological Surgery
Johns Hopkins University School of Medicine
Baltimore, Maryland

Nadine Bradley, RN, BSN
Children's of Alabama Section of Pediatric Neurosurgery
University of Alabama School of Medicine
Birmingham, Alabama

M. Ross Bullock, MD, PhD
Miami Project to Cure Paralysis
Miller School of Medicine
University of Miami
Coral Gables, Florida

Stephen S. Burks, MD
Department of Neurological Surgery
Miller School of Medicine
Lois Pope LIFE Center
University of Miami
Miami, Florida

S. Shelby Burks, MD
Department of Neurological Surgery
Miller School of Medicine
Lois Pope LIFE Center
University of Miami
Miami, Florida

Simon Buttrick, MD
Department of Neurosurgery
School of Medicine
University of Miami
Miami, Florida

Adriana L. Castano, APN-C, RNFA
Atlantic Neurosurgical Specialists
Morristown, New Jersey

Yi-Ren Chen, MD
Department of Neurosurgery
Stanford University School of Medicine
Stanford Health Center
Stanford, California

Cheng-Hsin Cheng, MD
University of California San Francisco
San Francisco, California

LeAnn DeRungs, BSN, MSN, APNP
School of Medicine and Public Health
Division of Geriatrics and Adult Development
University of Wisconsin
Madison, Wisconsin

Sanjay Dhall, MD
Department of Neurological Surgery
University of California
San Francisco, California

Marine Dididze, MD, PhD
Miami Project to Cure Paralysis
Miller School of Medicine
University of Miami
Miami, Florida

Gabriel Duhancioglu, MS
Chicago Medical School
North Chicago, Illinois

Yoshua Esquenazi, MD
Department of Neurological Surgery
University of Texas Health
Houston, Texas

Colleen M. Foley, MS, RN, ACNS-BC, AGPCNP-BC, APNP
UW Health
University of Wisconsin Madison
Madison, Wisconsin

Erika Freiberg, PA-C
Boulder Neurosurgical and Spine Associates
Boulder, Colorado

Tristan Fried, BS
Thomas Jefferson University
Philadelphia, Pennsylvania

Bruno V. Gallo, MD
Department of Neurology
University of Miami
Miami, Florida

Jamshid Ghajar, MD, PhD
Department of Neurosurgery
Stanford University School of Medicine
Stanford Health Center
Stanford, California

George M. Ghobrial, MD
Department of Neurological Surgery
Miller School of Medicine
Lois Pope LIFE Center
University of Miami
Miami, Florida

C. Rory Goodwin, MD
Department of Neurological Surgery
Johns Hopkins
Baltimore, Maryland

Odette A. Harris, MD, MPH
Associate Professor, Neurosurgery
Brain Injury
Stanford University School of Medicine
and
Rehabilitation
(Polytrauma, SCI/D, BRS, PM&R)
Defense Veterans Brain Injury Center
VA Palo Alto HCS
Palo Alto, California

James S. Harrop, MD, FACS
Department of Neurological Surgery
Thomas Jefferson University Hospital
Philadelphia, Pennsylvania

Rachel Hart, DNP, AGACNP-BC
UW Health
University of Wisconsin Hospital
Madison, Wisconsin

Roger Härtl
Department of Neurological Surgery
Weill Cornell Brain and Spine Center
Weill Cornell Medical College
New York, New York

Luke R. Hattenhauer, DNP, CRNA
Department of Anesthesiology
University of Wisconsin School of Medicine and
Public Health
Madison, Wisconsin

Alisabeth C. Hearron, DNP, ARNP-C
Miami Neurological Institute
Miami, Florida

Jeffrey Hernandez, BSN, RN, MSCN
Multiple Sclerosis Center of
Excellence
Miller School of Medicine
University of Miami
Miami, Florida

Daniel J. Hoh, MD
Department of Neurological Surgery
University of Florida
Gainesville, Florida

Honglian Huang, MD, PhD
Physical Medicine and Rehabilitation
Cleveland Clinic Foundation
Cleveland, Ohio

Christina Hughes, MMS, PA-C
Department of Neurological Surgery
Johns Hopkins
Baltimore, Maryland

Danielle Hulsebus, ACNP-BC
Department of Neurosurgery
University of Michigan
Ann Arbor, Michigan

Tricia Jette-Gonthier, APRN
Bone and Joint Center
Southern New Hampshire Medical Center
Nashua, New Hampshire

Eli Johnson, BS
Department of Neurosurgery
Stanford School of Medicine
Stanford Health Center
Stanford, California

Sara Kadlec, PA-C
Boulder Neurosurgical and Spine Associates
Boulder, Colorado

Rahul Kamath, MS
Chicago Medical School
North Chicago, Illinois

Megan Keiser, RN, DNP, CNRN, ACNS-BC, NP-C
Department of Nursing
University of Michigan–Flint
Flint, Michigan

John Kenneally, MSW, LCSW
University of Wisconsin Hospital
Madison, Wisconsin

Daniel Kim, MD
Department of Neurological Surgery
University of Texas–Houston
Houston, Texas

Alison Kirkpatrick, OTR
Department of Neurological Surgery
Miller School of Medicine
Lois Pope LIFE Center
University of Miami
Miami, Florida

Ricardo Komotar, MD
Department of Neurological Surgery
Miller School of Medicine
Lois Pope LIFE Center
University of Miami
Miami, Florida

Wendell B. Lake, MD
Department of Neurosurgery
University of Wisconsin School of
    Medicine and Public Health
Madison, Wisconsin

John Lee, MD
Physical Medicine and Rehabilitation
Cleveland Clinic Foundation
Cleveland, Ohio

Elizabeth Lee, RN, GNP, FNP, AANP
Department of Neurosurgery
Stanford Healthcare
Palo Alto, California

Allan D. Levi, MD, PhD
Miller School of Medicine
University of Miami
Miami, Florida

Yiping Li, MD
Department of Neurological Surgery
University of Wisconsin Medical School
Madison, Wisconsin

Dennis T. Lockney, MD
Department of Neurological Surgery
University of Florida
Gainesville, Florida

Karthik Madhavan, MD
Department of Neurological Surgery
Miller School of Medicine
Lois Pope LIFE Center
University of Miami
Miami, Florida

Janice Y. Maldonado, MD
Multiple Sclerosis Center of
  Excellence
Miller School of Medicine
University of Miami
Miami, Florida

Martha Mangum, ACNP-BC
Department of Neurosurgery
University of Michigan
Ann Arbor, Michigan

Álvaro Martín Gallego
Department of Neurosurgery
HRU de Málaga
Málaga, Spain

Eric Mayer, MD
Center for Spine Health
Cleveland Clinic
Cleveland, Ohio

Cristina Matthews, MSN, FNP-BC
Department of Neurosurgery
Massachusetts General Hospital
Boston, Massachusetts

Chelsie McCarthy
Department of Neurological Surgery
Weill Cornell Brain and Spine Center
Weill Cornell Medical College
New York, New York

Scott A. Meyer, MD
Atlantic Neuroscience Institute
Morristown Medical Center
  and
Atlantic Neurosurgical Specialists
Morristown, New Jersey

Jacques Morcos, MD
Department of Neurological
  Surgery
University of Miami
Coral Gables, Florida

Praveen V. Mummaneni, MD
Department of Neurological Surgery
University of California San Francisco
San Francisco, California

Valli Mummaneni, MD
Department of Anesthesiology
University of California San Francisco
San Francisco, California

Junichi Ohya, MD
Department of Neurological Surgery
University of California San Francisco
San Francisco, California

Solomon Ondoma, MD
Department of Neurological Surgery
University of Wisconsin Medical School
Madison, Wisconsin

Christine Orlina Macasieb, ACNP-BC
Department of Neurological Surgery
University of California San Francisco
San Francisco, California

Candice Osuga Lin, RN MSN ACNP-BC
Department of Neurosurgery
Stanford Healthcare
Stanford, California

Nelson M. Oyesiku
Neurosurgery
Emory University
Atlanta, Georgia

Paul Park, MD
Department of Neurosurgery
University of Michigan
Ann Arbor, Michigan

Sherri Patchen, ARNP
University of Miami
Miami, Florida

Nirav Patel, MD, MA
Department of Neurosurgery
Brigham and Women's Hospital
Boston, Massachusetts

Valentina Pennacchietti, MD
Dipartimento di Neuroscienze
Università degli Studi di Torino
Torino, Italia

Ruth Perez, ARAP
University of Miami
Miami, Florida

Laura Ellen Prado, MSN, NP
Atlanta Brain and Spine Care
Atlanta, Georgia

Sharad Rajpal, MD
Boulder Neurosurgical and Spine Associates
Boulder, Colorado

Daniel K. Resnick, MD
Department of Neurological Surgery
University of Wisconsin School of Medicine and
    Public Health
Madison, Wisconsin

Angela Richardson, MD
Department of Neurological Surgery
University of Miami
Miami, Florida

Brandon G. Rocque, MD, MS
Department of Neurosurgery
University of Alabama School of Medicine
Birmingham, Alabama

Cathy M. Rosenberg, ARNP
Department of Neurological Surgery
University of Miami
Coral Gables, Florida

Michael Safaee, MD
University of California
San Francisco, California

Carolina Sandoval-Garcia, MD
Department of Neurological Surgery
University of Wisconsin School of Medicine and
    Public Health
Madison, Wisconsin

Christina Sayama, MD, MPH
Department of Neurological Surgery
Oregon Health and Science University
Portland, Oregon

Gregory D. Schroeder, MD
The Rothman Institute
Thomas Jefferson University
Philadelphia, Pennsylvania

Danial M. Sciubba, MD
Johns Hopkins University School of Medicine
Baltimore, Maryland

Katie Shpanskaya, BS
Department of Neurosurgery
Stanford School of Medicine
Stanford Health Center
Stanford, California

Kristina Shultz, MSN, NP-C
Department of Neurosurgery
Massachusetts General Hospital
Boston, Massachusetts

Krishana Sichinga, MHS, PA-C
Department of Neurosurgery
Penn State Milton S. Hershey Medical Center
Hershey, Pennsylvania

Lauren N. Simpson, MD, MPH
Department of Neurological Surgery
Oregon Health and Science University
Portland, Oregon

Kern Singh, MD
Department of Orthopedic Surgery
Rush University Medical Center
Chicago, Illinois

**Sandra Stafford Cecil, RN, MSN, CNL,
    CRRN, CEN**
Polytrauma Rehabilitation
VA Palo Alto Health Care System
Palo Alto, California

Christie Stawicki, BS
Thomas Jefferson University
Philadelphia, Pennsylvania

Jasmin Stefani, FNP-C
Division of Neurological Surgery
Barrow Neurological Institute
St. Joseph's Hospital and Medical Center
Phoenix, Arizona

Gary K. Steinberg, MD, PhD
Department of Neurosurgery
Stanford Stroke Center
Stanford University School of Medicine
Stanford, California

Michael P. Steinmetz, MD
Chairman, Department of Neurosurgery
Cleveland Clinic Lerner College of Medicine
Cleveland, Ohio

**Andrea L. Strayer, MS, AGPCNP-BC,
    CNRN**
Department of Neurological Surgery
University of Wisconsin School of Medicine and
    Public Health
Madison, Wisconsin

Kyle Swanson, MD
Department of Neurosurgery
University of Wisconsin School of Medicine and
    Public Health
Madison, Wisconsin

Laura Sweeney, RN, CRNP
Department of Neurological Surgery
Thomas Jefferson University Hospital
Philadelphia, Pennsylvania

Khoi D. Than, MD
Department of Neurological Surgery
Oregon Health and Science University
Portland, Oregon

Nancy Thomas, PhD, NP
Department of Neurosurgery
University of Michigan
Ann Arbor, Michigan

Leticia Tornes, MD
Multiple Sclerosis Center of Excellence
Miller School of Medicine
University of Miami
Miami, Florida

Gregory R. Trost, MD, FAANS
Department of Neurological Surgery
University of Wisconsin School of Medicine and
    Public Health
Madison, Wisconsin

Luis M. Tumialán, MD
Barrow Neurological Institute
St. Joseph's Hospital and Medical Center
Phoenix, Arizona

Tammy L. Tyree, ACNP
Division of Neurological Surgery
Barrow Neurological Institute
St. Joseph's Hospital and Medical Center
Phoenix, Arizona

Timur M. Urakov, MD
Department of Neurological Surgery
Miller School of Medicine
University of Miami
Miami, Florida

Alexander R. Vaccaro, MD, PhD
The Rothman Institute
Thomas Jefferson University
Philadelphia, Pennsylvania

Joli Vavao, MSN, ACNP, CNRN
Department of Neurosurgery
Stanford Stroke Center
Stanford University School of Medicine
Stanford, California

Nancy E. Villanueva, PhD, CRNP, BC, CNRN
Department of Neurosurgery
Temple University
Philadelphia, Pennsylvania

Jennifer A. Viner, NP
University of California
San Francisco, California

Michael Virk, MD, PhD
Department of Neurosurgery
Cornell University
New York, New York

Nilesh A. Vyas, MD, FAANS
Inova Medical Group Neurosurgery
Inova Health System
Fairfax, Virginia

Kelly Walters, MSN, CRRN, CNP
Cleveland Clinic Foundation
Physical Medicine and Rehabilitation
Cleveland, Ohio

Amy Wang, OTR
Department of Neurological Surgery
Miller School of Medicine
Lois Pope LIFE Center
University of Miami
Miami, Florida

Michael Y. Wang, MD
Department of Neurological Surgery
Miller School of Medicine
Lois Pope LIFE Center
University of Miami
Miami, Florida

Patrick Wang
Department of Neurological Surgery
Miller School of Medicine
Lois Pope LIFE Center
University of Miami
Miami, Florida

Angela Wolfe, ARNP
Department of Neurological Surgery
University of Florida
Gainesville, Florida

PART I

Introduction

1

THE IMPORTANCE OF NEUROLOGICAL ILLNESSES, EMERGENCIES, AND TREATMENTS

S. Shelby Burks and Michael Y. Wang

Many neurological illnesses are debilitating, but within the discipline of neurosurgery there is a broad range of pathology. In a large majority of instances patients under the care of the neurology or neurosurgical service are going through one of the most impactful events in their lives. Families and patients will depend on vigilant providers to walk them through this complex landscape. The "high stakes" conditions that come with neurosurgical diseases stem from the unforgiving nature of the nervous system and its crucial role in human function. Understanding the nuances of such critical situations will make an enormous difference to patients seen in the emergency room, intensive care unit, hospital floor, and even outpatient setting. Currently, the largest expansion of providers in this area has been advanced practitioners, primarily nurse practitioners and physician assistants. For this reason, the practitioner treating these patients may need to be especially knowledgeable, vigilant, and compassionate.

A review of some common neurological and neurosurgical conditions is informative:

- Patients with severe traumatic brain injuries have high rates of mortality, up to approximately 40% in some series (Rosenfeld et al., 2012). In the acute setting, a failure to recognize an intracranial hematoma can lead to a vegetative state or death (Figure 1.1).
- After trauma, plain cervical spine radiographs can miss spinal fractures in up to 15% of cases (Griffen et al., 2003). Failure to order three-dimensional imaging such as a computed tomography (CT) scan or to use a detailed clinical examination to evaluate the patient can lead to a missed diagnosis and loss of neurological function, including paralysis (Figure 1.2).
- The concept of a "Stroke Alert" or "Brain Attack" was developed to emphasize the importance of rapid action when neurological tissues are at risk. Opportunities now exist with endovascular therapy and intravenous "clot busting" thrombolytics to provide blood supply in the setting of ischemic stroke. It has been shown that for every 3.2 patients treated emergently, one will have regained functional independence as a direct result of the intervention (Campbell et al., 2015). Hemorrhagic strokes also may require emergent treatment to stop active bleeding or to relieve elevated intracranial pressure (Figure 1.3).
- New-onset seizures in the middle-aged patient with headaches (consistent with elevated intracranial pressure) are often a presenting feature in primary or metastatic brain tumors (Figure 1.4). Many of these patients will go on to require surgery and adjuvant treatments. However, all will require intensive and balanced discussions through the process of achieving a diagnosis, formulating a treatment

3

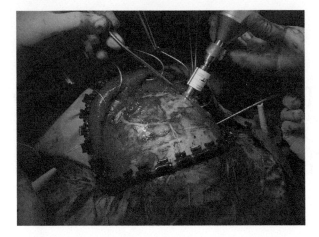

Figure 1.1 A patient undergoing an emergent craniotomy to evacuate a hematoma from head trauma.

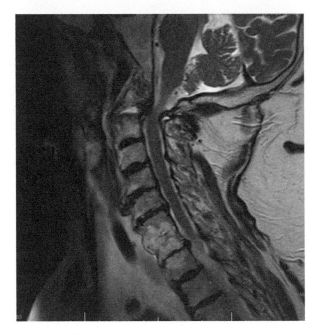

Figure 1.2 This 82-year-old man fell and suffered a C2 fracture of the odontoid. Failure to recognize it led to increasing instability and eventual partial quadriparesis due to compression of the spinal cord.

plan, and executing upon it. Many of these neoplasms, such as a glioblastoma, are uniformly aggressive and fatal.

• Traumatic spinal cord injuries are particularly devastating, largely because young, active males in the prime of their lives are the most commonly affected (Figure 1.5). In cases of cervical cord injury, the chance of conversion by at least one American Spinal Injury Association (ASIA) Grade is nearly 60% but the timing of spinal cord decompression plays an important role in optimizing recovery (Fehlings et al., 2012). Neurosurgical teams must work to get the patient to the operating room quickly and safely in order to impact outcomes.

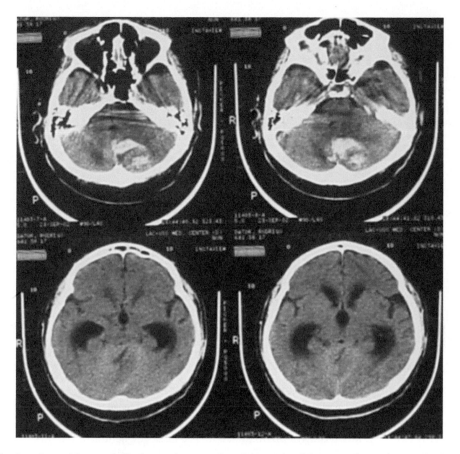

Figure 1.3 A patient with a cerebellar hemorrhage causing obstruction of the ventricles with acute hydrocephalus requiring emergent ventricular drainage to relieve life-threatening intracranial pressure.

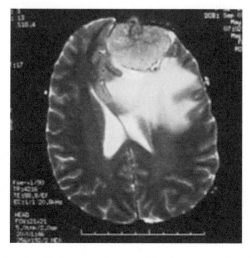

Figure 1.4 A 52 year old who developed seizures and personality changes was found to have this large right frontal extra-axial brain tumor with compression of the brain and surrounding edema.

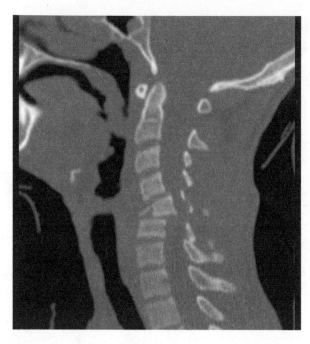

Figure 1.5 An 18-year-old male who fell from a tree and suffered a C5 fracture and accompanying ASIA Grade A (complete quadriplegia) spinal cord injury.

These facets of neurological and neurosurgical care have led to the concentration of specialization at tertiary care centers. In fact, one of the major differentiators in the designation of a level I trauma center versus a level II trauma center is the availability of 24-hour emergency neurosurgical care.

The formation of specialized treatment centers in the university setting has been the result of an increasing awareness of the disproportionate burden of neurological conditions on an ever aging population. Alzheimer's disease, Parkinson's disease, degenerative spinal arthritis, and peripheral nerve disorders all increase with age and have a disproportionate social, economic, and psychological impact on patient populations. The concentration of clinical expertise, basic research labs, and clinical trials in specific centers affords an economy of scale.

There are numerous impediments to neurological and neurosurgical care, including

- The need for highly trained personnel at all levels of the medical team
- Dependency on expensive capital equipment
- Specialized training of nurses, therapists, and ancillary support personnel to recognize and respond appropriately to nonintuitive clinical symptoms and signs
- Intensive rehabilitation programs and facilities
- Dedication to this challenging but rapidly advancing arena of medicine

In the practices of neurology and neurosurgery, the impact on the lives of patients and their families quickly becomes clear. This is especially pronounced in the situations mentioned above. Caring for these patients unifies practitioners and is extremely rewarding but requires dedication and effort.

Common pitfalls and medicolegal concerns

- Trusting the neurological exam by those unfamiliar with neurosurgical patients
- Finding a balance between swift and thorough care
- Recognizing secondary gain in the patient
- Advising the patient and his or her family of the risks associated with a particular procedure and confirming understanding

Relevance to the advanced practice health professional

Seamless communication between members of a neurosurgical team improves patient safety and outcomes. Understanding the importance of neurological illnesses, emergencies, and treatments allows the advanced practitioner to provide prompt attention and consider the potential disasters.

References

Campbell BC, Donnan GA, Lees KR, et al. Endovascular stent thrombectomy: the new standard of care for large vessel ischaemic stroke. *Lancet Neurol.* August 2015; 14(8):846–854.

Fehlings MG, Vaccaro A, Wilson JR, et al. Early versus delayed decompression for traumatic cervical spinal cord injury: results of the Surgical Timing in Acute Spinal Cord Injury Study (STASCIS). *PloS One.* 2012;7(2):e32037.

Griffen MM, Frykberg ER, Kerwin AJ, et al. Radiographic clearance of blunt cervical spine injury: plain radiograph or computed tomography scan? *J Trauma.* August 2003;55(2):222–226; discussion 226–227.

Rosenfeld JV, Maas AI, Bragge P, Morganti-Kossmann MC, Manley GT, Gruen RL. Early management of severe traumatic brain injury. *Lancet.* September 22, 2012; 380(9847):1088–1098.

2

NEUROLOGICAL DECOMPENSATION AND EMERGENCIES

Nirav Patel and Bianca Belcher

Decompensation and emergencies

We believe identifying and managing emergencies and neurological decline are among the most important skills for anyone taking care of neurologically injured patients; it is Neurosurgery 101, but this can take time to master. This short list of emergencies will serve you well when things go badly, and they *will* go badly.

We have to trust our examination, and that of our colleagues, especially in this day of hand-offs. For example, when the sign-out was "moving all fours" through the night, but the patient's left arm is weaker on morning rounds, we must believe this is a change that needs to be pursued right away. Furthermore, we should take exam changes seriously, ruling out the worst etiologies first, rather than attributing a change to a benign reason, such as "not sleeping well" or "maybe we should just give him time."

It is important to stay flexible in one's mind about the diagnosis of a patient when the patient's exam is changing. It is important to reevaluate a working diagnosis, even though it may be endorsed by others or in the chart since admission.

The emergencies listed below need swift, correct diagnosis and proper action. The exact etiology can be worked out later, since many etiologies converge in a common pathway of emergency (e.g., hematoma, brain tumor, and hydrocephalus if untreated lead to herniation). For this reason, we have listed the emergency, how it may present, and options for management, as well as provided a short explanation next to the recommendations.

When called about a change, I ask myself, "What's the worst mistake I can make here?" This way, I can rule out the life-threatening issues first.

"Need to know neurosurgical emergencies"

Brain herniation and coma

Herniation and coma happen when a mass (blood, cerebrospinal fluid [CSF], or tumor) is pushing on the brain causing dysfunction. The mass effect may force the brain to herniate out of a dural opening since the skull is unable to expand to accommodate the mass.

Red flag physical findings

- Motor changes such as hemiparesis due to compression of internal capsule.
- Pupillary changes due to compression of the third nerve against the tentorium.
- A decline in consciousness due to brainstem compression; may be subtle early in herniation and appear as confusion, or even anxiousness.

Treatment

- Elevate the head of the bed to greater than 30°.
  - *Reason*: By increasing venous outflow, there is a decrease in intracranial pressure (ICP).
- Osmotics: Administer mannitol 1 g/kg IV bolus (or 100 g as a rough dose) put in fast *or* 10–20 mL of 23.4% saline *or* give a bolus of 3% (250 mL) if the patient is hypotensive and mannitol is a less optimal choice.
  - *Reason*: These agents pull water out of the brain by increasing serum osmolality (OSM), which decreases ICP.
- Intubation and hyperventilation: The herniating patient will not be able to protect his or her airway and will have irregular breathing. Taking the PCO_2 to 25 is a short-term measure to decreased ICP as it constricts blood vessels.
- EVD: Placing a drain into the lateral ventricles will allow you to remove CSF, which will immediately decrease force on the brain by taking volume out of the skull.
- Sedation with propofol bolus, midazolam, and/or paralytics: These reduce metabolic demand.
- Pentobarbital 500 mg IV bolus: This medication is used to help get the patient to the operating room or to the computed tomography (CT) scanner.
  - *Reason*: It decreases metabolic demand of the brain, increasing cells' ability to survive with less blood flow or high ICP and acts directly to stabilize the cell membrane. It also leads to burst suppression on an electroencephalogram (EEG).
- Surgical decompression: Surgery can directly address herniation by relieving the rigid skull or by removing mass from inside the skull (brain, tumor, blood, or CSF).

Brain herniation is the most urgent neurosurgical emergency. It should be treated with the same urgency as a myocardial infarction or hypotensive shock. It requires immediate action as the patient has minutes until irreversible damage or death occurs. *Remember that the CT scan does not treat herniation or ICP.*

Often a patient's exam can be confounded or limited by sedating medications or paralytics, often right after being intubated. In these cases, one can rely more on pupillary findings (very few medications will dilate pupils) and imaging. Initial aggressive treatment should be considered rather than possibly missing the chance to treat at all. This concept can also be applied to younger patients with poor exams at presentation. We favor treating them aggressively to give them the best chance of survival rather than attempting to predict prognosis at such an early stage (Figures 2.1 and 2.2).

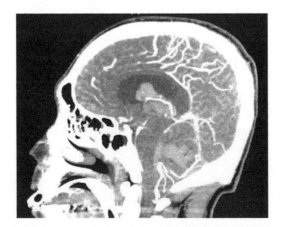

Figure 2.1 Sagittal CTA, a 20 year old with intracerebral hemorrhage from a posterior fossa arteriovenous malformation (AVM), found in dense coma. Note how the posterior inferior cerebellar artery (PICA) around the tonsil sags well below the foramen magnum. This illustrates tonsillar herniation.

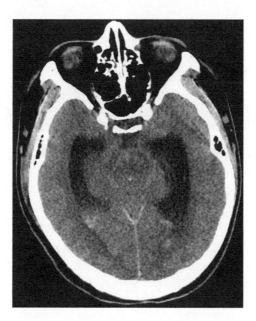

Figure 2.2   The same patient with ventriculomegaly from obstructive hydrocephalus. Critical management of tonsillar herniation included emergent placement of an EVD as well as surgical decompression. The patient went on to make a good recovery and returned to college.

Intracranial pressure emergencies with ICP monitoring

When a patient has a bolt or external ventricular drain (EVD) in place, we can measure ICPs. ICPs that are trending up and sustained above 20 should be treated. Under these conditions, the brain is not getting blood flow, and this will lead to permanent damage. Sudden increases in intracranial pressure (>20–25 mm Hg for 5 minutes) are life threatening and should be considered an acute ICP crisis. While considering an etiology is important, the first priority is to get the ICP down (remember getting a head CT image does not treat ICPs).

Treatment for rising ICP

- Elevate the head of the bed to 30°–40°.
  - *Reason*: By increasing venous outflow, there is a decrease in ICP.
- Control blood pressure.
  - *Reason*: Avoid hypotension (SBP < 90 mm Hg), which causes decreased cerebral perfusion (CPP = MAP – ICP).
- Maintain adequate oxygenation.
  - *Reason*: Avoid hypoxia (PO_2 < 60 mm Hg), which could cause ischemic brain injury.
- Troubleshoot the EVD or bolt.
  - Is the drain working? Is the ICP measurement real?
- Administer mild sedation with propofol or midazolam.
  - *Reason*: This decreases the metabolic demand of the brain, which decreases activity of the body, decreasing ICP.
- Stop seizures or prevent seizures.

- Reduce fever.
  - Fever increases the activity of the brain, which increases the ICP.
- Obtain a head CT.
  - *Reason*: Rule out a surgical cause for sustained increased ICP.

Acute ICP crisis (sustained ICP > 25 mm Hg)

- Manage the airway.
  - *Reason*: Check the airway and positioning of the intubation tube for obstructions.
- Sedate and consider paralyzing the patient.
  - *Reason*: Paralying the patient helps to reduce hypertension and sympathetic tone that are exacerbated by movement; sedation will decrease the metabolic activity of the brain.
  - Midazolam, morphine/fentanyl, and vecuronium may be used.
- Drain CSF by lowering EVD.
  - *Reason*: This immediately reduces ICP by reducing volume. Caveat: Do not plug up the drain by sucking up brain or blood.
- Mannitol 1 g/kg IV bolus (over <20 minutes) *or* 10–20 mL of 23.4% saline *or* give a bolus of 3% (250 mL) and titrate a gtt (drip) (start at 30 mL/hr) to increase the serum sodium to >150; 3% may be preferred in patients with subarachnoid hemorrhage (SAH) during spasm to avoid overall dehydration worsening spasm.
  - *Reason*: These agents pull water out of the brain by increasing serum OSM, which decreases ICP.
- Hyperventilation (Ambubag): Aim for $PCO_2 > 25$ mm Hg
  - *Reason*: Reducing PCO_2 decreases ICP for a short time.
- Cooling: Bring the patient's temperature down to at least normal (not febrile).
  - *Reason:* Decreasing the temperature will decrease the metabolism occurring in the brain, which decreases blood flow and CSF production. Fever needs to be controlled in patients with elevated ICPs.
- Pentobarbital 500 mg IV bolus: This is a "last resort" medication used to help get the patient to the operating room or to the CT scanner. It can also be used as a gtt, but only after other measures are exhausted. There are a number of side effects to the heart, liver, and potassium that one must keep in mind.
  - *Reason*: This decreases metabolic demand of the brain, increasing the cell's ability to survive with less blood flow or high ICP, and acts directly to stabilize the cell membrane. This will lead to burst suppression.
- Head CT: Obtain only when ICP has come down and the patient will tolerate being flat.
- If all measures fail, the patient will need to be surgically decompressed.

Spinal cord emergencies
Cauda equina syndrome

Cauda equina syndrome (CES) is a group of neuromuscular and urogenital symptoms that generally present acutely and are due to compression of the bundle of nerve roots located at the base of the spinal cord. The spinal cord begins to taper approximately at L1-L2 in most adults, and the roots can be compressed simultaneously before they have exited the spinal canal.

Red flags in patient history

- Hx of B-cell lymphoma
- Hx of metastatic cancer

- Low back trauma
- Recent spinal procedure/surgery
- Ankylosing spondylitis
- Acute complaints for extensive numbness, pain, and loss of motor function beyond one dermatome or myotome; urinary retention

Red flag physical findings

- Saddle anesthesia: sensory deficits in the region of the anus, perineum, lower genitals, buttocks, and the upper posterior aspect of the thighs
   NOTE: If there is total perineal anesthesia, the patient will likely have permanent bladder dysfunction.
- Sphincter disturbance: urinary retention, urinary/fecal incontinence, diminished anal sphincter tone
   NOTE: If the patient does *not* have urinary retention (tested by having the patient void and looking for residual volume on a bladder ultrasound), then there is a low likelihood that the patient has CES.
- Significant lower extremity motor weakness
   NOTE: This is generally not limited to a single nerve root.
- Sexual dysfunction
   NOTE: This may not be present initially.

Imaging

- Urgent lumbar magnetic resonance imaging (MRI), imaging of choice
- Myelography and CT myelography if MRI is not possible, but have disadvantage of being invasive techniques that may take longer

Treatment

- Urgent decompression, preferably in less than 24 hours.

Spinal cord injuries (trauma)

Spinal cord injuries should be considered an emergency for two reasons: Hypotension and possible worsening neurological function if the injury is not complete and the spine is unstable.

Hypotension should be treated with volume and dopamine (or another pressor). Studies have shown that by keeping the mean arterial pressure (MAP) greater than 80, neurological function can improve. Steroids are generally no longer used.

Physical exam: American Spinal Injury Association Score and Level

Closely examine the patient's motor strength, sensory level, reflexes, and rectal tone.

If the exam is not complete, then it matters how quickly the cord is decompressed. Examine all the motor groups, scoring 0–5 on both sides, for a total of 100 possible points. The sensory exam is related to dermatome to determine a sensory level.

Treatment

- Urgent decompression and stabilization, preferably in less than 6 hours

Status epilepticus

Status epilepticus is an acute, prolonged epileptic crisis (>5 minutes of seizure activity without the patient returning to baseline) that is life threatening.

Treatment for adults

1. Administer lorazepam (Ativan) 4 mg IV, slow infusion over 2 minutes; repeat q5 minutes.
    NOTE: Make preparations to intubate just in case respiratory rate drops.
2. Load with phenytoin (Dilantin) at the same time, and then check blood level.
    a. Patient on phenytoin at home: 500 mg
    b. Patient not on phenytoin at home: 1200 mg
    NOTE: Monitor blood pressure for hypotension and electrocardiogram for arrhythmias.
3. Administer phenobarbital IV, up to 1400 mg until seizures stop (infuse at <100 mg/min).
    NOTE: It can take 15–20 minutes to work. Monitor blood pressure, because phenobarbital is a myocardial depressant.
4. Instead of phenobarbital another option is intubation and propofol gtt at high doses to lead to burst suppression. This will *always* stop seizures.
    NOTE: Though evidence has been equivocal, Keppra is also used instead of Dilantin because it has a better side effect panel and does not require blood level testing.

Ischemic stroke

Brain cells require more blood and oxygen than any other cell in the body, and due to this they are unable to survive when blood flow is stopped more than minutes. Two million neurons die every minute when there is not enough blood flow. The ischemic stroke diagnosis is made by having a high suspicion and then obtaining imaging to confirm. The most important tenet is to act quickly when you suspect stroke, as you can make the difference between a poor patient outcome requiring 24/7 nursing home care versus a patient walking, talking, and going back to work. Nowhere else in neurosurgery have we made such strides in the past decade.

Two anatomic locations of stroke can be most effectively treated and reversed: Anterior stroke (middle cerebral artery [MCA] or internal carotid artery [ICA]) and posterior circulation (basilar tip).

Red flag physical findings

*   *Sudden exam changes*: Paresis, speech, vision, dizziness and syncope, to coma
*   *MCA stroke syndrome*: Hemiplegia, speech deficit if stroke is left sided, arm > leg, hemi-face weakness
*   *Basilar stroke*: Thrombus into the basilar artery leads to decreased flow to the brainstem; coma, pupil changes, hemiparesis, or tetraparesis

Imaging

*   Vascular study (computed tomography angiography [CTA] or magnetic resonance angiography [MRA]) will show lack of blood flow such as M1, carotid, or basilar cutoff (Figures 2.3 and 2.4).

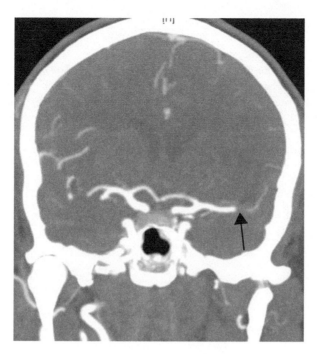

Figure 2.3 Coronal CTA depicting nonfilling of the left M1, commonly referred to as "cutoff."

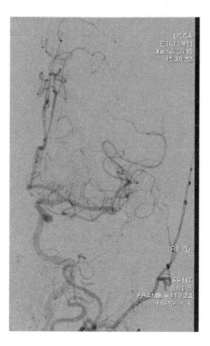

Figure 2.4 Neuroendovascular surgery was performed for clot retrieval. Following removal of the clot, the MCA has filling, though still slow in the M3. The patient improved from presenting right-sided hemiplegia and aphasia, to only mild deficits, ambulatory and verbal at discharge.

Treatment

- Administer IV tissue plasminogen activator (tPA).
- Endovascular treatment for clot retrieval is now the "gold standard," as five randomized controlled trials have concluded. The majority of acute large vessel occlusions can be reopened by endovascular neurosurgical techniques. The time window for intervention is extending past 6 hours and goes now to 24 hours (DAWN preliminary results) (Berkhemer et al., 2015; Campbell et al., 2015; Jovin et al., 2015; Saver et al., 2015).
  - Getting the patient to the neuroendovascular suite is an emergency.

Mental status checklist

It is important to complete the items in the chart simultaneously. *Take home message*: Take action when it is a neurological emergency.

Physical examination

- Evaluate for focal examination changes.
- A fast decline in neurologic status often translates to a more dangerous etiology.
- Obtain a head CT for suspicious anatomic causes.

Laboratory evaluation

- Sodium
  - Hyponatremia can be an etiology for brain edema as well as acute metabolic encephalopathy.
- White blood cell count
  - Evaluate for infection.
- Arterial blood gas
  - Hypercarbia and hypoxemia can lead to acute metabolic encephalopathy.
- Liver function
  - Hyperammonia can lead to acute metabolic encephalopathy.
- BUN/creat
  - Acute kidney injury can lead to acute metabolic encephalopathy.

References

Berkhemer OA, Fransen PS, Beumer D, et al. A randomized trial of intraarterial treatment for acute ischemic stroke. *N Eng J Med*. 2015;372(1):11–20. doi:10.1056/NEJMoa1411587

Campbell BC, Mitchell PJ, Kleinig TJ, et al. Endovascular therapy for ischemic stroke with perfusion-imaging selection. *N Eng J Med*, 2015;372(11):1009–1018. doi:10.1056/NEJMoa1414792

Jovin TG, Chamorro A, Cobo E, et al. (2015). Thrombectomy within 8 hours after symptom onset in ischemic stroke. *N Eng J Med*. 2015;372(24):2296–306. doi:10.1056/NEJMia1503780

Saver JL, Goyal M, Bonafe A, et al. Stent-retriever thrombectomy after intravenous t-PA vs. t-PA alone in stroke. *N Eng J Med*. 2015;372(24):2285–2295. doi:10.1056/NEJMoa1415061

3

THE NEUROINTENSIVE CARE AND NEUROMONITORING UNIT

Michael Safaee and Sanjay Dhall

Introduction

The neurointensive care unit (Neuro-ICU) is responsible for the management of critically ill patients with diseases of the central nervous system, specifically the brain and spinal cord. Patients in these units, particularly at trauma centers, are often unstable and require close attention to recognize and respond to acute changes in their neurologic status. Patients in the Neuro-ICU, can be roughly divided into two groups—those with acute neurologic injuries (e.g., stroke, head trauma, aneurysmal subarachnoid hemorrhage, and acute spinal cord injury) and those who are being observed after elective neurosurgical procedures. This chapter provides a brief introduction to the Neuro ICU with specific attention to the neurologic exam, neuromonitoring, and neuroimaging.

Neurologic exams

Close monitoring of the vital signs and the neurologic exam is an essential component of care in the Neuro-ICU. A change in the neurologic exam may be the first sign of an acute decompensation and prompt diagnostic or therapeutic interventions. Most patients require an hourly neurologic exam, which includes an evaluation of mental status, cranial nerves, motor strength, and sensation. This can be limited in patients who are intubated or require sedation for control of pain, agitation, delirium, or elevated intracranial pressure. Mental status is generally assessed through questioning to determine if patients are oriented to their surroundings with normal language and comprehension. The cranial nerve exam is focused on the pupillary response, extraocular movements, facial strength and sensation, hearing, and tongue movements. It is important to consider patients' preinjury conditions when performing the neurologic exam; for example, glasses and hearing aids should be used when appropriate and will also help minimize delirium during their stay in the ICU (Van Rompaey et al., 2009; Thomason et al.,2005). The motor exam should focus on upper and lower extremity strength, with special attention to the side or spinal level corresponding to the injury. Sensation is generally assessed by light touch; however, pain and temperature are useful in patients with spinal cord injuries. In patients who are sedated or comatose, brainstem reflexes are an important part of the exam and include the pupillary response, vestibule-ocular reflex, and cough and gag reflexes. Although historically evaluated by penlight, objective measures of pupillary response are now commonly obtained with pupillometers (Meeker et al., 2005, Zafar and Suarez, 2014). It is important to remember that as a whole, the clinical exam should often be tailored to the specific pathology, for example, the exam in a patient with an acute left-sided holohemispheric subdural hematoma will place special focus on mental status, language, pupillary exam, and right-sided strength. Learning to perform an accurate and reliable neurological exam is a cornerstone of care in the Neuro-ICU.

Neuromonitoring

In addition to close monitoring of vital signs and the neurologic exam, patients in the Neuro-ICU often require advanced neuromonitoring for continuous measurement of intracranial pressure (ICP), cerebral perfusion pressure (CPP), electroencephalography (EEG), brain tissue oxygenation, and brain tissue temperature (Brophy et al., 2012; Gelabert-Gonzalez et al., 2006; Kett-White et al., 2002; Maloney-Wilensky et al., 2009; Muralidharan, 2015; Schomer and Hanafy, 2015). The indications for placement of these devices will be discussed in later chapters, but in brief, they allow for continuous monitoring of intracranial physiology and often guide therapeutic interventions. One type of ICP monitor, the external ventricular drain (EVD), is a catheter placed in the lateral ventricle that allows for both measurement of ICP and drainage of cerebrospinal fluid (CSF) as a therapeutic intervention for elevated ICPs. ICP can also be measured using a fiberoptic catheter; however, these devices do not allow for drainage of CSF. The CPP is a measurement of cerebral perfusion calculated by subtracting the ICP from the mean arterial pressure (MAP). Placement of a radial arterial line allows for continuous monitoring of blood pressure and CPP. EEG is useful for identifying seizure activity, particularly in patients with nonconvulsive status epilepticus. Brain tissue oxygenation and brain tissue temperature are still under active investigation but can provide insight into cerebral metabolism and blood flow. All of these monitors are placed by neurosurgeons at the bedside using sterile technique and should be kept clean to minimize the risk of infection. Frequent calibration and close attention to head positioning should also be performed to ensure accurate measurements.

Neuroimaging

In cases of acute changes in a patient's vitals, neurologic exam, or neurophysiologic monitoring, imaging is often required to identify the cause of the change and determine the appropriate intervention. The most common modality for acute imaging of the brain and spinal cord is computed tomography (CT). Magnetic resonance imaging (MRI) provides valuable information but is limited by long acquisition times and as a result is not suitable for use for unstable patients. In the event of an acute change requiring imaging of the brain or spinal cord, patients are quickly transferred to the CT scanner where imaging can be acquired within minutes. If patients are too unstable for transfer to the CT scanner, many ICUs have portable scanners that can be moved into the patient's room and provide focused imaging without having to transfer the patient out of the ICU (Peace et al., 2010). Other imaging modalities provide limited information and thus CT is the workhorse of the Neuro-ICU. Ultrasound, such as transcranial Doppler (TCD), is a useful modality for evaluating vasospasm in patients with aneurysmal subarachnoid hemorrhage (SAH); however, these are often performed by specially trained technicians and may not be readily available (Frontera et al., 2009; Newell and Winn, 1990).

Polytrauma

Level I trauma centers will often care for patients with polytrauma and injuries to the brain or spinal cord. Multidisciplinary teams including neurosurgeons, trauma surgeons, orthopedic surgeons, and intensivists often manage such patients.

Special considerations

The Neuro-ICU provides care for some of the most critically ill patients and as a result communication between bedside nurses, nurse practitioners, and physicians is critical. Delirium is a common complication of ICU stay and as a result patients should be provided with frequent orientation and allowed access to their hearing aids or glasses when needed (Van Rompaey et al., 2009). This is particularly relevant given the increase in elderly patients with head trauma (Thompson et al., 2006). Patients in the Neuro-ICU may be comatose or sedated and as a result are at increased risk for pressure ulcers; thus, frequent repositioning and appropriate padding of pressure points are crucial (Anderson et al., 2015; Krupp et al., 2015). Given the severity of illness in these patients, frequent visits by family and friends are common. Ensuring good hand hygiene, particularly among visitors and health-care providers, is important to minimize risk of infection (Qushmaq et al., 2008; Tschudin-Sutter et al., 2010). Most importantly, communication between providers and family members is vital for ensuring comprehension of illness severity and overall prognosis, which promotes appropriate care and decision making (Mathew et al., 2015; Schubart et al., 2015).

Summary

The Neuro-ICU provides care to some of the most critically ill patients in a given hospital. These patients require close nursing care and frequent monitoring of their vitals, neurologic exam, and ICP when applicable. Patients may be sedated or comatose, and thus small changes in the exam may be the first sign of an acute decompensation. The CT scan provides fast and reliable imaging of the central nervous system; many Neuro-ICUs have portable scanners that allow for acute imaging in the ICU for patients who are unstable for transport. Patients with polytrauma are often managed by multidisciplinary teams and require constant communication for optimal management. Delirium is a common complication of prolonged ICU stay, and it is important to promote good sleep hygiene, provide frequent orientation, and ensure that patients are allowed to wear glasses and hearing aids when possible.

References

Anderson M, Finch Guthrie P, Kraft W, Reicks P, Skay C, Beal AL. Universal pressure ulcer prevention bundle with WOC nurse support. *J Wound Ostomy Continence Nurs.* 2015;42(3):217–225.

Brophy GM, Bell R, Claassen J, et al. Guidelines for the evaluation and management of status epilepticus. *Neurocrit Care.* 2012;17(1):3–23.

Frontera JA, Fernandex A, Schmidt JM, et al. Defining vasospasm after subarachnoid hemorrhage: what is the most clinically relevant definition? *Stroke.* 2009;40(6):1963–1968.

Gelabert-Gonzalez M, Ginesta-Galan V, Sernamito-García R, Allut AG, Bandin-Diéguez J, Rumbo RM. The Camino intracranial pressure device in clinical practice. Assessment in a 1000 cases. *Acta Neurochir (Wien).* 2006;148(4):435–441.

Kett-White R, Hutchinson PJ, Al-Rawi PG, Gupta AK, Pickard JD, Kirkpatrick PJ, Adverse cerebral events detected after subarachnoid hemorrhage using brain oxygen and microdialysis probes. *Neurosurgery.* 2002;50(6):1213–1221; discussion 1221–1222.

Krupp AE, Monfre J. Pressure ulcers in the ICU patient: an update on prevention and treatment. *Curr Infect Dis Rep.* 2015;17(3):468.

Maloney-Wilensky E, Gracias V, Itkin A, et al., Brain tissue oxygen and outcome after severe traumatic brain injury: a systematic review. *Crit Care Med.* 2009;37(6):2057–2063.

Mathew JE, Azariah J, George SE, Grewal SS. Do they hear what we speak? Assessing the effectiveness of communication to families of critically ill neurosurgical patients. *J Anaesthesiol Clin Pharmacol.* 2015;31(1):49–53.

Meeker M, Du R, Bacchetti P, et al. Pupil examination: validity and clinical utility of an automated pupillometer. *J Neurosci Nurs.* 2005;37(1):34–40.

Muralidharan R. External ventricular drains: management and complications. *Surg Neurol Int.* 2015;6(suppl 6): S271–S274.

Newell DW, Winn HR. Transcranial Doppler in cerebral vasospasm. *Neurosurg Clin N Am.* 1990;1(2):319–328.

Peace K, Wilensky EM, Frangos S, et al. The use of a portable head CT scanner in the intensive care unit. *J Neurosci Nurs.* 2010;42(2):109–116.

Qushmaq IA, Heels-Ansdell D, Cook DJ, Loeb MB, Meade MO. Hand hygiene in the intensive care unit: prospective observations of clinical practice. *Pol Arch Med Wewn.* 2008;118(10):543–547.

Schomer AC, Hanafy K. Neuromonitoring in the ICU. *Int Anesthesiol Clin.* 2015;53(1):107–122.

Schubart JR, Wojnar M, Dillard JP, et al. ICU family communication and health care professionals: A qualitative analysis of perspectives. *Intensive Crit Care Nurs.* 2015;31(5):315–321.

Thomason JW, Shintani A, Peterson JF, Pun BT, Jackson JC, Ely EW. Intensive care unit delirium is an independent predictor of longer hospital stay: a prospective analysis of 261 non-ventilated patients. *Crit Care.* 2005;9(4):R375–381.

Thompson HJ, McCormick WC, Kagan SH. Traumatic brain injury in older adults: epidemiology, outcomes, and future implications. *J Am Geriatr Soc.* 2006;54(10):1590–1595.

Tschudin-Sutter S, Pargger H, Widmer AF. Hand hygiene in the intensive care unit. *Crit Care Med.* 2010;38 (suppl 8):S299–305.

Van Rompaey B, Elseviers MM, Schuurmans MJ, Shortridge-Baggett LM, Truijen S, Bossaert L. Risk factors for delirium in intensive care patients: a prospective cohort study. *Crit Care.* 2009;13(3):R77.

Zafar SF, Suarez JI. Automated pupillometer for monitoring the critically ill patient: a critical appraisal. *J Crit Care.* 2014;29(4):599–603.

4

THE NEUROSURGICAL OPERATING ROOM

Erika Freiberg, Sara Kadlec, and Sharad Rajpal

Hazards in the neurosurgical operating room

The operating room (OR) is a highly specialized environment. As such, special considerations must be undertaken for the surgeon and surgical assistants.

Bovie smoke

Smoke from Bovie devices has been shown to contain carcinogenic compounds. These include hydrocarbons, nitriles, fatty acids, and phenols (Hensman et al., 1998). Human papillomavirus has even been found to be present in the smoke flume from electrocautery (Sawchuk et al., 1989), which causes concern for disease exposure. The National Institute of Occupational Safety and Health suggests that Bovie smoke be captured within 2 inches of the surgical site, and tubing and filters that contain the smoke be treated as infectious waste. When assisting, pay careful attention to rapid smoke removal by suctioning as close to the Bovie as possible.

Needlesticks

Needlesticks can occur often in the OR if one is not cautious. Although each hospital has protocols for handling needlesticks, the initial most important step following a needlestick exposure is to wash the area with soap and water. The risk of HIV exposure following percutaneous exposure is approximately 0.3% and 0.09% after mucous membrane exposure (Centers for Disease Control and Prevention, 2005). The average risk of contracting hepatitis C following percutaneous exposure is 1.9% (Centers for Disease Control and Prevention, 2001), and transmission rarely occurs from mucous membrane exposure. Ensure your hepatitis B vaccination is up to date. Double-gloving helps significantly reduce the risk of skin contamination by blood and body fluids and is recommended for all higher-risk cases (Gani et al., 1990).

Radiation

Long-term radiation exposure in the OR can lead to increased risk of cancer. The best way to reduce radiation exposure is distance. Standing at least 3 meters away from the radiation source drastically diminishes exposure. Radiation scatter is also a huge risk and occurs greatest at the beam source secondary to backscatter from the patient (McCormick, 2008). Next to distance, shielding is essential. The most effective lead apron is the wraparound two-piece garment. Minimizing time of exposure is also key to avoiding long-term consequences from radiation. Remember to use thyroid- and eye-shielding devices.

Noise

With drills, suctions, and anesthesia equipment, the OR can be a noisy place. Studies have measured elevated decibel readings in the OR that can potentially damage hearing (Fritsch et al., 2010). Minimize noise exposure, not only for hearing preservation, but also for effective communication during each case. Poor communication could pose a threat to patient safety (Hasfeldt et al., 2010).

Anesthesiology concerns

Know your patient's medical history to help ensure a smooth intraoperative course. Communicate to your anesthesiologist any concerns you may have regarding the patient prior to starting the case.

Blood availability

If there is risk of significant blood loss, a blood type and screen (TS) is important. If there is concern that a patient will require a blood transfusion, a type and crossmatch (TC) should be ordered. Type and screen refers to testing for ABO and Rh status, whereas TC refers to testing recipient blood against donor blood to investigate if any antibodies are formed. Often a TC can take up to an hour, so performing this ahead of time is important if a blood transfusion is anticipated. Closely monitor blood loss during surgery and communicate this with the entire OR team.

Blood pressure management

Blood pressure management is important intraoperatively to prevent end organ damage, minimize blood loss, and improve operating conditions. Failure to control blood pressure can increase morbidity rates (Laresen and Kleinschmidt, 1995). Blood pressure fluctuations can be seen during the induction of anesthesia, as well as with a sympathetic response due to pain, hypoxia, or volume overload (Varon and Marik, 2008). Adequate pain control and close monitoring of volume status deserve attention. However, low blood pressure can be even more hazardous for neurosurgical patients as the central nervous system is intolerant of hypoperfusion. A frequently used parameter is to maintain the mean arterial blood pressure (MAP) above 75 mm Hg.

Blood glucose

Elevated perioperative blood glucose levels have been implicated in increased infection rates. Studies have shown a serum blood glucose of 80–110 is optimal (Van den Berghe et al., 2006); however, risk of hypoglycemia is increased with such tight blood glucose control and can lead to other complications, including death (Duncan, 2012). Ensure blood sugars are adequately monitored and controlled intraoperatively.

Antimicrobial prophylaxis

Perioperative antibiotic prophylaxis is recommended to help reduce surgical site infections (SSIs). The American Society of Health-System Pharmacists recommends cefazolin as the first-line antibiotic for neurosurgical procedures. Alternatives for the cephalosporin-allergic patient are clindamycin or vancomycin. Single-dose antimicrobial prophylaxis should be given within 1 hour prior to incision time. Antimicrobials with a short half-life may require redosing during long procedures. Redose antibiotics at around two times the half-life of the agent in patients with normal renal function. For instance, cefazolin has a half-life of approximately 2 hours, and redosing is therefore recommended at 4 hours (Bratzler et al., 2013).

Access

Placements of relevant anesthesia lines are variable and depend on the surgical procedure. Invasive lines should only be used when indicated, as they can also increase the risk of adverse effects. Frequent potential lines that may need placement before starting surgery include: (1) a Foley catheter to help accurately monitor urine output; (2) an arterial line to help monitor blood pressure in real time and to obtain samples for arterial blood gas measurements; and (3) a central line in those instances that a patient requires rapid fluid resuscitation, frequent blood draws, or needs his or her central venous pressure measured.

Surgical tables, frames, and headrests

Operations on the lumbosacral spine often require the patient to be positioned in the prone or lateral decubitus position. A "Jackson" table allows for this and is commonly used because it allows for 360° rotation of patients during combined approach operations. It is also radiolucent and allows for easy intraoperative imaging (Schonauer et al., 2004). In the prone position, avoid abdominal compression, as this may cause high airway pressures, resulting in decreased cardiac output and increased systemic venous pressure. High venous pressure can decrease mean arterial pressure, thereby increasing the risk of neurological compromise. Supporting the patient on the table with the abdomen free decreases the likelihood of these complications (Schonauer et al., 2004). The "Wilson" and "Andrews" frames are commonly used for positioning of patients for lumbar spine surgery. The Andrews frame supports patients in an adapted knee-chest position. Padding protects the patient, and the frame can adjust to change the degree of hip flexion. Allowing for flexion, the adjustable Wilson frame has two arched sets of pads that support the chest and pelvis but allow for a pendulous abdomen (Schonauer et al., 2004). Studies have shown that adjusting the Wilson frame to increase kyphosis of the lumbosacral spine can improve exposure for transforaminal lumbar interbody fusion (TLIF) procedures (Cardoso and Rosner, 2010). Both frames allow for C-arm use (Schonauer et al., 2004).

Common cranial or cervical spine procedures typically involve a horseshoe headrest or "Mayfield" headholder. The Mayfield provides rigid skeletal fixation by pinning the skull with three or more fixation points and is secured to the surgical table. Any cranial flexion position requires a minimum of two fingers between the jaw and the chest to ensure adequate ventilation and venous return. Although the head may be axially rotated between 0° and 45°, it is critical to consider the patient's preoperative neck flexibility before any manipulation to avoid adverse outcomes (Rozet and Vavilala, 2007).

Surgical skin preparation

Surgical skin preparation impacts postoperative infection rates. Hair removal is typically performed prior to skin prep. Use electric clippers for hair removal as razors can damage the epidermis and can increase wound infection rates (Walcott et al., 2012). Several types of skin preparation solutions are available on the market. Make sure to discuss any potential preferences with your surgeon. Preoperative cleansing of the surgical site with a chlorhexidine-alcohol solution has been shown to be more effective than povidone-iodine cleansers (Walcott et al., 2012; Zinn et al., 2010).

- Povidone-iodine
  - Free iodine binds to bacteria and is highly effective against Gram-positive bacteria and slightly less effective against Gram-negative bacteria.
    - Binds with organic substances and is therefore less effective in the presence of blood.
    - Has moderate speed of action and low residual activity.
    - Is known to cause pain to the treatment area and may cause irritation (Zinn et al., 2010).

- Chlorhexidine gluconate (CHG)
  - Can be prepared with or without alcohol.
    - Disrupts cell membranes, causes cell death of both Gram-positive and Gram-negative bacteria.
    - Is not affected by the presence of organic materials.
    - Has moderately rapid activity and strong persistent activity.
    - Has contraindications for use that include use on brain, spinal tissues, eyes, ears, mucous membranes, genitalia, and sensitive patients.
    - Has potential for corneal damage, ototoxicity, and neurotoxicity.
    - May dry the skin and be made inert by saline solution (Zinn et al., 2010).

- Parachlorometaxylenol (PCMX)
  - Prevents uptake of essential amino acids, thereby disrupting cell membranes.
    - Has fair and good activity against Gram-negative and Gram-positive bacteria, respectively.
    - Is nearly 100% effective against methicillin-resistant *Staphylococcus aureus*.
    - Has moderate speed of action and continued activity.
    - Is not affected by blood or organic material; has continued activity in saline.
    - Is a safe choice for surgical sites that involve the mucous membranes.
    - May be less effective than other agents (Zinn et al., 2010).

- Alcohol
  - Shows strong activity against both Gram-positive and Gram-negative organisms.
    - Denatures proteins as its mechanism of action.
    - Has rapid germicidal action but fails to sustain continued activity (Zinn et al., 2010).

- Iodine with alcohol (DuraPrep)
  - Is more effective than these substances individually in reduction of surgical site infections.
    - Alcohol acts immediately, and iodine has better residual activity.
    - The alcohol base in DuraPrep increases the chance for surgical fires.
    - Ensure that any alcohol-based skin preparations have completely dried before starting the operation to avoid fires (Zinn et al., 2010).

Surgical hand scrub

Presurgical hand scrub by the surgeon and any assistants is a routine and critical aspect of the operation that could assist in the prevention of SSIs (Walcott et al., 2010). Hungarian physician Ignaz Semmelweis demonstrated in 1846 that handwashing with an antiseptic is superior to washing with soap and water. He achieved an immediate decrease in infection-related patient mortality after the introduction of hand disinfection in his practice (George, 2010). Gowns and gloves prevent the surgical team's skin from contacting the surgical field, but holes can allow transmission of microorganisms to the surgical site. Use of surgical scrub prior to operating reduces microbial load, which in turn can reduce the chance of transfer of the assistant's skin flora to the surgical site. Aqueous or alcohol-based rubs may be used. Alcohol rubs are at least equal to more traditional water-based scrubs. There is no clear consensus over which is superior. Alcohol rubs may improve compliance as they are potentially better tolerated and take a shorter amount of time. Several studies have suggested that chlorhexidine-based scrubs are preferred over povidone-iodine–based scrubs based on superior efficacy. The use of brushes/sponges has not been proven to reduce SSIs (Walcott et al., 2012). Refer to the package directions for specific surgical hand scrubs to maximize effectiveness.

Wound closure

Surgical wounds are closed by reapproximating layers of tissue, fascia, and muscle from deep to superficial. Absorbable sutures such as vicryl can be used for deeper layers. The skin may be closed with any of several different materials, including staples, nylon sutures, absorbable sutures like Monocryl, or tissue adhesives (glues). Sutures are superior to glues in preventing wound dehiscence. Tissue adhesives provide the advantages of quicker and more facile application (Coulthard et al., 1996). In the event of a contaminated or infected wound, monofilament sutures are preferred due to their more inert properties; multifilament sutures may shelter infectious microbes (Mackay-Wiggan et al., 2014). Suture sizes are variable and typically selected based on the smallest size that can provide a tension-free wound closure. In the event of a high tension wound, use of large-diameter sutures is preferred, as smaller-sized sutures may result in tissue damage. Match the strength of the suture to the tissue layer being sutured (Mackay-Wiggan et al., 2014). Familiarize yourself with the countless different types of sutures and their properties.

Surgical drains

Several types of drains are used in neurosurgery. After cranial procedures, intraventricular, subdural, or subgaleal drains may be left in place to drain cerebrospinal fluid or blood products. In a surgical procedure in which there is concern of potential cerebrospinal fluid leaks, a lumbar drain may be placed. Surgical drains in spine surgery are often utilized to reduce the chances of postoperative hematoma formation. Drains come in many shapes and sizes and may be made of silicone or latex. Poorman et al. (2014) found no difference in complications for patients who did or did not have a drain placed. The decision on whether to place a drain will ultimately depend on surgeon preference and the location and type of surgery completed.

Surgical dressings

Once the surgical wound has been closed, a dressing is typically applied. Dressings provide a more appealing look for the patient's wound and may possibly provide protection from microbes. Some theorize that a dressing may actually increase the risk of infection. Applying an antibiotic ointment rather than a dressing has shown to result in similar rates of infection. Typical dressing options include gauze, tissue adhesives, and silver-impregnated bandages. Octyl cyanoacrylate is a common tissue adhesive and provides a barrier against both Gram-positive and Gram-negative nonmotile organisms for at least 3 days. Use of silver-impregnated bandages has been shown to reduce infections after lumbar fusions (Walcott et al., 2012). Discuss dressing options and preferences with your surgeon.

How to best assist

Assisting is very surgeon specific, and time/experience is the best way to know how to efficiently assist your surgeon. Here are some tips to help you with any surgeon.

- Imaging studies
  - Ensure that any and all relevant images (CT, MRI, angiograms, etc.) are available for pre- and intraoperative viewing.
    - Ensure navigation workstations (if used) are functioning properly or related films are correctly loaded and available.
- Familiarize yourself with the microscope, and balance the microscope before surgery begins, ensuring that the optics are properly positioned.

- Protect all lines during patient manipulation, and make sure the patient is secured to the bed before any bed manipulation.
  - Avoid moving patients by yourself to prevent injury.
    - Never move a patient from an OR table to a hospital bed, or vice versa, without approval/readiness from your anesthesiologist.
- Keep the surgical field clean and dry.
  - Use suction and sponges to keep blood and Bovie smoke away from the area(s) of interest.
- Irrigation
  - Use irrigation, with or without antibiotics, periodically throughout the case to help decrease infection and keep the surgical field more visible and tissues moist.
- Learn your surgeon's preferences for suction sizes, settings on bipolar, Bovie, etc.
- Learn your surgeon's preference for closure of each procedure, and have sutures and drains opened and ready on the field to avoid delays.

Common patient complaints

Postoperatively, patients may complain of bruising or soreness from surgical positioning. When positioning, diminish interference with anesthesia, respiration, and circulation, and make attempts to avoid nerve injury and skin breakdown. Protect dependent pressure points. For example, breasts, penis, and/or pannus should receive extra attention to ensure no pressure is on these areas. They should not be occluded or obstructed with the table, cardiac monitoring devices, neuromonitoring, or Foley catheters. Any neck manipulation should avoid compression of the endotracheal tube or jugular vein. Check all sensitive areas prior to draping. Ask nursing staff to document any bruises/lesions that you notice on your patient prior to the operation starting. Reduce chances of nerve injury by careful limb/appendage placement and padding (Knight and Mahajan, 2005). Neuromonitoring needles, if used, can cause bruising postoperatively. Educate patients prior to the procedure about this possibility. Discuss postoperative care for needle sites with the neuromonitoring staff. Tape reactions are common patient complaints. Use as little adhesive as possible to accomplish your goals, and use caution when removing adhesive, particularly in elderly patients or those with poor skin quality.

Conclusion

Do not hesitate to discuss any concerns with your nursing staff or surgeon. The OR should be a safe environment for everybody involved, and this can only be achieved if everybody feels empowered to speak up.

References

Bratzler D, Dellinger E, Olsen K, et al. Clinical practice guidelines for antimicrobial prophylaxis in surgery. *Am J Health Syst Pharm*. 2013:195–283.

Cardoso M, Rosner M. (2010). Does the Wilson frame assist with optimizing surgical exposure for minimally invasive lumbar fusions? *Neurosurg FOCUS*. 2010;28(5):1–4.

Centers for Disease Control and Prevention. Updated U.S. Public Health Service guidelines for the management of occupational exposures to HIV and recommendations for Postexposure Prophylaxis. *MMWR*. 2005;54(No. RR-9):2.

Centers for Disease Control and Prevention. Updated U.S. Public Health Service Guidelines for the Management of Occupational Exposures to HBV, HCV, and HIV and Recommendations for Postexposure Prophylaxis. *MMWR*. 2001;50(No. RR-11):3, 6, 7.

Coulthard P, Worthington H, Esposito M, Elst M, Waes O. Tissue adhesives for closure of surgical incisions. *Cochrane Database of Syst Rev*. 1996.

Duncan AE. Hyperglycemia and perioperative glucose management. *Curr Pharm Des.* 2012;18(38):6195–6203.

Fritsch MH, Chacko CE, Patterson EB. Operating room sound level hazards for patients and physicians. *Otol Neurotol.* July 31, 2010;(5):715–721.

Gani JS, Anseline PF, Bissett RL. Efficacy of double versus single gloving in protecting the operating team. *Aust N Z J Surg.* March 1990;60(3):171–175.

George D. A guide to "scrubbing in." *Student BMJ.* 2010. doi:10.1136/sbmj.c3274

Hasfeldt D, Laerkner E, Birkelund R. Noise in the operating room-what do we know? A review of the literature. *J. Perianesth Nurs.* December 25, 2010;(6):380–386.

Hensman C, Baty D, Willis RG, Cuschieri. Chemical composition of smoke produced by high-frequency electrosurgery in closed gaseous environment. An in vitro study. *Surg Endosc.* August 1998;12(8):1017–1019.

Knight D, Mahajan R. Patient positioning in anesthesia. Continuing education in anaesthesia. *Crit Care Pain.* 2005;4(5).

Laresen R, Kleinschmidt S. Controlled hypotension. *Anaesthesist.* April 1995;44(4):291–308.

Mackay-Wiggan J, Ratner D, Sambandan D. Suturing Techniques. November 24, 2014. Retrieved June 14, 2015.

McCormick P. Fluoroscopy: reducing radiation exposure in the OR. *AANS Bulletin.* 2008;17(1).

Poorman C, Passias P, Bianco K, Boniello A, Yang S, Gerling M. Effectiveness of postoperative wound drains in one- and two-level cervical spine fusions. *IJSS Int J Spine Surg.* 2014;8:34–34. doi:10.14444/1034

Rozet I, Vavilala M. Risks and benefits of patient positioning during neurosurgical care. *Anesthesiol Clin.* 2007;25(3):631–653. doi:10.1016/j.anclin.2007.05.009

Sawchuk WS, Weber PJ, Lowry DR, Dzubow LM. Infectious papillomavirus in the vapor of warts treated with carbon dioxide laser or electrocoagulation: detection and protection. *J Am Acad Dermatol.* July 1989;21(1):41–49.

Schonauer C, Bocchetti A, Barbagallo G, Albanese V, Moraci A. Positioning on surgical table. *Eur Spine J.* 2004. doi:10.1007/s00586-004-0728-y

Van den Berghe G, Wilmer A, Hermans G, et al. Intensive insulin therapy in the medical ICU. *N Engl J Med.* February 2, 2006;354(5):449–461.

Varon J, Marik PE. Perioperative hypertension management. *Vasc Health Risk Manag.* 2008;4(3):615–627.

Walcott B, Redjal N, Coumans J. Infection following operations on the central nervous system: deconstructing the myth of the sterile field. *Neurosurgical FOCUS.* 2012;33(5). http://thejns.org/doi/pdf/10.3171t/2012.8. FOCUS12245. Accessed June 14, 2015.

Zinn J, Jenkins J, Swofford V, Harrelson B, McCarter S. Intraoperative patient skin prep agents: is there a difference? *AORN J.* 2010;92(6):662–674. doi:10.1016/j.aorn.2010.07.016

5

NEUROLOGICAL TRIAGE AND THE DIFFERENTIAL DIAGNOSIS

Krishana Sichinga

An immediate evaluation of the neurological patient who begins to deteriorate is crucial in recognizing conditions that may threaten the life of the patient or lead to irreversible neurological deficits. The initial patient assessment will identify if the patient is at risk for cardiopulmonary decompensation due to his or her evolving condition and if the patient may benefit from urgent surgical or medicinal intervention to arrest an acute process. As in any field of medicine, determining the etiology of a change in the neurological patient's exam begins with a detailed history and a focused physical examination. A thorough detailing of the events surrounding the patient's decline and a skilled neurologic examination will generally allow the clinician to identify the underlying process, and follow-up diagnostic tests and lab studies will simply confirm the diagnosis.

The patient admitted to the hospital with a neurologic or neurosurgical diagnosis may develop complications while hospitalized that will affect the patient's long-term outcome. Following are some of the most common changes that may occur in a neuroscience patient, a review of the important historical elements to assess, the neurologic exam to perform, and the diagnoses to consider.

Change in mental status

Approach to clinical assessment

- Determine if the patient is hemodynamically stable.
- Determine the patient's level of consciousness and associated neurologic deficits.

Highlights of the history (generally obtained from the bedside nurse or others with the patient)

- Characterize the mental status change: acute onset or gradual? Complete loss of consciousness, decreased alertness, or disorientation? Stable, fluctuating, or progressive decline in exam?
- Identify preceding or concurrent symptoms: Headache? Nausea or vomiting? Speech or language deficits? New numbness or weakness in an extremity? Fever?

Focused neurologic examination

- Assess hemodynamic stability and airway patency. Note blood pressure, heart rate and rhythm, and respiratory rate and pattern.
- Determine level of consciousness and a Glasgow Coma Score (GCS). In the verbal patient, assess orientation and note new dysarthria or aphasia.

- Evaluate the eyes for a gaze deviation or abnormal eye movements. Evaluate the pupils, comparing size and response to direct and consensual light.
- Assess motor function. In the unresponsive patient, assess the patient's response to painful stimuli bilaterally. In the patient able to follow commands, assess muscle tone and muscle strength in the bilateral upper and lower extremities, noting symmetry of responses.
- Assess additional brainstem reflexes in the unconscious patient, including bilateral corneal reflexes and cough and gag reflexes if the patient is intubated.
- In the cooperative patient, complete a cranial nerve exam, a sensory exam, and a reflex exam, noting new deficits and differences in responses bilaterally. Assess for a pronator drift and a positive Babinski.

Differential diagnosis

- *Acute intracranial hemorrhage*: A stat computed tomography (CT) will demonstrate the hemorrhage, commonly the result of conversion of an ischemic stroke, a complication following a recent cranial procedure, or an initial hemorrhage from or a rehemorrhage of a vascular lesion or a brain tumor.
- *Acute ischemic stroke or transient ischemic attack (TIA)*: A computed tomography angiography (CTA)/ computed tomography perfusion (CTP) may identify an area of stenosis or blockage and the area of ischemia/infarct. Consider an acute ischemic event in the patient admitted with large artery atherosclerotic disease or a cardiac source for emboli, or in the patient with a recent subarachnoid hemorrhage in the window for vasospasm.
- *Status epilepticus or postictal state.*
- *Increasing hydrocephalus*: A CT will identify enlarging ventricles, often in the patient admitted with a subarachnoid or intraventricular hemorrhage, or in the patient with meningitis or an intraventricular tumor. Any patient with a draining external ventricular drain (EVD) or shunt may also develop increasing hydrocephalus in the setting of device malfunction.
- *Increasing cerebral edema*: A CT scan may show increasing edema, often in a patient admitted with an ischemic stroke, an acute intracranial hemorrhage, a traumatic brain injury, or in the patient who has just undergone an intracranial surgical procedure.
- *Expanding or reaccumulating subdural hematoma*: A CT will demonstrate increasing thickness of the hemorrhage.
- *A new cerebrospinal fluid (CSF) infection*: If suspected, a CSF specimen must be obtained for culture and analysis. However, in cases of acute deterioration the empirical treatment of meningitis prior to CSF sampling may be indicated if lumbar puncture cannot be performed immediately.
- *Nonneurologic causes*: Acute pulmonary embolism, arrhythmia, myocardial infarction (MI), hypertensive encephalopathy, metabolic abnormality (hyponatremia, hypoglycemia or severe hyperglycemia, acid-base disorder), overdose of narcotics or benzodiazepines, infection of the blood or urine, and sepsis.

Headache

Approach to clinical assessment

- Determine if the patient has a change in his or her mental status or other focal neurologic deficits associated with the headache.
- Characterize the headache.

Highlights of the history

- Characterize the headache: Sudden onset or gradual? Constant in severity or fluctuating? Positional or nonpositional?
- Identify associated symptoms: Nausea or vomiting? Fever? Neck stiffness? Visual changes? Speech or language abnormalities? Gait difficulty or coordination deficits?

Focused neurological examination

- Survey the patient for a toxic appearance and obtain vital signs.
- Assess mental status for a decreased level of consciousness or disorientation, and listen to the patient's speech for a new dysarthria or aphasia.
- Complete a cranial nerve exam to identify associated deficits. Assess for a new visual field deficit. Do a fundoscopic exam to assess for papilledema if indicated.
- Complete motor and sensory exams to assess for hemiparesis or hemisensory loss. Check reflexes and assess for clonus or a positive Babinski if motor deficits are present. Assess for a pronator drift or dysmetria.

Differential diagnosis

- *Acute intracranial hemorrhage*: A noncontrast CT head may identify a new hemorrhage in the hospitalized patient with a recent intracranial hemorrhage, an ischemic stroke or status postcranial surgery, or in the patient with an unsecured intracranial aneurysm or on anticoagulation therapy.
- *Increasing hydrocephalus*: CT head shows enlarging ventricles, often secondary to an intraventricular brain tumor, a subarachnoid hemorrhage, or a malfunctioning EVD or shunt.
- *Increasing cerebral vasospasm*: CTA/CTP shows stenosed large vessels, most commonly in the patient admitted with a subarachnoid hemorrhage. Transcranial Doppler studies also demonstrate increasing velocities of blood flow within the cerebral arteries.
- *Meningitis*: CSF culture and analysis demonstrate infection, commonly in the hospitalized patient whose CSF has been accessed multiple times.
- *Uncontrolled pain following an open cranial procedure.*
- *Spinal headache*: May occur following a lumbar puncture or an intraoperative durotomy.
- *Uncontrolled muscle spasms*: Occur often following a posterior cervical surgery or a suboccipital procedure.
- *Nonneurologic causes*: These include accelerated hypertension, metabolic abnormality, systemic infection, medication side effect.

New speech or language deficit

Approach to clinical assessment

- Determine if there are associated neurologic deficits present.
- If associated neurologic deficits are identified, localize the central nervous system abnormality based on the deficits.

Highlights of the history

- Characterize the change in speech or language: Acute onset or gradual? Transient or persistent? Hoarseness, slurred speech, nonsensical speech, halted speech, repetitive speech, or no speech?
- Identify associated symptoms: Mental status changes? Visual changes? Facial weakness? Numbness or weakness in an extremity? Headache? Dizziness?

Focused neurological examination

- Observe vital signs, and assess mental status for decreased alertness or disorientation.
- Assess speech and language, noting voice volume, articulation of words, fluency, repetition, comprehension, naming ability, and perhaps reading and writing ability. Define the type of aphasia, if present. Aphasia is associated with anterior circulation lesions. Dysarthria without aphasia is associated with posterior circulation lesions.
- Evaluate for associated cranial nerve deficits. Assess for nystagmus or a new visual field deficit.
- Perform motor and sensory exams to identify an associated hemiparesis or hemisensory loss, and evaluate tendon reflexes in the setting of other focal findings. Assess for a pronator drift or dysmetria.

Differential diagnosis

- *Acute intracranial hemorrhage*: Noncontrast CT head will show a new hemorrhage. Associated neurologic deficits will help localize the hemorrhage.
- *Acute ischemic stroke or TIA*: A CTA/CTP may show occluded intracranial vessels and identify infarcted or ischemic territories. Physical exam findings aid in localization of the lesion.
- *Cerebral vasospasm following a subarachnoid hemorrhage*: CTA/CTP identifies cerebral vessels with significant stenosis and areas of ischemia within the brain. Transcranial Doppler study shows increasing velocities in cerebral arteries.
- *Active seizure activity or the postictal period*: An electroencephalogram (EEG) will demonstrate ongoing seizures.
- *Injury to a facial, recurrent laryngeal, or hypoglossal nerve*: Injury may be a complication following carotid endarterectomy or anterior cervical discectomy and fusion.
- *Overuse of narcotic pain medications*: This may be seen particularly in the postoperative patient.

Visual changes

Approach to clinical assessment

- Determine if the visual change involves a loss of vision, double vision, or another phenomenon, and determine if the change is bilateral or unilateral.
- Determine if there are associated neurologic deficits indicative of an acute intracranial process.

Highlights of the history

- Characterize the visual change: Sudden onset or insidious? Bilateral or unilateral? Double vision, vision loss, or other? Transient or persistent? Painful or painless? Associated redness or tearing? For double vision, horizontal or vertical images? Gaze in which double vision is worst?

- Determine associated neurologic symptoms: Headache? Speech or language changes? Numbness or weakness in the face or an extremity? Coordination or gait difficulties?

Focused neurological examination

- Assess mental status for decreased alertness or disorientation, and assess speech for dysarthria or a new aphasia.
- Examine the eye structure for visible corneal injection, tearing, or a new ptosis.
- Evaluate the pupils for anisocoria and note any asymmetry in the response of the pupils to direct and consensual light. Assess for an afferent pupillary defect.
- Assess visual acuity and test the extraocular muscles for dysconjugate movements or nystagmus. Assess visual fields by confrontation and define boundaries of deficits detected.
- Evaluate additional cranial nerves, and complete a motor, sensory, and reflex exam to determine associated neurologic deficits. Assess for a pronator drift or a positive Babinski.

Differential diagnosis

- *Postoperative corneal abrasion.*
- *Acute retinal artery occlusion*: This may be seen particularly in the patient with severe carotid artery disease or in the patient status post a carotid endarterectomy or cerebral angiography.
- *Homonymous hemianopsia or quadranopsia*: This occurs secondary to a new or evolving hemorrhage or infarct along the optic tract. Associated neurologic deficits help define the location of the lesion. CT and CTA/CTP are the initial imaging studies to obtain.
- *Horner syndrome*: This may occur following a carotid endarterectomy or ACDF, or due to a small brainstem or hypothalamus stroke or a carotid dissection.
- *Increasing intracranial pressure due to hydrocephalus.*
- *Migraine headache.*
- *Progressive myasthenia gravis or Guillain-Barré syndrome.*
- *Nonneurologic causes*: These include accelerated hypertension and hyperglycemia.

New weakness in an extremity

Approach to clinical assessment

- Determine if the patient is hemodynamically stable.
- Localize the lesion based on symptoms and physical exam findings.

Highlights of the history

- Characterize the weakness: Acute onset or gradual? Unilateral or bilateral? Upper extremity, lower extremity, or both? Stable or progressive? Associated pain in the affected extremity?
- Identify associated symptoms: Confusion or lethargy? New speech or language difficulty? Visual changes? Numbness or tingling in an extremity? Bowel or bladder dysfunction? Incoordination? Nausea or vomiting?

Focused neurological examination

- Assess hemodynamic stability of the patient.
- Evaluate for associated neurologic deficits suggestive of an acute stroke, including a mental status change, new facial droop, pupillary change, visual field deficit, gaze deviation, or neglect.
- Assess motor tone and strength in each individual muscle group in all extremities, comparing bilaterally. Assess for involuntary motor movements. Examine affected extremity and opposing extremity for ipsilateral or contralateral sensation deficits to light touch, temperature, or pain. Examine tendon reflexes in affected extremities bilaterally. Assess for a positive Babinski or the presence of clonus. Assess for a pronator drift or dysmetria.

Differential diagnosis

- *Acute intracranial hemorrhage or acute ischemic stroke*: This may include ischemia due to cerebral vasospasm following a subarachnoid. An urgent noncontrast CT will identify a hemorrhage, or a CTA/CTP may identify the occluded vessel and the ischemic or infarcted territory. Associated neurologic deficits aid in localization of the lesion.
- *Increasing intracranial edema*: This may occur following a head injury, intracranial surgery, or a large stroke. A CT head is the initial diagnostic study.
- *Expanding subdural hematoma*: CT imaging shows increased subdural collection.
- *Active seizure activity or postictal Todd paralysis*: EEG demonstrates continued seizing.
- *Spinal epidural hematoma*: This may be seen particularly following a spinal procedure. An urgent MRI or CT is needed, followed by surgical decompression.
- *Spinal cord ischemia or infarction*: MRI imaging is indicated.
- *Acute myelopathy secondary to a spinal cord tumor*: MRI imaging is indicated.
- *Progressive Guillain-Barré syndrome.*
- *Nerve root injury*: This may be transient or permanent, as a complication of a spinal procedure.

Increasing back pain

Approach to clinical assessment

- Determine if there are associated neurologic deficits in one or both lower extremities, and determine if the lesion is upper motor neuron or lower motor neuron.

Highlights of the history

- Characterize the back pain: Sudden onset or gradual? Localized or diffuse? Specific movements that aggravate pain or positions that relieve pain? Associated leg pain?
- Characterize radicular pain, if present: One leg or both? Pain located in a specific distribution?
- Identify other associated symptoms: Numbness, tingling, or weakness in an extremity? Associated bowel or bladder changes? New gait difficulty?

Focused neurological examination

- Assess if the patient is visibly distressed due to discomfort.
- Palpate the spine and paraspinal muscles for localized tenderness. Examine surgical incision or groin incision, if present, for signs of infection or a hematoma. Note flank bruising or excessive groin tenderness in the patient status post cerebral or spinal angiography.

- Complete a motor, sensory, and reflex exam. Note new muscle weakness in a specific muscle group, decreased sensation in a dermatomal distribution or saddle anesthesia, and specific reflexes that are decreased or absent. Compare bilaterally. Assess for clonus. Deficits, if present, may localize the level of compromise.
- Complete additional maneuvers such as straight leg raise and contralateral straight leg raise if useful in determining a diagnosis.

Differential diagnosis

- *Spinal epidural hematoma*: This may occur as a complication following a spinal procedure. Urgent MRI or CT imaging is indicated, followed by surgical decompression.
- *Nerve or nerve root injury*: This may be transient or permanent, as a complication of a spinal procedure.
- *Positioning of spinal hardware following a spinal fusion*: Plain x-rays are the initial study to assess placement.
- *Muscle spasms*: They may occur following a lumbar surgical procedure.
- *Retroperitoneal hematoma*: This may occur following cerebral angiography. Stat CT imaging of the abdomen and pelvis demonstrates the hemorrhage.
- *Nerve root compression due to edema*: This is associated with a spinal tumor or leptomeningeal disease, visualized on MRI imaging.
- *Nerve root irritation*: This may occur following a lumbar puncture or subarachnoid hemorrhage.
- *Localized infection*: This may be seen at a surgical incision.
- *Nonspecific back pain*: This may occur secondary to preexisting spinal disease and hospital immobility.
- *Nonneurologic causes*: These include renal calculi or severe urinary tract infection.
- *Aortic aneurysm*: This is a diagnosis that should not be missed, as a dissecting or rupturing aortic aneurysm is a surgical emergency that can lead to the patient's death.

PART II

Anatomy

6
NEUROANATOMY OVERVIEW
Part I: Cranial

Cristina Matthews

Skull

The skull is composed of eight cranial bones:

- Frontal bone
- Two parietal bones
- Two temporal bones
- Occipital bone
- Ethmoid bone
- Sphenoid bone

The skull base is divided into three sections consisting of the anterior cranial fossa, middle cranial fossa, and posterior cranial fossa (Figure 6.1). Each of these three sections houses different structures of the brain. The anterior cranial fossa houses the frontal lobes, the middle cranial fossa houses the temporal lobes and the pituitary gland, and the posterior cranial fossa houses the cerebellum, pons, and medulla.

Foramina and fissures

The foramina are openings within the skull through which the vasculature and/or the cranial nerves pass. The foramina also serve as valuable landmarks. Table 6.1 presents a partial list of the foramina, their locations, and the structures within them (Figure 6.2).

Brain

The average adult human male brain weighs approximately 1400 g with the female brain weighing approximately 100 g less. The covering of the brain (dura) is composed of three membranes.

Dura

Dura mater: The dura mater is the outermost layer of dense, fibrous, tough connective tissue. It is made up of two layers called the periosteal and meningeal layers. Sinuses are created where these two layers split to form a cavity for venous drainage.

Arachnoid: The arachnoid layer is a web-like, nonvascular membrane that sits just below the dura mater.

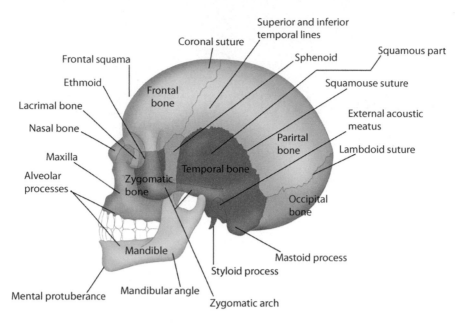

Figure 6.1 The skull.

Table 6.1 List of Foramina—Structures and Locations

Foramen	Location	Structures
Foramen cecum	Anterior cranial fossa	Emissary veins to superior sagittal sinus
Posterior ethmoidal foramen	Anterior cranial fossa	Posterior ethmoidal artery, posterior ethmoidal vein, posterior ethmoidal nerve
Optic canal	Anterior cranial fossa	Ophthalmic artery
Foramen ovale	Middle cranial fossa	Accessory meningeal artery, mandibular nerve (V3)
Foramen spinosum	Middle cranial fossa	Meningeal branch of the mandibular nerve (V3)
Jugular foramen	Posterior cranial fossa	Glossopharyngeal nerve (IX), vagus nerve (X), accessory nerve (XI)
Foramen magnum	Posterior cranial fossa; largest opening	Anterior spinal artery
		Posterior spinal artery, vertebral arteries, medulla oblongata

Subarachnoid space: The subarachnoid space lies between the arachnoid membrane and the pia mater. This layer is filled with cerebrospinal fluid (CSF) and houses the vasculature of the brain.

Pia mater: The pia mater is the innermost layer of connective tissue. The pia mater is adherent to the surface of the brain.

Blood–brain barrier

A delicate balance exists between the brain and the circulating blood. This is regulated by the blood-brain barrier. The blood-brain barrier is a cellular membrane made up of tight junctions. It regulates the exchange of water and solutes between the plasma and CSF.

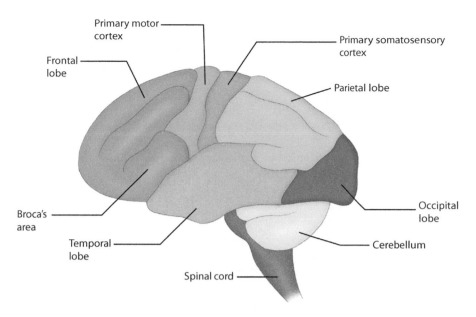

Figure 6.2 The brain.

The ventricles

The brain contains four ventricles: two lateral ventricles and a third and a fourth ventricle. The two lateral ventricles communicate through an intraventricular foramen (the foramen of Monroe), and the third and fourth ventricles communicate by way of a cerebral aqueduct (Sylvius).

Cerebrospinal fluid (CSF)

There are approximately 140 mL of circulating CSF volume in the ventricles, spinal cord, and subarachnoid space. Approximately 500 mL of CSF is made in a 24-hour period by the choroid plexus. CSF circulates through the brain and spinal cord and is reabsorbed by the arachnoid villi in the subarachnoid space and drained through the venous system.

The brain is divided into three main sections as follows:

1. *Brainstem:* The brainstem is made up of the medulla, pons, and midbrain. The brainstem controls basic body functions such as heart rate and respiration.
   a. *Medulla:* The medulla is the most inferior section of the brainstem. The medulla starts at the end of the pons and ends at the beginning of the spinal cord.
   b. *Pons:* The pons sits above the medulla.
   c. *Midbrain:* The midbrain sits above the pons. The midbrain is made up of the cerebral peduncles and corpora quadrigemina (inferior and superior colliculi).
2. *Cerebellum:* The cerebellum sits directly behind the brainstem. It is responsible for motor control, coordination, and balance.
   a. *Diencephalon:* The diencephalon sits on top of the midbrain and consists of the thalamus, the hypothalamus, and the pineal gland. The thalamus controls sleep and wake patterns; it also serves as a relay station for information.
   b. *Basal ganglia:* Basil ganglia include the caudate, putamen, and globus pallidus. These nuclei work with the cerebellum to coordinate fine motions, such as fingertip movements.

3. *Cerebrum:* The cerebrum is divided into two cerebral hemispheres (right and left) that are partially connected by the corpus callosum. The cerebral hemispheres are responsible for receiving, processing, and relaying information for sensory and motor integration. The left hemisphere is thought to be responsible for logic and mathematical reasoning, while the right hemisphere is believed to be more involved in the arts and creativity.

Cerebral cortex

The cerebral cortex is the surface of the brain consisting of the gray and white matter and is divided into the following two sections:

*   Outer cortex consisting of six layers of gray matter
*   Inner cortex consisting of the white matter

Gyri/Sulci

Gyri and sulci are groves and ridges on the surface of the brain. The central sulcus and the lateral sulcus are the two main sulci that provide the landmarks for demarcation of the lobes of the brain.

The four lobes of the brain are named for the bone under which they sit and are separated by lateral and central sulci as follows:

Frontal: The frontal lobe sits anterior to the central sulcus. It is responsible primarily for decision making, problem solving, and planning.

Parietal: The parietal lobe sits posterior to the central sulcus. Its primary function is sensory and motor input. The sensory cortex and the motor cortex are located in the parietal lobe.

Temporal: The temporal lobe is located inferior to the lateral sulcus. The primary functions of the temporal lobe are language, hearing, and memory.

Occipital: The occipital lobe is located posterior to the temporal and parietal lobes. Its primary function is vision.

Table 6.2 The Cranial Nerves

Cranial nerves	Sensory	Motor
I—Olfactory	Smell	
II—Optic	Visual acuity	
III—Ocular motor		Constricts pupil; eye movement (with cranial nerves IV and VI)
IV—Trochlear		Eye movement (with cranial nerves III and VI)
V—Trigeminal	Facial sensation	Chewing
VI—Abducens		Eye movement (with cranial nerves III and IV)
VII—Facial	Sensation of the face	Facial expression
VIII—Vestibulocochlear	Hearing/equilibrium	
IX—Glossopharyngeal	Pharyngeal sensation	Swallowing
X—Vagus	Pharyngeal sensation	Swallowing
XI—Accessory		Movement of neck/shoulders
XII—Glossopharyngeal		Tongue movement

Cranial nerves

There are 12 pairs of cranial nerves that are responsible for sensory, motor, or both sensory and motor function. Table 6.2 presents the cranial nerves and their corresponding sensory and/or motor functions.

Cerebrovascular

Circle of Willis

The circle of Willis is located at the base of the brain and provides blood supply to the brain. The internal carotid arteries (ICAs) and the vertebral arteries (VAs) anastomose create the circle of Willis (Figure 6.3).

Internal carotid arteries (ICAs)

The ICAs originate from the common carotid artery. The ICAs divide to form the middle cerebral artery (MCA) and the anterior cerebral artery (ACA).

Anterior circulation

The anterior circulation supplies the anterior portions of the brain.

Anterior cerebral artery (ACA)

The ACA runs along the interhemispheric fissure. The ACA supplies the medial and superior aspects of the brain.

Middle cerebral artery (MCA)

The MCA runs along the lateral sulcus. The MCA provides the greatest supply of blood to the lateral aspect of the brain.

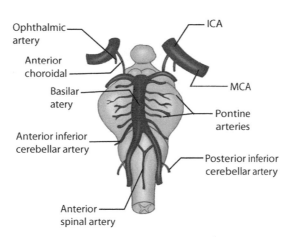

Figure 6.3 The cerebrovascular system.

Posterior circulation

The posterior circulation supplies the brainstem and cerebellum.

Vertebral arteries (VAs)

The VAs supply the posterior circulation of the circle of Willis. The VAs arise from the subclavian artery and join to form the basilar artery (BA).

Basilar artery (BA)

The BA is formed at the connection of the two VAs at the area of the pons. The BA splits at the midbrain into the posterior cerebral artery.

Posterior cerebral artery (PCA)

The PCA branches off the basilar artery. The PCA gives rise to the posterior communicating artery that connects the anterior and posterior circulation.

Posterior communicating artery (PComm)

The PComm connects the ICA to the PCA. The PComm connects the anterior circulation via the ICA to the posterior circulation via the vertebrobasilar artery. The PComm supplies the occipital lobes and inferior parts of the brain.

Cerebral venous drainage

All cerebral drainage ultimately terminates through the jugular veins. The confluence of sinuses is where the straight sinuses, the superior sinuses, and the occipital sinuses meet and then drain into the transverse sinus, which in turn drains into the sigmoid sinus, then into the cavernous sinus, to the superior petrosal sinus, then to the inferior petrosal sinus, and into the inferior jugular vein. This drainage system is unlike any other in the body as it operates without valves or muscles.

7

NEUROANATOMY OVERVIEW

Part II: Spine

Carolina Sandoval-Garcia and Daniel K. Resnick

The human vertebral column consists of 33 vertebral bodies, which provide the main support for the body. It is a complex three-dimensional structure governed by biomechanical principles and responsible for support of the head as well as stability and movement of the trunk.

For practical purposes, the human spine is subdivided in regions that share anatomic and functional similarities.

Normal configuration of the spine

As shown in Figure 7.1, rostrally, the cervical spine has a lordotic curvature and is composed of seven vertebrae designated C1 through C7. The thoracic region has 12 vertebrae from T1 through T12 and has added stability provided by the sternum and rib cage (Brasiliense et al., 2011). It has a kyphotic curve. The lumbar region has five vertebrae. These are the largest vertebrae owing to the accumulated load, and this region normally has a lordotic curvature (Yoganandan et al., 2004). Both in normal and pathologic conditions, these sagittal curves arise as an evolutionary response to ambulation and erect posture. They develop progressively over time after birth as the individual develops more complex body positions and motion (Izzo et al., 2013). The more caudal aspect of the spine is the sacrococcygeal area, composed of five fused sacral vertebrae and up to four separate coccygeal bones (Yoganandan et al., 2004).

Vertebrae

The bony elements of the spine are the vertebrae that are essentially composed of an anterior cylindrically shaped body and posterior elements arranged as a ring, also known as the neural arch, as the arch forms a canal containing the spinal cord and nerve roots. The vertebral bodies and posterior elements to a lesser degree are composed of a core of trabeculated cancellous bone with a surrounding shell of cortical bone. The posterior arch varies within the different regions of the spine but in general is composed of pedicles, laminae, facet articulations, and a spinous process. The pedicles are small tubular structures that connect the vertebral body to the laminae. The pedicle ends in the caudal portion of the superior articulating process of the facet. Transverse processes arise laterally at this junction point on either side and provide attachment sites for paraspinal musculature. The laminae are slanted plates that project posteromedially from the pedicle and join in the midline to form the spinous process.

Together with the intervertebral discs and spinal ligaments, the facets connect adjacent vertebrae and are responsible for mechanical stability, facilitate the transmission of loads in the spine as well as control

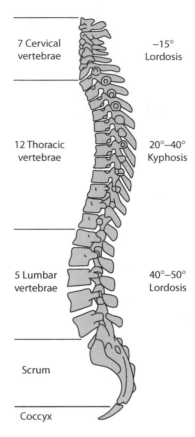

7 Cervical vertebrae — −15° Lordosis

12 Thoracic vertebrae — 20°–40° Kyphosis

5 Lumbar vertebrae — 40°–50° Lordosis

Scrum

Coccyx

Figure 7.1   Sagittal view of the human spine.

of the direction and amplitude of movement. Their orientation and configuration vary as with other spine elements, depending on the region and required motion. The facet articulation, also known as zygapophyseal joint, is formed by the inferior facet of the superior vertebra meeting the superior facet of the inferior vertebra. As such, each vertebral level has two superior and two inferior facets, and the bone segment between the superior and inferior facets is referred to as pars interarticularis. The facets are then symmetrically positioned relative to the midsagittal plane and have a ligamentous capsule that encloses the joint space (Jaumard et al., 2011).

The features of the vertebrae vary to some extent depending on the anatomic region and function. In the cervical region, the C1 vertebra also known as atlas is the transition from the head to the spine. It is a ring-like structure that connects the occipital region of the skull with the rest of the spine. It has an anterior and a posterior arch with no proper vertebral body. The second cervical vertebra (C2), also known as axis, is also unique. It has a distinct vertebral body configuration, having developed a superiorly projecting peg-like structure known as the dens or odontoid process. The vertebrae from C3 through C7 share a similar structure with short bodies that are larger in the transverse than in the anteroposterior diameter and increase in size gradually (Panjabi et al., 1991). The uncovertebral joints are also present only in C3-C6 and represent the upward curving of the most lateral aspect of the endplates in this region forming uncinate processes (Lu et al., 1998). The pars interarticularis in the cervical vertebrae is called the lateral mass. The articulating facets have a coronal orientation. The transverse processes are unique in the cervical vertebrae in that they contain the transverse foramen through which the vertebral artery ascends, usually between C6 and C2. The spinous processes tend to be bifid from C1 through C6.

46

The thoracic vertebrae share a similar configuration and increase progressively in size from T1 through T12. The spinous processes tend to be horizontally oriented on the first and last thoracic segments but adopt a vertical orientation and are longer and overlapping from T3 through T10. The laminae are also broader and somewhat overlapping, and the rib cage significantly adds to the thoracic spine stability compared to the other regions. The connection between each rib and the vertebrae occurs at costovertebral and costotransverse articular surfaces (Panjabi et al., 1991). The facets are oriented in the coronal plane rostrally and develop a more sagittal orientation in the lower segments.

The lumbar vertebrae continue the trend of caudal increase in size and share similar attributes from L1 to L5. Their laminae are broad and have minimal overlap; they have the largest transverse processes extending laterally and prominent spinous processes projecting dorsally, which increase in size peaking at around L3 and becoming slightly smaller in the lower two segments (Panjabi et al., 1992). The facets have a predominantly sagittal orientation. For a representation of the typical configuration of vertebrae at each particular region see Figure 7.2a–e.

The sacrococcygeal region is composed of the five fused sacral segments with a slight concave orientation and a small tail-like ending called coccyx which has two to up to four fully fused segments. In most adults the coccyx curves anteriorly and inferiorly (Woon and Stringer, 2012).

Vertebral endplates and discs

The vertebral endplates are the superior and inferior vertebral body surfaces and have a cartilaginous layer that is in intimate contact with the intervertebral discs. The discs are located between each pair of vertebral bodies from the C2-C3 level all the way down through L5-S1. The intervertebral discs account for one-third to one-fifth of the total height of the vertebral column (Yoganandan et al., 2004).

The discs are formed by an outer rim called annulus fibrosus and a core called nucleus pulposus. The annulus fibrosus is composed predominantly of collagen type I fibers arranged obliquely in a lamellar fashion, the orientation of the fibers within each layer is the same but changes by 30° within each section. The core region is a gelatinous structure with an irregular mesh of type II collagen fibers and high water content (Humzah and Soames, 1988; Rodrigues-Pinto et al., 2014).

Ligaments

The ligaments provide different degrees of stability to the spine depending on many biomechanical parameters beyond intrinsic strength or the number of segments each particular ligament spans (Izzo et al., 2013). The ligaments of the spine are shown in Figure 7.3.

The main ligaments include anterior and posterior longitudinal ligaments, which span the entire length of the spinal column as well as others with varying functions related to their moment arm, namely, interspinous, supraspinous, intertransverse, flavum, and capsular. The anterior longitudinal ligament begins in the occiput and travels down to the sacrum in longitudinally arranged fibers covering up to a third of the anterior surface of each vertebral body. The ligament is thickest over the vertebral bodies, and the more posterior layer actually binds the edges of the intervertebral discs. Of note, the ligament portion from occiput to C1 is also referred to as anterior atlantooccipital membrane.

The posterior longitudinal ligament also spans the entire column beginning as a tectorial membrane in its more rostral portion and extending down to the sacrum. The longitudinally oriented fibers attach more closely to the disc than to the bony surface at the most dorsal layer in each level. The ligament is thickest on the thoracic region but is overall thinner than its counterpart and is particularly thinnest and narrow at the vertebral level, spreading out laterally over the disc space (Yoganandan et al., 2004).

The interspinous and supraspinous ligaments are located as their names indicate, along the spinous processes. The interspinous ligament attaches from the base to the tip at each particular level from C2-C3 to

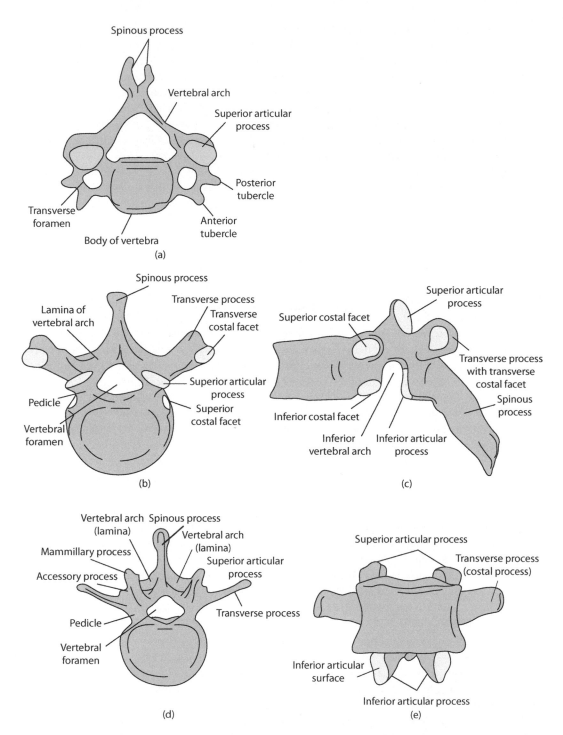

Figure 7.2 (a) Superior view of a cervical vertebra; (b) and (c) Superior and lateral views representative of thoracic vertebrae; (d) and (e) Superior and anterior views of a typical lumbar vertebra.

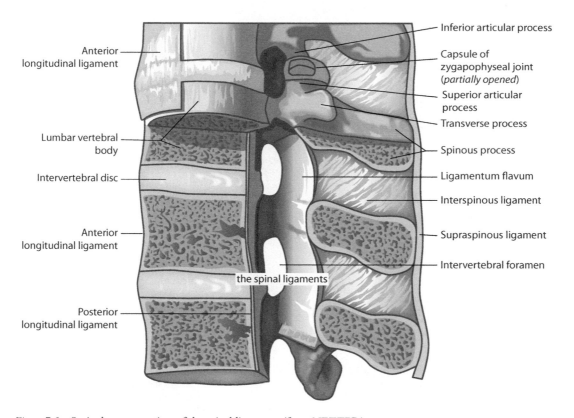

Anterior longitudinal ligament

Inferior articular process

Capsule of zygapophyseal joint (*partially opened*)

Superior articular process

Transverse process

Lumbar vertebral body

Spinous process

Intervertebral disc

Ligamentum flavum

Interspinous ligament

Anterior longitudinal ligament

Supraspinous ligament

Intervertebral foramen

the spinal ligaments

Posterior longitudinal ligament

Figure 7.3 Sagittal representation of the spinal ligaments (from NETTER).

L5-S1. The nuchal ligament working like a fibrous intermuscular septum spreads from the external occipital protuberance connecting the spinous process of all the cervical vertebrae (Kadri and Al-Mefty, 2007). The supraspinous ligament is the continuation of the nuchal ligament and connects the tips of spinous processes from C7 to the lowest lumbar segments.

The ligamenta flava (also known as yellow ligaments) are broad, paired interlaminar ligaments. As such, they insert in the inferior dorsal aspect of the rostral lamina and extend inferiorly toward the ventral and superior edge of the caudal lamina and are present bilaterally at all levels from C1 down to S1. They are considered the most elastic tissues in the body (Yoganandan et al., 2004).

The craniocervical region has an additional set of ligaments worth mentioning separately. Given the importance of maintaining stability while allowing for full mobility of the head in relationship to the rest of the body, one of the key ligaments in the occipitocervical junction is the cruciate ligament. The superior and inferior limbs that form this complex offer no significant support, but in turn, the transverse ligament is the strongest found in the cervical spine and maintains the odontoid process anteriorly against the dorsal surface of the anterior arch of C1 while separating it from the spinal cord. The alar ligaments start on the lateral aspects of the odontoid process and attach to the base of the skull and the apical ligament, also known as suspensory or middle odontoid, attaches the tip of the odontoid process to the basion. Dorsally, the posterior atlantooccipital membrane is a thin ligament spanning from foramen magnum to atlas. It is continuous with the posterior atlantoaxial membrane, which in turn becomes ligamentum flavum inferiorly (Tubbs et al., 2011). The ligamentous structures of the craniocervical junction are illustrated in Figure 7.4.

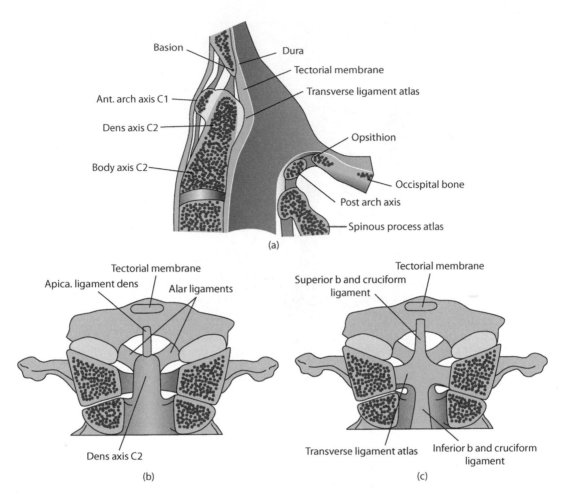

Figure 7.4 (a) Midsagittal posterior sections of coronal views of the craniocervical region ligaments.

Muscles

The musculature of the spine is believed to contribute significantly to active stabilization.

In the upper spine, the muscles responsible for extension are attached medially to the nuchal ligament, and they can be divided into three layers, the trapezius is the most superficial layer, the splenius capitis and cervicis constitute an intermediate layer, and finally the superficial and deep erector spinae muscles, some of which span the entire vertebral column, constitute the third layer (Dodwad et al., 2014).

In the thoracolumbar region, the most prominent muscle of the superficial group is the latissimus dorsi. It arises from the spinous process and extends laterally toward the axillary region.

In the lumbar spine, the psoas major acts as the primary flexor muscle, and the abdominal musculature acts in conjunction even though there are no direct insertions in the spine. The quadratus lumborum and lateral intertransversarii attach to the transverse process and act as lateral flexors. A long list of erector muscles (interspinales, intertransversarii mediales, multifidi, and lumbar erector spinae [longissimus and iliocostalis]) act as extensor muscles (Hansen et al., 2006).

Spinal cord

The spinal cord travels inside the spinal canal extending out the foramen magnum from the medulla, and it is covered by the same meningeal layers as the central nervous system (dura, arachnoides, and pia) The dentate ligaments arise from the pia and are bilateral structures that suspend the cord to the dura laterally.

The spinal cord is composed of 31 segments divided into five anatomic regions: 8 cervical, 12 thoracic, 5 lumbar, 5 sacral, and 1 coccygeal, which is mainly vestigial. The cord ends as conus medullaris around the level of L1-L2 on normal adults and continues intrathecally as cauda equina, which consists of the free floating nerve roots. The spinal nerves travel laterally into the spinal foramina as seen in Figure 7.5. Sensory nerves entering the spine have their cell bodies in the dorsal root ganglion and project to the dorsal root entry zone of the spinal cord. Motor fibers have their cell bodies in the ventral spinal cord, and after emerging from the cord they project to their target muscles. With the exception of C1 which has only a sensory root, all segments have motor and sensory divisions bilaterally, which exit through the corresponding neural foramina (Yoganandan et al., 2004).

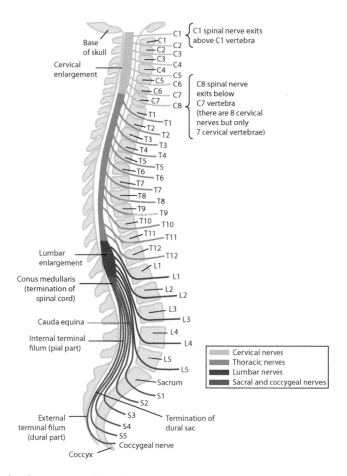

Figure 7.5 Spinal cord and nerve roots (Netter).

References

Brasiliense LBC, Lazaro BCR, Reyes PM, Dogan S, Theodore N, Crawford NR. Biomechanical contribution of the rib cage to thoracic stability. *Spine*. 2011;36(26):E1686-1693. doi:10.1097/BRS.0b013e318219ce84.

Dodwad S-NM, Khan SN, An HS. 2014. Cervical spine anatomy. In: Samartzis D, Fessler RG, Shen F, eds. *Textbook of the Cervical Spine*. Amsterdam, Netherlands: Elsevier Health Sciences.

Hansen L, de Zee M, Rasmussen J, Andersen TB, Wong C, Simonsen EB. Anatomy and biomechanics of the back muscles in the lumbar spine with reference to biomechanical modeling. *Spine*. 2006;31(17):1888-1899. doi:10.1097/01.brs.0000229232.66090.58.

Humzah MD, Soames RW. Human intervertebral disc: structure and function. *Anat Rec*. 1988;220(4):337-356. doi:10.1002/ar.1092200402.

Izzo R, Guarnieri G, Guglielmi G, Muto M. Biomechanics of the spine. Part I: spinal stability. *Eur J Radiol*. 2013;82(1):118-126. doi:10.1016/j.ejrad.2012.07.024.

Jaumard NV, Welch WC, Winkelstein BA. Spinal facet joint biomechanics and mechanotransduction in normal, injury and degenerative conditions. *J Biomech Eng*. 2011;133(7):71010. doi:10.1115/1.4004493.

Kadri PAS, Al-Mefty O. Anatomy of the nuchal ligament and its surgical applications. *Neurosurgery*. 2007;61(5)(suppl 2):301-304; discussion 304. doi:10.1227/01.neu.0000303985.65117.ea.

Lu J, Ebraheim NA, Yang H, Skie M, Yeasting RA. Cervical uncinate process: an anatomic study for anterior decompression of the cervical spine. *Surg Radiol Anat*. 1998;20(4):249-252.

Panjabi MM, Duranceau JMS, Goel V, Oxland TM, Takata K. Cervical human vertebrae quantitative three-dimensional anatomy of the middle and lower regions. *Spine*. 1991a;16(8):861-869.

Panjabi MM, Goel V, Oxland T, et al. Human lumbar vertebrae. Quantitative three-dimensional anatomy. *Spine*. 1992;17(3):299-306.

Panjabi MM, Takata K, Goel V, et al. Thoracic human vertebrae quantitative three-dimensional anatomy. *Spine*. 1991b;16(8):888-901.

Rodrigues-Pinto R, Richardson SM, Hoyland JA. An understanding of intervertebral disc development, maturation and cell phenotype provides clues to direct cell-based tissue regeneration therapies for disc degeneration. *Eur Spine J*. 2014;23(9):1803-1814. doi:10.1007/s00586-014-3305-z.

Tubbs RS, Hallock JD, Radcliff V, et al. Ligaments of the craniocervical junction. *J Neurosurg Spine*. 2011;14(6):697-709. doi:10.3171/2011.1.SPINE10612.

Woon JTK, Stringer MD. Clinical anatomy of the coccyx: a systematic review. *Clin Anat*. 2012;25(2):158-167. doi:10.1002/ca.21216.

Yoganandan N, Dickman C, Benzel E. Chapter 30: practical anatomy and fundamental biomechanics. In: Benzel E, ed. *Spine Surgery: Techniques, Complication Avoidance, and Management*. Vol 2. Philadelphia, PA: Churchill-Livingston; 2004, 1:267-289.

8

NEUROANATOMY OVERVIEW

Part III: Peripheral Nervous System

Marine Dididze and Allan Levi

Peripheral nerves

Basic structure of peripheral nerves

The major tissue components of a peripheral nerve can be divided into the following components. The covering layers include the following (Figure 8.1):

- *Epineurium:* The outer covering of the nerve, made of collagen and elastic fibers. External to epineurium is mesoneurium, a flimsy layer of tissue. The epineurium is continuous with interfascicular epineurium, which invests the different fascicles.
- *Perineurium:* Surrounds each fascicle. The perineurial cells have tight junctions and form the majority of the blood-nerve barrier.
- *Endoneurium:* Encircles each axon within a fascicle. Microvessels are found within the endoneurium. Their endothelial cells have tight junctions, which provide the second portion of the blood-nerve barrier.

The neural component of the peripheral nerve consists of the axons and their associated Schwann cells. Large fibers tend to be myelinated and the smaller ones ensheathed by the Schwann cell. The membrane of each Schwann cell wraps itself around an axonal segment, providing a myelin covering, leaving nodes of Ranvier in between. Nonmyelinated axons are wrapped by Schwann cells, but they do not produce myelin.

Axoplasm contains a bidirectional transport system that has both fast and slow (1–2 mm/day) components.

Brachial plexus

The brachial plexus is formed from the anterior and posterior divisions of cervical roots C5, C6, C7, and C8 and the first thoracic nerve root (T). The C5 and C6 roots merge into the upper trunk, C7 forms the middle trunk, and C8 and T1 form the lower trunk. Each trunk divides into an anterior and a posterior division (Figure 8.2). The anterior divisions of the upper and middle trunks form the lateral cord; the anterior division of the lower trunk forms the medial cord; and the posterior divisions of each trunk form the posterior cord of the plexus.

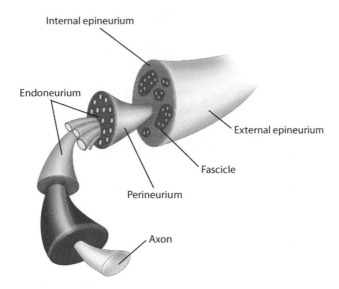

Figure 8.1   Layers of the peripheral nerve.

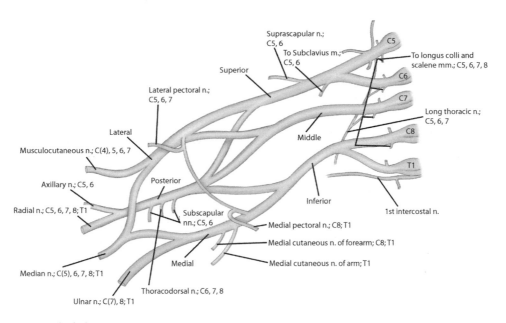

Figure 8.2   Brachial plexus.

Branches of the roots are as follows: (1) long thoracic nerve; (2) dorsal scapular nerve; and (3) nerve to the subclavius.

The branch of the upper trunk includes the suprascapular nerve. Branches of the lateral cord include the following: (1) lateral pectoral nerve; (2) musculocutaneous nerve; and (3) lateral head of the median nerve (C6, C7). Branches of the medial cord are as follows: (1) medial pectoral nerve; (2) medial head of the median nerve; (3) medial cutaneous nerve of the arm; (4) medial cutaneous nerve of the forearm; and (5) ulnar nerve. Branches of the posterior cord are as follows: (1) upper subscapular nerve; (2) thoracodorsal nerve; (3) lower subscapular nerve; (4) axillary nerve; and (5) radial nerve.

Median nerve

The median nerve arises from contributions from the "V" formed by the lateral and medial cords of the brachial plexus (C6, C7, C8, T1 [C5]) and courses slightly lateral to the third portion of the axillary artery and proximal brachial artery. The nerve remains closely applied to the brachial artery in the arm passing superficially to it from lateral to medial. It also passes directly to the antebrachial fossa (no branches in the arm) in the interval between the biceps and brachialis lying medial to these muscles.

In the antecubital fossa, the nerve lies medial to the brachial artery, which lies medial to the biceps tendon (TAN). Motor branches are given off to the pronator teres, the flexor carpi radialis, and the palmaris longus. The median nerve travels deep in the antecubital fossa to its apex and passes between the heads of the pronator teres. Deep to the pronator teres the anterior interosseus nerve is given off, which follows the anterior interosseous membrane and supplies the flexor pollicis longus, the flexor digitorum profundus, and the pronator quadratus. The main nerve passes beneath the flexor digitorum sublimis but on top of the flexor digitorum profundus directly to the carpal tunnel. In the forearm, the median nerve supplies flexors to digits II–V.

At the wrist, the median nerve lies lateral to sublimis tendons between the flexor carpi radialis and the palmaris longus. A palmar cutaneous branch leaves the nerve proximal to the carpal tunnel, and runs along the ulnar side of the flexor carpi radialis tendon superficial to the flexor retinaculum. The recurrent motor branch comes off the radial side of the median nerve at the distal border of the flexor retinaculum to supply the thenar muscles (see carpal tunnel). In the palm, sensory branches are given off to the thumb, index, and middle half of the ring finger, and motor branches to the two radial lumbricals are given off.

Branches

1. Arm—None
2. In forearm
    a. Pronator teres
    b. Flexor carpi radialis
    c. Palmaris longus
    d. Flexor digitorum sublimis (II–V)
3. Anterior interosseous nerve
    a. Flexor pollicis longus
    b. Pronator quadratus
    c. Flexor digitorum profundus (II-III)
4. In hand—Thenar eminence
    a. Abductor pollicis brevis
    b. Opponens pollicis
    c. Flexor pollicis brevis (all by recurrent branch)
    d. Lumbricals I and II

Ulnar nerve

The ulnar nerve arises from the medial cord (C8, T1) beneath the pectoralis minor. Three branches are given off before the ulnar nerve is formed:

1. Medial cutaneous nerve of arm
2. Medial cutaneous nerve of forearm
3. Medial root of the medial cord to the median nerve

It courses downward medial and posterior to the axillary and proximal brachial artery. In the middle of the arm it pierces the medial intermuscular septum and descends in front of the medial head of the triceps. In 70% of patients, the nerve passes under the arcade of Struthers (distinct from the ligament of Struthers), which is a flat, thin fibroaponeurotic band extending from the medial head of the triceps to the medial intermuscular septum. This is often found about 3 inches above the medial epicondyle. The arcade may be a point of kinking if anterior transposition of the ulnar nerve is performed without adequately dividing this arcade and the adjacent medial intermuscular septum.

At the elbow, the ulnar nerve travels in the ulnar groove posterior to the medial epicondyle. It passes between the humeral and ulnar heads of the flexor carpi ulnaris in the cubital tunnel. Motor branches to the flexor carpi ulnaris are given off proximal to the cubital tunnel.

In the forearm, the nerve passes beneath the flexor carpi ulnaris but superficial to the flexor digitorum profundus. A branch is given off to flexor digitorum profundus (IV and V), and to the flexor carpi ulnaris. A Martin-Gruber anastomosis may exist from the anterior interosseous branch of the median to the ulnar nerve in the proximal forearm.

At the wrist, the ulnar nerve passes into Guyon canal. Proximal to the canal, a palmar cutaneous branch is given off. There is also a dorsal cutaneous branch that separates deep to the flexor carpi ulnaris and passes around the medial dorsal border of the forearm to supply sensation to the ulnar aspect of the dorsum of the hand.

In the hand, the ulnar divides into superficial and deep branches:

1. Deep branch (hypothenar muscles)
   a. Abductor digiti minimi
   b. Flexor digiti minimi
   c. Opponens digiti
   The deep branch then turns laterally around the hook of the hamate to supply the
   d. Interossei
   e. Lumbricals III, and IV
   f. Adductor pollicis
2. The superficial branch supplies the palmar surface of ulnar 1 and 1/2 fingers

Summary of ulnar nerve branches

1. Arm—No motor branches (just sensory)
2. Forearm
   a. Flexor carpi ulnaris
   b. Flexor digitorum profundus (IV, V)
3. Hand
   a. Hypothenars
      – Abductor digiti minimi

       – Flexor digiti minimi
       – Opponens digiti minimi
  b.   Lumbricals III, IV
  c.   Interossei—Four dorsal, three palmar
  d.   Adductor pollicis

Radial nerve

Radial nerve in the axilla

The radial nerve originates as a terminal branch of the posterior cord of the brachial plexus, approximately at the level of the coracoid process. It contains within it fibers from C5 to C7, and a small contribution from C8. However, it is mainly from C7. It is possible to split the posterior cord into its major branches (nerve to lattisimus dorsi, axillary nerve) for several centimeters if this is necessary. Close to the radial nerve origin, a number of branches leave it to supply one or more of the three heads of the triceps. Also, while in the axilla, it gives off the posterior brachial cutaneous nerve supplying a small area on the posterolateral aspect of the arm. The nerve can be approached either medially or laterally to the axillary artery during surgery. If there is a lot of scarring, it is better to find the nerve in the axilla and dissect proximally. Branches of the axillary artery should be preserved, namely, the circumflex humeral vessels (along which the axillary nerve is found) and the profunda brachial artery, with which the radial nerve leaves the axilla. At this point, it is the thickest nerve in the axilla (thicker than the ulnar nerve and the medial cutaneous nerve of the forearm).

Radial nerve in the upper arm

Falling anteriorly across the subscapularis, teres major, and latissimus dorsi, it leaves the shoulder to enter the arm.

    The radial nerve travels in the arm by going through the triangular space along with the profunda brachii vessels (space bounded by the long head of triceps medially, humerus laterally, and teres major superiorly). The nerve crosses the medial head of the triceps to wind up in the spiral groove deep to the lateral head of the triceps. It travels sinuously in the spiral groove around the posterior aspect of the arm between the medial and lateral heads of the triceps, which it supplies. Supply to the anconeus is also given off here. In the spiral groove, the nerve is reduced to the least number of fascicles in its entire course (4–5). Prior to piercing the lateral intermuscular septum, two small cutaneous nerves are given off—the inferior lateral cutaneous nerve and the posterior antebrachial cutaneous nerve. It then pierces the lateral intermuscular septum to wind up in the anterior compartment of the arm. Here, it is separated from bone by brachialis, and descends into the intermuscular slit between brachialis and brachioradialis. It can be identified here by splitting these two muscles. A branch is given off to the brachioradialis and to extensor carpi radialis longus about 2–3 cm proximal to the elbow.

Radial nerve in the forearm

The radial nerve enters the antecubital fossa under the cover of extensor carpi radialis longus (ECRL) and brachioradialis. It then gives off the posterior interosseous branch, and a branch to extensor carpi radialis brevis (ECRB). The remainder is a slender, purely cutaneous nerve that retains the name superficial radial nerve, runs down the forearm on top of supinator, pronator teres, flexor digitorum superficialis, and flexor pollicis longus, beneath the cover of the brachioradialis, and lateral to the radial artery. It winds around the lower end of the radius deep to the tendon of brachioradialis, crosses the abductor pollicis longus, the extensor pollicis brevis, and the extensor pollicis longus (the anatomical snuff box) to reach the back of the hand. The posterior interosseus nerve (PIN) supplies all the extensor muscles on the back of the forearm with the exception of ECRL. It wraps around the head and neck of the radius (cf. common peroneal nerve) and passes between the two heads of the supinator. The supinator and extensor carpi ulnaris are supplied by the PIN before it dives in. The volar supinator forms an arch or "arcade" around the PIN known as the arcade of Frohse. The PIN then forms deep and ulnarly directed branches that supply the abductor pollicis longus, extensor pollicis brevis, extensor pollicis longus, and extensor indicis proprius, and superficial and radial directed branches supply the extensor digitorum communis, extensor digiti quinti proprius, and extensor carpi ulnaris. A terminal branch gives sensory fibers to the dorsal aspect of the wrist. In summary, muscles supplied by the radial nerve are as follows:

- Triceps
- Brachioradialis
- Anconeus
- ECRL
- ECRB
- Extensor carpi ulnaris
- Extensor digitorum communis
- Extensor digiti minimi
- Abductor pollicis longus
- Extensor pollicis longus
- Extensor pollicis brevis
- Extensor indicis

Axillary nerve

The axillary (circumflex) nerve (C5) exemplifies Hilton's law by supplying the deltoid, the shoulder joint, and skin over the joint (Figure 8.3). It passes backward through the quadrilateral space, lying above its artery and the vein, in contact with the neck of the humerus just below the capsule of the shoulder joint, which it supplies. The posterior branch supplies the teres minor and winds around the posterior border

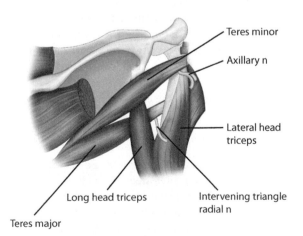

Figure 8.3 Quadrilateral space (posterior view), demonstrating the passage of the axillary nerve toward its final target—the deltoid muscle (not shown) and the radial nerve, which exits below the quadrilateral space as it courses toward the spiral groove.

of the deltoid to supply a small portion of it. The anterior (deep) branch lies on the humerus between the teres minor and the lateral head of the triceps and supplies the deltoid. The upper lateral cutaneous nerve of the arm supplies skin over the shoulder.

Quadrilateral space

- Laterally—Humerus
- Medially—Long head of triceps
- Superiorly—Teres minor
- Inferiorly—Teres major

Lumbosacral plexus

The lumbosacral plexus is composed of the T12, L1-L5, and S1-S3 spinal nerve roots; it innervates the muscles of the lower extremities (Figure 8.4). The major branches are as discussed in the following sections.

Femoral nerve

The femoral nerve arises from L2 to L4 and courses retroperitoneally through the psoas muscle and then distally in the groove between the iliacus and the psoas muscle, innervating the iliacus muscle. Then it courses deep to the inguinal ligament just lateral and adjacent to the femoral artery but separated from it by the iliopsoas fascia. After passing under the inguinal ligament, it branches into its many motor and sensory branches. It supplies the sartorius, the rectus femoris, the vastus lateralis, the vastus medialis, and the vastus intermedius, and gives rise to the saphenous nerve and the anteromedial and medial cutaneous nerves of the thigh.

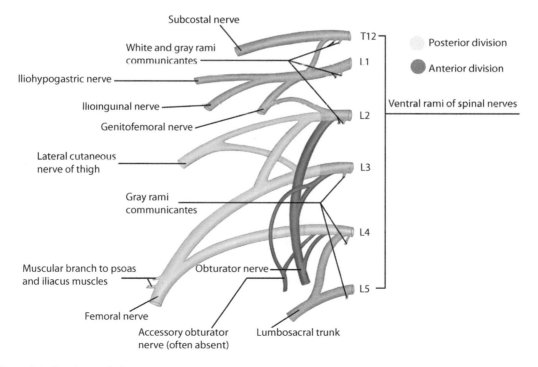

Figure 8.4 Lumbosacral plexus.

Lateral femoral cutaneous nerve

This nerve arises from L1 to L2 and courses obliquely through the pelvis lateral to the femoral nerve, but not as lateral as the ilioinguinal and genitofemoral nerves. It then courses anteriorly at the level of the lateral pelvic brim to exit the pelvis medial to the anterior superior iliac spine. It runs beneath and sometimes through some of the lateral fascia of the inguinal ligament. It supplies sensation to the skin of the lateral thigh in a "trouser pocket" distribution.

Obturator nerve

The obturator nerve arises from L2 to L4 and passes through the obturator foramen by passing through the psoas major muscle behind the common iliac vessels. It courses along the wall of the pelvis on the ala of the sacrum where it may be easily dissected free, lying in an areolar fatty channel. It is best identified intrapelvically by feeling for the obturator foramen.

The nerve passes through the foramen to divide into anterior and posterior divisions. The anterior segment supplies the adductor longus, the gracilis, the pectineus, and the adductor brevis. The posterior division supplies the obturator externus, adductor magnus. In effect, the adductors are all supplied by the obturator nerve except the presemimembranosus part of the adductor magnus.

Sciatic nerve

The sciatic nerve is the largest nerve in the body and arises from L4, L5, and S1–S3. It passes out of the pelvis through the greater sciatic foramen *below* the pyriformis muscle resting on the posterior surface of the ischium. It lies deep to the gluteus maximus muscle but superficial to the gemelli (superior and inferior), obturator internus, and quadratus femoris. The superior gluteal artery passes above the pyriformis; the inferior gluteal artery passes below the pyriformis, medial to the sciatic nerve. The sciatic nerve lies halfway between the greater trochanter and the ischial tuberosity. In the posterior thigh, the nerve travels on top of the adductor magnus and deep to the long head of the biceps femoris. The nerve then reaches the popliteal fossa (see common peroneal nerve and popliteal fossa) as the tibial nerve.

Branches

1. Articular—hip joint
2. Biceps femoris
3. Semitendinosus
4. Semimembranosus
5. Ischial head of adductor magnus

Tibial nerve

Initially lateral to the vessels in the upper popliteal fossa, the tibial nerve crosses to the medial aspect caudally. The vessels (artery, vein) lie deep to the nerve throughout. The nerve travels to the distal border of the popliteus and passes deep to the arch of the soleus. The nerve lies superficial to the tibialis posterior here, but then lies more superficial in the lower leg to reach the interval between the medial malleolus and the tendocalcaneus. It divides under the flexor retinaculum into the medial and lateral plantar nerves.

Branches

1. Articular, three branches following arteries to the knee joint.
2. Muscular
   Gastrocnemius
   Soleus
   Plantaris
   Popliteus
   Posterior tibial
   Flexor digitorum longus
   Flexor hallucis longus
3. Medial sural nerve—Forms the sural nerve
4. Calcaneal branches
5. Medial plantar nerve
   – Accompanies the medial plantar artery
   – Supplies the flexor digitorum brevis and the abductor hallucis
   – Has digital cutaneous branches supplying the medial 3 1/2 toes, plantar
6. Lateral plantar nerve
   – Crosses the sole obliquely deep to the first layer of muscles
   – Supplies the flexor accessorius and the abductor digit minimi
   – Has perforating branches through the plantar aponeurosis to the skin on the lateral side of the sole
   – Divides into superficial and deep branches near Vth metatarsal base
   – Has superficial branch that supplies IVth cleft, and little toe, and supplies the flexor digiti minimi, and two interossei of IVth
   – Has a deep branch that supplies the rest of the interossei and the transverse head of the adductor hallucis

Posterior tibial nerve

This terminal branch of the sciatic nerve descends vertically in the posterior aspect of the leg deep to the soleus muscle and enters the tarsal tunnel just behind the posterior tibial vessels.

The nerve divides either within the tunnel or at a distal border of the tunnel into three terminal branches:

1. *Calcaneal nerve*

   A purely sensory nerve with highly variable course. It may arise proximal to the ligament, may course through the ligament, may pass deep to the ligament, and usually supplies sensation to the heel.
2. *Medial plantar nerve*

   This nerve passes through an individual opening in the abductor hallucis muscle and may become compressed distal to the flexor retinaculum in the fibrous hiatus. It supplies motor to intrinsic foot muscles and supplies sensation to sole of foot (distribution similar to median nerve).
3. *Lateral plantar nerve*

   This nerve passes through individual opening in abductor hallucis muscle and may become compressed distal to flexor retinaculum in fibrous hiatus. It supplies the motor intrinsics to the foot and supplies sensation to the sole of the foot (distribution similar to the ulnar nerve).

Common peroneal nerve

The common peroneal nerve innervates the muscle of dorsiflexion, or extension of the foot. It is most commonly injured by athletic or automobile accidents related to trauma to the lateral aspect of the head of the fibula. Clinically, it is characterized by a foot drop.

Anatomy of the common peroneal nerve

The common peroneal nerve is the lateral component of the sciatic nerve and arises from the L4 to S2 nerve roots. It is one of the terminal branches of the sciatic nerve, branching along with the tibial nerve at a variable distance above the popliteal fossa. The common peroneal nerve travels along the medial margin of the biceps femoris muscle (giving off a cutaneous branch and the sural nerve), wraps around the head of the fibula, and dives deep to the peroneus longus muscle. At this point, the common peroneal nerve divides into three branches:

1. Recurrent articular branch (sensory to the knee, and tibiofibular joint).
2. Superficial peroneal branch (motor to peroneus longus and brevis, and sensory to lateral surface of the leg and dorsum of the foot). This nerve passes downward over the peronei and divides above the ankle into medial and lateral branches that supply the skin of the dorsum of the foot. The medial branch divides to supply the medial side of the dorsum of the great toe and the sides of the second cleft. The lateral branch divides to supply the third and fourth clefts.
3. Deep peroneal (anterior tibial) branch, which provides motor innervation to the four extensor muscles (extensor digitorum longus and brevis, extensor hallucis longus and brevis) as well as the tibialis anterior. It passes through the upper part of the origin of the extensor digitorum longus muscle to the lateral border of the tibialis muscle. Here in the anterior compartment of the leg on the anterior interosseous membrane, it travels along the lateral aspect of the anterior tibial artery and descends with it to the ankle. This nerve is involved in the ischemic condition known as the anterior tibial compartment syndrome. The nerve is exposed by dissecting between the tibialis anterior and extensor digitorum longus tendons superiorly (extensor hallucis longus tendon inferiorly) to expose the deep peroneal nerve lateral to the anterior tibial artery and vein.

The popliteal fossa

The diamond-shaped space behind the knee.

Boundaries:

- Superomedially—Semimembranosus and semitendinosus tendons
- Superolaterally—Biceps femoris tendon
- Inferomedially and inferolaterally—Heads of gastrocnemius
- Roof—Fascia lata
- Floor—Popliteal surface of the femur, the capsule of the knee joint and the popliteus muscle covered by fascia

Contents:

- Popliteal artery (lies deep and medial to the nerve)
- Popliteal vein (lies between the artery and the nerve)
- Tibial nerve
- Common peroneal nerve
- Popliteal lymph nodes

9

THE NEUROLOGICAL EXAMINATION

Part I: Cranial

S. Shelby Burks and Michael Y. Wang

A detailed neurological examination provides vital insight into which particular regions of the nervous system are impaired. This information will be critical in guiding treatment. Understanding the neurological examination and approaching it systematically allow for thorough patient care. The cranial neurological examination will be detailed below but should always start with assessment of a patient's level of consciousness. From this the examination can be focused. Taking a minute to confirm that the patient knows where he or she is and asking a few other simple orientation questions can be very important in considering pursuing further diagnostic studies, especially in the inpatient setting. Once the patient's level of consciousness is determined, go through the cranial nerves (CNs) from rostral to caudal. Keep in mind that you may be the first to perform a detailed cranial nerve exam in a patient new to the neurosurgery service.

Please note that if there is concern about one of your patients or in consultation of a new patient use the physical exam first before deciding on what type of diagnostic tests to pursue. In a patient with recent cranial surgery, especially that centered on the skull base, you should consider each cranial nerve.

Level of consciousness can be determined by asking for the patient's name, present location, and date. Asking a secondary question such as "who is the president of the United States?" "who is this sitting at your bedside?" or "why are you in the hospital?" will further elucidate the patient's cognitive function.

CN I—Olfactory nerve: A simple way to test this is to take a small bag of coffee beans or a bottle cap filled with cleaning detergent. The olfactory nerve is the only cranial nerve that does not have a nucleus in the brainstem. This CN can often be skipped unless there is specific concern. Certain tumors of the anterior skull base can impair the sense of olfaction as can intranasal pathology or transsphenoidal surgery.

CN II—Optic nerve: This CN must be assessed in multiple ways, namely, visual acuity, visual fields, and pupillary reactivity (note that this also tests CN III). Visual acuity (VA) is best assessed using a Snellen chart. These are easily carried in a white coat pocket and are highly recommended. Others prefer to use a smartphone. In the interest of time, ask the patient to begin with a line he or she can easily read and progress down from there. Assess each eye separately. Ask the patient to hold the chart (or phone) so that he or she can maintain it in a comfortable distance and position. The specific distance is detailed on the chart. The fraction grade for a patient's VA should be listed on the side of the chart. In the United States, it is standardized to 20 feet; in other countries, this is set at 6 meters. Document the patient's best acuity on each eye and note if vision is corrected or uncorrected. Adjust for letters missed, such as "20/30 −2" if two letters were incorrect. If the patient's vision is too poor and he or she cannot read the top letter of the Snellen chart, hold up your fingers and ask the patient to count at varying distances; 1, 2, or 3 feet. If unable to count fingers, determine if the patient can see your hand waving, and this is described as "hand movements" (HMs). Last, if unable to see hand movement, check for light perception (LP). NLP refers to "no light perception." OD refers to the right eye; OS refers to the left eye. OU refers to both.

Visual fields should be assessed by "confrontational exam." Basically you are determining if the patient can see in all of the four quadrants in each eye. Do this by aligning your left eye with the patient's right eye, or vice versa, so that your faces are about 2 feet apart. Have the patient cover one eye. Move your hand to each of the four quadrants asking the patient to count fingers. Use one, two, or five fingers as three and four will be somewhat ambiguous. It may be helpful to close one of your eyes to get a sense of where to place your hand. Note that this test can be especially important for pathology in the sella. The classic finding in tumors of the sella is a bitemporal hemianopsia (Figure 9.1). This may be subtle and not easily detected. One adjunct method is to wiggle your fingers in the periphery of a patient's vision, moving them toward the center slowly, asking the patient to note when he or she sees the motion.

CN III, IV, and VI—Oculomotor, trochlear, and abducens nerves: Extraocular movement can be easily assessed asking the patient to follow your finger as you move it up and down, left and right. Assess not only for obvious deviation or asymmetry, but also ask the patient if he or she notices double vision, as this will be more sensitive. For example, in the case of a CN III palsy, the affected eye will usually be directed down and out on forward gaze with a degree of ptosis (Figure 9.2a). CN III palsy must be characterized as either pupil sparing or pupil involving. CN III palsy with pupillary involvement is often the result of a compressive lesion, and one must consider a posterior communicating artery aneurysm. This is often referred to as the "surgical" third nerve palsy. CN IV palsy has the characteristic eye position of up and slightly in (Figure 9.2b). Patients will have worsening diplopia on downward and lateral gaze away from the affected eye. Head tilting to the affected side will also illicit diplopia. Acquired trochlear nerve palsies are often the result of head trauma. This nerve has the longest course of all cranial nerves and is thus the most susceptible to injury. Patients may complain of difficulty going down stairs. CN VI palsy manifests as inward deviation on resting position (Figure 9.2c). This nerve can be injured with high intracranial pressure.

After assessing extraocular movements, be sure to document any pupillary abnormalities, commenting specifically on the size in millimeters. Note that the Snellen chart typically has pupil measurements on the bottom. Use the "swinging flashlight" test to determine if an afferent pupillary defect is present. This would be the case in optic nerve pathology. A light source is moved back and forth from one eye to the other. A normal response in the eye not receiving the light would be to contract as the light is shined into the opposite eye. When it dilates after light is moved from that eye to the other, an afferent pupillary defect is presumed (see Figure 9.3).

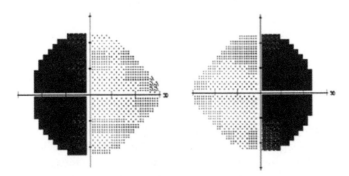

Figure 9.1 Bitemporal hemianopsia. Depicted are the typical visual field deficits for a patient with a mass in the sella compressing the optic chiasm. The shaded regions represent lack of vision. This corresponds to a lack of peripheral vision.

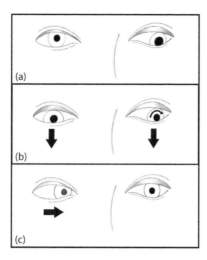

Figure 9.2 Typical abnormalities of extraocular movements. The baseline findings of a patient with a cranial nerve III, oculomotor, palsy on straight gaze are depicted on the top image with the pathologic pupil facing down and out. Note that the affected eye has a degree of ptosis (a). Middle image shows lateral rotation of the affected pupil on downward gaze. This represents a cranial nerve IV, trochlear nerve palsy (b). Finally, on the bottom image a patient with cranial nerve VI, abducens, palsy showing the affected eye cannot move laterally (c).

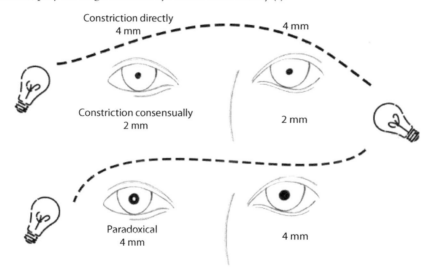

Figure 9.3 Swinging flashlight test. Depicted are the expected findings on a swinging flashlight test in the setting of optic nerve pathology. The light source is moved from the normal, left eye to the affected side, right eye, and the affected eye paradoxically dilates.

CN V—*Trigeminal nerve*: Facial sensation should be tested comparing light touch, pinprick, and temperature sensation across the face. Compare one side to the other, and determine which branch of the trigeminal nerve is involved as V1-3 have characteristic dermatomes (Figure 9.4). Note that the trigeminal nerve also supplies the temporalis muscles bilaterally as well as other muscles of mastication.

CN VII—*Facial nerve*: Facial nerve function can be assessed by looking at facial asymmetry. Ask the patient to smile and close his or her eyes tightly. Look for weakness on one side or the other. Determine if the facial weakness involves the forehead or eyebrows. If it does then the lesion is peripheral, but if it does

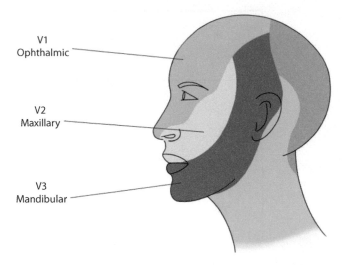

Figure 9.4 Dermatomal map of the trigeminal nerve. Here is a lateral image of the face with each shaded region representing a distinct distribution of a trigeminal nerve branch, V1-3.

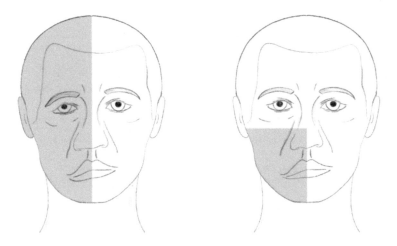

Figure 9.5 Facial palsy. A peripheral (left) versus central (right) facial paralysis is distinguished by involvement of the forehead. A central lesion will not impair a patient's ability to elevate their eyebrows.

not then the lesion is central (Figure 9.5). Peripheral facial palsy can be due to a fracture in the temporal bone or an acoustic neuroma, for example. Central facial palsy may be the result of an ischemic stroke. Note that the facial nerve also supplies taste to the anterior portion of the tongue.

CN VIII—Vestibulocochlear nerve: Test the patient's hearing by whispering into one ear and asking the patient to plug the other ear. Alternatively, you can rub fingers together near the external auditory canal.

CN IX and X—Glossopharyngeal and vagus nerves: These nerves mediate the gag reflex, which is described later in this chapter. You can also ask the patient about swallowing difficulty. Have the patient open his or her mouth and say "ahh," looking at the uvula determining if it elevates symmetrically; this is mediated by CN IX. The uvula will deviate away from the affected nerve.

CN XI—Spinal accessory nerve: The accessory nerve supplies the sternocleidomastoid (SCM) and the trapezius muscles. The SCM is tested by asking the patient to turn his or her head to one side or another while you hold resistance against the chin. Similarly, test the trapezius by having the patient shrug his or her shoulders against resistance.

CN XII—Hypoglossal nerve: Simply ask the patient to stick out his or her tongue. The tongue will deviate toward the side of the affected nerve.

In the *comatose patient*, the cranial nerve exam may be focused on cranial nerve reflexes. In these patients with impaired consciousness, the reflexes evaluate brainstem function.

Pupillary light reflex: Normally, the pupils constrict to light in both direct and indirect fashions. Look at the sizes of the pupils and their relative levels of reactivity. Their reaction may be "brisk" or "sluggish." Pupils that clearly do not react to light are called "nonreactive." A fixed, or nonreactive, pupil may be "blown," meaning maximally dilated, "midposition," or "pinpoint." A patient suffering from severe anoxic brain injury or untreated, obstructive hydrocephalus often presents with fixed and dilated pupils. Pinpoint pupils can be the result of pontine hemorrhage or ischemia but may also be seen in the overnarcotized patient. Asymmetric pupils may be caused by transtentorial herniation and must be recognized abruptly.

Vestibuloocular "doll's eye" reflex: This reflex looks at the communication between the vestibular system and eyes through multiple nuclei. To test this reflex, the head is quickly turned to one side or the other, and the pupils should move away from the head turn. If pupils stay midglobe, this is abnormal and a negative doll's eye. Be careful in trauma patients with cervical spine pathology.

Corneal reflex: This tests both CN V and CN VII. A patient's eye is opened, and a soft piece of cotton is gently touched to the cornea watching for a reflexive blink. Due to the risk of corneal abrasion, an alternative method is dropping saline in the opened eye.

Pharyngeal "gag" reflex: Here CN XI (efferent) and CN X (afferent) are tested. A patient with stimulus to the pharynx will cough. In an intubated patient, the small suction tubing can be passed into the proximal trachea and a cough elicited. Another variation is to apply gentle pressure to the laryngeal cartilage or to the endotracheal tube itself, watching for a cough.

Cerebellar signs can be assessed after cranial nerves. Assess whether the patient can maintain his or her balance in the seated position. If the patient appears to be falling to one side or another, this may be a type of truncal ataxia. Look then at the arms and legs, assessing fine motor movements. Hold a finger out and ask the patient to touch his or her nose and then to touch your finger, move your finger around and see if the patient has difficulty. In the lower extremities, ask the patient to run his or her heel up and down the opposite shin. Difficulty with these tests would be known as appendicular ataxia.

Pearls and pitfalls

As mentioned in the beginning of this chapter, the patient's level of consciousness should be noted, and then further going into subtle signs of confusion or agitation. Nowhere is this more important than in recognizing *hydrocephalus*. Hydrocephalus can be due to various intracranial pathologies. If secondary to a lesion in the posterior fossa, patients can present with hydrocephalus before other findings, and thus any change in consciousness in these patients should be taken very seriously.

Certain physical exam findings in the patient with suspected *meningitis* should be mentioned. Here assess for hypersensitivity to light and neck rigidity or stiffness. Usually to look at neck, or nuchal, rigidity, the patient is asked to touch his or her chin to the chest.

In patients with *pathology involving the sella*, a careful ophthalmic examination must be performed. These patients must have a documented visual acuity and visual field exam. Often, ophthalmology is called specifically for this purpose, but this varies across institutions. Note that if possible, these patients should see an ophthalmologist as an outpatient so formal visual field exams can be documented.

In the trauma or otherwise comatose patient, the importance of a *pupillary exam* should be stressed. Remember that you may be the only provider performing a cranial nerve exam. Documenting any baseline pupillary abnormality will be helpful.

Recalling the contents of the *cavernous sinus* is important in patients with skull base pathology. Cranial nerves III, IV, V (V1 and V2), and VI all run through the cavernous sinus and can be affected by associated pathology. The cavernous portion of the carotid artery also lives in this region.

Common grading systems

The *Glasgow Coma Scale* (GCS) was originally described to comment on the patient with head trauma, but it is helpful in all types of intracranial pathology. It has three portions contributing to a total score of 15—eyes (4), speech (5), and motor (6):

- *Eyes*: Spontaneous (4), opening to voice (3), opening to pain (2), closed (1)
- *Speech*: Normal and fluid (5), confused (4), inappropriate (3), moaning/sounds (2), none (1)
- *Motor*: Following commands (6), localizing (5), withdrawing or appropriate flexion (4), inappropriate flexion (3), extension (2), none (1)

Patients who are intubated will automatically receive a score of 1 on speech, signified with a "T" added to the score (i.e., GCS of 10T).

Localization is differentiated from flexion by the ability to cross the midline.

The *Hunt Hess Scale* is used to comment on the level of consciousness for a patient suffering from an aneurysmal subarachnoid hemorrhage. It is graded as 0 to 5 with 1 and 2 typically called "good grade," and 3 or above called "bad grade":

- Grade 0—Intact aneurysm
- Grade 1—Mild headache or neck stiffness
- Grade 2—Severe headache or cranial nerve palsy
- Grade 3—Drowsy or confused
- Grade 4—Stupor or hemiparesis
- Grade 5—Deep coma or abnormal posturing

The *House-Brackmann Grading Scale* looks at the severity of facial nerve weakness in association with acoustic neuromas. This is noted pre- and postoperatively:

- Grade 1—Normal facial function
- Grade 2—Mild asymmetry, complete eye closure, and normal at rest
- Grade 3—Moderate dysfunction, complete eye closure, asymmetric at rest
- Grade 4—Moderate to severe, incomplete eye closure
- Grade 5—Severe dysfunction with only subtle movement detected
- Grade 6—Complete paralysis

Relevance to the advanced practice health professional

Often the initial and comprehensive physical exam will be performed by an advanced practice professional. Occasionally confirmation of initial exam will be impossible when an emergency situation arises.

Understanding the cranial neurologic exam is paramount. Exam findings will often be the basis for surgical decision making.

Common phone calls, pages, and requests

Difficulty performing ophthalmologic examination or confirming some abnormality?

Consultation with ophthalmology—Establish a good relationship with ophthalmologists, particularly one specializing in neuroopthalmology.

Uncertain about your examination in the comatose or otherwise difficult to examine patient?

Consultation with neurology—This can be particularly helpful in patients in whom brain death confirmation is required.

Trauma patient with a GCS of 3?

Confirm there are no paralytics on-board—These are typically used by anesthesia for intubation and will undermine your exam.

10

THE NEUROLOGICAL EXAMINATION

Part II: Spine

Sherri Patchen and Ruth Perez

An initial spinal assessment should include a complete neurologic exam for baseline comparison; subsequent exams may be focal relevant to the current complaint. The complete neurologic exam is useful in screening patients for neurologic deficits. A screening exam is helpful in determining what other diagnostic tests are needed to focus on a particular aspect of the nervous system. The exam findings along with corroborating diagnostic test results are used to further diagnose the patient and begin treatment. The complete neurologic exam should include a thorough history as well as a physical exam that should consist, at minimum, of the following exams (Hickey, 1997; Seidel, 1997).

General examination

Visually assess the spine for normal lordosis versus kyphosis or scoliosis. Palpate for any tenderness or spasms. Assess cervical and lumbar range of motion in flexion, extension, and side-to-side bending. Note any limitations and if pain is present with movement.

Gait

Assess stride for smooth, regular movement when walking. Gait should be assessed for a minimum of 10 feet. Unexpected findings would include foot drop, unsteadiness, wide-based gait, ataxic; spastic; rigid, shuffling-type gait.

To assess tandem, have the patient walk heel-to-toe to assess balance. The test should be performed with eyes open and arms at the patient's side. The patient should be assessed for a minimum of 10 feet.

Assess the patient's ability to walk on his or her toes. Toe walking assesses plantar flexor strength. Note any difficulty in the ability to maintain plantarflexion while walking.

Assess the patient's ability to walk on his or her heels. Heel walking assesses dorsal flexor strength. Note any difficulty in the ability to maintain dorsal flexion while walking.

For the Romberg test, the patient stands with eyes closed, feet side by side and close together, and arms by the sides. Note the patient's ability or inability to maintain balance. A mild sway can be a normal variant.

Motor

Test the major muscle groups comparing side by side. Palpate the belly of the muscle while testing to assess effort and mass. Assess for atrophy or fasciculation that is often seen in lower motor neuron disease. Assess for increased tone or spasticity that is sometimes seen with central lesions. Differentiate between increased tone and rigidity. Increased tone causes resistance with passive movement of the extremity. Rigidity causes increased resistance with active and passive range of motion. When testing motor strength, position the patient so that he or she has the benefit of ease of movement. Note if the patient has any limitation in the range of motion of joints. Muscle bulk can decrease with age, especially in the intrinsic muscles of the hands and the feet.

When grading motor strength, use a muscle motor scale of 0–5:

5—Normal movement with full resistance
4—Normal movement with some resistance
3—Normal movement against gravity without resistance
2—Movement with gravity eliminated (side-to-side movement)
1—Only the muscle contracts; there is no movement of the joint
0—No movement; flaccid

Major muscle groups and associated nerve roots are as follows:

- Shoulder shrug CN XI
- Deltoid C5
- Bicep C5-C6
- Tricep C6-C7
- Wrist extensor C6-C7
- Wrist flexor C7-C8
- Hand intrinsics T1
- Finger flexors C8
- Hip flexor L2-L3
- Knee extensor L3-L4
- Knee flexor L5-S1
- Dorsiflexion L4-L5
- Extensor hallucis longus L5
- Gastrocnemius S1-S2

Sensory

The sensory exam should be performed with the eyes closed. Assess sensitivity to light touch and pinprick. Assess all dermatomes asking the patient to compare side to side (Figures 10.1 and 10.2). Light touch is assessed using a cotton wisp. Pinprick is assessed using a sharp pin, such as a Neurotip.

When testing vibratory sense, start distally and compare side to side. Vibratory sense is tested using a tuning fork. If vibration is absent in the most distal joint, one should assess the more proximal joint (i.e., thumb, wrist, and elbow in the upper extremities, and toe, ankle, and knee in the lower extremities).

Proprioception tests joint position. Hold the digit at the lateral aspect, starting in a neutral position before moving the joint up or down. Patient should have eyes closed, and after you move the joint, ask the patient in which direction the joint was moved.

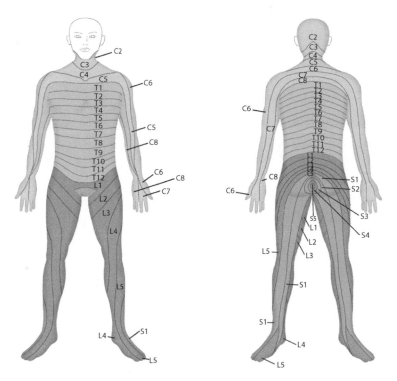

Figure 10.1 Dermatomal patterns.

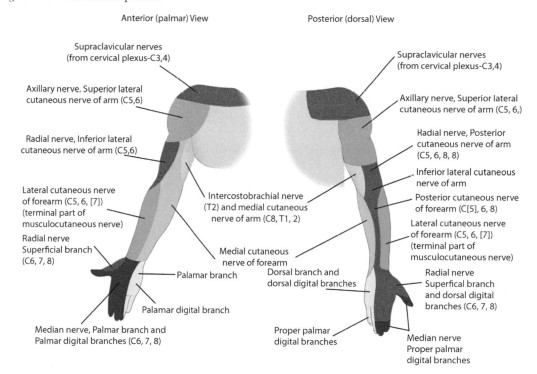

Figure 10.2 Peripheral nerve sensory innervation of the upper extremity.

Deep tendon reflexes

Absent—0
Hypoactive—1
Normal—2
Hyperactive—3
Clonus—4

Test reflexes at the bicep, tricep, brachioradialis, knees, and ankles. Assess the reflexes side by side. Hyperactive reflexes can be associated with a central nervous system problem. Hypoactive reflexes can be associated with a peripheral nervous system problem.

Hoffman sign

Assess for Hoffman sign. A Hoffman sign can be elicited by flicking the nail of the middle finger. The presence of a Hoffman sign can indicate spinal cord compression.

Babinski sign

Assess the plantar reflex for the Babinski sign. Stroke the sole of the foot firmly. If present, the big toe will move upward and the other toes fan out. This reflex is only normal in children up to 2 years old. An abnormal finding can be indicative of a central nervous system problem.

Straight leg raise

Straight leg raise can be used to assess nerve root compression or irritation in the lumbar spine. The test is performed while the patient is supine. The examiner raises the affected leg in a straight position. The leg is raised slowly to 90 degrees, and one should assess at what degree the patient experiences pain in the posterior aspect of the leg. The presence of pain in the affected leg at less than 60–70 degrees indicates nerve root compression or irritation.

Reference

Hickey JV. *The Clinical Practice of Neurological and Neurosurgical Nursing.* 4th ed. Philadelphia, PA: Lippincott; 1997.
Seidel HM. *Mosby's Guide to Physical Examination.* 5th ed. St. Louis, MO: Mosby; 1997.

11

THE NEUROLOGICAL EXAMINATION

Part III: Peripheral Nervous System

Yoshua Esquenazi and Daniel Kim

Introduction

The peripheral nervous system (PNS) consists of the structures that contain nerve fibers or axons that connect the central nervous system (CNS) with motor and sensory, somatic and visceral, end organs. These structures are the spinal nerves, the nerves of the extremities, and the cervical, brachial, and lumbosacral plexuses. Examination should be conducted in a comfortable room where both the patient and the examiner will be free from distraction. The nature and object of the test should be explained to the patient, as most patients will be unfamiliar with the procedures taking place during a neurological examination.

Motor testing

Inspection: Abnormal posture, wasting, and fasciculation with the limb at rest.

Power: Assessed by testing the strength of movement at a single joint. Movements chosen should be able to help differentiate upper from lower motor neuron lesions. They should be innervated by a single spinal root and peripheral nerve, in order to identify the affected nerve and the site of the injury.

Lower motor neuron versus Upper motor neuron

Lower motor neurons (LMNs) (first-order motor neuron): Cell bodies (soma) reside in the spinal cord (in anterior gray matter) or in the brainstem (for cranial nerve motor nuclei). Axons connect directly to the neuromuscular junction of muscles.

Upper motor neurons (UMNs) (second-order motor neurons): Somas may reside in the primary motor cortex or in the brainstem. Axons project to LMNs.

Medical Research Council Scale for Testing Muscle Strength

0. No contraction
1. Flicker or trace of contraction
2. Full range of active movement, with gravity eliminated
3. Active movement against gravity
4. Active movement against gravity and resistance
5. Normal power (O'Brien et al., 2010)

Common pitfalls and medicolegal concerns

Muscles are usually innervated by more than one nerve root, and the exact distribution varies between individuals. When testing a movement, the limb should be firmly supported proximal to the relevant joint in order to isolate the chosen muscle group.

Sensory testing

Sensory examination requires considerable concentration of both patient and examiner. It may be helpful to divide sensory testing into two groups: (1) those modalities that travel in the ipsilateral posterior columns of the spinal cord (light touch, vibration, and joint position sense) and (2) those that travel in the crossed spinothalamic tracts (pain and temperature). There is considerable overlap in the area of skin (dermatome) supplied by consecutive nerve roots.

Innervation, function, and evaluation of major muscles in the upper extremities

Serratus anterior muscle (Figure 11.1a)

- Innervation: Long thoracic nerve (C5–C7).
- Function: Abduction of scapula.
- Physical examination: The patient pushes against resistance (e.g., the examiner's hand or a wall). If the serratus anterior is paralyzed, winging of the scapula can be observed.

Rhomboid major and minor muscles (Figure 11.1b)

- Innervation: Dorsal scapular nerve (C4 and C5).
- Function: Adduction; rotation of scapula.
- Physical examination: The patient places a hand on his or her back and pushes backward against resistance. (Arrow: Muscle bellies can be seen.)

Levator scapulae muscle (Figure 11.1c)

- Innervation: Dorsal scapular (C5) and cervical (C3 and C4) nerves.
- Function: Raises scapula and inclines neck to corresponding side if scapula is fixed.
- Physical examination: The patient tries to shrug the shoulders (arrows) against resistance.

Supraspinatus muscle (Figure 11.1d)

- Innervation: Suprascapular nerve (C4, C5, and C6).
- Function: Initial abduction of shoulder joint.
- Physical examination: The patient abducts the shoulder (arrow) against resistance.

Infraspinatus muscle (Figure 11.1e)

- Innervation: Suprascapular nerve (C5 and C6).
- Function: External rotation of head of humerus at the shoulder joint.
- Physical examination: The patient externally rotates (arrow) the upper arm at the shoulder.

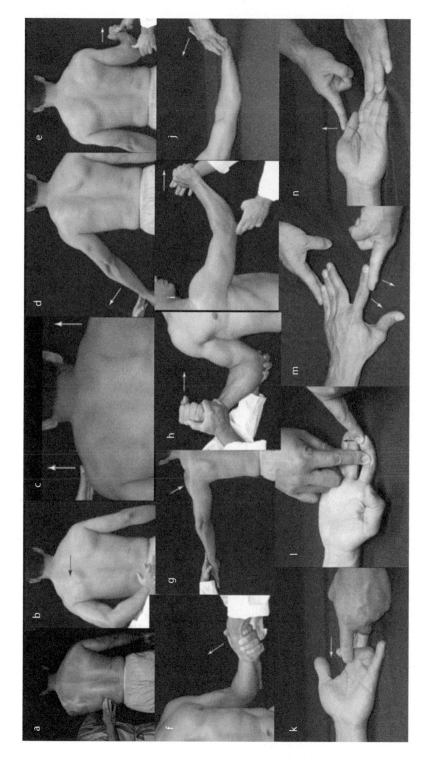

Figure 11.1 Evaluation of major muscles in the upper extremities. (From Kim DH et al., *Atlas of Peripheral Nerve Surgery: Expert Consult*, 2013, Elsevier [Saunders].)

Brachioradialis muscle (Figure 11.1f)

- Innervation: Radial nerve.
- Function: Flexion of elbow joint.
- Physical examination: The patient flexes the forearm (arrow) against resistance, with the forearm midway between pronation and supination.

Deltoid muscle (Figure 11.1g)

- Innervation: Axillary nerve (C5 and C6).
- Function: Abduction of shoulder joint.
- Physical examination: The patient abducts the shoulder (arrow) against resistance.

Biceps brachii muscle (Figure 11.1h)

- Innervation: Musculocutaneous nerve (C5 and C6).
- Function: Flexion at elbow joint and supination at forearm.
- Physical examination: When the patient flexes (arrow) the supinated forearm against resistance, the muscle can be seen.

Triceps brachii muscle (Figure 11.1i)

- Innervation: Radial nerve (C6 to C8).
- Function: Extension of elbow joint.
- Physical examination: The patient extends the elbow (arrow) against resistance.

Extensor digitorum muscle (Figure 11.1j)

- Innervation: Posterior interosseous nerve of radial nerve (C7 and C8).
- Function: Extension of medial four digits; assists in extension of wrist joint.
- Physical examination: While the patient's hand is firmly supported by the examiner's hand, extension at the metacarpophalangeal joints (arrow) is maintained against resistance.

Flexor digitorum superficialis muscle (Figure 11.1k)

- Innervation: Median nerve (C7-T1).
- Function: Flexion of middle and proximal phalanges of medial four digits; flexion of wrist joint.
- Physical examination: With the proximal phalanx fixed, the patient flexes the proximal interphalangeal joint (arrow) against resistance.

Flexor digitorum profundus muscle (Figure 11.1l)

- Innervation: Medial part: ulnar nerve (C8 and T1); lateral part: median nerve (C8 and T1).
- Function: Flexion of terminal phalanges of medial four digits after superficialis flexes third phalanges; flexion of wrist.
- Physical examination: The patient flexes the distal interphalangeal joint (arrow) against resistance while the middle phalanx is fixed.

Dorsal interosseous muscles (Figure 11.1m)

- Innervation: Ulnar nerve (C8 and T1).
- Function: Abduction of digits.
- Physical examination: The patient abducts the second finger from the middle finger (arrow) against resistance.

Abductor pollicis brevis muscle (Figure 11.1n)

- Innervation: Recurrent branch of median nerve (C8 and T1).
- Function: Abduction of the thumb at right angles to plane of palm.
- Physical examination: The patient abducts the thumb at the carpometacarpal joint (arrow), in a right angle plane to the palm.

Innervation, function, and evaluation of major muscles in the lower extremities

Iliopsoas muscle: Psoas and iliacus muscles (Figure 11.2a)

- Innervation: Upper part of iliac fossa to lesser trochanter (iliacus).
    - Psoas major: Lumbar nerves (L1, L2, and L3).
    - Iliacus: Femoral nerve (L2 and L3).
- Function: Flexion of hip joint.
- Physical examination: The patient lies supine with the leg flexed at the knee and hip and tries to flex the thigh against resistance.

Hip adductor muscles: Obturator externus, adductor brevis, adductor longus, and adductor magnus (Figure 11.2b)

- Innervation: Obturator nerve (L2, L3, and L4).
- Function: Adduction of the hip.
- Physical examination: The patient lies supine with the leg extended at the knee and tries to adduct the hip joint against resistance.

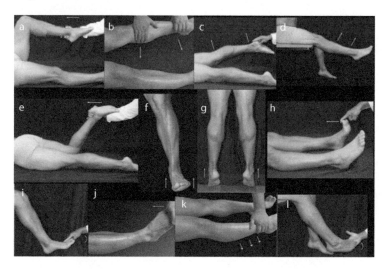

Figure 11.2   Evaluation of major muscles in the lower extremities. (From Kim DH et al., *Atlas of Peripheral Nerve Surgery: Expert Consult*, 2013, Elsevier [Saunders].)

Gluteus maximus muscle (Figure 11.2c)

- Innervation: Inferior gluteal nerve (L5, S1, and S2).
- Function: Extension of thigh and lateral rotation.
- Physical examination: The patient lies prone with legs extended and tries to elevate the leg against resistance.

Quadriceps femoris muscle: Rectus femoris, vastus medialis, vastus intermedius, and vastus lateralis muscles (Figure 11.2d)

- Innervation: Femoral nerve (L2, L3, and L4).
- Function: Extension of knee joint.
- Physical examination: With the leg flexed 90° at the knee, the patient attempts to extend the knee against resistance.

Hamstring muscles: Biceps femoris, semitendinosus, and semimembranosus muscles (Figure 11.2e)

- Innervation: Sciatic nerve (L5, S1, and S2).
- Function: Flexion of knee joint.
- Physical examination: The patient lies prone and tries to flex the leg at the knee against resistance.

Tibialis anterior muscle (Figure 11.2f)

- Innervation: Deep peroneal nerve (L4 and L5).
- Function: Dorsiflexion of ankle joint.
- Physical examination: The patient tries to dorsiflex the foot against resistance.

Triceps surae muscle: Soleus and gastrocnemius muscles (Figure 11.2g)

- Innervation: Tibial nerve (S1 and S2).
- Function: Plantarflexion of the ankle joint.
- Physical examination: The patient tries to plantarflex the ankle joint against resistance.

Extensor hallucis longus muscle (Figure 11.2h)

- Innervation: Deep peroneal nerve (L5 and S1).
- Function: Dorsiflexion of the ankle joint and extension of the metatarsophalangeal joint of the big toe.
- Physical examination: The patient tries to extend the metatarsophalangeal joint of the big toe against resistance.

Extensor digitorum brevis muscle (Figure 11.2i)

- Innervation: Deep peroneal nerve (L5 and S1).
- Function: Extension of metatarsophalangeal joints of the second through fifth toes.
- Physical examination: The patient tries to dorsiflex the proximal phalanges of the toes against resistance.

Gluteus medius, gluteus minimus, and tensor fasciae latae muscles (Figure 11.2j)

- Innervation: Superior gluteal nerve (L5 and S1).
- Function: Tension of iliotibial tract.
- Physical examination: The patient lies supine with the leg extended at the knee and tries to abduct the limb against resistance.

Tibialis posterior muscle (Figure 11.2k)

- Innervation: Tibial nerve (L4 and L5).
- Function: Plantarflexion of the ankle joint and inversion of the subtalar joint.
- Physical examination: The patient tries to invert the foot against resistance.

Peroneus longus and peroneus brevis muscles (Figure 11.2l)

- Innervation: Superficial peroneal nerve (L5, S1, and S2).
- Function: Plantarflexion of talocrural joint and eversion of subtalar joint.
- Physical examination: The patient tries to evert the foot against resistance.

References

Kim DH, Hudson AR, Kline DG. Upper extremity: Anatomy and function in the upper extremity; Anatomy and function in the lower extremity (Chapters 1 and 13). In *Atlas of Peripheral Nerve Surgery: Expert Consult.* 2nd ed. Amsterdam, Netherlands: Elsevier (Saunders); 2013.

O'Brien M. Introduction. In *Aids to the Examination of the Peripheral Nervous System.* 5th ed. Amsterdam, Netherlands: Elsevier (Saunders); 2010.

12

LESION LOCALIZATION

Jennifer A. Viner

Introduction

The brain is a complex organ. With our current understanding of its intricate layout, we are only able to understand general functions relative to specific structures. The concept of lesion localization in the brain has its basis in our understanding the basic anatomic structures, how they communicate with one another, and which structures they neighbor. The foundations of clinical neurology and neurosurgery that allow us to localize a lesion include anatomy and physiology, the patient history, the neurologic examination, and then use of this information to identify where in the nervous system the lesion is and then provide a differential diagnosis of what the pathology is. This information allows the clinician to formulate a plan to try and confirm the diagnosis, develop a treatment plan, and provide a prognosis. Nurses and advanced health-care providers can enhance their ability to care for neurologically compromised patients by knowing where in the brain their patient's lesion lies. This information allows for a better understanding of the patient's presenting symptoms and the expected clinical exam findings. A comprehensive treatment plan can then be tailored and executed. A brain lesion can include a variety of diagnoses that pertain to an area of dysfunction anatomically or physiologically. This could include aneurysm, vascular malformation, tumor, infection, inflammation, hemorrhage, demyelination, traumatic lesion, or congenital cyst.

Please refer back to previous chapters to review the basic anatomical structures, including the different areas of the brain and their functions. Also, review the cranial nerves and their anatomical location as they exit the skull. The reader needs to review how to perform a comprehensive neurological examination, and know what are normal and abnormal findings relative to each test. Physical examination findings during the neurological examination will assist with the lesion localization site in the brain.

Case studies

The following case study examples will help the reader practice his or her ability to understand the principles of lesion localization as they relate to the clinical scenarios. Each example describes the patient's presenting symptoms, pertinent positives or negatives in the medical history, and relevant clinical examination findings; each also provides a corresponding radiographic magnetic resonance image (MRI) revealing the lesion. Note that images on MRI are flipped left to right by convention so the patient's right side is marked with an R. The diagnosis will be presented, along with a short discussion of learning points. The goal is for the reader to understand that the lesion can be localized largely by the history and physical and that a lesion in the brain can affect more than one central nervous system function due to the size and nature of the lesion, and the topography of the brain. It is important to remember that some brain lesions can be discovered incidentally and do not have any related symptoms or clinical exam findings. Treatment may not be indicated for lesions that are suspected to be benign and those not causing any symptoms or neurological deficits. Clinicians need to understand the natural history of the lesion to determine if and when it is appropriate to intervene with treatment.

Case 12.1

A 56-year-old female with a history of breast cancer presents with a 3-day history of nausea and vomiting. She has a 3-week history of disequilibrium, falls, and headache. On examination, she has dysmetria with slower finger-to-nose tapping on the left, a positive Romberg test, and ataxic gait. She cannot walk heel-toe in a straight line.

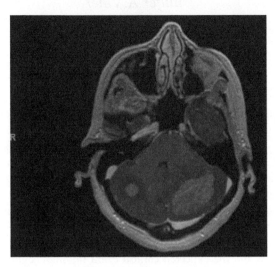

Diagnosis: Large left and smaller right cerebellar tumors; provisional diagnosis given prior medical history consistent with metastatic breast cancer.

Discussion: Breast cancer is one of the most common types of cancer that metastasizes to the brain (Devroom et al., 2004). The patient has multiple brain tumor metastases, but the largest one is the one located in the left cerebellum. This is the tumor causing her symptoms. The cerebellum's functions include coordination of motor movement, control of equilibrium, and control of muscle tone (Slazinski and Littlejohns, 2004). Clinical examination findings associated with cerebellar lesions are typically exhibited on the same side (Goldberg, 2010). The edema is contributing to mass effect and increased intracranial pressure, which explains the new-onset headache, nausea, and vomiting.

Case 12.2

A 69-year-old male presents with spatial disorientation and paresthesias on his right side. He also has intermittent involuntary jerking movements of the right upper extremity lasting a few minutes at a time, without loss of consciousness. His family notes that he leans to the right. He has a 6-month history of right lower extremity weakness. On examination, he has right-side neglect and altered proprioception. When asked why he was holding his right hand up in the air, the patient states this is not his right hand and that instead it belongs to somebody else. He has right lower extremity strength 3/5; he has active movement against gravity only but not to resistance (Hobdell et al., 2004). Right-side pronator drift is positive.

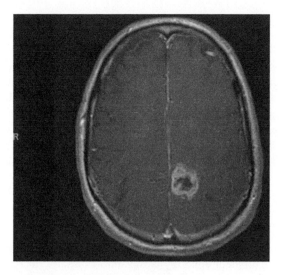

Diagnosis: Left parietal tumor; anaplastic astrocytoma.

Discussion: The tumor is in the left parietal lobe, causing contralateral somatotopic neglect. The patient is unable to recognize the contralateral side of his body as belonging to himself (Moscovitch and Behrmann, 1994). The primary sensory cortex is affected, and that is contributing to the presence of both paresthesias and weakness (Slazinski and Littlejohns, 2004). The episodes of involuntary motor movements of the right arm he describes are simple partial seizures with motor phenomena. These are synchronous cortical discharges resulting in symptomatology related to the brain region affected but without alteration in consciousness (Buelow et al., 2004).

Case 12.3

A 58-year-old right-handed female presents after a single generalized seizure and 2-week history of confusion. The family reports poor short-term memory and confabulation. On examination, she has a fluent aphasia. Calculation for simple numbers is impaired, naming 5/5 is correct, and repetition is intact. She cannot follow more than one simple command at a time. She is not oriented to day of week or year. During spontaneous speech and conversation she makes literal paraphasic errors. She has no abstract judgment.

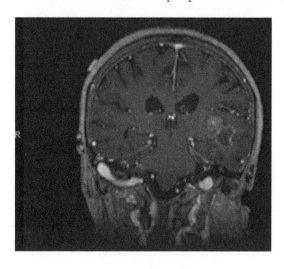

Diagnosis: Left temporal tumor; glioblastoma.

Discussion: The temporal lobes' functions include hearing, memory and learning, and receptive language function (Slazinski and Littlejohns, 2004). The tumor is in the left temporal lobe, an eloquent speech area. In most people, the left hemisphere is dominant for language (Goldberg, 2010). She has a Wernicke's aphasia, which is characterized by fluent speech, without meaningful content, use of paraphrasia, circumlocution, and reduced auditory comprehension (Hobdell et al., 2004). Wernicke's area functions to understand spoken language (Slazinski and Littlejohns, 2004). Lesions based in the temporal lobe and cortical-based lesions are most frequently associated with seizures (Devroom et al., 2004). A seizure can be the first symptom of a brain lesion (Devroom et al., 2004). A generalized seizure impairs consciousness and distorts the electrical activity involving both cerebral hemispheres (Buelow et al., 2004).

Case 12.4

A 67-year-old male presents with complaints that he has been in multiple minor car accidents in the last 2 months. His wife notes that he continuously bumps into things on his right side. On confrontational visual field examination, he is noted to have a right-side field cut with each eye.

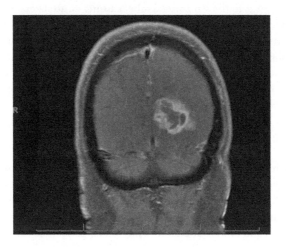

Diagnosis: Left occipital tumor; glioblastoma.

Discussion: The primary visual cortex is located in the occipital lobes (Slazinski and Littlejohns, 2004). Homonymous hemianopsia occurs because the left half of the brain has visual pathways for the right hemifield of both eyes, and the right half of the brain has visual pathways for the left hemifield of both eyes. When one of these pathways is damaged, the corresponding visual field is lost (Slazinski and Little-johns, 2004).

Case 12.5

A 46-year-old male presents with blurry vision, headaches, depression, low libido, weight gain, and fatigue. On ophthalmoscopic examination, he has papilledema. On confrontation, he has peripheral field cuts bilaterally. He has a flat, depressed affect.

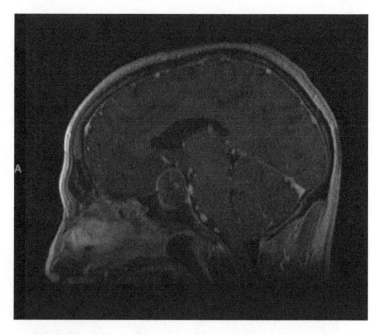

Diagnosis: Pituitary adenoma.

Discussion: The pituitary fossa, also known as the sella, is in a small, enclosed space with limited capacity to accommodate an expanding mass. The cells that may form the tumor can secrete hormones, causing hormone overproduction syndromes (McPhee and Ganong, 2006). The tumor is causing hypothalamic-pituitary axis dysfunction, visual disturbance by pressing on the optic chiasm, and hydrocephalus. The depression and flat affect are related to pituitary malfunction and neuroendocrine hormone insufficiency. The hypothalamus is affected as evidenced by the appetite increase, sexual dysfunction, and lack of motivation (McPhee and Ganong, 2006; Procyk, 2004).

Case 12.6

A 48-year-old male presents with rapid onset of symptoms and rapid clinical deterioration. He has a 2-week history of hoarseness, poorly articulated speech, and in the last few days, choking on food. Today he developed disequilibrium and shortness of breath. He was intubated upon arrival to the emergency room. On examination, he is able to follow commands and communicate his needs with pen and paper. He is moving all extremities well. Heart rate was sinus tachycardia in the 120s prior to intubation but now running in the 90s. He has difficulty raising his head off the pillow.

Diagnosis: Brainstem tumor; medullary glioblastoma.

Discussion: The brainstem is the part of the brain continuous with the spinal cord and comprising the medulla oblongata, pons, and midbrain. It is involved in many automatic functions, such as breathing, heart rate, body temperature, wake and sleep cycles, digestion, sneezing, coughing, vomiting, and swallowing. Ten of the twelve cranial nerves originate in the brainstem (Slazinski and Littlejohns, 2004; Goldberg, 2010). Therefore, lesions affecting the brainstem commonly present with multiple cranial nerve deficits. In this case, the lower cranial nerves are affected because of their position to the medulla. The history reveals rapid progression of symptoms suggesting an aggressive lesion. Because the patient was emergently intubated, the examiner cannot assess the quality of his voice, but the history reveals a change, which can be reflective of glossopharyngeal, vagal, and hypoglossal nerve dysfunction.

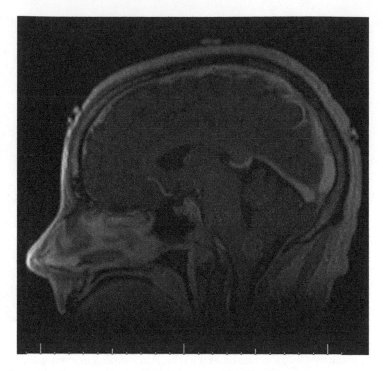

Swallow and gag have also been compromised. These could also reflect vagus nerve dysfunction. The sinus tachycardia could have been related to respiratory distress or direct involvement of vagus nerve dysfunction. The inability to lift his head from the pillow suggests spinal accessory nerve involvement. The tongue position and strength cannot properly be examined, but the history of dysarthric speech suggests hypoglossal nerve compromise (Slazinski and Littlejohns, 2004; Hobdell et al., 2004).

Case 12.7

A 58-year-old female presents with loss of smell 3 years ago, and a 40-pound weight loss in that same time period. She has progressive visual loss in the last 6 months to the point that now she cannot read fine print, and lighting always seems dim. Her family notes a personality change. She is now angry and irritable, and this is not her baseline. She quit her job abruptly about 6 months ago. The patient, however, states she is at her baseline

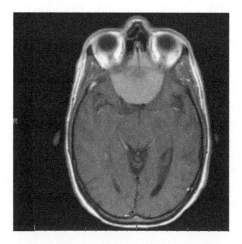

personality. On examination, she is abrupt, agitated, and uninhibited. She has bilateral optic nerve head atrophy on ophthalmoscopic exam. Visual acuity is 20/80. She cannot distinguish different odors.

Diagnosis: Anterior cranial fossa olfactory groove meningioma affecting CN I, CN II, and frontal lobe function.

Discussion: It often takes patients some time to note dysfunction of both olfactory nerves, causing loss of sense of smell. The flavor experience of food is influenced strongly by smell. Commonly, these patients lose weight as a result of simply not enjoying food anymore (Doty, 2009). The loss of vision really prompted her evaluation, and in this case, it is caused by the tumor compressing the optic nerves. The tumor is also compressing the frontal lobe. The frontal lobe regulates personality, affect, inhibition, judgment, reasoning, planning, and abstract thinking (Slazinski and Littlejohns, 2004). The family identifies the change in personality, not the patient, which is common in patients with a frontal lobe syndrome.

Case 12.8

A 65-year-old female presents with headache, nausea, and vomiting for 2 days. She has gradual loss of vision in the right eye for 2 years, and it is now blind. On examination, she is wearing sunglasses. When removed, she is found to have a grossly abnormal protruding right eye. She has a complete right-side ptosis; with effort, she cannot open the eyelid at all. The right eye has a fixed downward gaze and a dilated nonreactive pupil. The left pupil is sluggishly reactive to light, 4–2 mm. She has poor left-side vision and cannot distinguish facial features. While looking down, she can move the left eye laterally only. Gaze is disconjugate. Facial sensation and symmetry are intact.

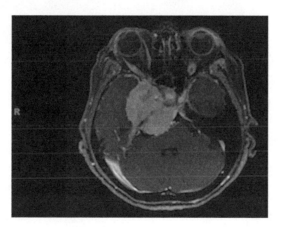

Diagnosis: Right cavernous sinus, middle fossa and petroclival meningioma affecting CN II, CN III, CN IV, and CN VI.

Discussion: The cranial fossae are divided into three large depressions in the skull base. They are the anterior, the middle, and the posterior cranial fossae (Slazinski and Littlejohns, 2004). This is an interesting case because even though the tumor is predominantly in the right middle and posterior cranial fossa, it is very large causing brainstem compression and right-to-left shift. The patient finally presented for care because of symptoms of headache, nausea, and vomiting, which are related to noncommunicating hydrocephalus caused by kinking of the cerebral aqueduct in the dorsal midbrain. Her vision had been affected several years prior, but she did not seek treatment. The optic nerves were damaged by the chronic papilledema due to elevated intracranial pressure from hydrocephalus leading to the loss of vision. The right oculomotor nerve has caused the eyelid to close, impairment of the pupillary light reflex, and impaired eye movement. The trochlear nerve and abducens nerve involvement is evident by her restricted eye movements down and in, as well as laterally (Hobdell et al., 2004).

Case 12.9

A 63-year-old male presents with severe "knife-like" sharp shooting pains along his right temple at the level of the eye down to the cheekbone. The pains are brief lasting a few seconds at a time, occurring about three times per day. He avoids brushing his teeth in the upper right corner as this has triggered the pain. The pain started several months ago and is progressively getting more frequent. On examination, he has weakness on the right jaw when clenching his teeth. He has diminished sensation on forehead, cheek, and jaw, on the right. He has absence of blinking on the right.

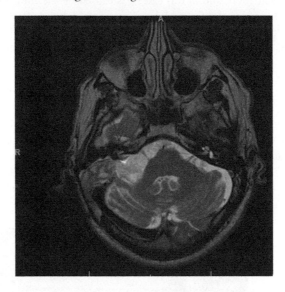

Diagnosis: Right cerebellar-pontine epidermoid cyst affecting CN V.

Discussion: The tumor completely encases the trigeminal nerve on the right. There are three major branches: the ophthalmic nerve (V_1), the maxillary nerve (V_2), and the mandibular nerve (V_3). The ophthalmic and maxillary nerves are purely sensory, and the mandibular nerve has sensory and motor functions (Leston, 2009). Trigeminal neuralgia is a very distinctive pain syndrome. The typical form of the disorder causes extreme, sporadic, sudden burning or shock-like facial pain in the areas of the face where the branches of the nerve are distributed. This includes the lips, eyes, nose, scalp, forehead, and upper and lower jaw. The pain episodes last from a few seconds to a few minutes. Triggers can include a light breeze or touch to the affected side of the face, talking, chewing, brushing teeth, or swallowing (Zakrzewska and Linskey, 2014). The masseter and temporal muscle weakness, loss of facial sensation, and absent corneal reflex are all indicative of right-side trigeminal nerve dysfunction (Hobdell et al., 2004).

Case 12.10

A 41-year-old male presents with a 2-year history of gradual hearing loss on the right. He initially thought the right side of his headphones was broken, but eventually he noted that he had no hearing on his right side. He has constant, low-pitched ringing in the right ear. In the last 6 months, he has had one episode of complete facial paralysis on the right, which resolved with a short course of steroid medication. He has disequilibrium and feels like he walks as though he were intoxicated. He has dizziness and has had three episodes of vertigo. On examination, he cannot repeat words whispered into his right ear. He has a flattened nasal labial fold on the right. He cannot close the right eyelid all the way. He has ataxic gait and requires a cane to ambulate. Saliva gathers out of the corner of the right side of his mouth. His voice is

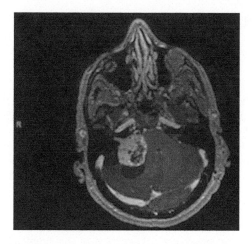

hoarse. The uvula and palate deviate away from the right when the patient is asked to say "ahhh." He has a decreased gag reflex.

Diagnosis: Right acoustic neuroma affecting CN VII, CN VIII, CN IX, and CN X.

Discussion: Lesions of the cerebellar pontine angle region can cause multiple cranial neuropathies and symptoms because of the various nerves and structures that are located in that region. Involvement of the facial nerve is demonstrated by the right-sided facial weakness and history of Bell palsy (Goldberg, 2010). The tumor extends down into the internal auditory canal along the course of the right vestibulocochlear nerve causing hearing loss, tinnitus, dizziness, imbalance, and vertigo (Hobdell et al., 2004). Extension down into the jugular foramen region is affecting lower cranial nerve function. The glossopharyngeal and vagus nerve dysfunction are characterized by the abnormal voice, hoarseness, palatal and uvula weakness, and decreased gag. This patient is at risk for aspiration (Hobdell et al., 2004).

Case 12.11

A 28-year-old female presents with blurry vision and restricted peripheral vision. She complains of daily headaches, progressively getting worse in the mornings. She also notes right shoulder weakness. On examination, she has decreased palate movement on the right. She has marked tongue atrophy with deviation to

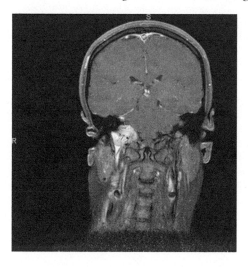

the right. There are fasciculations on the right side of the tongue. Speech is dysarthric. Her right sterno-cleidomastoid and trapezius muscles are weak. She cannot move them against resistance. On ophthalmo-scopic exam, she has profound papilledema with microhemorrhages.

Diagnosis: Right jugular foramen tumor with intracranial pressure elevation secondary to venous hypertension; affecting CN IX, CN X, CN XI, and CN XII.

Discussion: The visual complaints and headaches are the result of the increased intracranial pressure. The palatal weakness is related to glossopharyngeal nerve and vagus nerve dysfunction. The right shoulder weakness is attributed to spinal accessory nerve dysfunction. The right hypoglossal nerve is also involved. The deviation of the tongue to the paralyzed side and atrophy are key findings (Hobdell et al., 2004).

Summary

The brain has symmetrical, discrete localization of function in the cerebellum, brainstem, diencephalon, and thalamus. In the cerebral cortex, language localization is most often on the left while motor, sensory, and visual functions are represented symmetrically for each side of the body (Goldberg, 2010). Apart from the organization of function in the cerebral/cerebellar hemispheres and brainstem, disorders of the vascular system, cranial nerves, and skull base may influence neurologic function and hence the clinical presentation in each case. Understanding anatomy is the key to being able to localize pathology based on the history and physical exam. Special tests such as MRI help confirm the localization and provide additional information to help diagnose the pathology. When nurses and advanced health-care providers understand the anatomy of where the patient's brain lesion exists, they can better understand the natural history of the suspected condition and the specific care needed for the patient given the patient's limitations. The knowledge of being able to apply the principles of lesion localization fosters a more comprehensive ability to care for the neurologically compromised patient.

References

Buelow J, Long L, Rossi AM, Gilbert K. Epilepsy. In: Bader MK, Littlejohns LR, eds. *AANN Core Curriculum for Neuroscience Nursing*. 4th ed. St. Louis, MO: Saunders; 2004:586-617.

Devroom H, Smith R, Mogensen K, Clancey J. Nervous system tumors. In: Bader MK, Littlejohns LR, eds. *AANN Core Curriculum for Neuroscience Nursing Fourth Edition*. St. Louis, MO: Saunders; 2004:511-535.

Doty RL. The olfactory system and its disorders. *Semin Neurol*. 2009;29(1):74-81.

Goldberg S. *Clinical Neuroanatomy Made Ridiculously Simple*. 4th ed. Miami, FL: MedMaster; 2010.

Hobdell E, et al. Assessment. In: Bader MK, Littlejohns LR, eds. *AANN Core Curriculum for Neuroscience Nursing*. 4th ed. St. Louis, MO: Saunders; 2004:115-173.

Leston JM. Functional anatomy of the trigeminal nerve. *Neurochirurgie*. 2009;55(2):99-112.

McPhee SJ, Ganong WF. *Pathophysiology of Disease: An Introduction to Clinical Medicine*. 5th ed. New York, NY: Lange; 2006.

Moscovitch M, Behrmann M. Coding of spatial information in the somatosensory system: evidence from patients with neglect following parietal lobe damage. *J Cogn Neurosci*. 1994;6(2):151-155.

Procyk LF. Neuroendocrine. In: Bader MK, Littlejohns LR, eds. *AANN Core Curriculum for Neuroscience Nursing*. 4th ed. St. Louis, MO: Saunders; 2004:94-114.

Slazinski T, Littlejohns LR. Anatomy. In: Bader MK, Littlejohns LR, eds. *AANN Core Curriculum for Neuroscience Nursing*. 4th ed. St. Louis, MO: Saunders; 2004:30-86.

Zakrzewska JM, Linskey ME. Trigeminal neuralgia. *BMJ Clin Evid*. 2014;10:1207.

13

NEUROLOGIC EXAMINATION OF THE INFANT AND CHILD

Karthik Madhavan, George M. Ghobrial,
Stephen S. Burks, and Michael Y. Wang

Introduction

There is no substitute for a thorough neurologic examination in a newborn. It is essential to remember that children are not little adults. Focused imaging of the growing child will help minimize and prevent unnecessary exposure to radiation. The neurologic exam continuously changes as the newborn progresses to being an infant and then a toddler. It is important for the health-care professional to be aware of the specifics to tailor the examination based on milestones.

Overview

The neurologic examination begins with a good history. The knowledge of milestones and tethering of the exams to various tract developments are keys to the right interpretation of the examination and identification of developmental delays. All developmental milestones have an age range according to the confidence interval from population studies. The caveat is that mild developmental delays are often missed. The milestones are based on fine and gross motor skills, language, behavior, and social skills. There are several test sets that are used across the country, like the Bayley infant neurodevelopmental screen and Denver II. However, they are quite likely to overlook mild developmental delays, and there is growing evidence that parent-based questionnaires are more accurate in identifying mild developmental delays. This also provides an advantage over clinical examination of the child in the clinic, as the parents answer these questionnaires based on several interactions with the child as compared to one-time interpretation of neurologic exams in the clinic, which is confounded by the child's mood, behavior, and illness during that time.

As the infant progresses toward the toddler years and early schooling, several other milestones in learning abilities, attention, social skills, and intelligence become more important. The Wechsler Intelligence Scale for Children—Third Edition is commonly used, which is mainly an intelligence assessment. Psychological skills require additional separate testing, which is beyond the scope of this chapter.

Societal significance

Understanding milestones and delays enables the health professional to recommend appropriate education focused on overcoming or improving the deficits. Psychological confidence is provided to the child as specific skills improve over a period of time.

Basic biologic and physiologic processes

Neurologic development occurs cranial to caudal in all infants.

History

The examination starts with a detailed history beginning from the pregnancy, complications during pregnancy, and delivery. This is followed by a detailed history of the developments and neurologic issues noted by the parents. Mother's age, parity, maternal illness, medication, and drug use are noted. Birth history includes the mode of delivery, meconium staining, and Apgar score. Any new symptoms to be evaluated should be noted as static, progressing, or improving and acute, subacute, or chronic. Social history of being a single parent, education, and habits of the parent are important. Family history should include any neurodegenerative or neurocutaneous disorders, epilepsy, and autosomal dominant disorders.

Anatomic review

At the time of examination, the white coat is best avoided, and the child is examined in his or her most comfortable position. Complicated and uncomfortable examinations like fundoscopy and testing of the gag reflex are best avoided until the end of the exam. Stranger anxiety is common and a sign of normal development. Professionals are advised to develop a rapport with the child by offering a toy or shiny object to grab attention. Physical examination should include evaluation of the skin, nails, and hair, as they directly represent the ectodermal origin embryologically. Head-to-toe examination of the child starts with the head circumference. Neurocutaneous lesions are commonly found in certain syndromes, for example, ash leaf spots (tuberous sclerosis), café au lait spots (neurofibromatosis), angiomas (Sturge-Weber syndrome), axillary freckling (found in neurofibromatosis), adenoma sebaceum (?), or shagreen patches (?). A whorl of hair is seen if there is any abnormality underneath. A single palmar crease is commonly encountered in Down syndrome. A spinal examination should include evaluation of kyphoscoliosis, sacral dimples, tufts of hair, or small openings in the spine.

Head circumference—Measure along the forehead to the inion:

- 35 cm at birth
- 2 cm per month from 0 to 3 months
- 1 cm per month from 3 to 6 months

Any abnormality should prompt further evaluation into craniosynostosis or macrocephaly. Hydrocephalus is often asymptomatic except for an increase in head circumference, prominent scalp veins, splayed sutures, and bulging anterior fontanelle.

Head—The anterior fontanelle closes between 12 and 18 months. It is usually soft, slightly depressed, and diamond shaped. The posterior fontanelle closes at 2–3 months.

Caput succedaneum and cephalhematoma are often noted during the first visit. Cephalohematoma is a traumatic subperiosteal hematoma that occurs underneath the skin, in the periosteum of the infant's skull bone. Cephalohematoma does not pose any risk to the brain, as it is extracranial accumulation and is limited at the suture. Caput succedaneum is a neonatal condition involving a serosanguinous, subcutaneous, extraperiosteal fluid collection with poorly defined margins caused by the pressure of the presenting part of the scalp against the dilating cervix; it does not follow the suture lines.

If the fontanelle appears to be closed, the patient must be brought to the attention of the pediatrician or neurosurgeon for intervention to accommodate the growing brain.

Cranial nerve examination

Cranial nerve I—Smell (olfactory)

It is very difficult to assess smell sensation in a newborn. Once the child is more vocal, then clove and peppermint are used for testing smell sensation.

Cranial nerve II (ophthalmic)

Blink response to bright light is reliable in newborns and infants. It develops at the age of 30 weeks of gestation and is present for the rest of life. The pupillary response appears around the same time in gestation (29–30 weeks) and is consistent by 32 weeks. The blink reflex is not present until 3–4 months, and only 50% have it by 5 months. It should be present in 100% of infants by the age of 12 months. Direct and consensual responses are tested with a medium-bright flashlight. Light is shined from one side and the ipsilateral pupil is visualized, followed by the contralateral pupil for consensual response. The same is repeated on the opposite side. This examines both cranial nerves II and III. Small pupils are secondary to parasympathetic lesion, and larger pupils are from sympathetic palsy. Drooping eyelids (ptosis) are secondary to weakness of the levator palpebrae supplied by the third cranial nerve; partial ptosis is from Müller muscle paralysis from a sympathetic nerve injury.

At 6 months of age, vision is noted to be 20/20 when evaluated with visual evoked response.

Cranial nerves III, IV, and VI (oculomotor, trochlear, and abducens)

Visual fixation on an object or face starts at the age of 34 weeks of gestation. The third cranial nerve supplies all the extraocular muscles except the superior oblique (intorsion of the eye), which is supplied by the fourth cranial nerve, and the lateral rectus (lateral movement), which is supplied by the sixth cranial nerve. Any deviation in the eyes should be noted

In addition, vestibuloocular reflex is assessed by spinning the infant and observing the quick component of nystagmus in the opposite direction as soon as the rotation is halted. This is followed by visual fixation on an object. This enables evaluation of the vestibular system, extraocular muscles, and vision (cranial nerves II, III, IV, VI, and VIII) at the same time.

The doll's eye phenomenon can initiate extraocular movements in a comatose patient, but this is suppressed by cortical activity in patients who are awake. It requires a normal functioning connection to the brainstem for this reflex.

In older children, similar reflexes are present; however, there may be compensatory mechanisms like tilting the head in the fourth nerve palsy. Each eye should be covered to inspect the other eye to detect for phorias where the abnormal eye deviates.

Cranial nerve V (trigeminal)

The fifth nerve supplies the sensation of the ipsilateral face. Motor components include the temporalis and masseter muscles. Sucking and swallowing are evaluations of the masseter. Fine touch and corneal reflex check the ophthalmic branch of cranial nerves V and VII. In children, it is much easier to evaluate fine touch sensation with a cotton wisp.

Cranial nerve VII (facial nerve)

All the facial muscles are controlled by this nerve. Any facial asymmetry is concern for abnormality. Sensation of taste is delivered through the VII nerve by the chorda tympani branch. This can be tested in children over 1 year of age by applying salt or sugar solutions by cotton-stick applicators.

Cranial nerve VIII (auditory)

The cochlear component is tested with a response to voice, or any sound (like that of a bell) is easily tested in children older than 1 year of age. Repetition is included. Infants cannot localize sound until 4 months of age. However, in infants, a blink response to sharp sounds is noted. Vestibular function is as described above on the evaluation of cranial nerves III–VI.

Cranial nerves XI and X (glossopharyngeal and vagus)

The gag reflex is noted beginning from 30 weeks of gestation, which is a part of both cranial nerves XI and X. Cranial nerve XI is the afferent and X the efferent limb as it controls the muscles of the pharynx and elevation of the palate. An abnormal infant cry can also be a sign of weakness of pharyngeal and laryngeal muscles.

Cranial nerve XI (spinal accessory)

Head turning against resistance examines the ipsilateral sternomastoid. Head tilt can be a sign of weakness of the ipsilateral side unless the child is trying to compensate for abnormal extraocular palsy. Shrugging of the shoulders is tested only in older children (over 1 year of age) who can follow commands.

Cranial nerve XII (hypoglossal)

The tongue will deviate toward an affected side due to unopposed genioglossus on the unaffected side. Fasciculation and atrophy are signs of a neurodegenerative disorder.

Examination of the motor system

The motor examination performed should test posture, tone, and strength of the child. In an infant, posture is the key to identifying some of the neurologic problems. An infant starts by lifting his or her head off of the exam table by 2 months of age when positioned prone. The infant lifts his or her head and upper chest by 3 months. At about 5–7 months of age, an infant is able to sit unsupported and is able to reach for objects at around the same age. Crawling starts beginning from 9 months, and standing with support typically occurs around 12 months of age. Most children are able to walk between 12 and 15 months of age starting from a wide-based gait to a regular gait by 6 years. Hand preference is not usually seen before 2 years of age. If noted early, it is abnormal.

As the infant grows, hypertonia starts to decrease in the upper extremities followed by lower as the corticospinal tracts develop and optimize the tone. In addition, neck tone gradually increases. This can be tested by lifting the infant's outstretched arms and clasping the examiner's fingers. At 3 months, if the head lags behind, then it is hypotonia. Passive movement of the arm across the chest can reveal hypotonia if the elbow crosses the midline.

Muscle strength in infants can be examined when they grip the fingers of the examiner and their entire torso can be elevated. In older children, the muscle groups can be tested individually (Table 13.1).

Cerebellar function

The ability of the infant/child to reach an object can reveal coordination in the upper extremity. Older children can be tested similar to adults by being able to touch a point in space, alternating movements, and tapping.

Table 13.1 Testing the Muscle Groups

0	No muscle contraction
1	Flicker or trace of contraction
2	Active movement without gravity
3	Active movement against gravity
4	Active movement against gravity and resistance
5	Normal strength

Table 13.2 Testing Reflexes

Reflexes	*Grading*
1+	Hyporeflexic
++	Normal reflex
+++	Hyperreflexic
Clonus	Sustained >3 beats

Sensory examination

This includes pinprick, light touch, position, and vibration senses, which are appreciated by children who can understand and answer questions. Infants react by removing their extremity to a new sensation or present a startle response to sense of vibration. Cortical object discrimination is identified by writing a number or letter of the alphabet on the palm with a finger and the child being able to recognize it. This works only with much older children.

Reflexes

Reflexes are tested by gently tapping the corresponding tendon with a hammer. Usually in infants, this tap is done on the top of the examiner's finger on the tendon (Table 13.2).

Clonus is abnormal in all stages of life.

Common reflexes tested

- Jaw jerk (CN V)—Exaggerated in brainstem lesions, does not need to be tested every time
- Biceps (C5-C6)
- Triceps (C6-C8)
- Brachioradialis (C5-C6)
- Patellar (L2-L4)
- Ankle (S1-S2)

> *Babinski sign*—This response is elicited by stroking the plantar aspect of the foot with a semiblunt object, like the back of a pen. In an infant, dorsiflexion of the great toe and fanning of the toes show incomplete pyramidal tract development. This is suppressed with corticospinal tract development as the response changes to plantar flexion of the foot.

Primitive reflexes

These are seen in infants and are always present at the time of birth. As the brain and the corticospinal tracts develop, these reflexes are suppressed only to return in patients with severe dementia and frontal lobe injury.

Vertical suspension—The infant is suspended by holding the chest with both hands and lifting the patient in an upright position, with the legs dangling. Scissoring or hyperextension of the legs is present in spastic infants secondary to ailments like cerebral palsy.

Landau reflex—An infant normally has to hold up the trunk in a horizontal prone position, and if there is a U shape with the trunk and abdomen flopping around the examiner's hand, that is a sign of hypotonia.

Sucking reflex—This reflex is noted when flicking gently along the cheek or the edge of the mouth, the infant turns toward that side. Coordinated suck and swallow are well developed by 37 weeks.

Moro reflex—When the head is acutely hyperextended by an inch below the trunk, an infant normally opens his or her hands and extends and abducts the arms. This is followed by flexion of both arms and a cry. This is usually present at 28 weeks in all newborns and disappears before the age of 6 months.

Asymmetric tonic neck reflex (fencer's stance)—When the head of the infant is turned to one side while lying supine, the ipsilateral arm and leg are extended with flexion of the arm and leg on the contralateral side. It usually appears at 35 weeks' gestation and disappears at about 6–7 months of age.

Palmar and plantar grasp reflexes—These can be seen beginning at the age of 28–30 weeks of gestation and get stronger by 40 weeks' gestation. The palmar reflex is a vestibular response, where placing a finger on the palm leads to flexion of the head. It disappears by 6 months. The plantar grasp reflex disappears by 9–10 months. Any persistence beyond is abnormal.

Parachute response—This response usually appears at 8–9 months of age and is a vestibular function. It persists in various forms throughout life. It is elicited when the infant is bought down toward the floor, and the infant responds by extending arms and hands. Any abnormality noted in the parachute response indicates a delay in vestibular development reflected in balance-oriented skills like walking.

Stepping reflex—When the infant's sole of the foot is placed at the edge of the exam table, the infant responds with a stepping action. This reflex persists until 4–5 months of age.

Final comments

This chapter provides information to assist the health-care professional in distinguishing the normal from the abnormal during examination in the clinical setting. It is unlikely to present as any emergency situation that will need an overnight nurse to answer. Any concerns should be answered by performing a full neurologic exam to evaluate the full extent of the pathology in question. A good history and neurologic response can help the practitioner avoid unnecessary tests and radiologic workups.

PART III

The Team Approach

14

COLLABORATIVE PRACTICE WITH THE NEUROINTENSIVIST, NEUROLOGIST, AND NEUROSURGEON

Megan Keiser

Introduction

Collaborative practice between physicians and other health-care providers, including nurses and advanced practice health professionals (physician assistants [PAs] and nurse practitioners [NPs]), has been shown to improve the cost, quality, and outcomes of health care. To that end, the World Health Organization (WHO) published a document titled *Framework for Action on Interprofessional Education and Collaborative Practice* (2010), which explores the issues related to and ramifications of collaborative practice. One of the key messages found in the document states, "Collaborative practice strengthens health systems and improves health outcomes" (WHO, 2010, p. 7). One of the building blocks of collaborative practice is interprofessional education, which "enables effective collaborative practice which in turn optimizes health services, strengthens health systems, and improves health outcomes" (WHO, 2010, p. 18). What does this mean? It means that in order for health-care professionals to practice within an interdisciplinary team, they must first understand the scope of practice for each discipline. From the regulatory standpoint, the scopes of practice for physicians, nurses, NPs, and PAs vary by state, and all are required to obtain licensure and/or certification from the state in which they practice. From a more practical standpoint, the education, training, and roles of these health-care providers are briefly described in the following sections.

Physicians

Neurologist: A neurologist is a physician trained in the treatment and diagnosis of brain and central nervous system disorders and diseases. Doctors trained in neurology complete medical school, a 1-year internship in internal medicine, and a 3-year residency in neurology. They may complete a subspecialty fellowship in a specific clinical area such as stroke or epilepsy.

Neurosurgeon: A neurosurgeon is a physician who specializes in the diagnosis and surgical treatment of disorders of the central and peripheral nervous systems. Doctors trained in neurosurgery complete medical school, a 1-year internship in general surgery, and 5–7 years in a neurosurgery residency program. They may complete a fellowship after residency to specialize in a particular area such as skull base surgery or spine surgery.

Neurointensivist: The intensivist is the "primary care physician" of the intensive care unit (ICU). The required training for a neurointensivist includes board certification in critical care medicine or completion of an accredited critical care fellowship after board certification in another medical or surgical specialty. Most neurointensivists are board certified in neurology or neurosurgery and then complete a fellowship in critical care medicine.

Generally speaking, the role of the physician on the health care team is to oversee care and develop a plan of care for the patient, ideally in collaboration with other members of the health-care team.

Advanced practice health professionals

Nurse practitioner: An NP is a master's or doctorally prepared registered nurse with specialty certification and state licensure to practice in an advanced nursing role. Although few clinical residency programs exist for NPs, many obtain additional specialty nursing certification in a clinical area such as neuroscience or critical care. The level of independent practice for NPs varies by state, but they must practice in collaboration with physicians when in the inpatient environment.

Physician assistant: A PA is a health provider who has received postbaccalaureate education lasting 2–3 years in an accredited PA program culminating in a master's degree as a PA. The only recognized certification for PAs is through the National Commission on Certification of Physician Assistants (NCCPA). They then are licensed in their state of practice. The level of independent practice for PAs varies by state, but they must practice in collaboration with physicians when in the inpatient environment.

In the inpatient environment, NPs and PAs typically practice in similar roles. They, in collaboration with physicians and other members of the health-care team, determine the plan of care for the patient. They are responsible for the ongoing assessment and management of the patient to achieve the goals of care.

Effectiveness of a practice model utilizing advanced practice health professionals

While understanding the roles of different health-care providers is important to function in a collaborative manner, we must also value and respect the contributions of each member of the team. A recent study performed at the Cleveland Clinic was presented as an oral abstract at the Society of Critical Care Medicine Congress. The researcher studied the impact of care provided by NPs and PAs to 1054 patients in two medical ICUs at the Cleveland Clinic from July 2013 to April 2014. Keller (2015) noted that the survival rate among ICU patients cared for by PAs and acute care NPs was 92% compared with 88.6% among those cared for by a team of residents ($p = 0.047$), with all other variables controlled. He reported, "Our findings suggest the partnership of PAs and acute care NPs with pulmonary and critical care physicians and fellows can improve outcomes in the medical ICU and help alleviate the projected shortfall of bedside intensivists" (Keller, 2015). Keller (2015) suggested that collaborative practice between intensivists and advanced practice health providers holds an advantage in patient care outcomes, as these providers have longer experience in the ICU versus the residents who tend to rotate through 1 month at a time. Further, the ongoing, stable relationship between advanced practice health providers and the physicians in the ICU may result in improved communication as well as better patient handoffs.

Collaborative practice

Although collaboration between members of the health-care team has been a topic of study and discussion for several years, collaborative practice models for use in the acute and intensive care settings have been lacking. Prior research has shown that the utilization of PAs and NPs, as well as specialty trained nurses, in the inpatient setting can improve patient outcomes, but continuing to expand and improve this practice must be focused on specific key areas in order to provide comprehensive, knowledgeable, and professional care for patients. These key areas include the following:

- Enhancing clinical knowledge in the management of patients with neuroscience disorders with ongoing education and scholarly production (research and publication)
- Obtaining specialty certification in critical care, acute care, and neuroscience where available
- Understanding the scope of practice specific to the role as well as for the state in which practice occurs

These three key areas will allow advanced practice health providers to become recognized as specialists and allow their physician colleagues to see them as qualified to participate in the collaborative management of these often challenging patients.

Additionally, advanced practice health providers must understand the components of collaborative practice so that they can have an effective working relationship with the neurologist, neurosurgeon, and/or neurointensivist with whom they practice as well as with the other members of the collaborative health-care team. These components include the following:

- *Communication*: This includes both written and verbal communication. Medical documentation is also a medium of communication between all members of the health-care team. It provides a record of care delivery as well as medical decision making. When functioning as a collaborative team, meetings or rounds that include the entire team should happen regularly so that everyone understands the plan of care as well as the role of each member of the team in providing that care.
- *Goal setting*: The goals of care must be mutually agreed upon by the entire health-care team and must include the participation of the patient and their family.
- *Self-awareness*: Advanced health-care providers must have a clear understanding of their own strengths and weaknesses. They must know what they do not know. They must seek the assistance and support of other NPs, PAs, nurses, physicians, and other members of the health-care team when appropriate.
- *Trust and mutual respect*: Each member of the health-care team has an important role in caring for the patient. Trust that each member will perform his or her role and request clarification when necessary. Understanding each other's role and not usurping their duties will lead to mutual respect within the health-care team.
- *Delegation*: This is an art. Those directing the plan of care include physicians and advanced practice health providers. The physicians may delegate to the NPs or PAs who, in turn, may delegate to other members of the health-care team. Take care not to sound bossy or ask members of the team to perform duties and services that are outside of their scope of practice.
- *Role development*: Continuing education and development is the role of every member of the collaborative health-care team. This includes individual activities required for licensure and certification as well as group team-building activities. Understanding each person's role in a collaborative team is imperative to the optimal functioning of that team.

Common pitfalls and medicolegal concerns for nurse practitioners and physician assistants in collaborative practice

In collaborative practice with a neurologist, neurosurgeon, or intensivist, the following are common pitfalls and medicolegal concerns for NPs and PAs:

- *Understand your scope of practice*: Each individual state has some sort of document that directs the practice of NPs and PAs. Some call it a code; others call it a practice act. Regardless, in every state, there is a set of rules that govern practice. Every NP and PA must be acutely aware of the document that governs their practice as well as the scope of practice that they must follow. Practicing outside of your scope of practice can lead to serious consequences, including disciplinary action, revocation or suspension of the license, and, in some cases, civil or criminal liability.

- *Collaborative practice agreements*: Some states and most hospitals require that a collaborative practice agreement be in place when PAs and NPs are employed in the inpatient environment to act as physician extenders. This document should include a list of duties that will be delegated to the NP or PA by a physician as well as the level of supervision to be provided by the physician. This document should not be restrictive, and the NP/PA should be able to practice within the full scope of his or her licensure and education.
- *Billing for services*: One of the issues facing hospitals today is reimbursement. NP/PA services can and should be billed to insurance to improve the reimbursement that hospitals receive. NP/PA services are often billed at a lower rate than services provided by a physician. For this reason, NPs and PAs should discuss billing with their collaborating physician and determine what services each person will provide and bill for—this should be incorporated into the collaborative practice agreement.

Relevance to the advanced practice health professional

Working collaboratively with a neurologist, neurosurgeon, and/or neurointensivist is necessary when NPs and PAs practice in the inpatient setting and manage patients with neurologic conditions. More importantly, the remainder of the health-care team, the patient, and the patient's family must all be considered integral members of the team. Utilizing a comprehensive, collaborative approach to care has been shown to improve patient outcomes as well as patient satisfaction. Including advanced practice health professionals in the collaborative team provides a stable, ongoing bridge between the physician and the remainder of the health-care team. NPs and PAs also provide that link between the physician and the patient/family to improve communication and provide patient education related to the diagnosis and medical treatment plan. In order to prove the value of the advanced practice health professional in the inpatient setting, further research needs to occur to demonstrate the positive impact that this practice model has on patient outcomes as well as hospital reimbursement.

References

Keller J. ICU outcomes of physician assistants and acute care nurse practitioners compared to resident teams. Paper presented at *The Society of Critical Care Medicine 2015 Critical Care Congress,* January 2015; Phoenix.

World Health Organization. Framework for Action on Interprofessional Education and Collaborative Practice. http://www.who.int/hrh/resources/framework_action/en/. 2010.

15

OCCUPATIONAL, PHYSICAL, AND SPEECH THERAPIES

Amy Wang and Alison Kirkpatrick

Physical, occupational, and speech therapists each have a specific role as part of the neuroscience patient care team. Their interventions are integral in restoring optimal function to patients along the continuum of care, including in the home.

While physical, occupational, and speech therapists each address particular functional deficits, they work collaboratively, as part of a specialized interdisciplinary team. They each develop patient-centered functional goals; treat the patient; document progress toward goals; and address injuries to the bones, muscles, tissues, and nervous system.

Occupational therapy

Occupational therapy (OT) is a health profession dedicated to promoting and maintaining health and independence in all facets of a person's life. OT is provided from infancy to the elder years, treating physical or cognitive problems that interfere with a person's ability to perform activities of daily living.

Education

OT—Currently from a minimum of a master's degree to a PhD
OT Assistant (COTA)—2-year associate degree
OT aide—At least a high school diploma/general equivalency diploma (GED) and on-the-job training

OTs evaluate and treat the following:

Cognition—Memory, orientation, problem solving, concentration and attention span, initiation, sequencing, learning, insight, and safety judgement

Vision and perception—Interpretation of sensory information as it relates to spatial relations, position in space, figure ground, form constancy, right-left discrimination, depth perception, and neglect

Motor control and tone—Ability to move upper and lower extremities, coordination (gross and fine motor), balance, functional mobility, tone, and synergy patterns

Sensation and its effect on motor performance and patient safety—Range of motion (ROM) and need for exercises and/or splinting to increase this, decrease pain, or manage spasticity

Retraining in activities of daily living (ADLs)—ADLs include feeding, grooming, bathing, dressing, handwriting, cooking, and household tasks; also include access to leisure activities

Possible need for modalities (i.e., iontophoresis, ultrasound, electrical stimulation)

Pain management techniques
Assessment and training with assistive devices to improve independence with ADLs

Physical therapy

Physical therapists (PTs) evaluate and provide treatment utilizing a variety of techniques to reduce pain, restore function, promote mobility, and prevent disability.

Education

PT—Currently master's degree to PhD
PT Assistant (PTA)—2-year associate's degree
PT aide—At least high school diploma/GED and on-the-job training

PTs evaluate and treat the following:

- Motor control, ROM, movement patterns, strength, balance, and coordination evaluations
- Cardiopulmonary and vascular abilities and endurance evaluations
- Therapeutic exercise training
- Gait training and transfer training
- Vestibular/balance training
- Assistive devices for mobility assessment and training
- Wheelchair/seating evaluation
- Need for orthotics/prosthetics assessment
- Body mechanics and postural stability evaluation and treatment
- Modalities (i.e., iontophoresis, ultrasound, cryotherapy, hydrotherapy, phonophoresis, thermotherapy, biofeedback, electrical stimulation) use assessment and treatment
- Patient and family training

Speech therapy

Speech-language pathologists (SLPs), also referred to as speech therapists, provide assessment and treatment for disorders related to speech, language, cognition, communication, voice, articulation, fluency, and swallowing (dysphagia).

Education

SLP requires a minimum master's degree.

SLPs evaluate and treat the following (Table 15.1):

- Dysphagia/swallowing abilities and recommendations for safe food and drink consistencies (e.g., pureed, mechanical soft, nectar thick liquids, honey thick liquids, and need for alternate nutritional sources)
- Auditory processing disorders
- Cognition
- Speech/articulation difficulties
- Hearing deficits

Table 15.1 Examples of Communication Disorders

Aphasia: Difficulty naming objects
Anomia: Word-finding problems
Broca: Difficulty expressing: mild problems understanding complex syntax
Conduction: Difficulty in repetition of spoken language, word-finding pauses
Crossed: Transient; occurs in right-handed person with right hemisphere lesion
Global: Most common and severe: few stereotypical words/sounds; comprehension
reading and writing impaired
Subcortical: Dysarthria and mild anomia with comprehension deficits (thalamic)
lesions in thalamus, putamen, caudate or internal capsule
Transcortical: Spontaneous speech restricted, able to repeat, comprehend, and read
Wernicke: Apahasia; severe disturbance in auditory comprehension
Agraphia: Writing ability disturbed; lesions in frontal or postlanguage area
Aprosody: Disturbance of melodic quality change in intonation
Dysarthia: Loss of control of articulation muscles

- Adaptive communication devices
  - Communication board
  - Use of a speaking valve with a tracheostomy
  - Patient and caregiver education

Provider orders

Each discipline requires provider orders for assessment and treatment of each patient. These orders usually specify the following:

- *Which discipline*—OT/PT/Speech evaluation and treatment
- *Frequency and duration*—Based on patient's impairments and limitations
- *Level of activity*—Bed level only, out of bed (OOB) to chair, ambulate with assistance, swallow evaluation for oral intake, weightbearing status or use of equipment (OOB with back brace only); discharge planning recommendations (rehab, nursing home, home)

Scales and evaluations often used by therapists include the following:

1. *Tone*—Upper motor neuron (UMN) problems (UMN—brain and spinal cord) are associated with increased tone. Lower motor neuron (LMN) problems are associated with decreased tone.
   Reflex responses are graded as follows:
   0—No response
   1+—Diminished, low normal
   2+—Average normal
   3+—Brisker than normal
   4+—Very brisk, hyperactive (LMN is affiliated with 0 or 1; UMN is associated with 3+ or 4+)
   (Tables 15.2 and 15.3)

2. *Cerebellar function*—Muscle coordination and balance
   a. Finger-to-nose test
   b. Finger-to-finger test
   c. Tandem walking

Table 15.2 MMT (Manual Muscle Testing)

Grade	Description	Gravity	Range of motion	Resistance
5	Normal	Against	Full	Maximum
4	Good	Against	Full	Moderate
3	Fair	Against	Limited	None
2	Poor	Eliminated	Full	Minimal
1	Trace	Eliminated	Limited	None
0	None	Eliminated	None	None

Table 15.3 Sensory Testing

Pain—Sharp/Dull
Impaired by spinothalamic tract
Test method: Use a pin while patient's vision is occluded
Temperature—Impaired anterolateral tract.
Method: Test with hot and cold water in tubes/ice or warm compress
Light touch—Impaired nerve root injury, brain/brainstem, peripheral polyneuropathy
Method: Light brush of skin (monofilaments)
Position Sense/Kinesthesia
Impaired by joint or muscle receptors
Method: Passive joint placement
Vibration—Demyelinating neuropathy
Method: Post-tap tuning fork, apply to bony prominence
Graphesthesia—Writing difficulties
Impairment of dorsal column, parietal lobe, ventral post thalamus, medial lemniscus
Method: Tracing numbers with finger on surface of hand

Table 15.4 Rancho Los Amigos National Rehabilitation Center's Rancho Levels of Cognitive Functioning

Stage	Function
Stage 1	No response to stimulation
Stage 2	Generalized response to stimulation
Stage 3	Localized response to stimulation
Stage 4	Confused, agitated behavior
Stage 5	Confused, inappropriate, nonagitated behavior
Stage 6	Confused, appropriate behavior
Stage 7	Automatic, appropriate behavior
Stage 8	Purposeful, appropriate behavior

3. Romberg test
4. *Cranial nerves*
5. *Mental status*
   a. Level of awareness, attentiveness, orientation, speech and language, memory, higher intellectual function, mood and affect (Tables 15.4 and 15.5)

Table 15.5 FIM (Functional Independence Measure)

Self-Care	
1. Eating	5. Dressing lower body
2. Grooming	6. Toileting
3. Bathing/showering	
4. Dressing upper body	
Sphincters	
1. Bladder management	
2. Bowel management	
Mobility	
1. Transfers: Bed/wheelchair/commode	1. Locomotion: Walking/wheelchair commode
2. Transfers: Toilet	2. Locomotion: Stairs
3. Transfers: Bathtub/shower	
Communication	
1. Expression	
2. Comprehension	
3. Social interaction	
Cognition	
1. Problem solving	
2. Memory	

Note: Developed at the University of Buffalo, provides a uniform measurement for disability.

Levels of required assistance

7 Complete independence
6 Modified independence (use of device)
5 Supervision (subject = 100%)
4 Minimal assist (subject = 75%–99%)
3 Moderate assist (subject = 50%–74%)
2 Maximal assist (subject = 25%–49%)
1 Total assist (subject <25%)

Common concerns include the following:

• Length of patient stay in acute care hospital versus rehabilitation hospital
• Recommended placement for longer-term patients
• Communication with other rehabilitation team members
• Family level of participation and family training needs
• Identification of adverse conditions

Resource information

• American Physical Therapy Association: www.apta.org
• American Occupational Therapy Association: www.aota.org
• American Speech-Language-Hearing Association: www.asha.org
• Americans with Disabilities Act: https://www.ada.gov/

16

NEUROANESTHESIA

Cheng-Hsin Cheng, Junichi Ohya,
Praveen V. Mummaneni, and Valli Mummaneni

Pharmacology

Intravenous anesthetic agents

Most intravenous anesthetic agents increase the duration of opening of the γ-aminobutyric acid A (GABA$_A$)-dependent chloride channel by an agonist effect at the GABA$_A$ receptor. The exception is ketamine, which acts through antagonism of the excitatory receptor *N*-methyl-D-aspartate (NMDA). The prolonged time of channel opening allows increased passage of chloride ions, which may introduce membrane hyperpolarization and inhibition of neuronal transmission.

An "ideal" intravenous anesthetic agent for neuroanesthesia should:

- Have rapid recovery from consciousness in order to permit quick assessment of neurologic status
- Be easily and rapidly titratable
- Have minimal effects on organ systems (such as liver and kidney)
- Have analgesic effects
- Provide maintenance of cerebrovascular autoregulation and vasoreactivity to CO_2
- Not elevate the intracranial pressure (ICP)

Propofol

Propofol is commonly used for intravenous induction during neurosurgical procedures. It is also used for conscious sedation. It can provide smooth induction of anesthesia with minimal excitatory effects and rapid recovery.

Ketamine

Ketamine is an antagonist of NMDA receptors. Ketamine can increase ICP, so it is often avoided in cranial surgery. Ketamine is used in conjunction with opiates for opiate-tolerant spinal surgery patients. Common side effects include nightmares and hallucinations.

Volatile anesthetic agents

Volatile anesthetics are frequently an important component of anesthesia for complex neurosurgery. The most commonly used volatile anesthetic agents are desflurane and sevoflurane.

Desflurane

Desflurane has a low blood/gas partition coefficient, which enables the anesthetist to titrate it rapidly according to the patient's needs, level of surgical stimulation, or neuromonitoring requirements.

Sevoflurane

Sevoflurane has minimal effects on cerebral blood flow and also has a low blood/gas coefficient. Sevoflurane is nonpungent and can be used for inhalational induction in both pediatric and adult patients.

Opioids and neuromuscular blocking agents

Opioids

Opioid analgesics include morphine, fentanyl, sufentanil, remifentanil, and alfentanil. They are an important adjunct to sedative and hypnotic drugs.

Cardiovascular effects

Opioids can decrease sympathetic tone and increase parasympathetic tone. Moreover, all opioids are associated with bradycardia and hypotension in large doses.

Respiratory effects

A moderately large dose of opioids can inhibit respiratory drive and also decrease coughing in response to the presence of an endotracheal tube.

Other effects

There are many side effects of opioids. Problems with nausea and vomiting are due to stimulation of serotonin (5-HT3) and dopamine receptors in the chemoreceptor trigger zone. The use of longer-acting agents can cause impaired gastric emptying, ileus, constipation, pupillary constriction, and pruritus.

Neuromuscular blocking agents

Although succinylcholine has the potential to increase ICP, the effect is small and transient. The elevated ICP can be decreased by pretreatment with nondepolarizing neuromuscular blockers. Coughing, straining, and intolerance of the endotracheal tube often cause elevated ICP, which can be diminished by neuromuscular blocking agents. The neuromuscular blocking agents, however, inhibit motor evoked potential and neuromonitoring for spinal cases and should be held after the patient is intubated.

Neuroanesthesia

Anesthesia for cranial surgery

Preoperative management

Before surgery, obtain patient history and perform a physical, review labs and test results, check blood product availability, and perform American Society of Anesthesiologists (ASA) risk assessment.

Intraoperative management

The goals of general anesthesia include

- Smooth induction
- Hemodynamic stability (hypertension increases the risk for hemorrhage and vasogenic edema; hypotension can lead to ischemia in areas of impaired autoregulation)
- Lower ICP and a relaxed brain (to reduce the risk for retractor damage and for optimal surgical access)
- Rapid and smooth emergence after operation to allow early neurologic evaluation

Induction

An intravenous anesthetic agent, usually propofol or thiopental, is used for intubation. This is often combined with an opiate and a muscle relaxant after induction. In addition to standard anesthesia monitoring, an arterial line, large-bore IVs or central venous line (if significant blood loss is anticipated), and a urinary catheter may be indicated.

Maintenance of anesthesia

An intravenous agent (propofol) and an inhalational agent (sevoflurane, desflurane, isoflurane) in combination with an opioid may be used. Continuous muscle relaxation can be used if no neuromonitoring or only somatosensory evoked potentials (SSEPs) are monitored. The body temperature should be maintained at normothermia. The keys are to maintain cerebral perfusion while preventing increases in ICP (avoid hypercarbia and hypoxia and provide an adequate level of anesthesia) and to allow rapid emergence at the end of surgery.

Fluid management

The patients in routine neurosurgical procedures are provided with glucose free isoosmolar crystalloid and colloid solutions for maintenance and resuscitation fluids in order to prevent elevated ICP from hypoosmolality. High glucose levels can potentially cause cerebral edema.

Anesthesia for spinal surgery

The common indications for spinal surgery include decompression of the spinal cord or a nerve root, to remove a tumor, or to stabilize the spine. Spine surgery may be done with neuromonitoring (*electromyography*, SSEP, motor evoked potential), so anesthesia providers should avoid inhibiting neuromonitoring. The anesthetic technique should include a short-acting muscle relaxant, <0.5 MAC of inhalational agent combined with an intravenous agent and opioids.

Induction and maintenance of anesthesia spinal cord perfusion

The anesthetic plan should help preserve adequate spinal cord perfusion during the operation. If there is the potential for heavy blood loss, several large-bore venous cannulas and/or a central venous catheter are often used.

When spinal cord compression is significant or maintenance of adequate spinal cord perfusion is an issue, invasive blood pressure monitoring with an arterial line is often used. Central venous pressure may be monitored when significant blood loss is anticipated. In addition, a cell saver device should be considered if massive blood loss is encountered.

Airway

Patients are typically intubated with a glide scope or with fiberoptic intubation for those with difficult airway or poor C-spine mobility.

Maintenance of anesthesia

The intraoperative monitoring of SSEPs or motor evoked potentials (MEPs) may cause the limitation of agents for maintenance of anesthesia. Most anesthesiologists use propofol and opioid infusion, which allows spinal cord monitoring using both motor and sensory evoked potentials. Sensory evoked potential monitoring can be performed with low-dose volatile agents.

Preservation of normothermia with warming devices is important, because hypothermia, lower than 36°C, increases the risk for postoperative infection and also reduces the signals for MEP.

Positioning

It is important to position the neck in a neutral position in patients with cervical cord compression. Some centers may position the patient under general anesthesia using flouroscopic imaging to confirm correct spinal column alignment. Some surgeons use pre- and postposition SSEPs or MEPs, or both, to confirm the positioning is not stressing the spinal cord.

The patients in the prone position undergo dorsal spine and spinal cord surgery. The special mattress or support should be prepared below the patient and should allow free movement of the abdomen with ventilation. Any elevated intraabdominal pressure results in possible inferior vena cava compression and contributes to reduced cardiac output.

The impairment of vision is a rare but serious complication after surgery in the prone position. Ischemic optic neuropathy is the most common cause. Otherwise, direct pressure on the globe can cause visual deficits as well.

If a patient's arms need to be positioned beside the head to facilitate imaging during prone thoracic/lumbar surgery, care must be taken to avoid stretching of the brachial plexus.

Conclusion

Anesthetic plans for neurosurgery need to take into account ICP, perfusion pressure, and venous return issues. The use of neuromonitoring may preclude the use of certain agents. A discussion regarding the goals of surgery between the surgical team and the anesthesia team is helpful to create the anesthetic plan. Patients should be well padded to prevent pressure sores for long procedures.

Additional bibliography

Absalom AR, Struys MR. *An Overview of TCI and TIVA*. Belgium, Gent: Academic Press; 2005.

Constant I, Seeman R, Murat I. Sevoflurane and epileptiform EEG changes. *Pediatr Anaesth*. 2005;15:266–274.

Crabb I, Thornton C, Konieczko KM, et al. Remifentanil reduces auditory and somatosensory evoked responses during isoflurane anaesthesia in a dose-dependent manner. *Br J Anaesth*. 1996;76:795–801.

Engelhard K, Werner C. Inhalational or intravenous anesthetics for craniotomies? Pro inhalational. *Curr Opin Anaesthesiol*. 2006;19:504–508.

Fagerlund TH, Braaten O. No pain relief from codeine… ? An introduction to pharmacogenomics. *Acta Anaesthesiol Scand.* 2001;45:140–149.

Gupta AK, Gelb AW. *Essentials of Neuroanesthesia and Neurointensive Care: A Volume in Essentials of Anesthesia and Critical Care.* 1st ed. Saunders: 2008

Hemmings HC Jr, Akabas MH, Goldstein PA, et al. Emerging molecular mechanisms of general anesthetic action. *Trends Pharmacol Sci.* 2005;26:503–510.

Hirsch N. Advances in neuroanaesthesia. *Anaesthesia.* 2003;58:1162–1165.

Holmstrom A, Akeson J. Sevoflurane induces less cerebral vasodilation than isoflurane at the same A-line autoregressive index level. *Acta Anaesthesiol Scand.* 2005;49:16–22.

Kaisti KK, Langsjo JW, Aalto S, et al. Effects of sevoflurane, propofol, and adjunct nitrous oxide on regional cerebral blood flow, oxygen consumption, and blood volume in humans. *Anesthesiology.* 2003;99:603–613.

Martyn JA, White DA, Gronert GA, et al. Up-and-down regulation of skeletal muscle acetylcholine receptors. Effects on neuromuscular blockers. *Anesthesiology.* 1992;76:822–843.

Norris FH, Colella J, McFarlin D. Effect of diphenylhydantoin on neuromuscular synapse. *Neurology.* 1964;14:869–876.

Pandey CK, Navkar DV, Giri PJ, et al. Evaluation of the optimal preemptive dose of gabapentin for postoperative pain relief after lumbar diskectomy: a randomized, double-blind, placebo-controlled study. *J Neurosurg Anesthesiol.* 2005;17:65–68.

Petersen KD, Landsfeldt U, Cold GE, et al. Intracranial pressure and cerebral hemodynamic in patients with cerebral tumors: a randomized prospective study of patients subjected to craniotomy in propofolfentanyl, isoflurane-fentanyl, or sevoflurane-fentanyl anesthesia. *Anesthesiology.* 2003;98:329–336.

Randell T, Niskanen M. Management of physiological variables in neuroanaesthesia: maintaining homeostasis during intracranial surgery. *Curr Opin Anaesthesiol.* 2006;19:492–497.

Ravussin P, Guiard JP, Ralley F, Thorin D. Effect of propofol on cerebrospinal fluid pressure and cerebral perfusion pressure in patients undergoing craniotomy. *Anaesthesia.* 1988;43(suppl):37–41.

Ravussin P, Tempelhoff R, Modica PA, et al. Propofol vs thiopental-isoflurane for neurosurgical anesthesia: comparison of hemodynamics, CSF pressure, and recovery. *J Neurosurg Anesthesiol.* 1991;3:85–95.

Ravussin P, Wilder-Smith OHG. Supratentorial masses: anaesthetic considerations. In: Cottrell JE, Smith DS, eds. *Anaesthesia and Neurosurgery.* 4th ed. St Louis, MO: CV Mosby; 2001:297–318.

Raw DA, Beattie JK, Hunter JM. Anaesthesia for spinal surgery in adults. *Br J Anaesth.* 2003;91:886–904.

Roberts I, Yates D, Sandercock P, et al. Effect of intravenous corticosteroids on death within 14 days in 10008 adults with clinically significant head injury (MRC CRASH trial): randomised placebo-controlled trial. *Lancet.* 2004;364:1321–1328.

Sneyd JR. Propofol and epilepsy. *Br J Anaesth.* 1999;82:168–169.

Sponheim S, Skraastad O, Helseth E, et al. Effects of 0.5 and 1.0 MAC isoflurane, sevoflurane and desflurane on intracranial and cerebral perfusion pressures in children. *Acta Anaesthesiol Scand.* 2003;47:932–938.

Stoneham MD, Cooper R, Quiney NF, Walters FJ. Pain following craniotomy: a preliminary study comparing PCA morphine with intramuscular codeine phosphate. *Anaesthesia.* 1996;51:1176–1178.

Strebel S, Lam AM, Matta B, et al. Dynamic and static cerebral autoregulation during isoflurane, desflurane, and propofol anesthesia. *Anesthesiology.* 1995;83:66–76.

Summors AC, Gupta AK, Matta BF. Dynamic cerebral autoregulation during sevoflurane anesthesia: a comparison with isoflurane. *Anesth Analg.* 1999;88:341–345.

Tietjen CS, Hurn PD, Ulatowski JA, Kirsch JR. Treatment modalities for hypertensive patients with intracranial pathology: options and risks. *Crit Care Med.* 1996;24:311–322.

Van Hemelrijck J. Anaesthetic considerations for specific neurosurgical procedures. In: Van Aken H, ed. *Neuroanaesthetic Practice.* London, England: BMJ Publishing; 1995:214–239.

Werner C, Kochs E, Bause H, et al. Effects of sufentanil on cerebral hemodynamics and intracranial pressure in patients with brain injury. *Anesthesiology.* 1995;83:721–726.

17

NUTRITION AND SURGICAL RECOVERY

Marianne J. Beare and Nilesh A. Vyas

Nutritional assessment in surgical patients

Negative consequences of malnutrition

- Malnutrition has been associated with increased surgical complications, including poor wound healing, susceptibility to infection, compromised immune status, increased frequency of decubitus ulcers, alternation of flora in the gastrointestinal (GI) tract, impairment of organ function, and increased mortality (Mainous and Deitch, 1994, p. 659; Santos, 1994, p. 243; Kinney and Weissmanm, 1986, p. 19).
- Malnutrition was traditionally defined as inadequate intake or starvation, but surgery causes a systemic inflammatory response that promotes cytokine-driven protein catabolism of the skeletal muscle—a different type of malnutrition (Collier et al., 2012, p. 395).
- The Joint Commission recommends malnutrition risk screening within 24–48 hours of hospital admission, followed by nutritional assessment and timely intervention.
- Up to 40% of hospitalized patients are malnourished (Barker et al., 2011, p. 514).
- Patients undergoing major elective surgery are often moderately depleted of body protein preoperatively because of their disease process. They can lose 5% or 43 g/day of body protein during the first two postoperative weeks (Hill, 1998, p. 557).
- Stress of surgery or illness can result in hypermetabolism, loss of lean body mass, and increased morbidity and mortality (Wright, 2004, p. 273).
- Early nutritional support has been shown to blunt hypermetabolism, reduce complications from surgery, and reduce length of hospital stay (Marik and Zaloga, 2001, p. 2264).
- Wound healing requires an anabolic state. Appropriate nutrition necessary for wound healing includes vitamins A, C, E, and zinc as well as adequate caloric intake and protein (Sinno et al., 2011, p. 287; MacKay and Miller, 2003, p. 359).
- Early feeding in critical illness results in better outcomes in terms of survival and disability (Perel et al., 2006).

Malnutrition criteria

- The diagnosis of malnutrition requires two or more of the following: insufficient energy intake, weight loss, loss of muscle mass, loss of subcutaneous fat, localized or generalized fluid accumulation, and diminished functional status (Mueller et al., 2011, p. 16; White et al., 2012, p. 275).

History and physical examination for malnutrition evaluation

History and clinical diagnosis: Type and length of surgery, infectious process, specific nutrient deficiencies, history of weight loss or gain, use of dietary supplements, food allergies/intolerances, chronic medical illnesses, past medical and surgical history, social history, and family history

Physical exam: General loss of subcutaneous fat, vital signs including weight/height, fluid status, surgical wound integrity, tissue depletion, muscle function, loss of muscle mass, hair loss, bitemporal wasting, conjunctival pallor, thyromegaly, ecchymosis, petechiae, and pressure ulcers

Laboratory data: Serum albumin, prealbumin, C-reactive protein (CRP), complete blood count (CBC), basic metabolic panel (BMP), transferrin

Food/nutrient intake: Modified diet history, 24-hour recall of food intake, discussion of nutritional intake with patient and family if appropriate

Functional assessment: Presurgical state, timeline for decline of physical function (if relevant) (White et al., 2012, p. 280; Wright, 2004, p. 273)

Laboratory tests: Essential for determining the nutritional status and effectiveness of nutritional intervention

Protein status (albumin, transferrin, prealbumin)

Common pitfalls

The measurement of protein may be unreliable if creatinine clearance is <50 mL/min or if the patient is in renal or hepatic failure (Wright, 2004, p. 278).

Serum albumin: Long half-life of 14–20 days and reflects intake during the previous 3 weeks. Low albumin is reflective of a negative catabolic state, a predictor of poor outcomes (van Stijn et al., 2013 p. 37). Albumin levels may become unreliable after massive fluid resuscitation, or any disorder causing large protein losses such as ascites, liver disease, excessive burns, and inflammation. For every gram deficit of untreated hypoalbuminemia, there is approximately 30% increase in mortality (Goldwasser and Feldman, 1997, p. 693).

Normal: 3.4–5.5 mg/dL
Borderline: 2.1–3.3 mg/dL
Low: <2.1 mg/dL

Prealbumin: Plasma protein metabolized in the liver. The half-life is 2–3 days, but the level responds quickly to adequate protein intake. Levels will typically rise to low normal within 10 days of initiation of adequate feeding/refeeding. Levels can be decreased due to cirrhosis, inflammation, malignancy, zinc deficiency, and/or estrogen therapy/oral contraceptive pills (OCPs). Levels can be elevated due to alcohol intoxication, corticosteroid use, Hodgkin disease, nonsteroidal anti-inflammatory drugs (NSAIDs), and progestational drugs.

Normal: 20–40 mg/dL
Borderline: 16–20 mg/dL
Low: <16 mg/dL

Transferrin: Half-life of 8–9 days, reflecting protein status over the past 2–4 weeks. Transferrin is also indicative of iron status, but it is only an indication of protein status if serum iron is normal (Seres, 2005, p. 308).

Normal: 212–360 mg/dL
Mildly low: 150–211 mg/dL
Moderately low: 100–149 mg/dL
Severely low: <100 mg/dL

Renal function: Blood urea nitrogen (BUN) and creatinine (Cr) should be evaluated to check the overall fluid volume status and kidney function. BUN will often gradually decrease in malnourished patients but will increase with worsening renal function. Creatinine is derived from the metabolism of creatinine in skeletal muscle and from dietary meat intake. It is filtered across the glomerulus and is not reabsorbed or metabolized by the kidney. Elevated BUN and Cr may be indicative of renal dysfunction.

Normal BUN: 7–20 mg/dL
Normal creatinine: 0.5–1.2 mg/dL

Electrolytes and others: Check daily when nutritional therapy is initiated, and then check 3–5 times per week until a stable regimen is achieved (Wright, 2004). Also check sodium, potassium, magnesium, calcium, phosphorous, vitamin B_{12}/folate, and iron levels.

Tools

Predictive equations for energy expenditure

There are over 200 predictive equations to estimate energy expenditure. Predictive equations can offer "stress" factors to account for the specific nutritional needs of special populations.

Ideal body weight

Male: 47.7 kg for the first 5 ft plus 2.7 kg for each inch above 5 ft
Female: 45 kg for the first 5 ft plus 2.25 kg for each inch above 5 ft
>200% ideal body weight: morbidly obese
126%–199% obese
111%–125% overweight
90%–110% adequate energy reserve
90%–90% lean body habitus or mildly depleted energy stores
<79% moderate or severe depletion of energy reserve

Body mass index (BMI): Weight in kg divided by height in meters^2

>30 Obese
25–29.9 kg/m^2 Overweight
18.5–24.9 kg/m^2 Normal weight
< 18.5 kg/m^2 Underweight

Caloric requirements: Protein, carbohydrates, lipids

Special considerations for stress stratification estimates are as follows:
26 kcal/kg/d after craniotomy
40–50 kcal/kg/d for patients with Glasgow Coma Scale (GCS) of 4–5

30–40 kcal/kg/d for patients with GCS of 6–7

30–35 kcal/kg/d for patients with GCS 8–12

27 kcal/kg/d for paraplegic patients

23 kcal/kg/d for quadriplegic patients

6–10 kcal/day for patients with brain death

60 kcal/kg/d for patients in status epilepticus

15–18 kcal/kg/d for patients in barbiturate coma

Indirect calorimetry

The gold standard of nutritional assessment in the intensive care unit (ICU) is indirect calorimetry; it is the most accurate method for determining the energy expenditure of critically ill patients (Haugen et al., 2007, p. 377). An instrument called a metabolic cart measures the exchange of O_2 and CO_2 across the lungs for 15–30 minutes and is then estimated for 24 hours. It is underutilized because of expense and clinical expertise required to interpret results (Wooley and Frankenfield, 2012, p. 25).

Nutritional interventions

Indications for supplementation

Supplemental or alternative nutrient support is required if a patient is unable to take in adequate nutrients orally or an illness results in a malfunctioning GI tract.

Normal postoperative course

- Start with clear liquids unless there is suspected dysphagia. A clear liquid diet is intended for short-term use. Clear liquids include things like lemon-lime soda and Jell-O.
- Consult speech therapy prior to feeding if you have any concern about swallow function. Even mild dysphagia may require a diet modification.

Common pitfalls

Slow diet progression is not necessary for most postoperative patients. You may advance the diet as tolerated back to their normal diet (Jeffery et al., 1996, p. 167). If the patient is diabetic, take care to order a diabetic diet.

If the patient has difficulty swallowing, consider whether it is neurologic, such as a cranial nerve dysfunction after a craniotomy, a motility issue such as after an anterior cervical discectomy and fusion, or a sore throat from intubation during surgery.

Common phone calls, pages, and requests with answers

If the patient is not eating due to nausea, consider an antiemetic such as ondansetron or promethazine hydrochloride.

Can the patient remove a cervical collar to eat? The answer is "no," unless cleared with the neurosurgeon. Some minor cervical procedures use a cervical collar for comfort only, but in the case of cervical fractures and some fusions, the surgeon may want the collar on at all times.

Protein/Nutritional requirements postoperatively

Calories: Increase to 30–40 kcals/kg, patients on ventilator require only 20–25 kcal/kg
Protein: Increase to 1–1.8 g/kg
Fluid: Individualize fluid requirements

Enteral feeding: "Nutrition provided through the GI tract via a tube, catheter, or stoma that delivers nutrients distal to the oral cavity" (McClave et al., 2009, p. 277).

- Tube indications: Functional GI tract, along with a clinical situation in which oral intake is unsafe, insufficient, or impossible. If you suspect inability to eat or inadequate oral intake, consider enteral tube placement.
- ICU patients who require nonoral nutritional support due to intubation, altered mental status, or dysphagia should have a nutritional consultation for optimization.

Common pitfalls

You do not need to hear bowel sounds to initiate enteral feeding (McClave et al., 2009, p. 285).

Common questions/Pages

Check nasogastric (NG)/orogastric (OG) tube placement with chest x-ray. Check postpyloric tube placement with KUB (kidney, ureter, and bladder) x-ray.

Types of enteral tubes: Gastric versus postpyloric

- Decisions should be based on disease state, gastrointestinal function, duration of enteral nutrition support, and available expertise or access (Ukleja et al., 2010, p. 403).
- Short-term feeding can be done through a NG or OG tube into the stomach, post the pylorus (i.e., distal to the ligament of Treitz).
- Long-term feeding options include gastrostomy, jejunostomy, and gastrojejunostomy tubes, which are endoscopically or surgically placed.

Common pitfalls

Nasogastric tubes should not be used after endonasal, transsphenoidal surgery, or with multiple facial fractures or other skull base defects or surgeries.

You do not need to check residuals through postpyloric feeding tubes.

Gastric feeds: Continuous: start at a rate of 20–50 mL/hr, advance in increments of 10–25 mL q 4–24 hours up to goal, check gastric residuals q 4 hours. If >150 cc, hold tube feeds for 2 hours (Parrish, 2003, p. 76). This is the most common way to feed patients who require enteral eeding.

Promotility agents such as metoclopramide 10 mg q 6 hours may reduce gastric residuals. If residuals remain high, consider small bowel feeding.

Bolus feeds: Start with 100–120 mL bolus feeds and increase by 60 mL q bolus to goal volume. Typical bolus feeds occur every 3–8 hours.

Postpyloric/small bowel feeds: Continuous feeding only. Start at 20 mL/hr, advance in increments of 20 mL q 8 hours to goal. Residuals do not need to be checked. Use postpyloric feeds if the patient is unable to tolerate gastric feeding or if high residuals, or to minimize risk of aspiration.

Aspiration precautions: Keep head of bed (HOB) >30–45°. If aspiration is suspected, stop tube feeds and consult speech therapy for swallow evaluation. If patient is unable to tolerate HOB elevation, you may use reverse Trendelenburg positioning.

Common pitfalls

Order sets for enteral nutrition should include patient name, formula name, enteral access device and site, as well as administration method (bolus versus continuous) and rate.

Complications of tube feeding

Delayed gastric emptying: Nausea and vomiting
Malabsorption: Gluten sensitivity, Crohn disease, enteritis, pancreatic insufficiency, short gut syndrome

Transition to oral feedings

- Transition when swallowing evaluation is successful.
- Give supplemental tube feeds to provide 50% caloric/protein needs.
- Adjust tube feeds per oral intake.
- Discontinue supplemental tube feeds when oral intake >60%–70% of goal, normal prealbumin, and weight is stable.
- Place back on 24-hour tube feeds if intake is <70% goal, patient has declining prealbumin or weight loss.

Common pitfalls and medicolegal concerns

The patient's tube feed residual is >250: Stop the tube feeds for 2 hours and recheck residuals. If still >150, administer a promotility agent and hold the tube feeds for 2 additional hours. Restart tube feeds when residuals <150 mL. Remember that the stomach is a reservoir, so a certain amount of residual is still acceptable.

A gastric or postpyloric feeding tube has been placed: Check radiograph for placement; ask the nurse to mark the entry point in the mouth or nose prior to imaging.

The feeding tube was dislodged (patient pulled, fell out), do I need to recheck an x-ray? You may also confirm placement by checking for gastric pH (between 1 and 3). Nurses also commonly inject a small amount of air into the tube and listen for the air bubble over the stomach, but radiography remains the only reliable method of confirming adequate placement in the stomach or duodenum.

Types of tube feeding

- There are over 200 types of enteral feeding formulas. They are a combination of carbohydrates, fiber, fat, protein, vitamins and minerals, electrolytes, and water.

The following are examples of commonly used tube feeding formulas:

Polymeric (Jevity): Used for patients with normal to near-normal GI function
Monomeric (Perative, Optimental): Predigested nutrients—Low-fat or high medium-chain triglycerides for patients with severely impaired GI function

Disease specific (Nepro, Glucerna): Available for patients with pulmonary disease, diabetes, and renal/hepatic failure, and for those who are immunocompromised.

Parenteral-IV solution example: Total parenteral nutrition (TPN) or peripheral parenteral nutrition (PPN)

Enteral feeding is preferred over parenteral nutrition (McClave et al., 2009, p. 279).

When TPN is required, it is a hypertonic liquid mixture given into the blood intravenously and containing over 40 chemicals and all the protein, carbohydrates, fat, vitamins, minerals, and other nutrients needed by the body. The bag is made in the pharmacy, and the order needs to be written daily based on labs and fluid status.

Indications for parenteral nutrition

Failed enteral nutrition trial with postpyloric feeding.
Malnourished patient unable to eat enterally by postoperative day 10–14.
Severe GI dysfunction such as paralytic ileus, mesenteric ischemia, small bowel obstruction, fistula, or extensive abdominal surgery.

Administration and monitoring

TPN must be given through a central line, for example, peripherally inserted central catheter (PICC), surgical port, jugular, or subclavian.
PPN may be given through a peripheral intravenous catheter.
Daily electrolytes are used to adjust/modify TPN/PPN additives, Accu-Chek glucose q 6 hours, triglycerides within 24 hours of initiation, liver function weekly, prealbumin weekly, and acid-base balance.

Complications/Considerations

Complications (common) include: Hepatic steatosis, cholestasis, gastrointestinal atrophy, line sepsis
Considerations: Cost of TPN is >$1000/day, tube feeding costs $10–$20/day, tube feeding preserves intestinal function

Special considerations

Head injury/Traumatic brain injury (TBI)

Excessive free water can disrupt sodium balance in the central nervous system–injured patient who is already at risk of sodium imbalance issues.

Neuromuscular blockade can cause a 4%–5% decrease in caloric need by Harris-Benedict equation (McCall et al., 2003, p. 27). Barbiturate coma for refractory intracranial hypertension also decreases energy expenditure (Dempsey et al., 1985, p. 128).

Hypothermia (as long as shivering is prevented) will decrease the resting metabolic rate (Bardutzky et al., 2004, p. 153).

Swallowing difficulty will be experienced by 61% of patients with TBI (Mackay et al., 1999, p. 365).

Phenytoin suspension used to treat or prevent seizures is less effective when given with enteral tube feeds as compared to patients who swallow it. The exact reason for the interaction and decreased absorption is unknown. Hold enteral feeds 1 hour before and 1 hour after administration of phenytoin suspension.

Common pitfall

Propofol is prepared as a 10% lipid emulsion. The caloric content 1.1 kcal/mL of the propofol emulsifier must be considered to avoid overfeeding.

Conclusion

Relevance to the advanced practice health professional

Nutrition is integral to optimal neuroscience patient outcomes. Assessing for nutritional deficits; evaluating an ideal means for receiving nutrition; providing adequate nutrition; and monitoring response constitutes a collaborative effort between the advanced practice health professional, the bedside nurses, and the nutritionist.

References

Bardutzky J, Dimitrios G, Kollmar R, Schwab S. Energy expenditure in ischemic stroke patients treated with moderate hypothermia. *Intensive Care Med.* 2004;30:151–154.

Barker LA, Gout BS, Crowe TC. Hospital malnutrition: prevalence, identification and impact on patients and the healthcare system. *Int J Environ Res Public Health.* 2011;8(2):514–527.

Collier B, Cherry-Bukowec J, Mills ME. Trauma, surgery, and burns. In: Mueller C, ed. *Adult Nutritional Support Core Curriculum.* 2nd ed. Silver Spring, MD: ASPEN; 2012:392–411.

Dempsey DT, Guenter PA, Mullen JL, et al. Energy expenditure in acute trauma to the head with and without barbiturate therapy. *Surg Gynecol Obstet.* 1985;160(2):128–134.

Goldwasser P, Feldman J. Association of serum albumin and mortality risk. *J Clinic Epidemiol.* 1997;50(6):693–703.

Haugen HA, Chan L-N, Li F. Indirect calorimetry: a practical guide for clinicians. *Nutr Clin Pract.* 2007;22:377–388.

Hill GL. Implications of critical illness, injury, and sepsis on lean body mass and nutritional needs. *Nutrition.* 1998;14(6):557–558.

Jeffery KM, Harkins B, Cresci GA, Martindale RG. The clear liquid diet is no longer a necessity in the routine postoperative management of surgical patients. *Am J Surg.* 1996;62(3):167–170.

Kinney JM, Weissman C. Forms of malnutrition in stressed and unstressed patients. *Clin Chest Med.* 1986;7(1):19.

MacKay D, Miller AL. Nutritional support for wound healing. *Altern Med Rev.* 2003;8(4):359–377.

Mackay LE, Morgan AS, Bernstein BA. Swallowing disorders in severe brain injury: risk factors affecting return to oral intake. *Arch Phys Med Rehabil.* 1999;80:365–371.

Mainous MR, Deitch EA. Nutrition and infection. *Surg Clin North Am.* 1994;74:659.

Marik PE, Zaloga G. Early enteral nutrition in acutely ill patients: a systemic review. *Crit Care Med.* 2001;29(12):2264–2270.

McCall M, Jeejeebhoy K, Pencharz P, Moulton R. Effect of neuromuscular blockade on energy expenditure in patients with severe head injury. *J Parenter Enteral Nutr.* 2003;27(1):27–35.

McClave SA, Martindale RG, Vanek VW. Guidelines for the provision and assessment of nutrition support therapy in the adult critically ill patient. *J Parenter Enteral Nutr.* 2009;33(3):277–316.

Mueller C, Compher C, Druyan ME. American Society for Parenteral and Enteral Nutrition ASPEN clinical guidelines nutrition screening, assessment, and intervention in adults. *J Parenter Enteral Nutr.* 2011;35:16–24.

Parrish CR. Enteral feedings: the art and science. *Nutr Clin Pract.* 2003;18:76–85.

Perel P, Yanagawa T, Bunn F, Roberts IG, Wentz R. Nutritional support for head-injured patients. *Cochran Database Syst Rev.* 2006;4:CD001530.

Santos JI. Nutrition, infection, and immunocompetence. *Infect Dis Clin North Am.* 1994;8(1):243.

Seres DS. Surrogate nutrition markers, malnutrition, and adequacy of nutrition support. *Nutr Clin Pract.* 2005;20(3):308.

Sinno S, Deok-Soon L, Khachemoune A. Vitamins and cutaneous wound healing. *J Wound Care.* 2011;20(6):287–293.

Ukleja A, Freeman KL, Gilbert K, et al. Shuster. Standards for nutrition support: adult hospitalized patients. *Nutr Clin Pract.* 2010;25:403–414.

van Stijn MF, Korkic-Halilovic I, Bakker MS, van der Ploeg T, van Leeuwen PAM, Houdijk APJ. Preoperative nutrition status and postoperative outcome in elderly general surgery patients: a systematic review. *J Parenter Enteral Nutr.* 2013;37:37.

White JV, Guenter P, Jensen G, Malone A, Schofield M and Academy Malnutrition Work Group, A.S.P.E.N. Malnutrition Task Force, A.S.P.E.N. Board of Directors. Consensus statement: Academy of Nutrition and Dietetics and American Society for Parenteral and Enteral Nutrition: characteristics recommended for the identification and documentation of adult malnutrition (undernutrition). *J Parenter Enteral Nutr.* 2012;36(3):275–283.

Wooley JA, Frankenfield D. Energy. In: Mueller C, et al. (ed). *Adult Nutrition Support Core Curriculum.* 2nd ed. American Society of Parenteral and Enteral Nutrition: Maryland Silver Springs, MD: ASPEN; 2012, pp. 22–35.

Wright WL. Nutrition. In: Bhardwaj A, Mirski MM, Ulatowski JA, eds. *Handbook of Neurocritical Care.* Totowa, NJ: Humana Press; 2004:273–294.

18

SOCIAL SERVICES AND CASE MANAGEMENT

John Kenneally

Introduction

Patient and family centered care is at the heart of the social worker and case manager roles. Each with a unique perspective, the social worker provides counsel and guides patients as well as caregivers through the challenges of neurological illness and neurosurgical interventions. A case manager answers practical questions such as insurance coverage for a skilled nursing facility or options for home health. Both are experts in local, state, and federal resources available to the ill and injured. As collaborative members of the discharge team, they are patient-centered liaisons in a complicated health-care environment. They assist with transitions in care planning, are patient advocates, and act as liaisons to the interdisciplinary team discharge.

The social worker

Neuroscience social workers are educated at a master's degree level and are certified or licensed by the state in which they are employed. After completing an initial psychosocial assessment, the social worker utilizes the information to counsel and guide the patient/caregivers. The following are examples:

- Advocate on the patient's/caregivers' behalf to sensitize the treatment team as to the social and emotional impact of illness in this particular situation.
- Lead discussions of discharge options. Provide information and then referrals to rehabilitation facilities, outpatient rehabilitation clinics, or home health agencies.
- Identify and link to community resources such as senior centers, meal sites, home care providers, support groups, and mental health services (Craig et al., 2015, p. 430).
- Provide assistance to both the medical team and patient/caregivers during goals-of-care discussions.
- Initiate ethics consultations in difficult scenarios.
- Assist with disability and insurance issues. This may include coordinating a new Social Security disability application, completing an employer's short-term disability paperwork, and assisting in obtaining health insurance for the uninsured.
- Provide short-term counseling or crisis intervention, working in conjunction with mental health or spiritual care professionals.
- Contact law enforcement and local human services agency in either suspected or documented abuse or neglect cases.

Advance medical directives

Critical to the role of the social worker is verification of advance medical directives (health care power of attorney [HCPOA] or living will). If the patient has not completed a HCPOA, the importance of the document is explained (Umansky et al., 2011, p. 2). Assuming the patient is willing, assist with document completion and appropriate filing in the health record.

In some states, once the HCPOA is completed, the designated agent can make medical decisions for the patient. In other states, prior to the designated agent making decisions on the patient's behalf, the document is activated ("springing" the document) via physician or psychologist determination, documenting the patient's incapacity.

Medical decision-making capacity (capacity versus incapacity)

Formal determination of incapacity occurs through documentation by members of the treatment team. Dependent on the requirements of statutes, this could be the patient's primary care physician, psychiatrist, or geriatrician. At baseline, a patient should be able to incorporate informed consent into their decision-making process. Absent the ability to understand informed consent, a patient is usually determined to be incapacitated.

Should a patient not have the capacity to make medical decisions, the social worker can verify the existence of a guardian or assist in petitioning for a guardian if necessary, coordinating the necessary legal documentation from the medical team to be submitted to the court system.

The case manager

Ideally, registered nurses fulfill the case management role. Neuroscience case managers provide patient admission assessment, coordinate care, and serve as liaisons between the hospital and insurance payer (Thomas, 2008, p. 62).

Examples of a case manager's role include the following:

- Provide ongoing documentation to insurance payers.
- Assist in identifying options and services to meet an individual's and family's comprehensive health needs.
- Initiate communication with other case managers involved in the patient's care (i.e., community resources, insurance provider).
- Convey medical justification for the patient's hospital stay to the insurance provider.
- Clear and detailed communication from the medical team through chart documentation is imperative for the case manager to support the need for the patient's continued inpatient stay or discharge needs.
- Ensure satisfactory patient discharge outcomes for health-care facilities, in a cost-effective manner.
- Collaborate with the interprofessional team to coordinate discharge planning and identify patient status (inpatient, observation, outpatient short stay) as this relates to hospital reimbursement and discharge planning. This collaboration also works to identify readmission trends for patients, working to anticipate patient and caregiver needs. Identifying these trends (i.e., inability to obtain medications, adequate home support, posthospital follow-up) will decrease future readmission rates (Thomas, 2008).

Working together throughout the patient experience

Together the social worker and case manager will work with the advanced practice health professional as the patient and family move through the continuum of care (Shepperd et al., 2013, p. 2).

Home and outpatient

The social worker and case manager work in conjunction with the interdisciplinary team to develop an understanding of the patient's and caregiver's home situation. Understanding the type of home, the ability to navigate, who is able to provide meals, transportation, supervision, and hands-on care are critical to developing a discharge plan. Identifying and connecting with established community resources (home health, social service agencies, outpatient therapy services) may expedite discharge planning.

Planning ahead

The social worker and case manager will utilize the advanced practice health professional to clarify a patient's admission status and discharge needs (medications, outpatient therapies, clarification of discharge orders to a receiving facility). The advance practice health professional's relationship with the attending physician should enhance strong communication and planning. The patient's length of stay should meet the desired parameters, and satisfaction of stay will increase.

Common discharge planning issues

The following are patient/family issues that social workers, case managers, and advance practice health professionals can collaborate to ensure an appropriate, satisfactory, cost-effective hospital stay on the neuroscience unit.

Identify the type of patient stay (observation, inpatient, and outpatient short stay). Early, appropriate identification of the patient's admission order assists the social worker and case manager in defining the appropriate trajectory of the hospital stay. This has ramifications in insurance reimbursement and access to different outpatient resources.

Determine the existence of an advance medical directive (HCPOA, durable power of attorney, or living will) and the patient's ability to make decisions regarding his or her health care. The advance practice health professional may be able to determine the patient's ability to participate in medical decision making or assist in consulting the appropriate professional to make this determination. In the absence of an advance medical directive, the patient may already have a guardian, or a guardianship petition may need to be initiated. Rules regarding medical decision making will differ from state to state.

Initiate early verification of insurance and coverage of insurance to assist with discharge planning. This may influence the possible course of the patient's inpatient stay, options for rehab (including type and location), and medication coverage. Early identification of possible length of stay for a patient is necessary, as commercial insurance may require preauthorization of requested services at discharge; preauthorization can take 24–48 hours to complete.

If a hospital stay is planned, having a discussion with the patient and family prior to admission about anticipated length of stay and discharge needs will assist both social worker and case manager in coordinating services at the end of the hospital stay. The patient and family may be able to confirm preferred providers of services (outpatient or inpatient rehabilitation facilities). They may be able to visit these resources and identify preferences, thus allowing for a decreased length of stay, increasing greater control and satisfaction with the hospital stay.

Most importantly, establishing an understanding between patient/caregiver and care team regarding goals of care for the hospitalization is essential. This discussion is fluid, taking place prior to hospitalization for elective stays and during the inpatient stay.

Communication is the key

The roles of the social worker and case manager may appear to blend. However, each professional has distinct skills and responsibilities. Working collaboratively, each is often able to step in for the other to address patient needs. The most important skill utilized by both roles is effective communication. Whether it is through chart documentation or daily rounding, consistent and clear communication among the entire interprofessional team is crucial to accurately assessing a patient's progress toward discharge goals as well as the ongoing patient and family treatment plan and progress toward discharge goals communication.

References

Craig SL, Betancourt I, Muskat B. Thinking big, supporting families and enabling coping: the value of social work in patient and family centered health care. *Soc Work Health Care*. 2015;54:422–443. doi:10.1080/00981389.2015.1017074.

Shepperd S, Lannin NA, Clemson LM, McClusky A, Cameron ID, Barras SL. Discharge planning from hospital to home. *Cochrane Database Syst Rev*. 2013;(1):CD000313. doi:10.1002/14651858.CD000313.pub4.

Thomas PL. Case manager role definitions: do they make an organizational impact? *Prof Case Manag*. 2008;13:61–71.

Umansky F, Balck PL, DiRocco C, et al. Statement of ethics in neurosurgery of the World Federation of Neurosurgical Societies. *World Neurosurg*. 2011;76:239–247.

19

COORDINATING AND PREPARING FOR THE TRANSITION FROM THE ACUTE CARE SETTING

Andrea L. Strayer and Gregory R. Trost

Every patient leaves the hospital. Preparing for discharge begins prior to planned admissions and on presentation to the hospital for unplanned admissions. Professional team members collaborate, guiding the patient/caregiver through the hospitalization to transition. Leading the collaborative effort, communication among (often many) providers and the patient/caregiver is a vital role of the advanced practice provider (APP).

Discharge planning starts in the outpatient setting

Elective admission discharge or transition planning ideally starts as an outpatient, at the time the decision for surgery or a necessary medical admission is made. Managing patient/caregiver expectations will lead to a more positive perioperative experience. Counseling with the patient/caregiver includes discussing perioperative/recovery expectations; securing necessary postoperative recovery assistance/resources; if necessary, screening potential skilled nursing facilities (SNFs) for subacute rehabilitation; and completing/filing a health-care power of attorney.

A frank discussion of postoperative expectations includes the patient/caregiver verbalizing a clear understanding of the goals of the operative intervention, patient experience during the hospitalization, and anticipated recovery details. Specific topics for discussion include the following: perioperative routines/nursing care/therapies; how much pain is expected; pain management in the hospital and postdischarge; goals for discharge—voiding, flatus, adequate oral intake, mobilization, and pain management; expected length of stay; and care needs following discharge.

Anticipating postdischarge care needs will aid in a smooth transition. It is the patients' responsibility to plan ahead and secure recovery help. No longer are hospitals or insurance companies compensating for those who are medically ready for discharge and have not planned for necessary assistance. Guidance includes the following: Will the patient require 24/7 help? If so, for how long? If not, how much intermittent help will be needed? What if the patient lives alone? What will the patient's restrictions be? Work? Driving? How will this affect children, pets, or adults/other family they provide care for?

For those with rehabilitation goals after surgery (often older or with more extensive surgery), subacute rehabilitation in a SNF may be an ideal option. Discuss with the patient his or her social situation, and if this seems to be a likely option, please ask the patient to provide his or her top choices. While a SNF cannot "pre-admit" a patient prior to surgery, communication by the patient/caregiver with potential SNFs, will expedite the transition out of the hospital.

Often overlooked is the importance of a health-care power of attorney on file. No matter the diagnosis, every person 18 years or older should complete this document. Please refer to Chapter 18, "Social Services and Case Management."

Interprofessional team

Interprofessional team members gather daily to discuss each patient's progress toward discharge goals. Models include sitting as a group with patient/caregiver communication in a separate interaction, as well as "walking rounds" where the patient/caregiver is present. Professionals present their perspectives on progress as well as their opinions regarding transition disposition (home, SNF, inpatient rehab, etc.) that is safe and will provide the patient with the best opportunity for an optimal long-term outcome. In neuroscience acute care, team members are likely to consist of physical/occupational/speech/swallow therapy, social services/case management, pharmacy, nursing, nutrition, in some settings spiritual care or palliative care, and the medical/surgical team representative. For older adults with medical conditions, a discharge plan unique to the individual likely results in reductions in the hospital length of stay (LOS) and readmission rate (Shepperd et al., 2013, p. 1). An APP is an excellent representative for this venue. As a liaison with the medical/surgical attending physician, the APP offers a holistic and global view of the patient and the patient's unique situation. While group discussion regarding challenging patient transitions is of utmost importance, ultimately, the patient is under the attending physician's care.

Discharge disposition options

Neuroscience patient transition options include home, assisted living, SNF, inpatient rehabilitation (IR), and long-term acute care hospital (LTACH). The services provided vary, especially in an assisted living or SNF setting. A member of the team, often the case manager, will be in contact with the facility to confirm services. Following lumbar laminectomy, a retrospective review demonstrated 14.8% discharged to either IR/SNF and 67.3% discharged to home. Factors influencing discharge to IR/SNF included those who live alone, walked a shorter distance during their hospital stay, had poorer balance scores, and were less functional both prior to surgery and during hospitalization (Kanaan et al., 2014, p. 1). Therapists involved in the patient's care often have insight into ideal discharge disposition. However, it is crucial that the patient and caregiver be active participants in communication throughout the hospital stay regarding these options.

Communication

Health care is complex. Often overwhelmed, patients and caregivers require consistent communication for the transition from acute care (Lee and Hohler, 2014). Whiteboards in the room to communicate the attending physician name, reason for admission, plan of care, and anticipated discharge date were found to be very successful with statistically significant increase in all measures expect plan of care. Additionally noted was an increase in patient satisfaction with his or her overall hospital stay (Tan et al., 2013). Coordinating a smooth transition also involves communication with the receiving primary care and specialty providers.

Written communication via the discharge orders and summary provides a reference document; however, there is no substitute for a verbal handoff. Speaking with the provider or someone on the provider's team, such as support registered nurse/medical assistant, will alert of the inpatient stay, will alert to problems requiring follow-up, and will decrease lack of communication issues. Other professionals such as home health and outpatient therapists often receive communication on your behalf through the case manager.

Optimizing the transition

The actual transition (discharge) should be a well thought-out, consistent process. Key steps to assure safety are medication reconciliation, specific discharge instructions/orders, and patient/caregiver verbal and written communication. Therapists and case managers generally coordinate medical equipment needs. As discussed previously, communication with outside facilities and specialists completes the transition.

Medication reconciliation

Adverse drug events during transitions of care are often preventable. Medication reconciliation entails systematically reviewing each patient's medications carefully, resolving discrepancies, assessing for potential drug interactions, discontinuing unindicated medications, and thoughtfully assessing and problem-solving issues such as compliance due to cost or regimen. The patient and caregiver are involved and educated fully (U.S. Department of Health and Human Services, 2014).

Readmission avoidance

Surgical complications from cerebrospinal fluid (CSF) shunts, CSF leaks, and surgical site infections were noted to be the major reasons for 30-day neurosurgery readmissions over a 3-year period (Buchanan et al., 2014). Surgical site infection and wound complications accounted for 72% of all readmissions for common lumbar pathologies over a 90-day period; overall readmissions were 3.3% over 90 days (Akamnonu et al., 2015). However, brain tumor readmissions were noted to be 7.5%, within 30 days. The top three causes of readmission were neurological, infection, and venous thromboembolism (VTE). The authors' assessment was that 70.4% were preventable. Higher-functioning patients and patients discharged home were less likely to get readmitted (Dickinson et al., 2015). Ischemic stroke patients were noted to have an 18.8% readmission rate in the first 90 days in Norway. Early readmissions appeared to be related to infections, a recurrent ischemic stroke, or another cardiovascular event (Bjerkreim et al., 2015).

Opportunities to decrease a 14.4% readmission rate have been described as printed discharge instructions with a 24-hour contact number and common postoperative problems reviewed; nursing to complete "teach-back" with discharge instructions; a follow-up call in 24–48 hours postdischarge; and a follow-up appointment scheduled prior to discharge. Patients with postoperative problems are preferably seen in clinic on an urgent basis and are not referred to the emergency department (Vaziri et al., 2014).

Common pitfalls

- Making assumptions, lacking data
- Not knowing your team members, including the registered nurses
- Not being knowledgeable about your patient's clinical and psychosocial status
- Having inaccurate orders/summary or orders/summary that say nothing helpful
- Not communicating

Common pages

The social worker calls you: "I have an SNF that can take your patient today, can the patient go?"

Decision making

Has the patient met his or her discharge goals?
Is this a safe transition?
What are the chances of a readmission or poor transition?
Has the patient/family been involved in the decision making? Will this be a surprise?

The registered nurse calls, "Your patient thought (no preoperative teaching provided) they could go home alone after surgery—but they are taking oxycodone 10 mg every 3 hours, can't get their brace off/on, and need at least one person and a walker for mobilizing—what should we do?"

Decision making

> The patient will need therapy goals for SNF placement for subacute rehabilitation, if that is most appropriate.
> Assess if the patient is safe to go home. If not, explain the advantages of subacute rehabilitation.
> Ask the social worker/case manager to meet with the patient and assess insurance coverage.
> Evaluate pain management options. Oxycodone every 3 hours is not a safe plan for discharge.
> Encourage mobilization.

The interprofessional team updates you on a patient who has been in the neurosurgery intensive care unit for 23 days and is ready to transition to general care. The patient suffered a subarachnoid hemorrhage, currently has a tracheostomy (has not started downsizing) and a percutaneous endoscopic gastrostomy (PEG) tube for nutrition. The patient is making slow functional progress; however, their insurance has a maximum of 21 acute rehabilitation days. What is your counsel to their family?

Decision making

While there is no "good" answer, the best may be to save the 21 rehabilitation days until the patient can fully participate, receiving the very most benefit. The recommendation would be an LTACH setting for tracheostomy weaning, therapies, and increased endurance—in the hopes of transitioning to acute rehabilitation.

Every patient leaves the hospital. Planning and coordinating patient transitions of care is an ongoing process, unique for each patient and his or her caregiver. Implementing processes to assure counseling/ education are provided, the importance of the specialization of neuroscience interprofessional team members, and ongoing communication will break down a complex health-care event to a positive experience for the patient and his or her caregiver.

References

Akamnonu C, Cheriyan T, Goldstein JA, Lafage V, Errico TJ, Bendo JA. Unplanned hospital readmission after surgical treatment of common lumbar pathologies. *Spine.* 2015;40:423–428.

Bjerkreim AT, Thomassen L, Brogger J, Waje-Andreassen U, Naess H. Causes and predictors for hospital readmission after ischemic stroke. *J Stroke Cerebrovasc Dis.* 2016; 25(1):157–162.

Buchanan CC, Hernandez EA, Anderson JM, et al. Analysis of 30-day readmissions among neurosurgical patients: Surgical complication avoidance as key to quality improvement. *J Neurosurg.* 2014;121:170–175.

Dickinson H, Carico C, Nuno M, et al. Unplanned readmissions and survival following brain tumor surgery. *J Neurosurg.* 2015;122:61–68.

Kanaan S, Yeh H-W, Waitman R, Burton D, Arnold P, Sharma N. Predicting discharge placement and health care needs after lumbar spine laminectomy. *J Allied Health.* 2014;43:88–97.

Lee J, Hohler A. Communication challenges in complex medical environments. *Continuum (Minneap Minn).* 2014;20:686–689.

Shepperd S, Lannin NA, Clemson LM, McCluskey A, Cameron ID, Barras SL. Discharge planning from hospital to home (Review). *Cochrane Database Syst Rev.* 2013; (1): Article ID: CD000313.

Tan M, Hooper Evans K, Braddock CH III, Shieh L. Patient whiteboards to improve patient-centered care in the hospital. *Postgrad Med J.* 2013;89:604–609.

U.S. Department of Health and Human Services, Office of Disease Prevention and Health Promotion. *National Action Plan for Adverse Drug Event Prevention.* Washington, DC: Author; 2014.

Vaziri S, Bridger Cox J, Friedman WA. Readmissions in neurosurgery: A qualitative inquiry. *World Neurosurg.* 2014;82:376–379.

20
ADAPTIVE EQUIPMENT

Amy Wang and Alison Kirkpatrick

Occupational, physical, and speech therapists each assess a patient's specific needs to maximize independence and safety, making adaptive equipment recommendations. Adaptive equipment can be defined as devices utilized by individuals with physical impairments in activities of daily living (ADLs). Therapists also train and educate patients and their caregivers in the use of this adaptive equipment. In general, adaptive equipment falls into the categories discussed in the following sections.

Mobility devices

These are items utilized by an individual to enhance locomotion or provide transportation. This may include canes (single-point cane, quad cane, hemi-walkers), walkers (pick-up frame, rolling walkers, rollators, two-wheeled walkers, three-wheeled walkers, four-wheeled walkers, and walkers with a seat), crutches (axillar and Lofstrand/Canadian crutches), wheelchairs (manual and powered mobility and appropriate pressure-relieving cushions for positioning in a wheelchair), and prosthetic devices (artificial devices used to replace a missing body part as a result of birth defect, disease, or accident) (Figure 20.1).

Transfer equipment

Transfer equipment includes sliding boards, Hoyer lifts, gait belts, sit-stand lift devices, and trapezes (for pulling upright in bed). A tub/shower chair can be placed in a tub or shower to provide a seat for bathing. A tub transfer bench extends out of the tub for individuals with a weak lower extremity. (For example, a patient with paraplegia may transfer directly from his or her wheelchair to a bath bench to be able to sit for showering.)

Fall management

Examples of items used for patient safety, especially those with cognitive impairments, include fall alarms and wander alert systems, wall supports, bed side rails, and grab rails.

Specialty beds

A variety of options are available for control of positioning, use of support rails, and need for pressure relief:

Gatch bed—Has three cranks to raise and lower the bed
Electric bed—Patients are able to adjust the bed themselves
Low beds—Set about 8 inches from the ground to prevent harm from falls
Low air loss beds—For burn patients or circulatory/ulcer issues
Circo-electric bed—Rotates for spinal cord or burn patients who cannot be moved
Clinitron bed—Dry, warm air circulates to maintain skin integrity

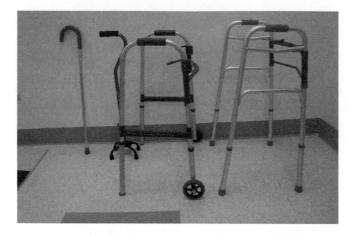

Figure 20.1 Single-point cane, quad cane, rolling walker, and standard walker.

Self-care devices for activities of daily living

Eating

Self-feeding can be a difficult task for those with quadriplegia, central cord syndrome, stroke, multiple sclerosis, or any other disability affecting the upper extremities.

Examples of tools to assist in self-feeding include long-handled utensils, long straws, nonskid bowls, mobile arm supports, plate guards, scoop dishes, weighted cups, universal cuffs, and rocker knives.

Grooming

Activities include tooth brushing, shaving, hair care, and makeup application.

Examples of tools to assist in grooming include one-handed denture brushes, adaptive shaving devices, special grips for toothbrushes, wash mitts, long-handled brushes, and universal cuffs.

Dressing

Dressing involves donning and doffing clothing from the upper and lower extremities. Patients have to be assessed for proper safety, balance, and strength. This may determine where the proper location for dressing should occur. For example, if a patient has weak trunk control such as higher-level paraplegia, the patient may need to perform tasks from a supported sitting/bed level. Shoe horns, sock aids, reachers, dressing sticks, and button hooks may be helpful. (Figure 20.2).

Helpful hints to provide to patients include utilizing Velcro or snaps instead of buttons and altering zippers by adding a pull made of fishing line or a key ring for those with weak hand musculature (such as C7 quadriplegia).

Bathing

Bathing is the process of maintaining self-cleanliness and can be modified based on the patient's physical status. The act can range from bed baths to special Hoyer lifts into modified bath areas. Items such as a bath mitt, long-handled sponge, handheld shower hose, tub benches and chairs, and grab bars may be used. Understanding the person's deficits is key to recommending products. For instance, if someone has temperature sensory loss, he or she may need a thermometer or a change in water temperature setting to prevent scalding of the skin.

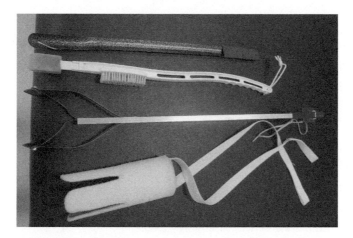

Figure 20.2 Top to bottom: Shoe horn, long-handled sponge, reacher, and sock aid.

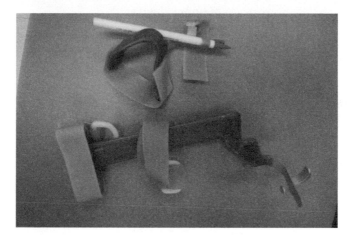

Figure 20.3 Writing aides to assist patients with limited hand strength.

Toileting

This involves the pulling down of clothing to allow bowel or bladder elimination, hygiene of the perineal area, and pulling up of clothin. Adaptive equipment may include bedside commode, bedpan, self-wiping aid, and the use of catheters.

Household tasks

Some simple adaptive equipment options that may assist a patient with increased participation in household tasks could include a jar opener, key holders, reachers/grabbers, and doorknob extenders.

Leisure activities

There is also a wide variety of adaptive equipment options for increased participation in leisure activities and adaptive sports from low-tech to high-tech devices. Examples include items such as card holders, book holders, and grasping cuffs (for pool sticks, bowling ball ramps, etc.). An occupational therapist, physical therapist, or recreation therapist may help a patient explore these options (Figure 20.3).

Communication devices

Augmentative and alternative communication (AAC) devices

Recommended by speech therapists, AAC devices may include electronic communication devices where an electronic voice is generated from a computerized input system, as well as communication or picture boards.

Braille

Braille is a system of raised bumps that allow a visually impaired person to read.

Hearing aids

These allow people with hearing deficits to amplify sound.

Memory devices

Multiple computerized apps exist, including calendars with reminders.

Assistive technology

This type of technology includes environmental control units (ECUs) and computer access devices (touch-screens, joysticks, head control, eye tracking, use of electrical muscle stimulation [EMS], etc.).

Other common rehabilitation equipment

Orthotic, Protective, and Supportive Devices

Cervical

Halo—Circular band of metal fixed to the skull
Philadelphia collar—Plastic collar that supports the chin and head
Soft foam—Minor motion control
Miami-J collar—Has a thoracic extension and a hole for the trachea
Thomas-type collar—Made from vinyl plastic and has ventilation
Aspen collar—Inner padding is breathable, has hole for trachea

Back

Thoracolumbosacral orthosis (TLSO)—Fitted to torso
Cervicothoracolumbosacral orthosis (Milwaukee brace)
Charleston Bending Brace—Worn while sleeping

Shoulder

Acromioclavicular separation splint—For AC separation
Hemiplegia sling—Post-cerebrovascular accident to prevent glenohumeral subluxation

Elbow

Elbow hinge for fracture bracing, contractures, and tendon/nerve repairs

Wrist

Static resting splint
Carpal tunnel splints

Knee

Cho-Pat rubber strap for patellofemoral tendon
Controlled motion knee brace
Palumbo patellar stabilization brace

Ankle

Ankle-foot orthosis (AFO)—Compensates for weak lower extremity muscles

Miscellaneous

Compression garments—For vascular support and pain management
Helmet—Orthotic device often recommended for use during any out-of-bed activity for a patient
who has had a bone flap removed from his or her skull
Passy-Muir Valve—A prosthetic device consisting of a one-way valve that is placed on the hub of a
tracheostomy tube to allow for inspiration and supports

Modalities

Biofeedback
Hot/cold therapy
Electrotherapy/ultrasound
Hydrotherapy
Portable electrotherapy
Paraffin therapy
Iontophoresis

Rehabilitation supplies

Items such as weights, balls, pulleys, TheraPutty, exercise bands, and tubing are utilized to regain strength
for functional recovery (Figure 20.4).

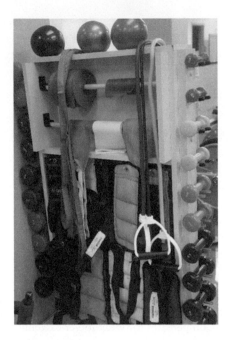

Figure 20.4 Rehabilitation supplies such as weights.

The lists of adaptive equipment and companies that provide the equipment are extensive and ever changing. Here are a few companies that can provide information on appropriate devices:

- www.thewright-stuff.com
- www.agingcare.com
- www.alimed.com
- www.pattersonmedical.com
- www.ncmedical.com

21

SHORT- AND LONG-TERM DISABILITY

Sandra Stafford

The rehabilitation journey after neurological insult can be an arduous and frustrating process for both patients and their families. Cognitive, behavioral, and physical changes can become life-altering events, and successful recovery is dependent on multiple variables including degree of injury, prior level of health and functioning, early goal-directed therapies, and family/social support systems. This chapter explores short- and long-term disabilities and best practices for return to maximal functional independence.

Case study

JS is a 24-year-old active duty Army corporal injured in Afghanistan when an improvised explosive device detonated under the Humvee in which he and three other soldiers were riding. JS was the sole survivor. He sustained bilateral subdural hematomas and multiple lower extremity fractures. Upon extrication, tonic-clonic seizures were noted with positive loss of consciousness. Initial Glasgow Coma Scale (GCS) score was 3. JS received an emergent tracheostomy in the field and was then stabilized for transport to a nearby Army medical facility. There he underwent a suboccipital craniotomy and hematoma evacuation on the right and multiple open reduction and internal fixation (ORIF) procedures for right ankle, tibial, and femur fractures. JS also received a percutaneous gastrostomy tube for feeding. As he was weaned off the ventilator, JS began to exhibit behaviors consistent with Rancho Three level functioning on the Rancho Levels of Cognitive Functioning scale, a 10-level rating scale developed by the Rancho Los Amigos National Rehabilitation Center to assess individuals after a closed head injury, based on cognitive and behavioral presentations as they emerge from coma (Hillegass, 2009, p. 151). JS would blink in response to strong light, turn to the sound of his name being called, and grimace in response to physical discomfort. Physical, occupational, and speech therapy were initiated, and he would inconsistently respond to commands, even occasionally smiling. The family remained hopeful for a complete recovery.

On postoperative day 10, JS's behavior changed. He became agitated and aggressive, striking out at staff during therapy or care, and attempting to pull at both his tracheostomy and gastrostomy tubes. He required scheduled and as-needed sedation and 24-hour constant observation at bedside. The family became frustrated when their efforts to calm JS were unsuccessful. The staff continued to provide education on the course of traumatic brain injury (TBI) recovery, and family therapists were involved to provide additional support. On day 16, JS self-decannulated and the decision was made to not re-insert the tracheostomy tube. His trach site was covered, and speech therapy focused on increased vocalization. JS gradually began to participate in social conversation, but his verbalizations were often inappropriate. His attention span improved, and he became more oriented, although he remained amnesic to the blast event. On day 21, JS passed a swallowing evaluation, and PO trials were begun.

Short-term disability

Neurological insult, of which TBI is a component, can have profound effects for individuals and their families. According to the Brain Trauma Foundation, TBI is the leading cause of death and disability in Americans aged 1–44 years of age. It also accounts for at least 5.3 million people (2% of the U.S. population) currently living with disabilities (Brain Trauma Foundation, 2015). In the short term, focus is placed on prevention of medical complications from immobility, skin breakdown, and alteration in nutritional status. Medical management may also include adequate pain control; patient safety measures if the patient is impulsive, perseverative, or lacks safety judgement; and family education on the usual course of brain injury recovery.

- Loss of functional mobility can place the patient at risk for deep vein thrombosis (DVT). The neurological injuries sustained by this patient place him at high risk for complications caused by immobility, such as thrombosis, contractures, and muscular atrophy. Orthopedic fractures and subsequent non-weight-bearing precautions require primary prevention and early risk reduction. Anticoagulation medications including low molecular weight heparin injections should be initiated in the immediate postoperative period (may need to delay initiation until after removal of external ventricular drain) to prevent the formation of lower extremity DVT.
- Sequential compression devices (SCDs) should also be ordered to limit the development of DVT and peripheral edema in immobile patients (Morris and Woodcock, 2004). An SCD, also known as a lymphedema pump, consists of an air pump connected to a disposable sleeve by a series of air tubes. The sleeve is placed around the patient's leg. Air is then forced into different parts of the sleeve in sequence, creating pressure around the calves and improving venous return.
- Pressure-relieving ankle-foot orthosis (PRAFO) splints/boots may also be indicated to prevent equinovarus contractures (Farmer and James, 2001).
- A physical therapy consult for passive range of motion and muscle activation can help to preserve circulation and prevent additional contractures even in the critical care setting, and as the patient's medical stability increases, continued physical therapy will improve the strength, balance, and coordination required for neuromuscular reeducation.

Common pitfalls

Any reports of pain, redness, warmth, or edema in the lower extremities should be investigated by ultrasound to rule out DVT formation. Avoid mobilization in therapies, and halt SCD use until negative imaging results are obtained.

- *Compromised nutritional status*—Ensuring adequate caloric and protein levels is essential for wound healing, endurance, and support of regulatory functions (Barker et al., 2011). Initial management includes a nutritional assessment by a dietary consultant, which can help guide selection of gastrostomy feeding formulas to best optimize target weight. Traditional recommendations to consider include adequate hydration, strict intake and output monitoring, and supplemental fiber medications, which may be necessary to promote bowel function.

A swallowing evaluation by a trained speech-language pathologist will help determine oral motor and cognitive readiness for PO trials, while preventing aspiration pneumonia. Speech therapy may also provide staff and family with swallowing tips, such as reminding the patient to alternate sips of fluid with bites of food, swallow twice after each mouthful, use portion-control cups or utensils, and modify food or liquid textures. Nutritional supplement shakes with meals may also be considered to improve daily caloric intake.

Free water boluses may need to be calculated in 24-hour intake goals to ensure adequate hydration if the patient is tube-fed dependent. If able to tolerate oral fluids, iced liquids are generally more easily tolerated, and involving the patient and family in food and beverage choices boosts compliance.

- *Bowel and bladder control*—Independent management of elimination functions is important for the preservation of skin integrity, dignity, and social appropriateness. Placing patients on a scheduled daily or every 12-hours bowel program may help regulate function and avoid incontinence. Bisacodyl or glycerin suppositories should be considered and bowel programs timed after meals to take advantage of the gastrocolic reflux. Adding bulk fiber solutions such as HyFiber to formula feeds can help with both constipation and diarrhea, and adding non-habit-forming laxatives such as psyllium powder (nonsystemic, made from ground psyllium seed husks) may also promote regularity. Again, adequate hydration is important, and fluid intake should be measured daily. Timed voids every 2–4 hours should be initiated to prevent urinary incontinence, and placing patients in an upright position (males may prefer to stand if safe) will contribute to improved bladder emptying and less urinary leakage.

Avoid prolonged indwelling catheters and consider condom catheters. Bladder scanning after voids may be necessary to measure postvoid residuals, especially if neurogenic bladder is suspected.

Any alteration in skin integrity must be evaluated. The development of trophic ulcers (decubitus or pressure sores) over bony prominences is a potentially disabling complication that can be prevented with frequent assessments and early interventions. Because neurologically impaired patients may have decreased sensation or ability to report pain, inspect the patient's skin every 4–8 hours to assess for redness, moisture, edema, bruising, or breakdown. If possible, bathe daily and protect frequently moist skin with creams or ointment to prevent breakdown.

Plastic tubing and straps from SCDs, splints, braces, slings, PRAFO boots, and other supportive immobilization devices may cause significant skin irritation and breakdown. Order the patient's position to be changed every 2 hours and remove all devices every 1–2 hours to examine skin appearance underneath.

Case study continued

JS continued to make rehabilitation progress. His nocturnal sleep patterns improved, and although he still required rest periods in the late morning and afternoon, fatigue during treatment sessions became less of a barrier. He could follow simple directions and engage in goal-directed behavior with assistance. He began to participate more meaningfully in therapy. He had difficulty learning new tasks, but he responded to short, clear commands and frequent repetition. He would become agitated by too much stimulation, and the family was educated about reducing environmental distractions by turning off the television and computer, having only one person speaking at a time, and lowering the lights. Working with neuropsychology, JS began to recall past events but remained amnesic regarding the blast injury. Family members were encouraged to motivate JS with praise for his accomplishments and explanations for the need for continuing rehabilitation. Occupational therapy focused their efforts on helping him perform his activities of daily living (ADLs) in an independent manner. He continued to have trouble with money management, got lost easily, and worried about his ability to care for his child and return to work. He began to show signs of depression and anxiety. Four months had passed since the accident.

Long-term disability

For JS in the long term, focus is placed on cognitive functioning, recapturing lost skills, building independence in ADLs, and promoting coping strategies with a realistic plan for posthospital life.

- *Cognitive deficits*—Mental status is an overlap between affective and cognitive function (Perry and Potter, 2004, p. 1105). The return of neurological function can continue for years, although the greatest period of recovery is usually in the first three months following injury (Teasell and Hussein, 2013). Impaired memory and chronic confusion place the patient at an increased safety risk, both at home and in the community. Discharge placement may require 24-hour supervision, which is often difficult for families to provide. Continuing outpatient occupational and speech therapy for ongoing cognitive retraining and memory enhancement should be ordered.

Common pitfalls

Controversy surrounds the use of neurostimulants, such as Amantadine, for long-term use. Amantadine is a reasonable option for improving cognition and reducing agitation following a TBI, but confirmatory evidence of the efficacy of the drug is necessary. Improved alertness may be short lived and actually impair long-term neuron regrowth. Use of the drug may also increase sleep disturbances and suicidal ideation (Leone and Polsonetti, 2005).

- *Mental health issues*—As the patient gains new insight into the severity of his or her deficits, depression, anxiety, and low self-esteem may result. Feelings of hopelessness and powerlessness can lead to ineffective coping, suicidal ideation, and risk of substance abuse. Early intervention with mental health providers and frequent follow-up as an outpatient are recommended. Family counseling may help with adjustment to new roles and reduce the risk of impaired parenting and caregiver strain. Benzodiazepines are contraindicated in brain-injured patients, and other central nervous system depressants should be used with caution. Selective serotonin reuptake inhibitors, such as Citalopram and Sertraline, may be effective in the treatment of depression.

Common pitfalls

Patients should be counseled to avoid alcohol use and to refrain from driving and other activities requiring alertness, as drowsiness is a frequently reported side effect of many antidepressants.

- *Chronic pain*—Neuropathic pain can continue for months or years following neurological injury. Initial treatments may include nonsteroidal anti-inflammatory drugs, long-acting morphine, antiepileptic drugs such as gabapentin, antidepressants such as amitriptyline, physical therapy, and complementary alternative medicine options including acupuncture, biofeedback, and massage therapy.

Common pitfalls

Chronic pain may be difficult to manage in the acute setting. Consultation with a pain specialist or physiatrist may be indicated.

- *Vocational loss*—Physical, cognitive, and behavioral changes may prevent return to previous employment. This can have long-term effects on financial stability, as well as a personal loss of identity. Social workers, occupational therapists, and case managers should be consulted to help identify community resources including state, federal, or local vocational rehabilitation programs, companies with special employer incentives, apprenticeships, and volunteer work experiences. Assistance may also be necessary for returning to school and for job-seeking skills. Adaptive equipment and assistive technology should be considered, as these may provide the cognitive aids the patient needs to manage time and priorities. If unable to return to driving, training in the use of public transportation or access to free or reduced-cost shuttle services can also promote independence.

Summary

An interdisciplinary team within a dedicated rehabilitation program may provide the best outcomes for patients who have sustained neurological insult. Active therapy involvement, skilled rehabilitation nursing and medical services, intensive social work, case management, and psychological support providers can prevent and minimize short- and long-term disability. This improves the quality of life for both patients and families.

References

Barker LA, Gout BS, Crowe TC. Hospital malnutrition: prevalence, identification and impact on patients and the healthcare system. *Int J Environ Res Public Health*. February 2011;8(2):514–527. Published online February 16, 2011.

Brain Trauma Foundation. *MD News*. May/June 2015, Cleveland Edition.

Centers for Disease Control and Prevention. https://www.cdc.gov/traumaticbraininjury/index.html, May 2015.

Farmer SE, James M. Contractures in orthopaedic and neurological conditions: a review of causes and treatment. *Disabil Rehabil*. 2001;23(13):549–558.

Hillegass EZ. *Rehab Notes*. Philadelphia, PA: F.A. Davis; 2009.

Leone H, Polsonetti BW. Amantadine for traumatic brain injury: does it improve cognition and reduce agitation? *J Clin Pharm Ther*. April 2005;30(2):101–104.

Morris RJ, Woodcock JP. Evidence-based compression, prevention of stasis and deep vein thrombosis. *Ann Surg*. February 2004;239(2):162–171.

Perry A, Potter P. *Clinical Nursing Skills and Techniques*. St. Louis, MO: Mosby; 2004: 1105.

Teasell R, Hussein N. Background concepts in stroke rehabilitation. In: *Evidence-Based Review of Stroke Rehabilitation*. 2013. http://www.ebrsr.com November 2013.

22

SCIENTIFIC RESEARCH AND CLINICAL TRIALS

Lauren N. Simpson, Christina Sayama, and Khoi D. Than

Clinical trials involving neurologic disorders, particularly those requiring critical care, can be very challenging to design and interpret for many reasons. Multiple treatments or interventions are frequently required to work in concert with one another, therefore complicating determination of the effect of one treatment alone. Action often must occur in an emergent fashion, and there can be wide variation in management between practitioners. Furthermore, many patients have an impaired level of consciousness, which can complicate obtaining consent, thus creating ethical considerations. Over the past few decades, emphasis on evidence-based medicine has caused a paradigm shift in our field. While we used to rely primarily on anecdotal evidence, case reports, and retrospective clinical series, now we use a diverse plethora of study designs and statistical methods to draw conclusions depending on the clinical question. This has resulted in improvement in neurologic outcomes and substantial public health impact (Alves and Skolnick, 2006). As health-care professionals, it is our responsibility to use scientific research and clinical trials in our decision making to provide the best care for our patients and improve outcomes.

Scientific research components

Scientific research begins with developing a protocol for the research study. The study protocol typically specifies the research question and its significance, the study design, the subject selection, data collection, planned statistical analysis, and a primary hypothesis. Study protocols then may be submitted for institutional review board (IRB) approval and grant fund applications. After study implementation, the data must be collected in either a prospective or retrospective fashion depending on the type of study being conducted. After sufficient data collection is performed, data analysis ensues, and the results of the study must be interpreted with the goal of drawing inferences from the findings. Internal and external validity of the study should be considered during protocol development and readdressed during study implementation and interpretation. Internal validity refers to the extent to which the inferences drawn from a study are warranted based on the study design and implementation. A study with strong internal validity draws conclusions that accurately reflect the causal relationships being studied. External validity refers to the generalizability of the study findings. A study with strong external validity draws conclusions that can be applied to people and events outside of the study (Haines and Walters, 2006, p. 2-13). Quality research provides health-care practitioners with evidence-based medicine to help guide clinical decision making.

Research question

The objective of scientific research is to answer a question on a treatment, risk factor, causation, natural history, prognosis, clinical assessment, or diagnostic test (Haines and Walters, 2006, p. 12-13). A literature review to determine the background and relevance of that topic helps to provide context and rationale and can lead to further shaping of the scientific question and development of a hypothesis (Hulley et al., 2013, p. 2-3). The type of clinical question being asked will largely determine the most appropriate study design.

Study designs

1. A *case report* is a study that describes a subject's exposures, characteristics, presentation, and the clinical course. It may also include the individual's natural history and/or outcomes to an intervention. Case reports are qualitative analyses used for describing rare and/or poorly understood diseases.

2. A *case series* is a collection of case reports. The subjects' exposures, characteristics, presentation, and the clinical course are described and compared across cases in order to hypothesize potential risk factors, prognostic factors, and treatment (Hulley et al., 2013, p. 87).

3. *Systematic reviews* evaluate the results of multiple studies addressing a particular research question. Inclusion criteria for a systematic review must be well defined. Meta-analysis refers to pooling the data from a systematic review for statistical analysis. These study designs can be useful in resolving conflicts in the literature (Hulley et al., 2013, p. 197).

4. *Cross-sectional studies* measure disease prevalence, exposure distribution, and other variables at one point in time. They allow for assessment of the relationship between disease prevalence and status of exposures. In some cases, they can be considered a proxy for longitudinal data (Rothman, 2002, p. 89-91).

5. *Cohort studies* measure disease occurrence in a group of subjects followed over time. Subjects are stratified by an exposure category that defines the cohorts. Prospective cohort studies identify an exposed group and an unexposed group and follow them forward for disease occurrence. Retrospective cohort studies identify an exposed group in whom disease has already occurred and compares them to an exposed group in whom the disease has not occurred. Cohort studies assess relative risk, prevalence, incidence, induction time, and natural history. They allow for examination of rare exposures but not rare diseases. Multiple effects of exposure can be studied, but the study design requires time for follow-up (Rothman, 2002, p. 57-73).

6. *Case control studies* measure the distribution of exposure in cases and controls (or subjects with and without disease, respectively) from the same source population. Case control studies compare the disease exposure relationship using odds ratios. This study design requires that control subjects be sampled independent of exposure status in order to estimate incidence rate ratio (Rothman, 2002, p. 73-94).

7. The *randomized clinical trial* (RCT) is the "centerpiece of clinical epidemiology." RCTs prospectively measure outcomes of a given treatment or intervention in a cohort of subjects with a disease in order to determine causation and associations. Randomization is used to minimize confounding by indication, and to compare how baseline characteristics may affect the outcome between cohorts. Baseline characteristics are measured at the time of randomization and treatment assignment. Control subjects resemble treatment subjects in all manners with the exception of the intervention. The gold standard intervention typically represents the control intervention. RCTs are often double-blinded to minimize bias (i.e., the evaluator and subject are both unaware of the treatment assignment). Subgroup analysis can determine effect modification or interaction in subgroups. Similarly, if a treatment is widespread in use and/or is considered the best option, then randomization is deemed unethical, because it would necessitate withholding the "standard of care" treatment from a group of subjects. Rare outcomes are not properly evaluated by RCTs, as it is nearly impossible to power a study in the case of a rare disease or outcome. RCTs can be time intensive and costly, particularly related to

maximizing follow-up and ensuring adherence to protocol. Crossover and noncausal associations require careful analysis of RCT data and results (Rothman, 2002, p. 60-61, 206-213).

a. Treatment efficacy and effectiveness. The ability of an intervention to result in the best outcome is referred to as efficacy within the controlled milieu of an RCT. Once efficacy has been demonstrated, effectiveness can be determined by the ability to produce the best outcome in real-world practice (Haines and Walters, 2006, p. 14).

b. Clinical trials for regulatory approval of new interventions advance through phases after preclinical studies with cell cultures, tissues, and animals have been completed (Hulley et al., 2013).

    i. Phase I assesses safety, toxicity, and pharmacokinetics in a small number of healthy volunteers. Testing in this phase is typically unblinded and uncontrolled.

    ii. Phase II assesses optimal dosing, tolerability, and efficacy on clinical outcome or biomarkers via relatively small randomized or time series trials.

    iii. Phase III compares the efficacy and adverse events of the new treatment to the efficacy and adverse events of the best available treatment and/or placebo in a relatively large randomized blinded trial.

    iv. Phase IV assesses rare and/or long-term adverse effects and additional therapeutic uses following U.S. Food and Drug Administration (FDA) approval. Large trials or observational studies are conducted.

Subject selection

Study subjects should be representative of the population of interest to improve the generalizability of the study findings relevant to the research question.

1. Inclusion criteria should be shaped by the target population's demographic, clinical, geographic, and/or temporal characteristics. Broadening inclusion criteria can increase generalizability and minimize random error. If statistical testing for effect modification between groups is desired, then there must be enough subjects in each group.

2. Exclusion criteria should describe factors that are likely to interfere with treatment adherence, follow-up success, data quality, and safety for subjects. Recruitment of a sufficient sample size minimizes the potential for statistically significant findings due to random error or chance (Hulley et al., 2013, p. 23-31).

Variables and bias

Research studies assess associations between variables. Most observational studies examine the relationship between many predictor variables and several outcome variables. Randomized clinical trials determine the effects of an intervention, which acts as the predictor variable, on one or more outcome variables with randomization to minimize the influence of confounding variables. Continuous variables are superior to categorical variables because they provide additional information, which can improve statistical efficiency and flexibility for interpretation of associations. There are two broad types of error afflicting epidemiological studies: (1) Systematic error, which is commonly referred to as bias, and (2) random error, or chance. Random errors can be reduced to zero in an infinitely large study, whereas systematic errors cannot (Rothman, 2002, p. 98).

1. Precision is the measure of the reproducibility, reliability, and consistency of a variable. It provides value to the study by increasing its power to detect effects. Random error, or chance, reduces the precision of a test.
   a. For continuous variables, precision is expressed as within-subject standard deviation or coefficient of variation (within-subject standard deviation divided by the mean).
   b. For categorical variables, precision is expressed as percent agreement, interclass correlation coefficient, or kappa statistic (Hulley et al., 2013, p. 35-36).

2. Accuracy is the measure of the trueness of a variable. It provides value to the study by increasing the validity of conclusions. Systematic error, or bias, reduces the accuracy of a variable (Hulley, 2013, p. 36-37).

3. Validity is the measure of how well a variable represents the phenomena it is meant to represent. For example, the validity of an IQ test may be measured as its ability to represent intelligence. Another example is the short form 36 health survey questionnaire (SF-36), which has been validated as a measure of health status (Hulley, 2013, p. 38-39).

4. There are several types of bias or systematic error that should be considered in the context of subject selection, variable consideration, and data collection:
   a. Confounding is systematic error that mixes effects, and thus confuses causal relationships and associations. Confounding variables are factors that have an effect on outcome and are unbalanced between comparison groups (Rothman, 2002, p. 101-109).
   b. Sampling bias is systematic error that occurs when determinants of outcome differ between subjects and the population of interest. Sampling bias must be considered when considering how to recruit subjects (Hulley, 2013, p. 9-10).
   c. Selection bias is systematic error that occurs when determinants of outcome differ between subjects in different comparison groups. Randomization is the ultimate tool to minimize selection bias (Rothman, 2002, p. 97-98).
   d. Recall bias introduces systematic error in case control studies because control subjects may be less likely to adequately recall an exposure. For cases, the disease often serves as a stimulus to consider potential causes, whereas controls have had no comparable stimulus (Rothman, 2002, p. 97-98).
   e. Chronology bias is introduced by the passage of time and can be minimized with the use of contemporaneous controls.
   f. Observation bias is introduced by unequal opportunities for observation and can be minimized by blinding investigators who are collecting and/or analyzing the data.
   g. Measurement bias is introduced by differing measurement or data collection methods between groups.
   h. Susceptibility bias is introduced by different susceptibility to a disease or treatment. When known factors affect or predict susceptibility to a disease or treatment under study, subjects should be stratified as they enter the study according to these known factors. Stratification is most effective at minimizing susceptibility bias at study entry as opposed to during data analysis.
   i. Compliance bias is introduced by intentional and unintentional deviation from protocol by subjects. Careful study design with mechanisms for monitoring and reporting compliance can minimize compliance bias (Haines and Walters, 2006, p. 10-11).

Statistical principles

1. The hypothesis is the research question that provides a basis for testing statistical significance. The null hypothesis states that there is no difference in outcome between groups. The alternative hypothesis states that there is a difference in outcome between groups.

a. Type I error, or false-positive error, occurs when the investigator rejects a null hypothesis that is true in the population (i.e., states that there is a difference when none exists). The maximum probability of a type I error is called α (alpha). Typically, $\alpha = 0.05$.

b. Type II error, or false-negative error, occurs when the investigator fails to reject a null hypothesis that is false in the population (i.e., states that there is no difference when one actually exists). The maximum probability of a type II error is called β (beta). Typically, $\beta = 0.20$.

c. Power $(1-\beta)$ is the probability of correctly rejecting the null hypothesis (i.e., the ability to detect a difference between groups). Increasing the number of subjects in a study increases the power of a study. The number of potential outcomes, compliance between treatment groups, and expected effect size influence the power of a study (Hulley, 2013, p. 43-53).

d. It is important to distinguish between clinical significance and statistical significance. A clinically significant finding may not be statistically significant if a study is not adequately powered. In the same way, statistically significant findings may not be clinically significant.

2. Measures of disease occurrence

a. The incidence of a disease quantifies the rate of disease occurrence, or the number of new cases of a disease in a population over a specified time period.

b. The prevalence of a disease quantifies the number of existing cases of a disease in a population at one point in time. The prevalence is determined from the incidence of the disease and the duration of the disease.

3. Measures of effect or risk

a. Absolute risk is the probability of an outcome in a population.

b. Absolute risk reduction is the difference in probability of an outcome between exposed and unexposed groups.

c. Number needed to treat is a measure of the number of subjects who need to be treated (or exposed) in order to prevent one bad outcome. It is often used in clinical trials comparing medications and is defined as the inverse of the absolute risk reduction.

d. Attributable risk is calculated by taking the risk difference between exposed and unexposed groups and dividing it by risk in the exposed group. It is a measure of the proportion of an outcome among exposed people that is caused by that exposure.

e. Number needed to harm is a measure of the number of subjects who need to be exposed to a risk factor in order to cause harm to one subject. It is calculated by taking the inverse of the attributable risk.

f. Relative risk or risk ratio (RR) is the risk of an outcome or incidence in an exposed group compared to the risk of an outcome or incidence in an unexposed group. The relative risk quantifies the strength of the association between exposure and outcome by comparing the likelihood of an outcome or disease based on exposure status. If RR > 1, then exposure and disease have a positive association. If RR < 1, then exposure and disease have a negative association. If RR = 1, no association exists. Relative risk can be calculated from cohort studies.

g. Odds are defined as the number of people who develop an outcome compared to the number of people who do not develop that outcome.

h. Odds ratio (OR) is the odds of exposure among those with an outcome compared to the odds of exposure among those without that outcome. Odds ratios are used to quantify the strength of the association between exposure and outcome in case control studies by comparing the likelihood of exposure based on disease status. The odds ratio approximates the relative risk when disease incidence is low (i.e., in rare diseases).

i. Confidence interval (CI) is the range of values in which a parameter is expected to fall. The number of subjects to produce acceptably narrow confidence intervals is used to determine sample size in descriptive studies. Generally, the 95% CI is used. If the 95% CI between groups overlaps, then the difference is not statistically significant. If the RR or OR 95% CI does not include 1, then there is a statistically significant difference between groups (Rothman, 2002, p. 24-33).

4. Measures of prognosis
   a. Case fatality rate is the percentage of people with a disease who die within a specified time frame.
   b. Kaplan-Meier curves are used to demonstrate survival in a cohort of patients with a disease by determining the average time between presentation, diagnosis, or intervention initiation and outcome (e.g., death, recurrence).
5. Measures of diagnosis
   a. Sensitivity is the probability that a patient with a disease will have a positive test result, sign, or symptom. High sensitivity is desirable for screening tests (to "rule out").
   b. Specificity is the probability that a patient without a disease will have a negative test result, sign, or symptom. High specificity is desirable for determination of a likely diagnosis (to "rule in").
   c. Positive predictive value is the probability that a patient with a positive result truly has a disease. Tests with high specificity have a high positive predictive value. Positive predictive value also increases in populations with high disease prevalence.
   d. Negative predictive value is the probability that a patient with a negative test does not have disease. Tests with high sensitivity have a high negative predictive value. Negative predictive value also increases in populations with low disease prevalence.
   e. Likelihood ratios are more comprehensive performance measures comparing the probability of a result in people with disease to the probability of the same result in people without disease (Hulley, 2013, p. 171-187).

Common pitfalls and medicolegal concerns

Funders and academic institutions typically do not allow heavy stakeholders of an intervention to serve as principal investigators of a clinical trial due to conflict of interest. In some cases, closer monitoring and modification of the stakeholder's role can be utilized.

Relevance to the advanced practice health professional

Health-care reform will have an impact on trends in scientific research, clinical trials, and funding. Patient outcomes, which are interconnected with high quality and low cost, will ultimately drive reimbursement. Research on cost-benefit analysis and quality improvement metrics will become increasingly relevant in our modern health-care environment.

Common phone calls, pages, and requests with answers

1. If a patient is cognitively impaired, is the patient competent to provide informed consent?
   a. To be competent, a patient cannot be psychotic or intoxicated. A patient must comprehend his or her medical situation enough to make medical decisions in agreement with his or her values.
2. Who can sign informed consent for incompetent patients?
   a. Designated surrogate decision makers and/or next of kin can sign informed consent for incompetent patients.
3. If a treatment is found to cause adverse outcomes during clinical trial implementation, what happens?
   a. The trial is deemed unethical and is stopped. Patients who received the treatment are informed with full disclosure.

References

Alves W, Skolnick B. *Handbook of Neuroemergency Clinical Trials*. San Diego, CA: Elsevier Academic Press; 2006.

Haines S, Walters B. *Evidence-Based Neurosurgery*. New York, NY: Thieme Medical Publishers; 2006.

Hulley S, Cummings S, Browner W, Grady D, Newman T. *Designing Clinical Research*. 4th ed. Philadelphia, PA: Lippincott Williams & Wilkins; 2013.

Rothman K. *Epidemiology: An Introduction*. Oxford: Oxford University Press, 2002.

PART IV

Monitoring the Patient

23

SERIAL NEUROLOGIC EXAMINATIONS

Adriana L. Castano and Scott A. Meyer

Introduction

The neurologic examination is an essential tool for clinicians who participate in the care of patients with an injury or disorder involving the nervous system. The examination is challenging and complex, but if performed in a systematic and orderly way can potentially save a patient's life or prevent permanent neurologic injury. Serial neurologic examinations are an important part of the clinical armamentarium that enables clinicians to follow the progress of a patient and identify neurologic stability, deterioration, or improvement. The foundation of the serial neurologic examination is the baseline examination. The baseline acts as a starting point that will be referred to with all additional examinations in order to determine the trajectory of a patient's condition. Subsequent examinations are timed based on the acuity or potential acuity of the ongoing process.

Baseline neurologic examination

The initial patient encounter represents an opportunity in some cases to gather information from family or friends as to any existing deficits or conditions. Following a thorough history, attention is turned to the neurologic examination. The examination in general includes an assessment of mental status, cranial nerves, followed by motor system, sensory system, coordination, and gait. (Victor et al., 2001) It is best to record one's findings, because clinical changes can be subtle; therefore, attention to detail is important. The examination is often tailored to the surrounding circumstances and frequently not every aspect of the exam is able to be completed secondary to the condition of the patient. There are obvious modifications when examining a comatose patient, and there are certain parts of the neurologic examination that are not able to be carried out. Establishing a baseline when you first see the patient makes it possible to determine any deviations from baseline allowing you to address a neurologic decline promptly. Imaging such as computed tomography (CT) and magnetic resonance imaging (MRI) are important adjuncts to the clinical exam but are not a substitute for a detailed neurologic examination.

Mental status measures the patient's level of consciousness, orientation, speech and language, memory, fund of information, insight and judgment, abstract thoughts, and calculations. Level of consciousness is the patient's awareness of self and environment where the patient can be anywhere from comatose to fully awake. If the patient is not fully awake, response to minimum stimuli is noted. The examiner elicits a number of stimuli to test a response from the patient: Verbal commands or brief, painful stimulus. The patient's response to the stimuli: Eye opening, reaching for, or pushing away the stimulus indicates the level of consciousness (Glick, 1993).

Orientation is examined by asking the patient to state his or her full name, location, and the time. Speech is assessed by articulation, rate, and rhythm. Language is evaluated by observing the content of the patient's verbal and written output, responses to spoken command, and the ability to read.

Memory is analyzed in three categories: immediate, short-term, and long-term. This is tested by three-object recall and how well the patient is able to provide history of his or her personal events in the proper chronological order. Fund of knowledge is appreciated by asking questions about major historical events or current events. Insight and judgment are analyzed by how the patient responds to certain questions during the interview, and you can also ask to see how the patient responds to a scenario that has a variety of outcomes; for example, "What would you do if you found a wallet on the street?" Abstract thought is examined by asking the patient to describe certain similarities between various objects or concepts. The patient's ability to perform calculations is tested by having the patient do certain computations like simple arithmetic or serial subtraction from seven (Spillane and Bickerstaff, 1996).

Cranial nerves can be assessed with a minimal exam including the visual fields, pupil size and reactivity, extraocular movements, and facial movements. A more detailed cranial nerve examination is described elsewhere in the book and is an important part of the baseline neurologic examination.

Motor examination involves checking for muscle atrophy and extremity tone. The patient can be assessed for a pronator drift, and strength in the wrist and fingers tests upper extremity strength. Asking the patient to walk on his or her heels and toes evaluates lower extremity strength. And finally, tap the biceps, patellar, and Achilles reflexes. When possible, strength is evaluated across all muscle groups in the upper and lower extremities and documented with the use of a five-point scale as detailed in Chapter 11.

Sensory examination is evaluated, but it is quite difficult to quantify and is purely subjective. Patients must be compliant in order to perform the exam and yield reliable results. In the uncooperative patient, this test is useless. Ask the patient whether he or she can feel light touch and the temperature of a cool object in the distal extremity.

Coordination is examined by testing rapid alternating movements of the hands and the finger-to-nose and heel-knee-shin maneuvers. Gait is evaluated by carefully observing the patient while walking normally, on heels, toes, and along a straight line.

Clinical case example

A 37-year-old female was brought by emergency medical services to the emergency department. She was down on the ground for an unspecified period of time and found by her family. She was lethargic but opened her eyes to voice. She followed simple commands moving her left side without difficulty but had no movement on the right side with 0/5 strength. She was oriented to person but not place or time. She was not a candidate for intravenous tissue plasminogen activator (IV-TPA) or mechanical thrombolysis. She underwent a CT scan of the head that demonstrated a large left cerebral infarct extending from the anterior to the middle cerebral artery territory (Figure 23.1). She was admitted to the neurologic intensive care unit for close monitoring and serial neurologic examinations.

Serial neurologic examinations

The exact frequency of the examinations will largely be determined based on the severity of the injury and the potential for deterioration. At least initially with any serious neurologic condition that has the potential for a rapid deterioration, frequent neurologic examinations are recommended. Patients who require frequent examinations are generally placed in the intensive care unit. Intracranial pressure (ICP) monitors are used in circumstances where there is a severe traumatic brain injury or concern for elevated ICP and can provide continuous monitoring of ICP. When a patient has been stable for a suitable period of time, the frequency of the neurologic examinations can be reduced. All subsequent examinations must be compared to the initial baseline examination in order to recognize subtle signs of deterioration.

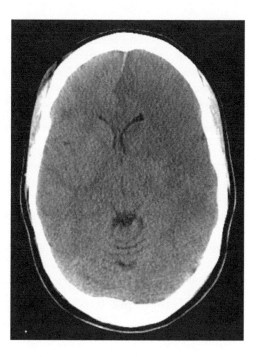

Figure 23.1 Noncontrast CT scan of the head demonstrating a well-demarcated left anterior cerebral artery and middle cerebral artery infarction with minimal mass effect.

Changes in a neurologic exam can be subtle or in some cases obvious. The examiner should complete the same evaluation as was performed for the baseline examination in each subsequent evaluation. If there is an obvious change that warrants urgent imaging or intervention, it is at times not necessary to complete the entire examination, as it may waste critical time. One of the first signs of impending deterioration in patients with a cerebral injury or process is a change in the mental status of the patient. In patients with spinal pathology, a more detailed motor and sensory exam is often required to identify changes from baseline. In spinal patients, the change may initially involve a sensory distribution or may affect urination, which can be overlooked in patients with a urinary catheter.

It is important to note that there are many variables that affect mental status that may give a false sense of neurologic decline. One must keep in mind that the causes for altered mental status include hypoxia, hypotension, seizure activity, hypoglycemia, and medications such as sedatives and opiates. If a patient has had a change in his or her level of consciousness, the nurse is often a valuable resource to see if there has been concern for seizure activity or if a medication was recently given that could have altered the examination. It is imperative that a fast-acting sedative is used in order to be able to turn off the medication and have an accurate neurologic examination. When a neurologic deterioration is confirmed, adjuvant imaging is obtained to assess for any radiographic changes that could explain the change. It is important that the patient's ability to protect the airway be assessed so as to avoid loss of his or her airway when obtaining imaging. If an ICP monitor is present, an elevation in pressures will often precede a clinical deterioration. When a change in ICP is not present and imaging does not demonstrate a cause for the deterioration, nonconvulsive seizures should be considered.

Clinical case example

On subsequent examination, the patient was found to be more lethargic. She did not open her eyes to voice and grimaced only to noxious stimuli. She had weak withdrawal of her left upper extremity. She had not received additional medication. She was intubated for airway protection, and a CT scan of the head was obtained, which demonstrated increased mass effect with midline shift and uncal herniation (Figure 23.2). Based on the findings and the patient's deterioration, an operating room was prepared for a left hemicraniectomy. On her way to the operating room, she was no longer responsive to noxious stimuli and her left pupil was fixed and dilated at 6 mm, nonreactive to light. She underwent a left hemicraniectomy to remove some of the mass effect (Figure 23.3) and ultimately made a good clinical recovery to her initial baseline of right hemiplegia, and with only a mild expressive aphasia.

Common pitfalls

- Imaging does not replace the neurologic examination; avoid defaulting immediately to repeat imaging when there is a change in the neurologic examination.
- Inadequate baseline examination or documentation removes the foundation and comparison for all subsequent examinations.
- Listen to the nurse taking care of the patient, as he or she is often the first one to pick up subtle changes.

Relevance to the advanced practice health professional

Serial neurologic examinations play a critical role in the care of patients with neurologic conditions. Utilizing a thorough baseline neurologic examination and subsequent serial examinations to identify important clinical changes improves neurologic outcomes and saves lives.

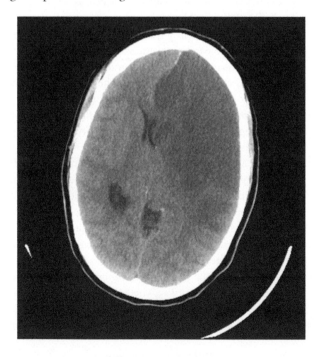

Figure 23.2 Noncontrast CT scan of the head demonstrating an increase in the extent of mass effect from the previously seen infarct with midline shift and uncal herniation.

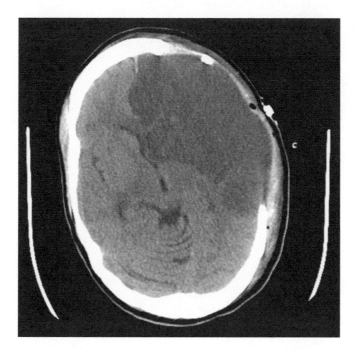

Figure 23.3   Noncontrast CT scan of the head demonstrating a left hemicraniectomy with interval improvement in the mass effect and midline shift.

Common phone calls, pages, and requests with answers

- The patient has generalized convulsions.
  - Immediate assessment is crucial. The treatment of status epilepticus in a timely fashion can be lifesaving. Treatment with a first-line medication such as lorazepam is indicated. It is important to ascertain if the patient is on an anticonvulsant and if so if the level is in a therapeutic range. Once the seizure is under control, imaging should be considered to rule out a hemorrhage or other cerebral cause. Video electroencephalography can also be utilized if continued seizure activity is suspected.
- A patient with a subarachnoid hemorrhage following a ruptured right posterior communicating artery aneurysm develops left-sided weakness 7 days after a coil embolization.
  - After assessing the patient, a CT scan of the head should be obtained to evaluate for hemorrhage or hydrocephalus. In the absence of hydrocephalus, a clinical diagnosis of cerebral vasospasm should be considered. The triad of hypertension, hypervolemia, and hemodilution is a common first line of therapy in symptomatic vasospasm.
- An intubated patient with a traumatic brain injury has sustained elevated ICP.
  - After assessing the patient for any neurologic changes, increasing the sedation level may help with elevated ICP. If a ventriculostomy is being utilized, opening or lowering the level of the ventriculostomy may also help with the ICP. After initial trouble-shooting, imaging should be obtained to rule out a space-occupying lesion that might need to be addressed surgically.

References

Glick TH. *Neurologic Skills: Examination and Diagnosis*. Boston, MA: Blackwell Scientific Publications; 1993.

Spillane JA, Bickerstaff ER. *Bickerstaff's Neurological Examination in Clinical Practice*. Oxford and Cambridge, MA: Blackwell Science; 1996.

Victor M, Ropper AH, Adams RD. *Adams and Victor's Principles of Neurology*. New York, NY: Medical Pub. Division, McGraw-Hill; 2001.

24

INTRACRANIAL PRESSURE MANAGEMENT

Eli Johnson, Yi-Ren Chen, Katie Shpanskaya, Jamshid Ghajar, and Odette A. Harris

Case vignette

A 31-year-old man is involved in a motor vehicle collision with a tree and is found to have a Glasgow Coma Scale score of 3. He is rushed to the nearest hospital where imaging reveals extensive right frontal bone fracture, bilateral frontal contusions, and nasal fracture (Figure 24.1). The patient is considered for possible organ donation and transferred to another hospital, where he was noted to have movement on his right side. An external ventricular drain was placed to monitor the intracranial pressure and provide drainage. He subsequently undergoes a bilateral decompressive craniectomy. After an extended stay in the hospital, the patient returns home and is regularly seen by a neurologist for complications of his brain trauma. One month after discharge, the patient is noted to be alert and oriented ×3 with right cranial nerves III and VI palsy. He is able to follow simple and complex commands with no gross sensory or motor deficits.

Case Figure

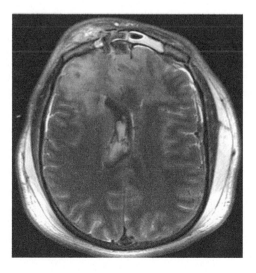

Figure 24.1   T2 magnetic resonance image, axial view, demonstrating diffuse frontal lobe hemorrhage. Shifting of the midline (falx cerebri) and compression of the left lateral ventricle are suggestive of elevated intracranial pressure. Additionally, the image shows right-sided fluid leakage through a fractured frontal bone.

Overview
Epidemiology

Elevated intracranial pressure (ICP) is a life-threatening complication of neurologic injury and is associated with nearly 20% mortality (Luks, 2009; Fakhry et al., 2004). Prompt recognition and rigorous monitoring of elevated ICP are critical in many conditions, including trauma, hydrocephalus, encephalitis, stroke, and central nervous system (CNS) neoplasm (Robertson et al., 1999). Normal intracranial pressures range from 0 to 15 mm Hg in supine adults and become pathologic at pressures ≥20 mm Hg. Children have lower physiologic ICP, and infants may have pressures below 0 mm Hg (Welch, 1980). Clinical signs of elevated ICP vary based on the primary location affected, but most often include headache, loss of consciousness, blurred vision, and vomiting. Clinical findings, medical history, and imaging studies are used in the diagnosis of elevated ICP (Kuo et al., 2006).

Societal significance

Numerous neurologic conditions can be complicated by increased ICP. Rising pressures can cut off the blood supply to delicate brain tissue, resulting in severe and potentially irreversible brain injury; this can happen without fracturing the skull. In cases of traumatic brain injury, inadequate ICP monitoring can lead to a slow progression into a comatose state or even death. Initially these individuals do not display any symptoms because their bodies can compensate for the increased ICP. As the pressure rises beyond the compensation threshold, patients become at risk for harm in their decompensated state (Figure 24.2). Contact sport athletes and motor vehicle accident victims are at increased risk (Field et al., 2003; Eisenberg et al., 1990).

Additionally, elevated ICP can be a sign of child abuse. The most common example is shaken baby syndrome, which requires appropriate comprehensive medical and social/case management follow-up. Elevated ICP following traumatic brain injury is one of the leading causes of death in children (Kukreti et al., 2014). Other common etiologies include meningitis and encephalitis in adolescents and young adults.

Basic biologic and physiologic processes

ICP is a measure of the pressure contained within the skull. Brain tissue, cerebral blood, and cerebrospinal fluid (CSF) are the compartments that contribute to the ICP. During early stages of neurologic injury, these compartments compensate for abnormal increases in pressure in a process called *autoregulation*. This compensation is critical for maintaining adequate cerebral blood perfusion.

Pathologic changes such as obstruction of venous or CSF return, cerebral edema, hemorrhage, or mass lesions can surpass the compensatory capacity of autoregulation and lead to a significant rise in ICP (Monro, 1783). Subsequent damage to brain tissue will arise due to decreased cerebral perfusion pressure (CPP) or to compression of the brainstem and brain parenchyma (Ghajar, 2000). CPP is a well-established surrogate marker for the adequacy of cerebral perfusion. It is indirectly measured by subtracting ICP from the mean arterial pressure (MAP) (Equation 24.1). Decreased CPP can result in devastating diffuse or global ischemia (Robertson, 2001). Therefore, the goal of ICP management is to improve the health-care team's ability to maintain optimal CPP and ICP (Robertson, 2001; Carney et al., 2016).

$$CPP = MAP - ICP \qquad (24.1)$$

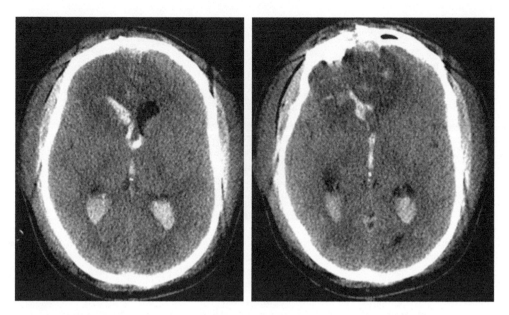

Figure 24.2　Noncontrast head CT, axial view, demonstrating extensive interventricular hemorrhage as well as diffuse effacement of the sulci and basal cisterns. Diminished gray and white matter differentiation can also be seen.

Anatomical review

Common physical examination findings

- Global symptoms
  - Headache
  - Depressed consciousness
  - Vomiting

- Additional signs
  - Papilledema (Figure 24.3)
  - Cranial nerve VI palsies
  - Cushing triad (bradycardia, respiratory depression, hypertension)—the presence of this finding requires urgent intervention (Kaye, 2001)

Relevant diagnostic tests

- Invasive ICP monitoring is indicated in patients who are (1) comatose with a Glasgow Coma Scale (GCS) <9, (2) in need of aggressive medical care, or (3) at high risk for elevated ICP (Robertson, 2001). Four main anatomical sites are used for ICP monitoring (Figure 24.4). Known bleeding disorders are the only contraindication for ICP monitor placement, but it is otherwise a low-risk procedure. Complications include catheter-related hemorrhage (4%–22%) and infections (1%–12%) (Pfausler et al., 2004).
  - Intraventricular drain—This is considered the "gold standard" of ICP monitoring catheters. However, infection can occur in up to 20% of patients. Risk of infection increases with duration of placement (Mayhall et al., 1984; Holloway et al., 1996).

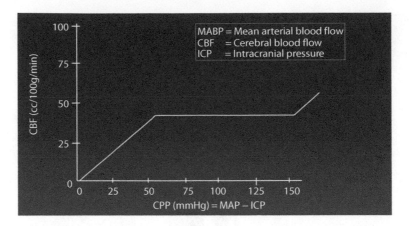

Figure 24.3 Autoregulation. Despite changes in the cerebral blood flow, CPP remain constant from 50 to 150 mmHg. Beyond these ranges brain damage occurs.

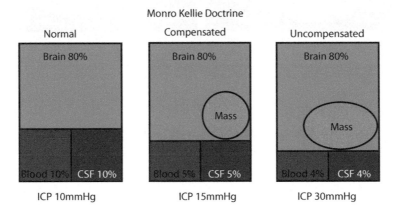

Figure 24.4 Monro Kellie Doctrine. ICP is a measure of the pressure in the skull. In the compensated state, any increase in one component of the ICP can be mitigated by a decrease in the other components. In the uncompensated state, mitigation does not restore the ICP below 15mmHG.

- Intraparenchymal fiberoptic catheter—This carries a much lower risk of infection and hemorrhage (<1%). However, CSF is unable to be drained, and the reliability of the device is debated (Ghajar, 1995; Ostrup et al., 1987).
- Subarachnoid bolts—Rarely used and have low accuracy (Brain Trauma Foundation et al., 2007).
- Epidural monitors—These are used in the management of coagulopathic patients with hepatic encephalopathy complicated by cerebral edema (Eisenberg et al., 1990).
- Imaging computed tomography (CT) or magnetic resonance imaging (MRI)
  - Look for evidence of mass lesions, midline shift, or effacement of the basilar cisterns (Figure 24.5). However, ICP may still be elevated without these manifestations (Eisenberg et al., 1990).

Noncontrast head CT, axial view, demonstrating extensive interventricular hemorrhage as well as diffuse effacement of the sulci and basal cisterns. Diminished gray and white matter differentiation can also be seen.

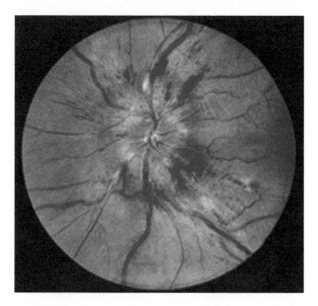

Figure 24.5 Papilledema is optic disc swelling that is caused by increased intracranial pressure. Its presentation is usually bilateral.

Principles of management

Elevated ICP is treated by addressing the underlying cause of increasing pressures and/or increasing the volume available for expansion of injured tissue. This can be accomplished by

1. Reducing the volume of another intracranial fluid compartment:
   CSF—by ventricular drainage
   a. Cerebral blood volume—by hyperventilation or hyperosmolar therapy
   b. Brain tissue edema—by mannitol
2. Increasing cranial volume by decompression
3. Removing swollen or irreversibly damaged brain tissue
4. A detailed outline of elevated ICP management is presented in Figure 24.7 (Rosner and Rosner, 1993; Chowdhury et al., 2014)

Treatment goals

A recommended target for ICP levels is below 22 mm Hg, as pressures above this threshold have been associated with an increased risk of mortality (Carney et al., 2016). Determination of an optimal CPP threshold is more challenging and may depend on the patient's autoregulatory capability. In general, CPP values above 60–70 mm Hg favor survival and improved outcomes (Carney et al., 2016).

Several factors may influence a patient's limit of autoregulation including preexisting hypertension, prior brain injury, and the pattern of injury. Chronically hypertensive patients will experience diminished brain perfusion at higher levels of CPP. Similarly, previous injury may reduce brain tolerance to hypotension and increase brain tissue susceptibility to hypoxia. CPP is a global measure of perfusion; however, focal areas of ischemia may occur without significant change to CPP. These factors should be considered when setting a patient's CPP goal.

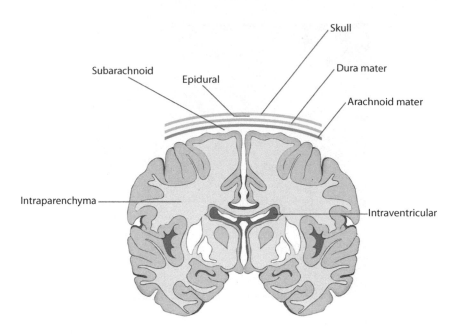

Figure 24.6. Invasive ICP monitoring sites.

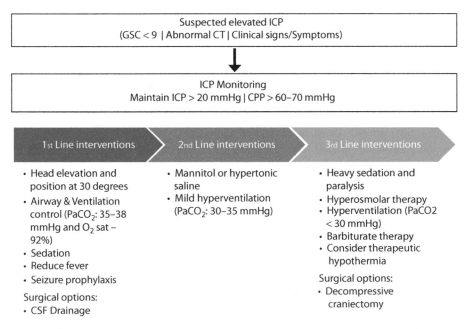

Figure 24.7. A detailed outline of elevated ICP management is shown (Rosner and Rosner, 1993; Chowdhury et al., 2014).

Family Counseling

Prognosis

Raised ICP results from various causes, such as trauma, encephalitis, stroke, and CNS tumor. The management of each diagnosis will differ. The prognosis of increased ICP strongly depends on the underlying etiology and the extent of neurological injury. Sudden elevated ICP is often life-threatening. Prompt intervention greatly reduces mortality. Focal neurologic deficits may result from irreversible tissue death.

Common questions

What signs should we look for?

There is always the risk that some bleeding may occur due to the initial injury or medical interventions. Families should look for signs of lethargy, vomiting, headache, and focal neurologic deficit.

For which medications are prescriptions likely?

After hospitalization with an elevated ICP complication, patients may be prescribed antiepileptic drugs like Dilantin (Phenytoin). Other medications vary based on the extent and location of damage. As discussed above, the underlying etiology of the elevated ICP will also strongly influence the necessary medications.

What are the long-term complications of increased ICP?

The long-term sequelae of elevated ICP depend on the underlying condition that caused the increased pressure in the brain. The patient is likely to be more susceptible to future brain trauma or any neurologic events that may decreased blood flow to the brain.

Common pitfalls and medicolegal concerns

In the early management of neurologic injury, it is important that patients be comprehensively evaluated and all etiologies be evaluated before a patient is declared brain dead. A patient may present with a low GCS score that may be explained by confounding factors, such as a postictal state, hypothermia, or significant electrolyte imbalance (Durant and Sporer, 2011).

Additionally, child and elder abuse are potential causes of elevated ICP. These cases warrant medical and social/case management follow-up to ensure the safety of the patient.

Relevance to the advanced practice health professional

Successful treatment of patients with elevated ICP relies on prompt recognition. Advanced practice health professionals are integral members throughout all stages of patient management and are uniquely positioned to intervene when signs of elevated ICP are noted. Furthermore, familiarity with ICP management is paramount in assessing the efficacy of therapeutic treatments.

Common phone calls, pages, and requests with answers

- Neurocritical care can be helpful in managing seizures or providing prognostication.
- Neuropsych evaluation can also be considered for rehabilitation, in addition to physical and occupational therapy

References

Brain Trauma Foundation, American Association of Neurological Surgeons, Congress of Neurological Surgeons, et al. Guidelines for the management of severe traumatic brain injury. VII. Intracranial pressure monitoring technology. *J Neurotrauma*. 2007;24 (Suppl 1):S45.

Carney N, Totten AM, O'Reilly C, et al. Guidelines for the management of severe traumatic brain injury, Fourth edition. *Neurosurgery*. 2016;80:6–15.

Chowdhury T, Kowalski S, Arabi Y, Dash HH. Pre-hospital and initial management of head injury patients: An update. *Saudi J Anaesth*. 2014;8:114–120.

Durant E, Sporer KA. Characteristics of patients with an abnormal glasgow coma scale score in the prehospital setting. *West J Emerg Med*. 2011;12:30–36.

Eisenberg HM, Gary HE Jr, Aldrich EF, et al. Initial CT findings in 753 patients with severe head injury. A report from the NIH Traumatic Coma Data Bank. *J Neurosurg*. 1990;73:688.

Fakhry SM, Trask AL, Waller MA, Watts DD. Management of brain-injured patients by an evidence-based medicine protocol improves outcomes and decreases hospital charges. *J Trauma*. March 2004;56(3):492–499; discussion 499-500.

Field M, Collins MW, Lovell MR, et al. Does age play a role in recovery from sports-related concussion? A comparison of high school and collegiate athletics. *J Pediatr*. 2003;142:546–553.

Ghajar J. Intracranial pressure monitoring techniques. *New Horiz*. 1995;3:395.

Ghajar J. Traumatic brain injury. *Lancet*. September 2000;356(9233):923–929.

Holloway KL, Barnes T, Choi S, et al. Ventriculostomy infections: the effect of monitoring duration and catheter exchange in 584 patients. *J Neurosurg*. 1996;85:419.

Kaye AH. *Brain Tumors: An Encyclopedic Approach*. 2nd ed. New York, NY: Churchill Livingstone; 2001:205.

Kukreti V, Mohseni-Bod H, Drake J. Management of raised intracranial pressure in children with traumatic brain injury. *J Pediatr Neurosci*. 2014;9:207–215.

Kuo JR, Yeh TC, Sung KC, Wang CC, Chen CW, Chio CC. Intraoperative applications of intracranial pressure monitoring in patients with severe head injury. *J Clin Neurosci*. February 2006;13(2):218–223.

Luks A. Critical care management of the patient with elevated intracranial pressure. *Critical Care Alert*. September 2009: 44–48.

Mayhall CG, Archer NH, Lamb VA, et al. Ventriculostomy-related infections. A prospective epidemiologic study. *N Engl J Med*. 1984;310:553.

Monro A. *Observations on the Structure and Function of the Nervous System*. London: Gale ECCO, 1783.

Ostrup RC, Luerssen TG, Marshall LF, Zornow MH. Continuous monitoring of intracranial pressure with a miniaturized fiberoptic device. *J Neurosurg*. 1987;67:206.

Pfausler B, Beer R, Engelhardt K, Kemmler G, Mohsenipour I, Schmutzhard E. Cell index—A new parameter for the early diagnosis of ventriculostomy (external ventricular drainage)-related ventriculitis in patients with intraventricular hemorrhage? *Acta Neurochir (Wien)*. May 2004;146(5):477–481.

Robertson CS. Management of cerebral perfusion pressure after traumatic brain injury. *Anesthesiology*. 2001;95:1513–1517.

Robertson CS, Valadka AB, Hannay HJ, et al. Prevention of secondary ischemic insults after severe head injury. *Crit Care Med*. 1999;27:2086–2095.

Rosner MJ, Rosner SD. Cerebral perfusion pressure management of head injury. In: Avezaat CJJ, van Eijndhoven JHM, Maas AIR, et al. eds. *Intracranial Pressure VIII*. Berlin: Springer-Verlag; 1993:540–543.

Welch K. The intracranial pressure in infants. *J Neurosurg*. 1980;52:693.

25

ELECTROPHYSIOLOGY

Danielle Hulsebus, Martha Mangum, and Paul Park

Which is more important, the brain or the heart? Despite the continued debate among experts in each respective field, science does not have the answer; however, we do know that each organ can affect the other. In this chapter, a quick review of electrophysiology is presented. Though basic, this will help the reader feel more confident in dealing with common cardiac rhythms that may occur in patients with neurologic conditions.

As first reported in a study completed in 1947, electrocardiographic (ECG) changes may occur in up to 90% of patients with cerebrovascular disease (Saritemur et al., 2013). Serious arrhythmias may occur in approximately 5% of patients with subarachnoid hemorrhage—most commonly atrial fibrillation or atrial flutter (Katsanos et al., 2013). Other ECG changes to be aware of include inverted T waves, prolonged QT interval, ST elevation or depression, supraventricular tachycardia, and ventricular fibrillation (Greenberg, 2006). Though there is no definitive reason why these changes occur, it is likely related to the sympathetic nervous system being activated by a surge of catecholamines during the initial neurologic injury (Saritemur et al., 2013). This provides support for the idea that cardiac monitoring may be beneficial in alerting the medical team to abnormalities, and that the team should be familiar with common cardiac rhythms that may occur.

Cardiac monitoring review

A P wave represents atrial depolarization and contraction. Typically, P waves are positive (upright) in leads I, II, aVF, V4–V6, usually positive but may vary in leads III and aVL, and are generally negative (inverted) in lead aVR (Jacobson et al., 2007).

A QRS complex represents depolarization of ventricular myocardium/beginning of ventricular contraction. Typically the complex is positive in leads I, II, III, aVR, aVF, V4–V6, negative in aVR, V1–V2, and biphasic in V3 (Mills, 2005). A significant Q wave (at least 0.4 seconds or more in duration) may indicate myocardial infarction has occurred (Mills, 2005).

The ST segment is the horizontal segment of the baseline that follows the QRS complex. This represents the initial phase of ventricular repolarization. Acute ST segment elevation or depression is usually a sign of serious pathology (Dubin, 2000). This should prompt further workup and consideration of consultation by the cardiology service. Consultation is important, because elevation or depression of the ST segment may represent injury to the myocardium or can indicate myocardial ischemia (Jacobson et al., 2007).

The T wave represents the final phase of ventricular repolarization (Jacobson et al., 2007). It is usually positive in leads I, II, V2–V6, negative in aVR, and variable in leads III and V1 (Mills, 2005). Inverted T waves are considered the characteristic sign of myocardial ischemia (Dubin, 2000). Tall, peaked, or tented T waves may represent hyperkalemia or myocardial injury (Mills, 2005).

Sinus rhythm

Sinus rhythm is characterized by normal P waves and a normal QRS (Figure 25.1). The rate is between 60 and 100 beats per minute. These beats are typically regular but can vary with respiration or can occur early if a premature atrial contraction (P wave) occurs. This can be a normal variance, and there is no need for treatment.

Sinus bradycardia

Sinus bradycardia is characterized by a rate of less than 60 beats per minute, although in certain individuals, such as extreme athletes, a rate less than 60 may be normal. ECG characteristics will be similar to sinus rhythm but at a slower rate (Figure 25.2). Possible causes include hyperkalemia, hypothyroidism, hypothermia, Valsalva maneuver, obstructive sleep apnea, and acute myocardial infarction. Medications such as opiates, beta-blockers, and calcium channel blockers may also be contributing factors to bradycardia. Two important causes to consider, especially in neurosurgical patients, are spinal shock and increased intracranial pressure (ICP). Increased ICP should be considered when sinus bradycardia occurs in patients with altered neurologic function. Bradycardia can occur in the later stages of progressive elevated ICP as part of the Cushing response (Hickey, 2003). Cushing triad includes hypertension, bradycardia, and respiratory irregularity. Although the full triad is seen in only approximately 33% of patients with increased ICP (Greenberg, 2006), it is important to fully assess the patient when you receive a call regarding bradycardia.

Sinus bradycardia is usually asymptomatic. However, symptoms such as hypotension, altered mental status, dizziness, blurred vision, chest pain, or syncope may occur. Intervention is usually not necessary as long as the patient is asymptomatic and the other vital signs are stable. If present, consider obtaining a 12-lead ECG, chest x-ray, and laboratory workup including electrolytes and thyroid studies; assess the patient for the above symptoms. The medication list should be reviewed. If the patient is symptomatic, identify and correct the underlying cause (Mills, 2005). Medications to increase heart rate may be required if the patient is symptomatic.

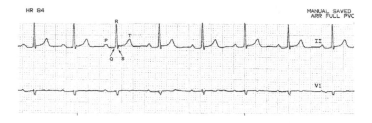

Figure 25.1   Sinus rhythm.

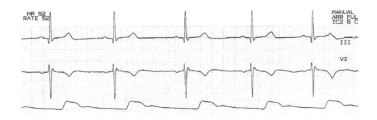

Figure 25.2   Sinus bradycardia.

Sinus tachycardia

Sinus tachycardia can be a common finding in hospitalized and postsurgical patients. ECG characteristics include uniform P waves, fixed P-R intervals, and a rate of greater than 100 beats per minutes (Figure 25.3). P waves may increase in amplitude as the heart rate increases, and the P wave may be superimposed on the preceding T wave, making it difficult to identify (Mills, 2005). Sinus tachycardia is often a response to a systemic illness (Marino, 2007). Possible causes include infection/inflammation, hypovolemia, bleeding/anemia, pain, hyperthyroidism, anxiety, pulmonary embolism, hypotension, shock, or adrenergic drugs.

Sinus tachycardia is often asymptotic, but it is important to assess the patient for signs/symptoms related to the above causes. If you receive a page regarding tachycardia in a patient, assess the patient for symptoms including dizziness, syncope, shortness of breath, chest pain, and palpitations. The primary goal of management is to identify and treat the associated illness (Marino, 2007). Although it usually occurs without serious adverse effects, prolonged tachycardia can be serious, as it may lower cardiac output (Mills, 2005).

After assessing the patient, consider obtaining a 12-lead ECG, as well as a laboratory workup including complete blood count (CBC), electrolytes, troponin, thyroid studies, blood cultures, and urinalysis. Also consider obtaining scans for deep vein thrombosis, and chest imaging to rule out pulmonary embolus. It is also important to review input/output status and the patient's medication list.

Atrial fibrillation

Atrial fibrillation is the most common cardiac arrhythmia in the general population, and approximately 15% of patients have no predisposing conditions (Figure 25.4) (Marino, 2007). ECG characteristics of atrial fibrillation include absent P waves, a wavy baseline, and an irregular QRS response (Dubin, 2000). Causes of atrial fibrillation may include failure to resume beta-blocker therapy after surgery (Marino, 2007), valvular heart disease, hyperthyroidism, coronary artery disease, acute myocardial infarction, hypertension, and chronic obstructive pulmonary disease (Mills, 2005). It may also occur in someone who is fatigued or under stress (Mills, 2005). Symptoms may include hypotension, lightheadedness, and chest pain.

If atrial fibrillation is uncontrolled, the patient can be at risk for heart failure, myocardial ischemia, or syncope. If left untreated for a period of time, atrial fibrillation can lead to thrombus formation,

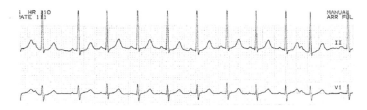

Figure 25.3   Sinus tachycardia.

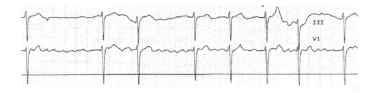

Figure 25.4   Atrial fibrillation.

putting the patient at risk for systemic atrial or pulmonary embolism (Mills, 2005) and ischemic stroke (Marino, 2007). Acute management should focus on controlling the heart rate. Other treatment strategies may include cardioversion and anticoagulation. Preferred agents for rate control include calcium channel blockers and beta-blockers. When called to assess a patient with an irregular rhythm (if not on a monitor), a 12-lead ECG should be obtained, and consider moving the patient to a telemetry bed. The patient should be assessed for chest pain, lightheadedness, and shortness of breath. Obtain a laboratory workup to include CBC, electrolytes, and thyroid studies. A surface echocardiogram should also be considered, as well as a cardiology consult. Since anticoagulation may be contraindicated, primary management will focus on rate control. However, since these patients may require anticoagulation at some point, it is important to have this discussion with the attending provider.

Ventricular tachycardia

Ventricular tachycardia (VT) is characterized by a widened QRS without significant P waves, as the origin of each beat is not originating from the sinus node (Figure 25.5). The rate is typically greater than 100 beats per minute and is regular in presentation. Possible causes include underlying electrolyte abnormalities or underlying cardiac disease. As previously mentioned, some studies link certain neurologic conditions to reversible ventricular systolic dysfunction (Saritemur et al., 2013). There may often be difficulties in distinguishing whether the presenting rhythm is truly VT. The QRS pattern should be analyzed and compared to the QRS pattern previously seen in sinus rhythm. If the QRS pattern is altered in the suspected rhythm, then it is suggestive of VT. If the rhythm is able to be captured in all leads, there should be concordance of the QRS waves, which is diagnostic of VT.

Prior to a detailed assessment, it is necessary to assess the patient and determine if the individual is stable (without symptoms) or unstable (with symptoms or have lost consciousness). If the patient is unstable, Advanced Cardiac Life Support (ACLS) guidelines should be initiated and followed. If the patient is stable, obtain an ECG, laboratory workup for electrolyte and troponin levels, and expert advice for further management. An echocardiogram will determine if the patient's myocardium has decreased function.

Common pitfalls

- Not visually assessing the patient at bedside
- Forgetting to review patient history, not reviewing medications/labs that could be causing electrophysiologic changes, not looking at entire clinical picture including net fluid balance
- Not comparing new ECGs/rhythm strips to previous ones (Dubin, 2000)
- Not consulting other medical teams if further help is needed

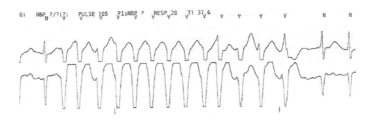

Figure 25.5 Ventricular tachycardia.

Relevance to the advanced practice health professional

It is important to have an understanding of ECG changes that can affect neurology and neurosurgery patients. A basic knowledge of electrophysiology and what to do when changes occur will better prepare advanced practice providers and members of the medical team in caring for these patients.

Common phone calls, pages, and requests with answers

- *Sinus bradycardia*: Assess symptoms and signs of patient including elevated ICP, vitals, and ECG; review medications.
- *Sinus tachycardia*: Assess symptoms and signs of patient including pain, vitals, ECG, and fluid status; review/obtain labs.
- *Atrial fibrillation*: Assess symptoms and signs of patient, vitals, and ECG; review/obtain labs (especially electrolytes); initially focus on rate control; and consider cardiology consult and surface echocardiogram.
- *Ventricular tachycardia*: Assess symptoms and signs of patient—if symptomatic, proceed with ACLS guidelines; if asymptomatic, obtain ECG, labs (especially electrolytes and troponins), and echocardiogram; consider cardiology consult.

References

Dubin D. *Rapid Interpretation of EKG's: An Interactive Course*. 6th ed. Tampa, FL: Cover Publishing; 2000.

Greenberg MS. *Handbook of Neurosurgery*. 6th ed. New York, NY: Thieme; 2006.

Hickey JV. *The Clinical Practice of Neurological and Neurosurgical Nursing*. 5th ed. Philadelphia, PA: Lippincott Williams & Wilkins; 2003.

Jacobson C, Marzlin K, Webner C, Cardiovascular Nursing Education Associates. *Cardiovascular Nursing Practice: A Comprehensive Resource Manual and Study Guide for Clinical Nurses*. Burien, WA: Cardiovascular Nursing Education Associates; 2007.

Katsanos AH, Korantzopoulos P, Tsivgoulis G, Kyritsis AP, Kosmidou M, Giannopoulos S. Electrocardiographic abnormalities and cardiac arrhythmias in structural brain lesions. *International Journal of Cardiology*. 2013;167:328–334.

Marino PL. *The ICU Book*. 3rd ed. Philadelphia, PA: Lippincott Williams & Wilkins; 2007.

Mills EJ, ed. *ECG Interpretation: A 2 in-1 Reference for Nurses*. Ambler, PA: Lippincott Williams & Wilkins; 2005.

Saritemur M, Akoz A, Kalkan K, Emet M. Intracranial hemorrhage with electrocardiographic abnormalities and troponin elevation. *American Journal of Emergency Medicine*. 2013;31:e5–e7.

26

CEREBROSPINAL FLUID DRAINAGE

Vincent J. Alentado and Michael P. Steinmetz

Case vignette

During your daily rounds, you check on the lumbar drain from a patient who is now 1 week postop from a lumbar laminectomy. His postoperative course was complicated by a cerebrospinal fluid (CSF) leak at the site of the surgical wound. The nurse tells you now that the drainage system has been collecting cerebrospinal fluid at a constant 10 mL/hr. You ask the patient about any postural headaches or focal weaknesses. When he denies any complaints, you examine the patient, being careful to inspect for any continued drainage from the cerebrospinal fluid cutaneous fistula (Figure 26.1).

Epidemiology

Cerebrospinal fluid (CSF) leaks are a relatively rare clinical manifestation for neurosurgical patients. Cranial CSF leaks are most commonly caused by head trauma, especially basilar skull fracture. Ten percent of head injuries are associated with basilar skull fracture, and 2% are associated with CSF leaks (Lewin, 1954, p. 1). Thus, the occurrence of CSF leak following basilar skull fracture is not infrequent. Traumatic cranial CSF leaks typically occur within 48 hours of injury, and 95% are recognized within 3 months of injury (Zlab et al., 1992, p. 316). In children, the incidence of CSF leak occurs in only 1% of closed head injuries due, in part, to the lack of development of air sinuses in children (Shulman, 1972). In regard to the spine, most CSF leaks are postoperative following incidental durotomy. The incidence of CSF leak requiring reoperation following spinal surgery is 0.3%, but this rate increases following more complex operations (Mayfield, 1976, p. 435).

Societal significance

Persistence of CSF leaks may lead to multiple complications, thereby significantly increasing patient morbidity and possibly mortality. CSF leaks may result in meningitis, pseudomeningocele formation, intracranial hypotension, neural element herniation, cranial nerve compression, fistula formation, and wound infection. Both cranial and spinal CSF leaks are usually treated with lumbar drainage. CSF leak requiring lumbar drainage is associated with prolonged hospitalization and increased health-care costs. When nonoperative management fails, CSF leak often requires surgical repair, which is associated with further increases in costs and a significant psychosocial burden on patients. Furthermore, a delay in lumbar drainage allows better formation of the fistula and increases risks for infection.

Basic biologic and physiologic processes

The pressure within the subarachnoid space exceeds that of nearby tissues, thereby causing CSF to drain into surrounding tissues when there is a defect in the dura. In the spine, this fluid often creates a fistula

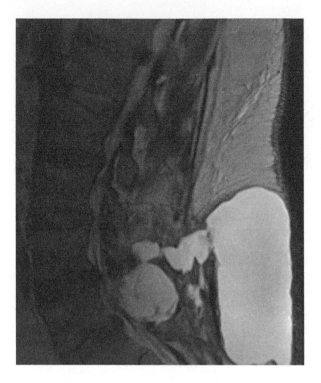

Figure 26.1 Postoperative CSF leak following lumbar laminectomy.

with the skin. In the cranium, the fluid usually flows through the porous sinuses within the skull. By draining CSF at a similar rate that it is being made, pressures within the central nervous system (CNS) are kept lower, and the path of least resistance for fluid becomes the catheter drainage site, rather than the area of the original defect. This allows the arachnoid and dura mater time to repair themselves without high-pressure fluid keeping the defect patent.

Anatomical review

Three layers of meninges cover the central nervous system. The outermost layer is the dense, fibrous dura mater. Intracranially, the dura mater is connected at several points to the cranial periosteum. The dura also descends through the foramen magnum to cover the spinal cord. The arachnoid mater is the middle sheath that loosely joins the dura mater. There is a potential space between the dura and arachnoid layers called the subdural space. The pia mater creates the innermost layer of the meninges. The pia mater is connected to the arachnoid mater by fine trabeculae. Between the arachnoid and pia mater is a true space called the subarachnoid space. The subarachnoid space is filled with CSF, which provides protection and nutrition to the CNS.

Common physical examination findings

During CSF drainage, it is extremely important to assess for signs of continued CSF leak from the fistula site. Some common physical exam signs associated with persistent CSF leak are as follows:

- The reservoir sign, or the ability for a patient to produce CSF by positioning the head in a certain way, is specific, but not sensitive, for a CSF leak with pooling in the sphenoid sinus.

- The target sign refers to a pseudochromatographic pattern produced by the differential diffusion of CSF admixed with blood or other serosanguinous fluid on absorbent surfaces. CSF has a tendency to migrate farther away from the leakage site, while blood remains more central.
    - This may be unreliable in cranial CSF leaks because nasal secretions admixed with blood exhibit the same phenomenon.
- Intracranial hypotension from persistent CSF leak may produce headache relieved by reclining, anosmia, optic nerve lesions, impaired vestibular function, facial nerve palsy, and cochlear damage.

Patients with lumbar drainage should be examined for signs of meningeal irritation such as nuchal rigidity, photophobia, and headache. Other tests for meningeal irritation include Kernig and Brudzinski signs.

- Kernig sign is positive when the hip and knee are bent at a 90° angle, and extension of the knee is painful.
- Brudzinski sign is positive when lifting the head of a supine patient causes flexion of the hips.

Warmth or redness around the leak is concerning for superimposed wound infection.

Relevant diagnostic tests

1. **Laboratory**
    - Glucose in CSF is equal to or exceeds 50% of serum glucose concentrations except in periods of meningitis, after subarachnoid hemorrhage, and a few select other cases.
    - Beta-2 transferrin is a specific marker for CSF.
2. **Vascular/Electrophysiologic**
3. **Radiologic**
    - Typically, no radiographic examination is required for monitoring CSF drainage. However, a variety of imaging modalities may be used to monitor for persistence of CSF leak or formation of pseudomeningocele.
    - Contrast cisternography with computed tomography or magnetic resonance imaging can be used to provide dynamic flow information.

Review of relevant interventional procedures and surgeries

Persistent CSF leaks are associated with significant morbidity and neurologic deficit and therefore must be treated aggressively. Initial management includes proper patient positioning. In intracranial leaks, the patient should have his or her head elevated from 40° to 75°. In spinal leaks, the patient should lay flat in bed. If these initial measures are unsuccessful after a predetermined period of time, often 24–72 hours, CSF diversion is often the next step in management. This intervention is usually curative; however, if the etiology of the leak is secondary to mass effect or hydrocephalus, the drain is only a temporizing measure.

The treating physician places a lumbar drainage catheter when indicated. In order to insert a lumbar drainage catheter, a 19-gauge catheter is threaded percutaneously through a 17-gauge Tuohy needle that has been inserted into the lumbar subarachnoid space. After 10–20 cm of the catheter tubing has been threaded rostrally, the needle may be removed over the catheter. The proximal end of the catheter should be connected to a closed, sterile drainage system. An occlusive dressing should be applied to the drainage site, and the catheter should be taped to the patient to prevent disconnection. After percutaneous insertion of the subarachnoid drain, 120–360 mL of CSF is drained per day for 3–5 days.

Drainage should be continued 3–5 days after stoppage of the leak to allow for adequate healing. If leakage reoccurs or does not improve with drainage, operative repair is indicated. The use of antibiotics in these clinical situations remains controversial. Daily samples of CSF may be acquired, cultured, examined by Gram stain, and analyzed by cell count with differential, glucose, and protein. This practice, however, is not standard.

After removal of the catheter, a single stitch can be performed to prevent a new CSF-cutaneous fistula. A new leak at the site of drainage can also be sealed with an injection of 10–20 mL of autologous blood, known as an epidural blood patch.

Common grading schemes

There are no well-recognized grading schemes for CSF drainage. Rather, drainage rate is based on the amount of CSF production. Typically, the brain creates and absorbs 20 mL of CSF per hour. Therefore, the typical rates for draining CSF are 7.5–15 mL/hr.

Family counseling

Prognosis

CSF drainage alleviates a CSF leak in 90%–100% of cases (Shapiro and Scully, 1992, p. 241). However, there are some associated complications with this procedure. The risk of infection following drain placement is roughly 10%; 2.5% of patients develop meningitis; 5% acquire discitis; and 2.5% develop a wound infection (Shapiro and Scully, 1992, p. 241). Transient nerve root irritation occurs in 24% of patients, but this often resolves after drain removal. Catheter blockage has been reported in 10% of patients (Findler et al., 1977, p. 456). However, this has become less common with the development of Teflon and silicone catheters.

Common question

How long is CSF drainage continued before operative intervention is required?

Depending on the etiology of the original CSF leak, the length of drainage will vary. If the leak is due only to a defect in the dura, a trial of 2–3 days is usually warranted to assess for any decreases in CSF leakage at the original site before surgical intervention is required.

Pitfalls

An important factor in alleviating CSF leaks through lumbar drainage is early detection of the original leak. After the leak has been identified, appropriate drainage monitoring is key in successful treatment. Overdrainage of CSF can cause life-threatening pneumocephalus, while underdrainage can cause persistence of the leak. Furthermore, acute reduction of CSF pressure may result in headache, nausea, and vomiting. This can typically be prevented through gradual lowering of the pressure and increasing drainage to the target rate over the course of several days.

Common pitfalls and medicolegal concerns

- Early detection of CSF leaks and early insertion of lumbar drainage catheter are key factors in improving prognosis in patients with CSF leaks.
- An abnormal CSF content on laboratory analysis should prompt administration of broad-spectrum antibiotics. This is not standard and is considered optional.

Relevance to the advanced practice health professional

An important factor in achieving favorable outcomes following CSF drainage is early detection of the CSF leak, and early catheter placement. Advanced practice health professionals are often the first health-care providers to examine postoperative wound drainage, so a high index of suspicion is needed for detecting CSF leakage. Patient interviews and physical exams are then paramount in monitoring adverse effects of CSF drainage, such as meningitis or other infection.

Common phone calls, pages, and requests with answers

- *How can the rate of CSF drainage be changed?*
  - Depending on devices available at your institution, drainage rates are determined by a rate-controlling device on the CSF receptacle itself or by gravity alone. To adjust drainage rates in a gravity-controlled device, the device may be moved lower down or higher to increase or decrease flow, respectively.
- *Does a patient with a lumbar drain need to be kept on his or her side to prevent disruption of the drain?*
  - Fortunately, patients with lumbar drains may remain lying on their backs with the lumbar drain in place. If this causes the patient discomfort, the patient may be resituated, or padding can be placed between the patient and the drainage hose.
- *How can a headache during lumbar drainage be treated?*
  - When a patient has a significant headache during lumbar drainage, it is first important to rule out secondary causes of the headache, such as infection. If the headache is directly related to the CSF drainage, medical management such as caffeine and nonnarcotic pain medications should be attempted first. If these fail to alleviate the headache, drainage rates may be temporarily lowered and increased again over the next several hours, as tolerated by the patient.

References

Findler G, Sahar A, Beller AJ. Continuous lumbar drainage of cerebrospinal fluid in neurosurgical patients. *Surg Neurol.* 1977;8(6):455–457.

Lewin W. Cerebrospinal fluid rhinorrhoea in closed head injuries. *Br J Surg.* 1954;42(171):1–18.

Mayfield FH. Complications of laminectomy. *Clin Neurosurg.* 1976;23:435–439.

Shapiro SA, Scully T. Closed continuous drainage of cerebrospinal fluid via a lumbar subarachnoid catheter for treatment or prevention of cranial/spinal cerebrospinal fluid fistula. *Neurosurgery.* 1992;30(2):241–245.

Shulman K. Late complications of head injuries in children. *Clin Neurosurg.* 1972;19:371–380.

Zlab MK, Moore GF, Daly DT, Yonkers AJ. Cerebrospinal fluid rhinorrhea: a review of the literature. *Ear Nose Throat J.* 1992;71(7):314–317.

27

SPINE SURGERY WOUND AND DRAIN MANAGEMENT

Christine Orlina Macasieb and Praveen V. Mummaneni

Most incisions are closed under primary intention. For skin closure, staples, sutures, Steri-Strips, and surgical adhesive are commonly used. In some cases a drain may be inserted in a location separate from the surgical incision. Common drains utilized in neurosurgery are closed-suction drains, gravity drains, lumbar subarachnoid drains, extraventricular drains, and subgaleal drains. Theoretically, the general purpose of drains is to remove excess exudate and blood products in order to prevent formation of fluid collections. Another purpose of drains is to eliminate dead space to prevent infection. Fluid collections and infection both have potential to cause neurological compromise.

Wounds should be kept under sterile dressing for the first 24–48 hours after surgery and kept dry to heal. Wounds should be checked periodically for symptoms of infection. Proper hand hygiene and aseptic technique before and after subsequent dressing changes should be observed (Mangram et al., 1999, p. 114; Owens and Stoessel, 2008, p. 8.) Topical antimicrobials are not recommended for surgical wounds closed by primary intention. It is advisable to wait 48 hours after surgery for showering. If wound cleansing is indicated, it should be done so with sterile saline (National Collaborating Centre for Women's and Children's Health, 2008).

When a drain is utilized, the amount of suction should be determined based on the site of the drain, and it is imperative to evaluate in the acute postoperative period, the patient's neurosensory motor exam, incision checks, patency, and duration of drain. Depending on the medical facility, an x-ray may be necessary to check for any retained foreign bodies after drains are removed.

Common pitfalls and medicolegal concerns

There is no gold standard regarding drain management. Surgeons place drains based on the type of the surgery, length of operating time, and patient variables such as anticoagulation medications; however, use of drains remains primarily at the discretion of the surgeon (von Eckardstein et al., 2015). The use of drains has not conclusively shown to be advantageous in decreasing complications such as infection rates or hematoma formation (Sohn et al., 2013, p. 582; Walid et al., 2012; Kanayama et al., 2010, p. 2692; Poorman et al., 2014). Some studies suggest an association between drains and acute blood loss anemia and frequency of blood transfusion postoperatively (Walid et al., 2012, p. 566). There are no guidelines regarding the use of antibiotics for drain prophylaxis. Some suggest prolonged duration of drain use may be an independent risk factor for surgical site infections after spinal fusion (Rao et al., 2011, p. 689).

Relevance to the allied health-care professional

With much variability in practice, it is important for the allied health-care professional (AHP) to understand and identify trends in the standards of practice of the surgeon, the health-care facility, and the specific patient population. Early identification of wound and drain complications are of utmost concern to the AHP. Common complications related to wound healing and drain management include the following:

- Wound infection, dehiscence
- Hematoma and seroma formation
- Cerebrospinal fluid leak and/or pseudomeningocele formation
- Neurological or hemodynamic compromise (Walid et al., 2012)

Common phone calls, pages, and requests with answers

1. *The patient calls on postoperative day 7 with concern for erythema around the wound. There is serosanguinous drainage from the incision as well as swelling and increased warmth around the wound.*

   Surgical site infections are of utmost concern to the AHP. The incidence of surgical site infections ranges from 1% to 14% (Radcliff et al., 2015, p. 337). Surgical site infections are also the most common cause of readmission (McCormack et al., 2012, p. 1261). Ultimately, surgical site infections increase length of stay and hospital costs (De Lissovoy et al., 2009; Owens and Stossel, 2008, p. 4). Many guidelines can be referenced in regard to perioperative care and prevention and treatment of surgical site infections. It is important to identify your hospital protocols regarding measures to prevent surgical site infections, such as preoperative showering, hair removal with clippers, and perioperative antibiotic prophylaxis (NCCWCH, 2008). It is also vital for the AHP to identify patient factors that can increase the risk of surgical site infection such as diabetes, nicotine use, chronic steroid use, age, poor nutritional status, coincident remote site infections, prolonged hospital stay, and perioperative transfusion of blood products (Mangram et al., 1999, p. 105). According to Werner et al. (2011, p. 143), clinical presentation and diagnostic workup involves the following:
   - Inspecting the wound for increased pain, erythema, and drainage.
   - Evaluating for any constitutional symptoms such as fever or chills.
   - Asking patients about pets in the home. Remind patients and caregivers to avoid close contact with animals until the sutures are removed. For instance, do not sleep with dogs, cats, or any other pets.
   - Pursuing lab workup, including white blood cell count (WBC), C-reactive protein (CRP), and erythrocyte sedimentation rate (ESR). Obtain a wound/fluid culture if indicated.
   - Obtaining magnetic resonance imaging (MRI) if indicated.
   - Considering empiric antibiotic treatment if infection is suspected. According to a review by Meredith et al. (2012, p. 440), *Staphylococcus aureus* and coagulase-negative staphylococcus are the most common causative bacteria causing surgical site infections. Equally important is to consider local resistance patterns and microbiologic data when choosing empiric therapy (NCCWCH, 2008).
   - Ensuring a follow-up incision check is scheduled for the patient.
   - Consulting a wound care specialist if applicable.
2. *It is postoperative day 3, and the patient complains of new-onset positional headaches. On examination, the patient is diaphoretic. Pain improves when the patient lies flat. Drain output appears clear or straw colored. Incision remains dry and intact.*

Intraoperatively, most dural tears are identified and repaired. The onset of cerebrospinal fluid (CSF) leak symptoms may be delayed. In addition to postural headache, CSF leak symptoms include photophobia, nausea, and vomiting.

- Rule out etiologies such as orthostatic hypotension, dehydration, migraine, and caffeine withdrawal.
- Evaluate labs, medications, and drain output trends.
- Consider testing drain fluid for beta-2 transferrin to differentiate CSF leak.
- Consider MRI evaluation of CSF leak.
- Use initial conservative treatment including hydration, caffeine, and bed rest. A lumbar subarachnoid drain may be inserted to divert CSF (Khazim et al., 2015).

3. *It is postoperative day 1 and the nurse notes that the dressing is saturated and drain output is high, greater than 50 mL/hr of sanguinous fluid. Vital signs indicate tachycardia and hypotension. Additionally, the patient is somnolent and appears pale.*
- Inspect the wound and ensure drains are patent and functioning properly.
- Strip drains per hospital protocol, as clots can develop and fluid may track around the drain or through the incision.
- Review past medical history and laboratory evaluation for anemia, coagulopathy, and nutritional deficiencies. High drain output can be associated with age, number of level, nicotine use, length of surgery, and corpectomies (Basques et al., 2014, p. 730).
- Reconcile medications taken presurgery, such as nonsteroidal anti-inflammatory drugs (NSAIDs), and anticoagulants.
- Trend daily labs and transfuse as indicated for acute blood loss anemia.
- Consider taking JP drains off suction and, instead, drain to gravity if the patient develops acute blood loss anemia.

4. *Does my patient need to be on antibiotic prophylaxis while drains are in place?*

Preoperative broad-spectrum antibiotics are recommended to decrease risk for infection in neurosurgery. However, there are currently no evidence-based data regarding dosing regimens or the recommended duration of antibiotics intraoperatively and postoperatively (Watters et al., 2009, p. 144.) First-generation cephalosporins such as cefazolin are effective against staphylococcus bacteria, and vancomycin can be used for those with an allergy to penicillins or those colonized with methicillin-resistant *S. aureus* (MRSA) (Meredith et al., 2012, p. 441). There is insufficient evidence in and around antibiotic prophylaxis for wound drains (Shaffer et al., 2013). It is the authors' practice with drain use to administer cefazolin prophylaxis until postoperative day 3. Drains are typically removed by postoperative day 3.

References

Basques BA, Bohl DD, Golinvaux NS, Yacob A, Varthi AG, Grauer JN. Factors predictive of increased surgical drain output after anterior cervical discectomy and fusion. *Spine*. 2014;39(9):728–735.

De Lissovoy G, Fraeman K, Hutchins V, Murphy D, Song D, Vaughn BB. Surgical site infection: incidence and impact on on hospital utilization and treatment costs. *Am J Infect Control*. 2009;37:387–397.

Kanayama M, Oha F, Togawa D, Shigenobu K, Hashimoto T. Is closed-drainage necessary for single-level lumbar decompression?: review of 560 cases. *Clin Orthop Relat Res*. 2010;468(10):2690–2694.

Khazim R, Dannawi Z, Spacey K, et al. Incidence and treatment of delayed symptoms of delayed symptoms of CSF leak following lumbar spinal surgery. *Eur Spine J*. 2015;24(9):2069–2076. http://link.springer.com/article/10.1007/s00586-015-3830-4/fulltext.html.

Mangram AJ, Horan TC, Pearson ML, Silver LC, Jarvis WR, The Hospital Infection Control Practices Advisory Committee. Guideline for prevention of surgical site infection. *Am J Infect Control*. 1999;27(2):97–134.

McCormack RA, Hunter T, Ramos N, Michels R, Hutzler L, Bosco J. An analysis of causes of readmission after spine surgery. *Spine J*. 2012;37(14):1260–1266.

Meredith DS, Kepler CK, Huang RC, Brause BD, Boachie-Adjei O. Postoperative infections of the lumbar spine: presentation and management. *Int Orthop*. 2012;36(2):439–444.

National Collaborating Centre for Women's and Children's Health (UK). *Surgical site infection: prevention and treatment of surgical site infection*. London: RCOG Press. http://www.ncbi.nlm.nih.gov/books/NBK53739/(accessed August 26, 2017). Published October 2008. (NICE Clinical Guidelines, No. 74) 7, Postoperative phase.

Owens CD, Stoessel K. Surgical site infections: epidemioloogy, microbiology, and prevention. *J Hosp Infect*. 2008;70(suppl 2):3–10.

Poorman CE, Passias PG, Bianco KM, Boniello A, Yang S, Gerling MC. Effectiveness of postoperative wound drains in one- and two-level cervical spine fusions. *Int J Spine Surg*. 2014. http://www.ncbi.nlm.nih.gov/pmc/articles/PMC4325495/.

Radcliff KE, Neuser AD, Millhouse PW, et al. What is new is the diagnosis and prevention of spine surgical site infections. *Spine J*. 2015;15:336–347.

Rao SB, Vasquez G, Harrop J, et al. Risk factors for surgical site infections following spinal fusion procedures: a case-control study. *Clin Infect Dis*. 2011;53(7):686–692.

Shaffer WO, Baisden JL, Fernand R, Matz PG. An evidence-based clinical guideline for antibiotic prophylaxis in spine surgery. *Spine J*. 2013;13:1387–1392.

Sohn S, Chung CK, Kim CH. Is closed-suction drainage necessary after intradural primary spinal cord tumor surgery? *Eur Spine J*. 2013;22:577–583.

Von Eckardstein KL, Dohmes JE, Rohde V. Use of closed drain suction devices and other drains in spinal surgery: results of an online, Germany-wide questionnaire. *Eur Spine J*. 2015;25(3):708–715. http://link.springer.com/article/10.1007%2Fs00586-015-3790-8.

Walid MS, Abbara M, Tolaymat A, et al. The role of drains in lumbar spinal fusion. *World Neurosurg*. 2012;77(3–4):564–568.

Watters WC, Baisden J, Bono CM, et al. Antibiotic prophylaxis in spine surgery: an evidence-based clinical guideline for the use of prophylactic antibiotics in spine surgery. *Spine J*. 2009;9:142–146.

Werner BC, Shen FH, Shimer A. Infections after lumbar spine surgery: avoidance and treatment. *Semin Spine Surg*. 2011;23:142–150.

28

NEUROLOGIC MONITORING

Michael Y. Wang and Gregory Basil

Case vignette

A 24-year-old patient was involved in a fall from scaffolding. He initially presented with a Glasgow Coma Scale (GCS) score of 14 (E = 4, M = 6, V = 4) and was conversant and following commands in the emergency room. Because of a left temporal skull fracture and large scalp hematoma, he was admitted to the close neurologic monitoring unit. Three hours after admission, he was found by the nursing staff to be minimally responsive with a GCS of 6 (E = 2, M = 3, V = 1), and his left pupil was blown.

An emergency computed tomography (CT) scan was obtained (Figure 28.1) showing a large epidural hematoma. The patient was taken emergently to surgery for a craniotomy for hematoma evacuation. Due to the early detection of neurologic decline, he made a rapid recovery and was discharged with a GCS of 15 to rehab due to gait instability.

Introduction

The care of neurologic, neurosurgical, and spinal patients differs markedly from the care of other critically ill hospital patients. While the layperson and generally trained health professional are likely well aware of the need to monitor respiratory and cardiac functions, the monitoring of neurologic function remains less well appreciated or understood. This is due to several factors, including the following:

1. The automation of standard cardiac and respiratory functions (e.g., heart rhythm and oxygen saturation monitors) with defined parameters for alerting abnormalities in physiologic deviation is common, but this is extremely difficult with neurologic function.
2. The subtleties in neurologic dysfunction are often detectable only with experience or attention to detail.
3. There is a wide variety of baseline neurologic function, and the interpretation of an examination in the appropriate context requires clinical judgment.
4. The neurologic examination will vary for any given patient depending on numerous factors (e.g., fatigue, intoxication, and medication).

Nevertheless, the onset of neurologic deterioration is in no way less important or impactful, as minutes and hours of delay can lead to devastating loss of function or even death (e.g., "brain attack" or "stroke alert").

Thus, many tertiary care hospitals have enveloped neurologic monitoring units. These have been classified variably as step-down units, close neurologic monitoring units, and neuroepilepsy monitoring units, just to name a few (Atkinson et al., 2012). The shared competency in these units is an experienced

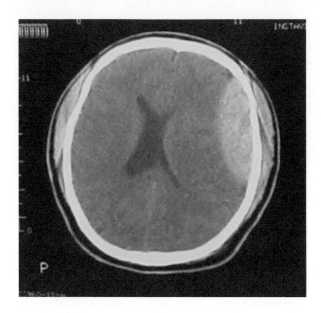

Figure 28.1   Large left-sided epidural hematoma.

nursing team that can recognize early deterioration in neurologic function to allow for early intervention. These units may also possess competencies in epilepsy recording, seizure prevention and treatment, bedside CT scanning (Figure 28.2), tracheostomy care, neurologic rehabilitation, transcranial Doppler recording (Figure 28.3), ventricular and lumbar drain management, mobilization (Kocan and Leitz, 2013), and hemodynamic support. Furthermore, the widespread need for acute postoperative pain control and the sedative effects of opioids make this a common setting for the postoperative spinal patient.

While the intensive care unit (ICU) setting is clearly indicated for particular patients, the close monitoring unit also serves a critical role in the tertiary care hospital. Particular conditions that require close neurologic monitoring include the following:

*   Step-down from a higher level of care such as a Neuro-ICU setting (due to acuity and bed constraints or lack of long-term care for a comatose patient)
*   Monitoring for intracranial hypertension
*   Assessment of a hematoma at risk of expansion
*   Management of lumbar or ventricular drain
*   Care of chronic subdural drain
*   Care of tracheostomy
*   Monitoring for cerebral vasospasm after subarachnoid hemorrhage
*   Care of the spinal patient requiring special pain control or at risk of epidural hematoma
*   Use of video epilepsy recording (Figure 28.4)
*   Monitoring for minor procedures requiring sedation

Monitoring protocols

While somewhat variable, the typical neurologic examination takes place every 4 hours. More frequent checks may be needed, but generally checks every 2 hours would militate for ICU level of care. That being

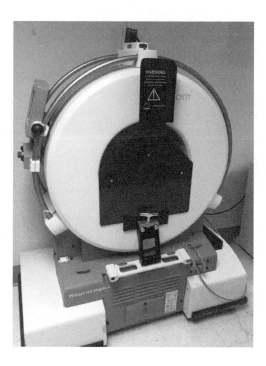

Figure 28.2   The portable mini-CT scanner, which allows patients to undergo a head CT without need for transport out of the safety of the Neuro-ICU.

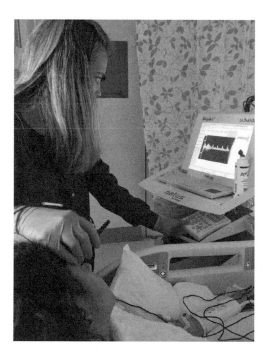

Figure 28.3   Transcranial Doppler ultrasound performed at the bedside daily to monitor for vasospasm following aneurysmal subarachnoid hemorrhage.

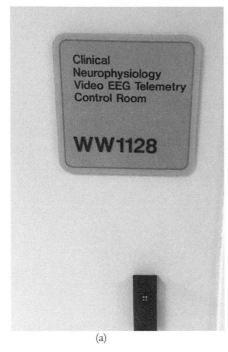
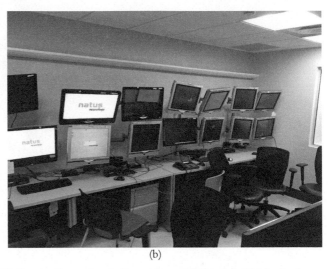

(a)　　　　　　　　　　　　　　　　　　　　　　(b)

Figure 28.4 (a) Video electroencephalogram (EEG) recording unit at Jackson Memorial Hospital. (b) Monitoring stations (without patient data being shown). The multiple flat-screen panels allow live monitoring and recording of a patient's vital signs, EEG tracings, and video of the actual patient.

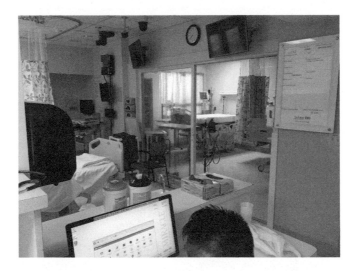

Figure 28.5 This neuromonitoring unit is typical with its "open" architectural structure that allows one nurse to simultaneously watch continuously over four beds.

said, the monitoring unit often places patients in an "open space" so that nearly constant observation is possible from a limited nursing staff. Much as a cardiac monitor functions continuously, this allows the nursing staff to detect neurologic emergencies such as a seizure with a minimum of delay (Figure 28.5). These units have become very popular as they allow for dual use as a close observation unit as well as a video EEG monitoring unit where seizure activity can be recorded, studied, and even induced in order to direct individualized patient treatments (Sethi et al., 2014).

Common pitfalls and medicolegal concerns

- Because the setting of a step-down unit shares features with the ICU (high patient acuity and risk of neurologic deterioration) yet often lacks the resources of an ICU (nurse-to-patient ratios and specialized monitoring equipment), the unit can be a high-stress environment for staff.
- Because minor procedures are commonplace, nursing and support staff are often asked to participate in the consent process under emotional and time pressures with family members. Nurses should be well-versed in the particulars of this process.

Relevance to the advanced practice health professional

Increasingly, advanced practice personnel are being asked to perform in an intermediary role in these settings. Whereas house staff were previously relied heavily upon, the expansion of neurologic care coupled with the reduction of training MD work hours has required midlevel providers to assume an ever more proactive and leadership role in these settings.

Common phone calls, pages, and requests with answers

- The intermediary role of the neuromonitoring unit requires that many decisions be made regarding triage. It is common that a request will be made to move a sick ICU patient into the unit, or to move a sick patient from the ward who needs an ICU bed into the unit. This requires decision making and prioritization. In addition, as an intermediary unit, when an ICU patient is moved in, another patient from the unit is often moved to the regular ward to make room. This doubles the amount of nursing effort (accepting a patient at the same time one is being transferred out). Flexibility is required in the decision making.
- Ventricular and lumbar drain management often become areas of contention. Your hospital will likely have a policy specifying whether these devices require ICU, step-down, or regular ward bed levels of nursing. In particular, there are issues with ventricular drain access for sampling (which should only be performed by those qualified for access) and lumbar drain kinking or dysfunction. Furthermore, like with many drains, care must be exercised to avoid inadvertent overdrainage by leaving them open, as they are a conduit directly to the central nervous system.
- In general, as presented in the case vignette, the monitoring unit will house patients who are at risk for deterioration. The fact that these patients are not in the ICU can make them especially vulnerable to complications. Thus, it is often best to err on the side of caution when assessing these patients. One should have a low threshold of going to see and examine them personally when called, or to order the appropriate imaging study.

References

Atkinson M, Hari K, Schaefer K, Shah A. Improving safety outcomes in the epilepsy monitoring unit. *Seizure.* 2012;21(2):124–127.

Kocan M, Leitz H. Special considerations for mobilizing patients in the neurointensive care unit. *Crit Care Nurs Q.* 2013;36(1):50–55.

Sethi N, Rapaport B, Solomon G. An audit of continuous EEG monitoring in the neurological-neurosurgical intensive care unit. *J Clin Neurophysiol.* 2014;31(5):416–417.

29

THE POST-ANESTHESIA CARE UNIT (PACU) ENVIRONMENT AND THE NEUROSURGICAL PATIENT

Luke R. Hattenhauer

Assessment of the neurosurgical patient in the PACU

Frequent and continued assessment of ABCs (airway, breathing, circulation)

- Airway reflexes, respiratory drive, and circulatory function may be reduced due to residual anesthetic agents and narcotics.
- ABCs may also be affected by neurosurgical pathology and/or surgical technique.
- The head–up position (15–30°), if appropriate, may improve oxygenation and facilitate venous drainage, thereby reducing intracranial pressure (ICP) (Bendo et al., 2001, p. 763).

Hemodynamic profile

- Blood pressure and heart rate abnormalities
- Cushing triad (hypertension, bradycardia, and respiratory disturbances)
- Invasive lines, catheters, and monitors

Neurologic assessment

- Mental status
- Neuromotor function (all extremities assessed), particularly important following spinal surgery
- Motor strength in the setting of recovery from neuromuscular blockade intraoperatively; incidence of postoperative weakness following neuromuscular blockade remains high despite routine pharmacologic antagonism by anesthesia clinicians
- Sensation
- Possibility of meningeal irritation (Windle, 2004, p. 810)
    1. Nuchal rigidity
    2. Light sensitivity (photophobia)
    3. Kernig sign: painful knee extension in setting of hip and knee flexion at 90° (Windle, 2004, p. 810)
    4. Brudzinski sign: passive flexion of neck results in hip and knee flexion (Windle, 2004, p. 810)

- Glucose monitoring: tight glucose control to assure accurate neurologic assessment (hypoglycemia) and prevent neuronal cell injury due to increased lactate production in setting of hyperglycemia (Bendo et al., 2001, p. 763)

Assessment of intracranial pressure

- Ongoing communication with neurosurgery and anesthesia regarding ICP readings in the PACU is imperative.
- There is a potential for rapid fluctuations in ICP during emergence from anesthesia due to pain, agitation, etc.
- Frequent adjustments may need to be made to the external ventricular drain (EVD) to maintain acceptable ICP readings.

Intake/Output

- Electrolyte derangements following neurosurgery are not uncommon and may be detected by close monitoring of intake/outputs.
- Diabetes insipidus and syndrome of inappropriate secretion of antidiuretic hormone (SIADH) can occur due to intracranial pathology or surgery near the pituitary stalk and/or hypothalamus.

Surgical site examination and location

- Certain spine and intracranial procedures are performed with the patient's head in tongs or pins.
- The patient may have multiple smaller surgical sites in addition to the main incision.
- A hematoma at the operative site may result in neurologic compromise and evolving neurologic deficits in the PACU (Windle, 2004, p. 811).

PACU Issues and the neurosurgical patient

Hypoventilation: Identify cause and manage accordingly

- Most general anesthetics cause some degree of hypoventilation. Ensure the airway is patent, and support ventilation with supplemental oxygen until the patient has completely emerged from anesthesia.
- Opioids cause significant respiratory depression. Conservative titration of opioids is imperative in the neurosurgical patient to provide for a reliable neurologic examination. If generous dosages of opioids have been administered, naloxone may be considered for reversal and improvement in ventilatory status.
- Severe elevations in ICP can manifest as irregular and/or inadequate respirations. This is often an ominous sign and may suggest impending brain herniation, requiring immediate attention (Morgan et al., 2002, p. 797).
- Central apnea can occur following posterior fossa surgery in which the respiratory centers have been damaged. This may require controlled mechanical ventilation (Bendo et al., 2001). Injuries to respiratory centers almost always manifests with hemodynamic changes as well.

Hypotension/Hypertension

- Strict blood pressure control in the PACU is important in the neurosurgical patient to maintain adequate cerebral perfusion pressure (CPP).
- It is particularly important to avoid hypertension following aneurysm repair (coiling or clipping).
- Neurosurgical patients often receive a conservative amount of IV fluid intraoperatively to reduce the risk of brain edema, particularly if elevations in ICP are present. This can occasionally result in an intravascular volume deficit and hypotension in PACU. Isotonic crystalloid fluid boluses may be administered in coordination with neurosurgery and anesthesia.
- Hypertension most commonly is the result of postsurgical pain and/or sympathetic nervous system activation resulting from surgery and anesthesia. This can be complicated in patients with chronic hypertension.
- Use diligent opioid titration if patient assessment suggests pain as the cause of hypertension.
- Elevations in ICP may result in a compensatory rise in blood pressure. Evaluate ICP, and treat accordingly.
- Bladder distension. If a urinary catheter is not in place, consider placement.
- If there is no identifiable cause of hypertension, blood pressure lowering agents may need to be administered. Consider beta-blockers, sodium nitroprusside, and nicardipine.

Agitation

- Postoperative agitation is not uncommon in the PACU and can be the manifestation of multiple factors, including the anesthesia itself.
- It is imperative that agitation be ameliorated as soon as possible to prevent associated elevations in ICP (and blood pressure).
- During emergence from anesthesia, pain, bladder distention, hypoxemia, surgical complication, and electrolyte abnormalities can often manifest as agitation.
- Ensure a calm, quiet environment.
- Avoidance of sedating pharmacologic agents in PACU is preferred to allow for continued neurologic assessment.
- Physical restraints may be needed to prevent the patient from dislodging drains and lines.

Nausea and vomiting

- Nausea and vomiting is a common problem following general anesthesia.
- Often, it is a side effect of opioids, volatile anesthetic gasses, and/or vagal stimulation.
- It can also be a sign of elevated ICP and/or meningeal irritation.
- It is important caution to consider a neurologic etiology of nausea and vomiting in this patient population.
- The act of vomiting can raise ICP to dangerous levels in the neurosurgical patient; thus, it is important to treat nausea aggressively.
- $5HT_3$ serotonin receptor antagonists (ondansetron, dolasetron) are effective at treating nausea and are nonsedating.
- Other antiemetics such as droperidol can cause significant sedation, limiting their use in the neurosurgical patient.

Shivering

- Shivering may result from hypothermia and/or volatile anesthetic agents. Other mechanisms are poorly understood but may be related to derangements in thermoregulation.
- Shivering less commonly can be due to neurologic abnormality, transfusion reaction, or allergic reaction.
- Shivering increases oxygen consumption and sympathetic nervous system activity, which may be harmful in patients with cardiopulmonary disease.
- Use warming blankets and warming lights.
- Meperidine 10–50 mg IV is very effective at reducing shivering; however, careful titration to avoid unwanted sedation is important.

Central diabetes insipidus (DI)

- Surgery and/or lesions near the hypothalamus and/or pituitary stalk can cause DI postoperatively due to alterations in ADH secretion.
- DI should be suspected in patients with polyuria (occasionally >6 L/day) with normal serum glucose and urine osmolality less than plasma osmolality.
- Treatment is with vasopressin or desmopressin (DDAVP), a synthetic analogue of ADH.

Scenarios in PACU with the neurosurgical patient

Acute ICP elevation

- It is imperative to pay close attention to ICP in the PACU.
- The patient may or may not report common clinical symptoms of elevated ICP due to residual anesthetic agents—headache, nausea, and vomiting (Rangel-Castillo et al., 2008, p. 524).
- Generally, ICP readings above 15 mm Hg are concerning and warrant prompt communication with neurosurgical and anesthesia teams.
- Ascertain that the monitor is set up and reading appropriately.
- If an EVD is present, check that the transducer is level at the external auditory meatus.
- Check that the EVD drainage point is at the appropriate level (per neurosurgical team order).
- Check for ICP waveform on the monitor.
- If not contraindicated, the head of the bed should be raised to 30° to promote drainage.
- Consider causes of elevated ICP: agitation, pain, straining, vasogenic edema, bleeding, cerebrospinal fluid (CSF) obstruction, and fluid shifts secondary to metabolic abnormality (Morgan et al., 2002, p. 568).
- Treatment is dependent on the suspected cause of elevated ICP.
- CSF may need to be drained via EVD.
- If mechanically ventilated, ventilator settings may be adjusted if hypercapnia is present.
- Bleeding may require a return to the operating room.
- Pain and agitation may be carefully treated with and without pharmacologic agents.
- Vasogenic edema may respond to corticosteroids (Morgan et al., 2002, p. 568).
- Osmotic diuresis with mannitol may be considered, along with furosemide, which also may decrease CSF production.
- Recent consideration has been given to the possibility that cervical collars may contribute to a rise in ICP due to the physical impedance of venous drainage caused by the collar (Stone et al., 2009, p. 102).

- ICP could also theoretically be elevated due to discomfort from the collar itself (Stone et al., 2009, p. 102).
- It is important to have an appropriately sized and well-fitted cervical collar to minimize the risk of raising ICP.

Recurrent laryngeal nerve injury

- Hoarseness in the PACU due to palsy of recurrent laryngeal nerve (RLN) following anterior cervical spine surgery may be observed.
- The RLN innervates the vocal cords and is involved in phonation.
- The cause of injury to the nerve may be multifactorial but is thought to be related to the position of surgical retractors intraoperatively (Jung et al., 2010, p. 12).
- RLNs originate bilaterally from the vagus nerves.
- Unilateral RLN injury may cause hoarseness to be seen in the PACU.
- Bilateral RLN injury may cause stridor and respiratory distress due to compromised innervation of the vocal cords.
- Injury or palsy to the nerve may be acute and resolve or may be permanent.
- Support of respiration and consultation with neurosurgery, anesthesiology, and ear, nose, and throat (ENT) may be needed.

Ophthalmologic injury

- Eye pain related to corneal abrasion can occur perioperatively due to lines or drapes coming into contact with the cornea while the patient is anesthetized.
- Patients often rub their eyes during emergence from anesthesia, inadvertently causing injury.
- Neurosurgical patients are sometimes positioned prone intraoperatively, which can increase the likelihood of an eye injury.
- Patients complaining of severe eye pain warrant communication with the anesthesia team, and may require a consultation with ophthalmology.
- Corneal abrasions generally heal relatively quickly but can be extremely painful depending on the severity.
- Ischemic optic neuropathy (ION) is much more severe and devastating, resulting in permanent vision loss postoperatively.
- ION is caused by ischemia to the optic nerve intraoperatively and may be related to hypotension and anemia due to blood loss.
- The prone position during spine surgery and prolonged surgical duration have also been implicated in ION.

CSF leak

- CSF leak can occur postoperatively anytime the dura is punctured intraoperatively.
- Any swelling at the surgical site should be investigated.
- Swelling could be due to hematoma or CSF leak.
- CSF leak following hypophysectomy may drain from the nose and appear as clear fluid.
- Suspicion of a CSF leak should prompt urgent communication with the neurosurgical team.

Autonomic dysreflexia

- Nonacute spinal cord injury (SCI) patients may exhibit autonomic dysreflexia in the PACU.
- Autonomic dysreflexia is generally seen in patients with transections at T5 or higher, while it is uncommon in those with injuries below T10.
- Eighty-five percent of SCI patients with injury above T5 will develop autonomic dysreflexia (Horlocker and Wedel, 2001, p. 1109).
- Stimulus below the level of injury can result in intense sympathetic activity without the inhibition from higher central nervous system centers.
- Surgical incision and distended bladder may cause autonomic dysreflexia.
- Severe vasoconstriction and hypertension associated with bradycardia are classic signs.
- Treatment mainstays are removal of stimulus, if possible, and administration of vasodilators.

Seizure

- Seizures occurring postoperatively in neurosurgical patients are often the result of insult to the neurologic tissue by surgery or pathology and/or metabolic derangements.
- Most general anesthetic agents used raise the seizure threshold.
- Onset of seizures in PACU can be an indicator of worsening neurologic condition.
- Selected neurosurgical patients will be given pharmacologic seizure prophylaxis perioperatively to reduce the risk of seizure.
- Prompt recognition and treatment of seizures in the PACU and support of airway, breathing, and circulation are imperative.
- Acute treatment of seizures in the PACU can be accomplished by administration of a benzodiazepine such as lorazepam. Phenytoin or fosphenytoin may also be considered.

Final considerations

- The condition of neurosurgical patients can change rapidly in the PACU.
- All caregivers must be extremely vigilant of the patient in the PACU.
- Communication with and among the neurosurgical and anesthesia teams is imperative regarding the patient's condition.
- The PACU team must be prepared to transport the patient emergently to the computed tomography scanner or other diagnostic locations should the patient's condition worsen acutely.

References

Bendo A, Kass I, Hartung J, Cottrell J. Anesthesia for neurosurgery. In: Barash P, Cullen B, Stoelting R, eds. *Clinical Anesthesia*. 4th ed. Philadelphia, PA: Lippincott Williams & Wilkins; 2001:743–781.

Horlocker T, Wedel D. Anesthesia for orthopedic surgery. In: Barash P, Cullen B, Stoelting R, eds. *Clinical Anesthesia*. 4th ed. Philadelphia, PA: Lippincott Williams & Wilkins; 2001:1103–1118.

Jung A, Schramm J. How to reduce recurrent laryngeal nerve injury in anterior cervical spine surgery: A prospective observational study. *Neurosurgery*. 2010;67(1):10–15.

Rangel-Castillo L, Gopinath S, Robertson C. Management of intracranial hypertension. *J Clin Neurol*. 2008;26(2):521–541.

Stone S, Tubridy C, Curran R. The effect of rigid cervical collars on internal jugular vein dimensions. *Acad Emerg Med*. 2009;17(1):100–102.

Windle, P. Neurologic surgery. In: Quinn D, Schick L, eds. *PeriAnesthesia Nursing Core Curriculum*. 1st ed. St. Louis, MO: Saunders; 2004:763–813.

PART V

Clinical Pathologies and Scenarios: The Brain

30

MILD TRAUMATIC BRAIN INJURY

S. Shelby Burks, Patrick Wang, and George Ghobrial

Case vignette

A 17-year-old female playing soccer goes for the ball and accidentally collides with a member of the opposing team. She does not lose consciousness but appears dazed. The coach calls her to the sideline. She becomes nauseated, then vomits. On questioning, she is answering questions appropriately but does not recall why she is on the field. She vomits a second time and is taken to the hospital where a computed tomography (CT) scan of the brain without contrast demonstrates a small area of traumatic hemorrhage in the left frontal lobe (Figure 30.1).

The patient is placed in observation, and a repeat scan done 6 hours later shows no changes. She is discharged and prescribed a 1-week course of prophylactic antiepileptic medication and short-interval follow-up with Neurology. She is able to return to school and normal activity in 1 month.

Overview

Epidemiology

Mild traumatic brain injury (mTBI) has been defined by multiple different organized bodies. This reflects the common nature of mTBI and range of medical personnel requested to treat patients with concussion. Probably the simplest definition comes from the American Academy of Neurology who defined concussion as "any trauma induced alteration in mental status that may or may not include a loss of consciousness" (Quality Standards Subcommittee, 1997). The Centers for Disease Control and Prevention (CDC) estimates anywhere from 1.6 to 3.8 million mTBIs occur annually. Of these about 10% will require hospitalization. About one-fifth of these head injuries can be attributed to sports; thus, a large proportion of patients are young. Other major contributors to mTBI include motor vehicle accidents, falls, and assaults.

Societal significance

In the last decade concussion has gained attention in mainstream media, specifically American football falling under scrutiny (Schulz et al., 2004). One group estimated U.S. football players to suffer from 1.5 concussions annually (Bailes and Cantu, 2001). Football has received much attention. but many other sports contribute to concussion in young people, and over half of high schoolers participate in organized sports. There is some evidence that younger age may be a factor contributing to worse outcomes after concussion, with high school athletes having memory impairment for 1 week and college athletes returning to normal within 24 hours (Field et al., 2003). Though evidence is not perfect, most experts believe the effects of concussion are additive. Athletes suffering from two or more concussions perform significantly worse on neurocognitive testing than their peers.

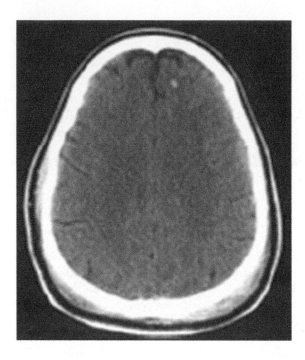

Figure 30.1 Noncontrast CT of the brain, axial view, demonstrating a small focal area of traumatic hemorrhage in the left frontal lobe. Gyri and sulci are easily identified as is the gray-white junction, suggesting there is no global edema. This finding can be seen in diffuse axonal injury.

Basic biologic and physiologic processes

Following a head injury, there is a brief, transient period of excitatory activity lasting for a few hours. This is followed by a metabolic depression lasting up to 1 month, and this has been demonstrated with positron emission tomography (PET) imaging studies (Bergsneider et al., 2000). Besides metabolic dysfunction, there is, unfortunately, a component of structural damage with mTBI (Raghupathi et al., 2000). This would fall on the spectrum of diffuse axonal injury, in which axonal shearing occurs on a microscopic level. With magnetic resonance imaging (MRI) scans, these diffuse axonal injuries can be detected; MRI scans are not routinely ordered in concussion (Figure 30.2).

Common physical examination findings

- The Glasgow Coma Scale (GCS) is commonly employed in evaluating TBI patients (see below). Mild TBI can be defined by GCS 13–15.
- In the case of basilar skull fractures, patients should be assessed for signs of cerebrospinal fluid leak. These may manifest as rhinorrhea or otorrhea, spinal fluid leaking from the nose or ear, respectively. Assistance from ear, nose, throat (ENT) colleagues will be especially helpful here—if a cerebrospinal fluid (CSF) leak is noted, these patients should be directed to the emergency room, as the risk of meningitis is high.
- After initial assessment and stabilization, whether in the field, clinic, or hospital, a neuropsychiatric assessment should be performed.

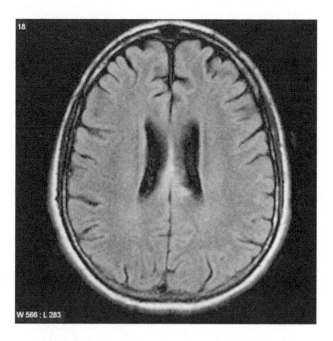

Figure 30.2 Fluid-attenuated inversion recovery (FLAIR) sequence MRI, axial view, showing hyperintensity in the corpus callosum (arrow). This can be seen in concussion and mTBI but is more common with moderate and severe brain injury. This is an example of diffuse axonal injury.

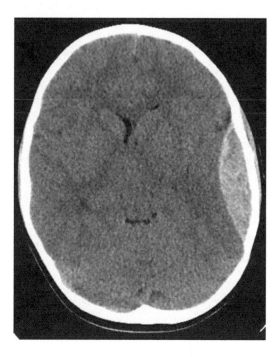

Figure 30.3 Epidural hematoma noted on plain CT of the brain. In certain cases of mTBI, following a lucid interval, patients can rapidly progress into a delayed coma with signs of herniation. Suspect development of an epidural hematoma.

Relevant diagnostic tests

- The first diagnostic decision in mTBI patients will be whether to obtain a head CT without contrast. Typically this decision will be based on patient comorbidities and neurologic exam. In a patient with a high-energy mechanism (motor vehicle collision [MVC], fall from height, assault, etc.), any neurologic deficit, or preexisting neurologic condition, it is likely safest to obtain a CT scan. Similarly in older patients or those taking antiplatelets or anticoagulants, a CT should be obtained.
- If the initial CT or exam raises suspicion for skull base fracture—a CT dedicated to the temporal bone should be obtained along with ENT consultation. Patients with temporal bone fractures require a dedicated otology exam and delayed audiogram.
- Routine laboratory testing can be performed on a case-by-case basis. Typically, at our institution, prothrombin time/international normalized ratio (PT/INR), partial thromboplastin time (PTT), basic metabolic panel (BMP), and complete blood count (CBC) are obtained in patients for whom a CT scan is ordered. Any abnormality in PT, PTT, or platelet function may need correction depending on CT findings. A platelet function assay (PFA) can be obtained in patients where platelet dysfunction is suspected. Note that routine laboratory analysis is important in workup of concussion.

Relevant interventional procedures and surgeries

- Fortunately, mTBI patients do not usually require any type of intervention.
- Certain types of hematomas can be seen in mTBI but are more common with moderate and severe injury. Usually in patients with concussion, small subdural or epidural hematomas are observed and do not require surgery, though the patient should undergo repeat CT scan to ensure no progression occurs (Figure 30.3).
- The use of an intracranial pressure monitor or external ventricular drain is not used in concussion. These devices are typically reserved for severe TBI.

Common grading schemes

The GCS is used to quickly convey information about a patient's clinical status/neurologic status after a head injury. The score runs from 3 to 15 and is scored as shown in Table 30.1.

Table 30.1 The Glasgow Coma Scale

Points	1	2	3	4	5	6
Motor	None	Extensor posturing	Flexor posturing	Withdraw *or* appropriate flexion	Localize	Following commands
Verbal	None	Moaning	Incomprehensible words	Confused	Appropriate speech	
Eye opening	None	Open to pain	Open to voice	Open spontaneously		

Family counseling

Prognosis

Typically, the prognosis for patients with mTBI is excellent, but there are certain issues patients should be aware of. Neurologic deterioration from a delayed hemorrhage is possible after concussion, but rare. In young patients, after they are observed for one night, the risk of delayed hemorrhage is exceptionally low. In older patients, mTBI can lead to formation of a chronic subdural hematoma, and in those patients with persistent headache or other progressive symptoms, CT imaging should be obtained. Parents of school-age children should be referred to a neurologist or primary care physician as students can develop headaches and concentration and memory difficulties. These are fortunately self-limited, and a full recovery should be expected.

Common questions

What should a parent watch out for after concussion? In the first 24 hours there is a small risk of delayed development of a hematoma that may require intervention. Family/parents should watch for lethargy, focal neurologic deficits, and persistent vomiting. Additionally, as previously mentioned, there is a small chance of basilar skull fracture with mTBI, which may present as CSF otorrhea or rhinorrhea, hearing loss, or possibly meningitis.

Is there any medication to prescribe? There is no medication to ameliorate the effects of concussion. In the case of any intracranial blood detected on CT, our practice is to prescribe AED for 1 week for seizure prevention.

When can the patient return to work? This depends on the age of the patient, severity of the injury, and nature of the work. In the case of a high school student, as mentioned previously, parents should wait about 2 weeks to 1 month before returning to full workload. This should be delayed if headache or cognitive difficulties present. Patients should be eased back into their workload.

Pitfalls

After mTBI, patients can typically be monitored for less than 24 hours, avoiding a costly hospital admission. If there is any concern such as neurologic deficit or lack of family support, there should be a low threshold of observational admission to a hospital with neurosurgical support.

Common pitfalls and medicolegal concerns

- Delayed hemorrhage may develop in a patient neurologically intact after mTBI, suggesting a role for further monitoring either at home or in the hospital.
- Any patient with coagulopathy or taking anticoagulant or antiplatelet medications should be evaluated in the hospital with a plain CT of the head, as these are high-risk patients.
- Skull fractures with CSF leak can lead to a disastrous development of meningitis if not recognized.

Relevance to the advanced practice health professional

The advance practice health professional will certainly play a role in evaluating the mTBI patient in the field, the emergency room, later in clinic, or over the phone answering questions. The ability to triage these patients will be immensely valuable, as they very seldom require neurosurgical intervention. Repeated mTBI must also be recognized as a disease that may lead to progressive long-term loss of neurologic function.

Common phone calls, pages, and requests with answers

- Neurology evaluation for assistance with the management of cognitive difficulties, headaches, or postconcussive epilepsy, as needed.
- Neuropsychiatric evaluation is routinely obtained in our institution after mTBI requiring admission, as are physical and occupational therapy.
- Patients with concussion should be discharged with appropriate pain medications, typically Tramadol or Tylenol with codeine can be used once the patient is deemed safe for discharge.

References

Bailes JE, Cantu RC. Head injury in athletes. *Neurosurgery.* 2001;48:26–45.

Bergsneider M, Hovda DA, Lee SM, et al. Dissociation of cerebral glucose metabolism and level of consciousness during the period of metabolic depression following human traumatic brain injury. *J Neurotrauma.* 2000;17:389–401.

Field M, Collins MW, Lovell MR, et al. Does age play a role in recovery from sports-related concussion? A comparison of high school and collegiate athletics. *J Pediatr.* 2003;142:546–553.

Quality Standards Subcommittee: American Academy of Neurology. Practice parameter: the management of concussion in sports. *Neurology.* 1997;48:581–585.

Raghupathi R, Graham DI, McIntosh TK. Apoptosis after traumatic brain injury. *J Neurotrauma.* 2000;17:927–938.

Schulz MR, Marshall SW, Mueller FO, et al. Incidence and risk factors for concussion in high school athletes, North Carolina, 1996-1999. *Am J Epidemiol.* 2004;160:937–944.

31

SEVERE TRAUMATIC BRAIN INJURY

George Ghobrial, Karthik Madhavan, and S. Shelby Burks

Case vignette

Subdural hematoma

A 40-year-old male arrived at an emergency department via ambulance. His vital signs are stable. Severe soft tissue bruising is evident on the left scalp. He was found down outside of a bar. The patient is withdrawing to painful stimuli without eye opening or verbal response. A decision was made to intubate the patient for airway protection. Given the poor neurologic examination with a correlative Glasgow Coma Scale (GCS) score of 6, computed tomography (CT) of the brain was obtained, revealing evidence of a small acute subdural hematoma on the left side, measuring 5 mm wide at the largest dimension at the level of the foramen of Munro, with 3 mm of rightward midline shift (Figure 31.1a). Subsequent attempts to wean the patient from sedation and wake the patient up from a neurologic exam were unsuccessful. A repeat CT scan was obtained, revealing enlargement of the subdural hematoma, measuring over 2 cm in diameter and 1 cm of resultant midline shift (Figure 31.1b).

Hyperosmolar therapy was administered, and the patient was taken immediately for a left-sided hemicraniectomy and evacuation of the subdural hematoma. An intraparenchymal monitor was also placed, and the patient was kept in the intensive care unit for cerebral perfusion pressure monitoring.

Diffuse axonal injury (DAI)

A 28-year-old male involved in a high-speed motor vehicle collision arrived in the emergency room by ambulance. A GCS of 4 was assessed at the site of the accident, which was in the automobile, where the individual was extricated. Intubation was performed onsite to ensure immediate airway protection. On examination in the emergency room, his pupils were sluggish, but reactive to light, with a symmetric response. No gag reflex was elicited. Extensor posturing to painful stimuli was evident. CT scan of the head was obtained (Figure 31.2a). No additional injuries were noted on secondary survey.

An intracranial pressure (ICP) monitor in the form of an external ventricular drain was placed. Aggressive ICP management and hyperosmolar therapy were instituted in the neurologic intensive care unit to maintain a cerebral perfusion pressure of 60–80 mm Hg. Neurologic recovery is variable and can occur over a period of months.

Epidemiology

Traumatic brain injury (TBI) is one of the most common causes of death in younger patients (Langlois et al., 2006). There are about 300 cases per 100,000 head injuries annually (Langlois et al., 2006). In the United States alone, 100,000 patients per year may require surgical intervention (Bullock et al., 2006). As

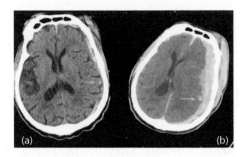

Figure 31.1 Computed tomography of the head, axial views, upon arrival (a, left) and 1 hour later (b, right) demonstrating growth in a left-sided acute subdural hematoma. Enlargement of a left posterior temporal contusion can be seen as well (arrows). Enlargement of a left-sided scalp hematoma can also be seen.

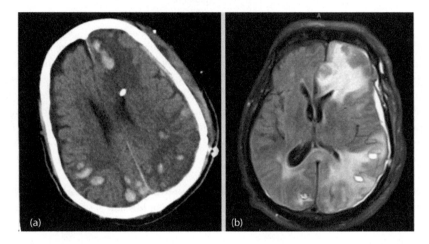

Figure 31.2 (a) Changes suggestive of diffuse axonal injury on noncontrasted CT, axial view, and magnetic resonance imaging (MRI). (b) MRI, fluid-attenuated inversion recovery (FLAIR) sequence study demonstrating multiple left-sided regions of hyperintensity corresponding to contusions.

per the Centers for Disease Control and Prevention (CDC), in 2010 there were 2.5 million emergency department (ED) visits for head injuries, 87% of which ($n = 2,213,826$) were evaluated and discharged directly from EDs, and 11% (283,630) were discharged from an inpatient setting. The mortality rate was estimated to be 2% (52,844). In addition, 34% are unable to return to work in 3–6 months. Depending on methodology, approximately $56 billion in medical expenses are thought to relate to TBI.

Societal significance

TBI affects all health and social aspects, including cognition, behavior, and physical abilities. CDC data note that about 3.2–5.3 million persons in the United States are living with a TBI-related disability (Langlois et al., 2006; Newacheck et al., 2004). Adolescents and adults affected by moderate or severe TBI who were discharged from rehabilitation facilities were more than twice as likely to die 3.5 years after injury compared to persons in the general population of similar age, sex, and race (Newacheck et al., 2004; Potoka et al., 2000). About 2 in 10 adolescents died at 5 years postinjury, and nearly 4 in 10 deteriorated from their level of function.

Basic biologic and physiologic processes

There are four types of associated pathologies that underlie severe TBI:

1. Subdural hematoma is most often due to venous injury of bridging veins found between the arachnoid and dura mater (Figure 31.3).
2. Epidural hematoma results from arterial injury superficial to the dura mater. Therefore, arterial injury is often related to middle meningeal artery injury and its distal branches. This is often related to squamous temporal bone fracture (Figure 31.4).
3. Traumatic subarachnoid hemorrhage is the most common form of hematoma related to TBI, resulting from venous injury between the pia and arachnoid mater, in the subarachnoid space. It is important to understand that rarely, aneurysmal subarachnoid hemorrhage could be masked by the trauma setting, and these findings should be recognized.
4. Diffuse axonal injury is one of the most severe forms of TBI where there is disassociation between the axons and the cell bodies, revealed as loss of gray-white differentiation. This also produces elevated ICPs but can be controlled with medical management. The recovery is often very prolonged (Figures 31.4 and 31.5 and Table 31.2).

Common physical examination findings

Examination of patients sustaining severe TBI is mainly directed by the GCS. This affords a quick and efficient communication between emergency practitioners. When assessing a patient's response to stimuli,

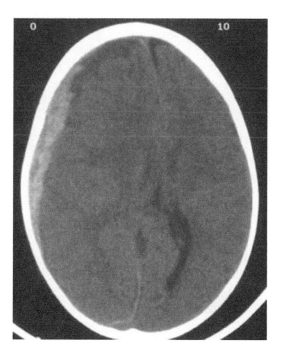

Figure 31.3 CT, axial view; right subdural hematoma is evident. These hematomas are described as "crescentic" in shape and layer the entire surface of the brain and are not bound by suture lines.

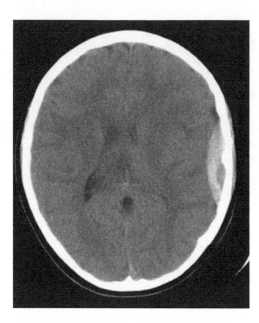

Figure 31.4 Computed tomography, axial view of the head, demonstrating an epidural hematoma (EDH). EDH is usually associated with a temporal bone fracture with damage to the middle meningeal artery. EDH is classically described as "lentiform" in shape as they do not cross suture lines, giving them a biconvex shape.

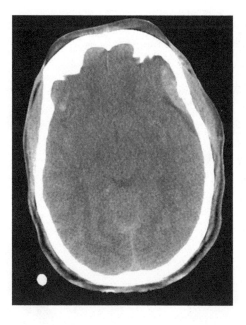

Figure 31.5 CT, axial view of the head, showing loss of gray–white differentiation. The junction between the gray and white matter is less evident due to diffuse cerebral swelling. Sulcal effacement and effacement of the basal cisterns describe conditions at which spaces that normally are filled with cerebrospinal fluid are not visible because of brain swelling, an indirect measure of elevated ICP.

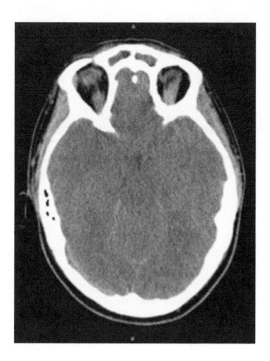

Figure 31.6 CT, axial view of the head, demonstrating effacement of basal cisterns. No visible cerebrospinal fluid (CSF) spaces are clearly seen.

central stimulation should precede peripheral stimulation via the supraorbital notch or sternum. A full examination of the neurologic patient is beyond the scope of this chapter.

It is essential to understand that a poor neurologic exam, which can be defined as less than or equal to a GCS of 8, may necessitate the placement of an ICP monitor. The inability to wean sedation or even in a timely manner to allow for a full and reliable physical examination should prompt the examiner to consider ICP monitor placement (Table 31.1).

Table 31.1 Glasgow Coma Scale

	1	2	3	4	5	
Eye	Does not open eyes	Opens eyes in response to painful stimuli	Opens eyes in response to voice	Opens eyes spontaneously	N/A	N/A
Verbal	Makes no sounds	Incomprehensible sounds	Utters incoherent words	Confused, disoriented	Oriented, converses normally	N/A
Motor	Makes no movements	Extension to painful stimuli (decerebrate response)	Abnormal flexion to painful stimuli (decorticate response)	Flexion/ withdrawal to painful stimuli	Localizes painful stimuli	Obeys commands

Note: The corresponding numeric value from each row is added to obtain a total score between 3 and 15.

Relevant diagnostic tests

Laboratory

Complete blood count is performed to evaluate his hemoglobin, white count, and platelets. Also coagulation and liver profile need to be checked, as patients who are alcoholic or have clotting deficiencies need consideration. Patients with poor hepatic and renal functions will not be able to clear drugs from their systems, potentially leading to prolonged muscle blocking agent action. Serum basic metabolic profile must be acquired to see the sodium, potassium, and renal function with creatinine and blood urea nitrogen. Consider a platelet function assay (PFA) if the patient takes antiplatelet medications or has a history of liver dysfunction.

Vascular/Electrophysiologic

Along with a plain CT scan of the brain, routine vascular imaging of the arteries in the head and neck can be done to rule out any underlying dissection or rupture. This should be considered for high-energy mechanisms such as a fall from a building or a motor vehicle collision. Nontraumatic findings such as arteriovenous malformations and aneurysms can be excluded, when indicated. Electrophysiologic monitoring is not performed unless there is a concern for subclinical seizure activity, or if the sustained injury does not correlate with the magnitude of the examination findings. Muscle twitch monitors can be utilized to determine whether a patient with no motor response is still under the effect of paralytic agents, often used prior to intubation.

Radiologic

All patients with a history of head injury presenting to the emergency department require a CT scan to evaluate the brain. In the presence of radiographic findings suggestive of any of the aforementioned pathologic findings, a cervical spine CT should be obtained as well, in the opinion of the author, regardless of GCS. Numerous literature reports document a high incidence of concomitant cervical spine injury in the setting of TBI. MRI of the brain is not necessary in the management of TBI. MRI may be performed later, however, to evaluate DAI (see Case 2). Edema in the corpus callosum or white matter tracts, along with punctate hemorrhaging, is suggestive of DAI on CT and is usually seen on MRI, regardless of CT findings. This is best appreciated on FLAIR sequence of the MRI, which is a fluid-attenuated sequence as shown in Figure 31.2b.

Review of relevant interventional procedures and surgeries

Neurosurgery is a critical element in the management of severe brain injury. In a patient with a GCS less than 8, an ICP is often required. External ventricular drains can be inserted at the bedside using sterile technique (Table 31.4).

The other major intervention performed in severe TBI is a decompressive craniectomy where the bone is left out of the head. These are often done from subdural hematoma with midline shift in a comatose patient. With epidural hematomas, on the other hand, the bone can often be replaced as injury to the underlying brain is not usually as severe.

Common grading schemes

Table 31.2 Grading of Diffuse Axonal Injury

DAI grade	Description
Mild	• Coma >6–24 hours, followed by mild-to-moderate memory impairment, mild-to-moderate disabilities, moderate coma
Moderate	• >24 hours, followed by confusion and long-lasting amnesia; mild-to-severe memory, behavioral and cognitive deficits severe
Severe	• Coma lasting months with flexor and extensor posturing; cognitive, memory, speech, sensorimotor, and personality deficits; dysautonomia may occur

Table 31.3 Marshall Grading of Brain CT after Trauma

Type	CT finding
Diffuse type I	• No visible pathology on CT imaging
Diffuse type II	• Cisterns present and <5 mm of midline shift
	• No mass lesion >25 mL
Diffuse type III	• Cisterns compressed or absent
	• Midline shift 0–5 mm
	• No mass lesion >25 mL
Diffuse type IV	• Midline shift >5 mm
Type V	• Any lesion surgically evacuated
Type VI	• Mass lesion >25 mL

Table 31.4 Management of Intracranial Pressure—American College of Surgeons Guidelines

	Elevated intracranial pressure (>20 mmHg)
Tier 1	• Ensure PCO_2 35–45
	• Normothermia
	• Elevate head of bed to 30°
	• Ensure appropriate analgesia and sedation with benzodiazepines and opioids
	• Evaluate abdomen and legs to ensure venous return not compromised
	• Drain CSF
	• Repeat CT head (CTH)
Tier 2	• Hyperosmolar therapy
	• Consider lowering PCO_2 goal 30–35
	• Repeat CTH
	• Neuromuscular paralysis
Tier 3	• Decompressive hemicraniectomy
	• Barbiturate coma
	• Hypothermia

Family counseling

Prognosis

Multiple factors help determine the prognosis of patients suffering from severe TBI. From a large cohort of TBI patients, the strongest predictors of outcome included age, postresuscitation GCS score, pupillary reactivity, portion of time with ICP above 20 mm Hg, presence of hypotension, and initial findings on CT brain (Ruff et al., 1993; Becker et al., 1997). Early death within 48 hours of injury has been correlated with the following: age over 65, posturing on examination, fixed and dilated pupils, presence of shock, and a Marshall grade greater than III on CT scan (Table 31.3) (Boto et al., 2006).

Common questions

Typically, families will ask about prognosis and return to function. Using some of the above criteria in patients who are young without evidence of hypotension who are able to follow commands at some point after their injury can usually be expected to have a reasonable recovery. Patients over age 65 who came into the emergency room hypotensive and extensor posturing have a much lower likelihood of returning to function.

Pitfalls

Families very often want numbers and specifics about their loved one. Health-care practitioners can make assessments and estimates but can run into issues with definitive predictions. All severe TBI is dangerous and potentially deadly; thus, family should know this.

Common pitfalls and medicolegal concerns

1. Patients can deteriorate in the after severe TBI and should be monitored in the intensive care unit.
2. Hypotension can be disastrous, and a mean arterial pressure of 80–100 is recommended to prevent ischemia. In the presence of an ICP monitor, cerebral perfusion pressure between 60 and 80 is desired. The cerebral perfusion pressure is defined as the mean arterial pressure minus the intracranial pressure.
3. An ICP monitor should be placed in patients with a GCS of 8 or less or who will not have an exam for an extended period of time in the setting of acute trauma with TBI. One common example is for a patient with the presence of a nonoperative intracranial hemorrhage in need of immediate stabilizing surgery, often in the trauma setting. In this scenario, ICP monitoring would be one way to continue monitoring the patient while receiving anesthesia.
4. Identification of coagulopathy from family or patient-provided history or from routine laboratory testing of coagulation should be obtained as expediently as possible prior to any neurosurgical intervention.

Relevance to the advanced practice health professional

Advanced practice health professionals can play an important role in the management of severely head injured patients. These particular patients require constant attention and will be a shared responsibility between all members of the neurosurgical team. Understanding the importance of having a continuous neurologic exam in the acute setting is important. A continuous neurologic exam can mean that the patient is readily able to have a neurologic exam without a prolonged wait or is able to be monitored by ICP monitoring.

Common phone calls, pages, and requests with answers

1. Common phone calls from any team member aiding in the multidisciplinary support of these patients. It is important that the needs of every member of the team be relayed to the primary team leader, patient (when able), and the main family contact. Often, confusion due to lack of communication between teams during the evolving acute care period is unavoidable to a degree.

2. Pages from emergency room departments, nursing staff, the trauma bay, radiology, and critical care teams require a prompt reply to ensure that care is expedited.

3. Intensive care teams evaluating the severe TBI patient will spend a significant amount of time with these patients. They will have calls to update the plan of care. It is important that this care be relayed to the primary team, and vice versa.

References

Becker DP, Miller JD, Ward JD, Greenberg RP, Young HF, Sakalas R. The outcome from severe head injury with early diagnosis and intensive management. *J Neurosurg.* October 1977;47(4):491–502.

Boto GR, Gomez PA, De La Cruz J, Lobato RD. Severe head injury and the risk of early death. *J Neurol Neurosurg Psychiatry.* September 2006;77(9):1054–1059.

Bullock MR, Chesnut R, Ghajar J, et al. Surgical management of acute subdural hematomas. *Neurosurgery.* March 2006;58(suppl 3):S16–24; discussion Si-iv.

Langlois JA, Rutland-Brown W, Wald MM. The epidemiology and impact of traumatic brain injury: a brief overview. *J Head Trauma Rehabil.* September–October 2006;21(5):375–378.

Newacheck PW, Inkelas M, Kim SE. Health services use and health care expenditures for children with disabilities. *Pediatrics.* July 2004;114(1):79–85.

Potoka DA, Schall LC, Gardner MJ, Stafford PW, Peitzman AB, Ford HR. Impact of pediatric trauma centers on mortality in a statewide system. *J Trauma.* August 2000;49(2):237–245.

Ruff RM, Marshall LF, Crouch J, et al. Predictors of outcome following severe head trauma: follow-up data from the Traumatic Coma Data Bank. *Brain Inj.* March–April 1993;7(2):101–111.

32

CHRONIC SUBDURAL HEMATOMA MANAGEMENT

Aminul I. Ahmed and M. Ross Bullock

Case vignette

Mr. Jones, an 88-year old gentleman, was climbing up some steps and lost his balance, hitting the side of his head. He sustained a small right-sided scalp laceration and had a slight headache, but given his fiercely independent nature, did not seek any medical help. His headache improved, and he continued with normal activity.

Two weeks later, Mr. Jones noticed a return of his headache. Over the course of the next 3 days, the severity increased, and he noticed that he was getting increasingly clumsy with his left hand. The next day, his family noticed he was dragging his left foot at times. They noticed a lack of concentration and some intermittent confusion. He was taken to the emergency room (ER), where the physician requested a computed tomography (CT) scan based on the history of trauma and symptoms. Imaging revealed a right-sided chronic subdural hematoma (CSDH) (Figure 32.1), and he was transferred to the neurosurgical ward. He was taken to the operating room for burr hole evacuation of his CSDH.

Overview

Epidemiology

CSDH is the most common neurosurgical disorder. Its incidence is around 1–2 per 100,000 per year, but this is predicted to grow to 17 per 100,000 per year by 2030 (Balser et al., 2015). More than four-fifths of patients are over 40 years old, and the peak incidence of the disease is in the eighth decade. Operating on CSDH is one of the most effective neurosurgical treatments in those over 80 years old.

Societal significance

Although acute subdural hematomas are regarded as neurosurgical emergencies, CSDH is regarded as a benign disease of the elderly. It is the most common neurosurgical procedure, and with an aging population, will increase in the coming years. This is coupled with an increased use of anticoagulants and the increased risk of falls in an elderly population. Patients who have an increased alcohol intake have a greater risk, since alcohol-associated brain atrophy is coupled with liver dysfunction, impaired coagulation, and frequent falls. An actual trauma is remembered by two-thirds of patients or their families. Due to age and frailty, patients may not be easily discharged to home and therefore may require placement in a skilled nursing facility or acute inpatient rehabilitation.

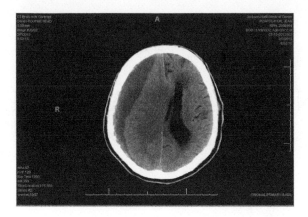

Figure 32.1   Axial CT scan shows a right-sided CSDH. Mass effect results in midline shift.

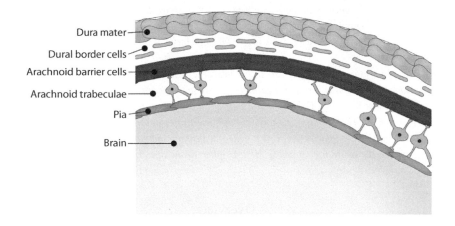

Figure 32.2   The meningeal layers. Between the tough dura mater and the arachnoid barrier cells is the dural border cell layer. Cells in this layer are loosely connected, and it is into this layer where a subdural hematoma typically forms.

Basic biologic and physiologic processes

CSDH is most common in the elderly. This is partly due to brain atrophy with aging. The bridging veins from the dura to the brain surface become taut. Hence, they are vulnerable to tearing and bleeding following mild trauma, especially if the patient is on anticoagulants. The most common layer into which the blood tracks is the loose dural border cell layer, and it can track freely across the whole hemisphere. As the space fills with blood, the bleeding is tamponaded and the blood clots. The acute clot triggers fibroblast migration and the forming of membranes around the clot, which walls off the hematoma. The membrane consists of an inner membrane against the brain surface, and a thicker vascular outer membrane against the dura. Over the coming weeks, the solid clot liquefies, and the membrane stabilizes (Cecchini, 2017). The new vessels in the outer membrane are thought to intermittently hemorrhage leading to perpetuation of the hematoma. The liquid clot can exert a mass effect leading to symptoms, and the patient may require surgical intervention (Figures 32.2–32.4).

Anatomical review

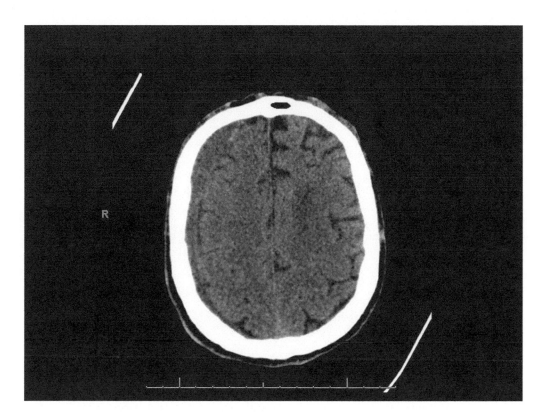

Figure 32.3   The CSDH is typically cresenteric in shape.

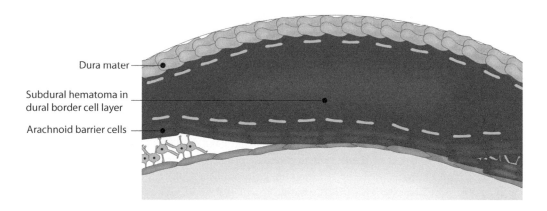

Figure 32.4   The CSDH forms in the dural border cell layer.

Common physical examination findings

Similar to stroke but has gradual onset:
- Contralateral hemiparesis (arm or leg)
- Gait problems
- Confusion, lack of concentration
- Speech problems (if CSDH over dominant hemisphere)
- Pronator drift—sensitive test

Rarely (less than 10%)
- Drowsiness
- Falling Glasgow Coma Scale (GCS)

Relevant diagnostic tests

1. Laboratory studies
    a. Complete blood count (CBC)
    b. Full chemistry (include liver function tests [LFTs] if alcohol abuse suspected)
    c. Coagulation panel
    d. Type and screen
    e. ECG
    f. Cardiac echo (if cardiac dysfunction)
2. Radiologic
    a. Noncontrast CT head
    b. Rarely, magnetic resonance imaging (MRI)

Review of relevant interventional procedures and surgeries

Treatment is occasionally conservative with serial CT scans. This would be indicated for small CSDH with no symptoms and no evidence of mass effect or midline shift on CT. The potential use of oral steroids, such as oral dexamethasone, is currently not standard practice but may be used. It has to be weighed against the risks of the medication (e.g., gastrointestinal bleeds or hyperglycemia), especially in the elderly population. Several trials are underway to confirm if dexamethasone is of benefit (NCT02111785 on clinicaltrials.gov and 13/15/02 on www.nets.nihr.ec.uk). Serial imaging can be employed every few weeks to determine resolution. Elderly patients, who are unfit for surgery, would also be managed conservatively.

If there are any symptoms or signs, or there is significant mass effect with midline shift, then surgical intervention is warranted. Surgical options are threefold and can be performed under local or general anesthesia. If a patient is at risk for general anesthesia, is compliant and not confused, local anesthesia is an option.

The first, least invasive method is a twist drill craniostomy (Chari et al., 2014), which can be performed at the bedside. It is least invasive but has the highest chance of recurrence and reoperation. A twist drill is used to make a craniostomy in the skull, usually at the most rostral portion of the CSDH. A drain is placed in the subdural space and left for up to 7 days under gravity. One such device is the Subdural Evacuating Port System (SEPS) (Chari et al., 2014), which is designed for use at the bedside.

The most common procedure is the burr hole evacuation of the CSDH. Burr holes are typically 10–30 mm in diameter. Usually, two are performed, one frontal and one parietal (but dependent on the exact location of the CSDH). This allows irrigation of the CSDH with warm saline. This is by far the most common method, since it balances the recurrence rate and invasive nature of the operation. Evidence suggests that a drain for 2 days reduces the subsequent recurrence risk (Santarius et al., 2009). If the patient is compliant, or perhaps too sick for a general anesthesia, this can be performed under local anesthesia, although a general anesthesia is the preferred option.

The third method, which is sometimes used, is a mini-craniotomy (>20 mm). This is usually under a general anesthetic and used if there is a recurrence (10%–20%), if the SDH is not fully liquid, or if there are multiple membranes. This is the most effective but is more invasive resulting in a higher morbidity.

Common grading schemes

The definition between acute, subacute, and chronic subdurals is arbitrary. In the Brain Trauma Foundation guidelines, an acute subdural is less than 14 days postinjury, with anything greater than that classified as a chronic subdural. On CT imaging, an acute subdural is hyperdense, a subacute subdural is isodense to the brain parenchyma, and a chronic subdural is typically hypodense.

Family counseling

Prognosis

The prognosis for CSDH is excellent. Postoperatively, flat bed rest (24–48 hours usually) is indicated. Often patients are confused so prove a challenge for the nursing staff. Regular contact and a familiar face help attenuate this.

Common questions (based on personal experience)

- When (if at all) they should restart anticoagulation after a CSDH. This is variable, but generally, low molecular weight heparin (LMWH) can be commenced for prophylaxis the next day, with 6 weeks a rough rule of restarting oral anticoagulation (usually after a late interval scan).
- When can the staples or sutures come out? Usually after 5 days.
- When can they fly? When there is no air on the CT scan. Usually after 10 days.
- Do we need a rescan? Only if there are symptoms. But some physicians prefer an interval scan especially if anticoagulation is to be restarted.
- Are there alternatives to surgery?

Pitfalls

Beware queries regarding anticoagulation. Deep vein thrombosis (DVT) prophylaxis will likely start postoperatively but may seem counterintuitive to the family. An explanation of balancing the risks may be advised.

Common pitfalls and medicolegal concerns

- Anticoagulation (warfarin, heparin, rivaroxaban, dabigatran).
- Elderly population.
- Complications include reaccumulation, tension pneumocephalus, seizures, empyema, wound infection, and an acute SDH.
- The recurrence rate is 10%–20%.

- If patients are routinely imaged after the operation, there is likely to be a persistent collection at 10 days. If the patient has improved clinically, it is not necessary to routinely scan. Scan if the patient deteriorates clinically or fails to improve after surgery.
- Keep the drain below head level so as to drain out fluid and prevent a pneumocephalus. It is a sub-dural-external drain, with *no* suction, and a closed drainage system. If the drain output is less than 25–30 mL in 24 hours, then it can be removed.

Relevance to the advanced practice health professional

The patient course postoperatively usually entails flat bed rest while the drains remain in situ (48 hours usually), primarily to facilitate expansion of the brain, encourage drainage, and reduce the accidental removal of the drain. In a confused patient, this may prove challenging for the nursing staff. Regular contact and a familiar face help attenuate this. After drain removal, the patient can be sat up and gently mobilized, and discharged when safely mobilizing (if this was achievable pre-CSDH). Immediately postoperatively, ensure judicious use of pain relief, especially opiates. Since patients are often frail, be aware that early nutrition, removal of lines and catheters, skin checks, and chest physiotherapy can avoid secondary complications.

Common phone calls, pages, and requests with answers

- *There has been a change in conscious level, the patient is sleepier.*
  - Were any pain medications given? What is the neurologic finding, including pupils, GCS, speech, and motor function? If there is a drop in neurologic function, the patient needs to be examined by the doctor.
- *When can the patient transfer out of the intensive care unit?*
  - If the patient is stable and alert, and can be managed with a lower level of nursing care.
- *When can the medications stop?*
  - If the patient is on antiepileptic medication, and if the patient has had a seizure, a neurology appointment needs to be arranged after discharge prior to stopping. If the medication is prophylactic, it can stop after 1–2 weeks. Stopping prophylactic anticoagulants is variable and at the discretion of the attending physician.
- *The drain is not draining.*
  - Even if there is no drainage, ensure that the drain is below the patient's head level, a minimum of 24 hours with the drain is recommended, with the strongest evidence suggesting 48 hours (Santarius et al., 2009).

References

Balser D, Farooq S, Mehmood T, Reyes M, Samadani U. Actual and projected incidence rates for chronic subdural hematomas in United States Veterans Administration and civilian populations. *J Neurosurg.* 2015;123:1209–1215. doi:10.3171/2014.9.JNS141550.

Cecchini G. Chronic subdural hematoma pathophysiology: a unifying theory for a dynamic process. *J Neurosurg Sci.* 2017;61(5):536–543.

Chari A, Kolias AG, Santarius T, Bond S, Hutchinson PJ. Twist-drill craniostomy with hollow screws for evacuation of chronic subdural hematoma. *J Neurosurg.* 2014;121:176–183. doi:10.3171/2014.4.JNS131212.

Santarius T, Kirkpatrick PJ, Ganesan D, et al. Use of drains versus no drains after burr-hole evacuation of chronic subdural haematoma: a randomised controlled trial. *Lancet.* 2009;374:1067–1073. doi:10.1016/S0140-6736(09)61115-6.

33

ACUTE HEMORRHAGIC STROKE

Elizabeth Lee and Odette Harris

Case vignette

Patient SC is a 74-year-old right-handed male who presents in the emergency room (ER) with an acute onset of a severe left-sided headache followed by progressive right-sided weakness, slurred speech, and mild right facial weakness. Two months prior to admission, SC was diagnosed with atrial fibrillation, and he was placed on warfarin anticoagulation. In the afternoon of admission, he complained of a rapid onset of right-sided clumsiness with slurred speech associated with headache. By the time he came to the emergency room, the right-sided weakness and speech improved. Computed tomography (CT) imaging obtained in the ER revealed a left basal ganglia hemorrhage stroke.

Overview

- Hemorrhagic stroke occurs when a blood vessel in the brain leaks or ruptures, resulting in an intracerebral hemorrhage (ICH).
- ICH constitutes 10%–15% of all strokes with a higher risk of morbidity and mortality than cerebral infarction or subarachnoid hemorrhage (Fewel et al., 2003).
- Hemorrhagic stroke accounts for about 13% of stroke cases, and this is related to a significant number of deaths worldwide.
- Volume of the hematoma correlates with morbidity and mortality (Broderick et al., 1993).
- Hypertensive bleeds can occur anywhere, but commonly occur in the basal ganglia.
- A cerebral angiogram is recommended except for patients over age 45 with preexisting hypertension and ICH in thalamus, putamen, or posterior fossa.
- Medical treatment with rFVIIa.
- The role of surgery may consist of craniectomy or craniotomy.

Risk factors

- Hypertension—Chronic hypertension causes changes in blood vessel integrity; certain drugs cause increased blood pressure (BP).
- Increased cerebral blood flow
  - Following carotid endarterectomy (Piepgras et al., 1988).
  - Following repair of congenital heart defects in children (Humphreys et al., 1975).

Table 33.1 Risk Factors for Hemorrhagic Stroke

Hypertension	Family history of strokes or previous stroke	Race—Blacks and Asians higher risk[a]
Anticoagulant medications	Diabetes, high cholesterol, obesity, and sedentary lifestyle	Gender male > female
Cerebral aneurysms/AVMs	Liver dysfunction Hemostasis may be impaired from thrombocytopenia, reduced coagulation factors, and hyperfibrinolysis[b]	Age—increased incidence >55, doubles with each decade until >80, then 25 times greater than previous decade
Substance abuse alcohol acute or chronic street drugs	Coagulopathies	Vascular anomalies

Table 33.2 APP History Checklist for ICH

Hypertension	Acute increased cerebral blood flow	Vascular anomalies (AVMS, cavernomas, aneurysms)
Brain tumor—primary or metastatic	Coagulation or clotting disorder	CNS infection
Drugs—stimulants, supplements, anticoagulants, ASA use	Posttraumatic—recent trauma	Pregnancy related—eclampsia or preeclampsia
Idiopathic	Leukemia	Previous stroke

- Following a previous cerebrovascular accident (CVA) (embolic or hemorrhagic): hemorrhagic transformation may occur in up to 43% of CVAs in the first month (Hornig et al., 1986).
- During or following a migraine (rare).
- Following surgery to remove an arteriovenous malformation (AVM): perfusion pressure changes or possibly from an incomplete resection.
- Physical factors such as increased exertion.
- Vascular anomalies: AVM, aneurysm, or venous angioma rupture.
- Arteriopathies:
  - Amyloid angiopathy: usual leads to lobar hemorrhages.
  - Fibrinoid necrosis (Lammie et al., 2000, p. 1427).
  - Cerebral arteritis.
- Brain tumor (primary or metastases).
- Coagulation or clotting disorders.
  - Iatrogentic: anticoagulation therapy, thrombolytic therapy, acute myocardial infarction (MI) or other thrombosis (Kase et al., 1990).
  - Risk increased with higher doses than recommended alteplase (recombinant tissue plasminogen activator [rt-PA]), in elderly, and adjunctive heparin (Hart et al., 1995).
  - Acetylsalicylic acid (ASA) combined with warfarin increases risk of ICH (Hart et al., 1999).
  - Leukemia.
  - Thrombocytopenia: thrombotic thrombocytopenia purpura, anaplastic anemia
- Central nervous system (CNS) infection: fungal, granulomas, herpes simplex encephalitis.
- Dural or venous thrombosis.
- Drug related:
  - Substance abuse: alcohol—more than three drinks a day increases risk of ICH approximately sevenfold; stimulant drugs such as cocaine (Martin-Schild et al., 2010).
  - Drugs that raise BP: alpha-adrenergic agonists, phenylpropanolamine.

- Ephedra alkaloids (ma huang) used to suppress appetite and increase energy associated with hypertension, ICH, subarachnoid hemorrhage, seizures, and death (Morgenstern et al., 2003).
- Posttrauma.
- Pregnancy related: Most commonly seen with eclampsia and preeclampsia with mortality approximately 6%, ICH being most frequent direct cause (Drislane and Wang, 1997, p. 197).
- Idiopathic.
- Hypertensive strokes can occur anywhere, but at least 35% occur in the basal ganglia (Figure 33.1).
- ICH patients have a high risk of hemorrhage expansion and neurologic deterioration within the first few hours.
- Prognosis is based on multiple factors including volume and location of hemorrhage, age, level of consciousness, presence of intraventricular hemorrhage, and warfarin use.
- Clinical presentation is more of a smooth progression, compared to embolic CVA where deficit is greatest at onset. ICH symptoms usually include headache, vomiting, and changes in level of consciousness.
- Hemorrhagic strokes and accompanying edema may disrupt or compress adjacent brain tissue, leading to neurologic deficit, and may cause elevation in intracranial pressure and potentially fatal herniation syndromes.
- An infarct will raise the intracranial pressure slowly as the edema worsens. A bleed raises it rapidly and can cause hydrocephalus by obstructing the ventricular outflow with a blood clot, or by

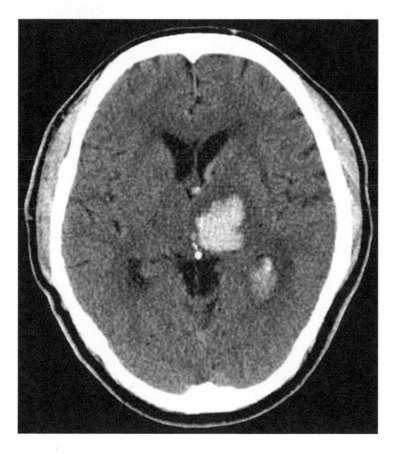

Figure 33.1 Acute left basal ganglia hemorrhagic stroke.

impairing the cerebrospinal fluid (CSF) resorption from the arachnoid granulations. Hydrocephalus raises the intracranial pressure further.

- Bleeds below the tentorium rapidly elevate the local intracranial pressure, possibly resulting in brain herniation.
- Brain tissues in the area of a hemorrhage are generally not totally destroyed, as opposed to an infarct. Viable brain tissue can be found amid the blood, which explains why neurologic deficits usually resolve more rapidly as the hematoma is resorbed.

Common ICH locations and symptoms

- Putamen—Contralateral hemiplegia, hemisensory loss, hemianopia, slurred speech
- Thalamic—Contralateral hemiplegia, hemisensory loss, small poorly reactive pupils, decreased level of consciousness
- Pontine—Locked-in syndrome, coma
- Cerebellar—Occipital headache, ataxia, dizziness, headaches, nausea, vomiting
- Lobar—Mimics cerebral infarct (e.g., contralateral motor and sensory signs)
- SC left basal ganglia hemorrhage

The goal of treatment is then to preserve whatever brain tissue remains viable in the area of hemorrhage. Persistent intracranial hypertension must be treated to prevent secondary damage to the brain tissue in and surrounding the hematoma.

Relevant diagnostic tests

Radiographic

CT—Provides rapid imaging and can be highly sensitive in identifying ICH (Zavier et al., 2003). Blood appears as a high-density lesion within the brain parenchyma immediately after a bleed.

> After 48 hours, large hematomas tend to show fluid levels, indicating they have not yet solidified (Mayer et al., 2006).
> Mass effect is common.
> Clot volume can have a prognostic significance.

MRI—Usually not the best study for ICH within the first few hours.

> It is best for evaluating ischemic events.
> Diffusion-weighted MRI is a measurement of edema; perfusion-weighted MRI will evaluate global cerebral blood flow.
> May be more useful later to identify cerebral amyloid angiopathy.
> ICH appearance is dependent on the age of the clot (Bradley, 1993).
> Localize and differentiate hemorrhages (extra- or intraaxial)—if intraaxial, locate the specific neuroanatomic site.
> Determine age of hemorrhage.

Cerebral angiography—Difficult to reliably differentiate mass effect of ICH from infarct or tumor.

> May demonstrate vascular blush in some cases of tumor.
> ICH Score by Hemphill et al. (2001) assigns points based on five features, then points are added for the ICH score to determine 30-day mortality.

CT perfusion or CT xenon scan—Information to evaluate cerebral blood flow.
PET/SPECT—Assess abnormal function of the brain.
EEG—Can be conducted at bedside to evaluate seizure activity.
Transcranial Doppler—Check for vasospasms, cerebral circulatory arrest, and emboli.

Laboratory

Coagulation profile—Correct coagulopathies, platelets for thrombocytopenia, and patients on platelet-inhibiting drugs. Start with 6 units of platelets.
Biochemical profile—Aggressively treat hyperglycemia, insulin drip if necessary, watch for syndrome of inappropriate secretion of antidiuretic hormone (SIADH).
Hematologic profile—Complete blood count with differential, platelets, evaluate for sepsis and anemia.
CK-MB—Isoenzymes for cardiac issues.
Drug screen—If suspected.
Lumbar puncture—Measures CSF pressures and obtains specimen check for elevated protein, low glucose, and elevated white blood count.

Medical management

Hypertension must be treated. There is controversy as to how to manage hypertension, as it may contribute to further bleeding, while BP must be maintained for cerebral perfusion. Suggested BP = 140/90; avoid overcorrection.

If the systolic BP (SBP) >200 mm Hg or mean arterial pressure (MAP) >150 mm Hg, aggressive BP reduction is considered.
IF SBP >180 mm Hg or MAP >130 mm Hg with possible elevated ICP, reduce BP with concurrent ICP monitoring to keep cerebral perfusion pressure (CPP) at 60–80 mm Hg.
If SBP >180 mm Hg or NAO >130 mm Hg and no suspicion of increased ICP, reduction of MAP to 110 mm Hg or 160/90 should be considered.
NovoSeven (recombinant activated coagulation factor VII [fFVIIa]).
Give IV within 4 hours of onset to reduce risk of clot enlargement (Mayer et al., 2006).
Forms a complex with tissue factor resulting in thrombin production.
Converts factor X to its active form, Xa, on the surface of activated platelets resulting in a "thrombin burst" at the site of damage (Mayer et al., 2006).
Expensive at approximately $10,000 per dose.
Steroids are controversial, no benefit with potential significant side effects (Poungvarin et al., 1987). Consider if significant perihemorrhage edema on imaging. Then 4 mg dexamethasone IV q 6 hrs, ruptured over 7–14 days.
Intracranial hypertension can be treated with mannitol and/or furosemide as tolerated. Consider ICP monitor if significant problems with increased ICP.
Anticoagulation following ICH.

For patients at risk (e.g., embolic disease), recommend 1–2 weeks off anticoagulation with mechanic heart valves.
Probability of ischemic CVA at 30 days following cessation of warfarin is approximately 2.6% for atrial fibrillation, 2.9% for patients with prosthetic valve, and 4.8% for those treated for cardioembolic stroke (Phan et al., 2000).
Anticonvulsants are optional prophylaxis. Treat if patient has seizure activity. Refer to Chapters 40 and 65.

Deep vein thrombosis (DVT) prophylaxis—Immobile state due to weakness predisposes ICH patients for DVT and pulmonary embolism (PE). Intermittent pneumatic compression devices and elastic stockings on admission. Low-dose heparin on hospital day 2 to prevent thromboembolic complications found to lower incidence of PE with no increase in rebelling (Boeer et al., 1991)

Intubate if stuporous or comatose for airway protection.

Interventional procedures and surgeries

Interventional embolization, coiling, and radiosurgery are not used for hemorrhagic strokes.

Craniotomy

- Evacuation of the bleed and resultant decompression of the brain.
- Removal of lesion with marked mass effect, edema, or midline shift on imaging.
- Removal of lesions where the symptoms appear to be due to increased ICP or mass effect (Juvela et al., 1989).
- Clinical rapid deterioration.
- Surgery for moderate to large hematoma (10–30 cc). Small clot (<10 cc) usually not clinically significant. Large clot (>30 cc) associated with poor outcome. Massive clot (>60 cc) with GCS <8: 90% mortality (Broderick et al., 1993, p. 990).
- Randomized prospective studies for patient with GCS 7–10 treated surgically indicated lower mortality rate. However, patients were all severely disabled (Juvela et al., 1989).

Craniectomy—Marinkovic et al. (2009) revealed that decompressive craniectomy performed up to 24 hours revealed lower mortality, better neurologic outcome, and more favorable behavioral outcome.

Ventriculostomy or external ventricular drainage (EVD)

Used if extension of blood causes acute obstruction of the third ventricle. The EVD is placed in the lateral ventricle contralateral to the hemorrhage.

Tissue plasminogen activator (rt-PA)

Intraventricular rt-PA may help lyse clot and maintain catheter patency or reopen a clotted catheter—2–5 mg of rt-PA in NS is administered through an intraventricular catheter. The IVC is closed for 2 hours after injection. Some centers repeat the procedure daily up to 4 days prn.

Family counseling

- Prognosis depends on the severity of the bleed and subsequent neurologic injury.
- Realistic expectations of physical, occupational, cognitive, and speech therapies into inpatient rehabilitation and in the home.
- Help patient and family adjust to pain or the loss of mental or physical function—ongoing referrals and renewals of therapies needed.
- Case management is critical in the inpatient period to help family organize resources for the patient, research inpatient rehab facilities, home care, etc. Effects need to be reviewed with patient and family. Safety measures in the patient home as directed by physical therapist and occupational therapist.

Common questions—long- and short-term disability, time frame on recovery, changes in family dynamics, supportive care for spouse, activity restrictions (driving, working, in-home needs, exercise, sex). Emotional support long term—issues with isolation, hopelessness, depression, and anxiety regarding current and future prognosis. Need ongoing follow-ups to address these issues long term.

Common pitfalls and medicolegal concerns

Pitfalls include the inability to go back to work, financial hardships, costs of care, inability to work, work retraining, etc. Social services referral is warranted to help family with in-house support. Depression with patient given recovery period and neurologic deficits. Assess patient's support system, access to transportation, and compliance with follow-up care.

If patient experienced seizures, discuss driver's license revocation. Provide clear documentation of conversations in medical chart to clarify restrictions in patient's ability including work and driving.

Thorough assessments and care throughout hospitalization and rehabilitation are necessary to avoid additional complications and or reinjury associated with ICH. Stress careful monitoring of BP, aggressive therapy to maximize recovery, family teaching and supportive care, and addressing any medical issues that were delinquent leading to hospitalization such as unhealthy habits. Ensure communication with primary care provider to ensure good local follow-up and coordination of care.

Finally, the discussion of withdrawing support for patients with severe brain injury related to an hemorrhagic stroke needs to be carefully evaluated by team members. Withdrawal of support in these patients will invariably lead to death. Family counseling to the durable power of attorney is crucial in order to do what is best for the patient. Careful documentation per the hospital's policy needs to be enforced for this particular issue.

Relevance to the advanced practice health professional

The advanced practice health professional offers significant benefits in managing and treating hemorrhagic stroke patients. Acute care nurse practitioners were found to improve clinical and financial outcomes by identifying patients at risk, monitoring for complications, and overall managing the patients (Russell et al., 2002). Coordination of care with consulting teams including neurology, neurosurgery, intensivists, physiatry, physical therapy, occupational therapy, speech therapy, social work, rehabilitation facilities, and case management are crucial to these patients. This is in addition to making sure their discharge planning meets the needs of the patient and family. The patient's primary care doctor and other specialists need to be aware of the patient's current condition and need for follow-up on discharge from the inpatient setting. Of course, the patient will follow up with the advanced practice provider in his or her preferred clinic following inpatient discharge.

Common phone calls, pages, and requests with answers

- Family members and/or family seeking information—Follow the Health Insurance Portability and Accountability Act (HIPAA) rules.
- Follow-up plans after discharge from hospital or rehab center—Discharge teaching critical to avoid confusion, reinforced with discharge paperwork outlining the same plan.
- Disability forms for EDD and short- and long-term disability for the patient's work.
- Family and Medical Leave Act (FMLA) forms for family members providing care for patient.
- Calls or pages from consulting teams regarding coordination of care.
- Contacting the primary care provider and having all necessary documents sent to their office regarding the patient's recent hospitalization.

References

Ariesen MJ, Claus SP, Rinkel GJ, Algra A. Risk factors for intracerebral hemorrhage in the general population. *Stroke*. 2003;34:2060–2065.

Blumenfeld H. *Neuroanatomy through Clinical Cases*. Sunderland, MA: Sinauer Associates; 2002.

Boeer A, Voth E, Prange HW. Early heparin in patients with spontaneous intracerebral hemorrhage. *J Neurosurg Psychiatry*. 1991;54:466–467.

Bradley WG. MR appearance of hemorrhage in the brain. *Radiology*. 1993;189(1):15–26.

Broderick J, Brett TG, Duldner JE, Tomsick T, Huster G. Volume of intracerebral hemorrhage. A powerful and easy to use predictor of 30 day mortality. *Stroke*. 1993;24(7):987–993.

Delacourt C, Huang Y, Arima H, et al. Hematoma growth and outcomes in intracerebral hemorrhage: the INTERACT1 study. *Neurology*. 2012;79(4):314–319.

Dowlatshashi D, Demchuk AM, Flaherty ML, Lyden PL, Smith EE. Defining hematoma expansion in intracerebral hemorrhage. *Neurology*. 2011;76(14):1238–1244.

Drislane FW, Wang AM. Multifocal cerebral hemorrhage in eclampsia and severe pre-eclampsia. *J Neurol*. 1997;224(3):94–198.

Fewel ME, Thompson BG, Hoff JT. Spontaneous intracerebral hemorrhage: a review. *Neurosurg Focus*. 2003;15(4):E1.

Fujii Y, Takeuchi S, Tanake R, Koike T, Sasaki O, Minakawa T. Liver dysfunction in spontaneous intracerebral hemorrhage. *Neurosurgery*. 1994;35(4):592–596.

Gonzalez-Perez A, Gaist D, Wallander MA, McFreat G, Garcia-Rodriguez LA. Mortality after hemorrhagic stroke: data from general practice (The Heath Improvement Network). *Neurology*. 2013;81(6):559–565.

Hart RG, Benavente O, Pearce LA. Increase risk of intracranial hemorrhage when aspirin is combined with warfarin: a meta-analysis and hypothesis. *Cerebrovasc Dis*. 1999;9(4):215–217.

Hart RG, Bradley SB, Anderson DC. Oral anticoagulants and intracranial hemorrhage. *Stroke*. 1995;26:1471–1477.

Hemphill JC, Bonovich DC, Besmertis L, Manley GT, Johnston SC. The ICH grading score: a simple, reliable grading scale for intracerebral hemorrhage. *Stoke*. 2001;32(4):891–897.

Hornig CR, Dorndorf W, Agnoli AL. Hemorrhagic cerebral infarction: a prospective study. *Stroke*. 1986;17(2):179–185.

Humphreys RP, Hoffman HJ, Mustard WT, Trusler GA. Cerebral hemorrhage following heart surgery. *J Neurosurg*. 1975;43(6):671–675.

Juvela S, Heiskanen O, Poranen A, et al. The treatment of spontaneous intracerebral hemorrhage: a prospective randomized trial of surgical and conservative treatment. *J Neurosurg*. 1989;70(5):755–858.

Kase CS, O'Neal AM, Fisher M, Girgis GN, Ordia JI. Intracranial hemorrhage after use of tissue plasminogen activator for coronary thrombolysis. *Ann Intern Med*. 1990;112(1):17–21.

Kaye AH. *Essential Neurosurgery*. Malden, MA: Blackwell Publishing; 2005.

Lammie GA, Lindley R, Keir S, Wiggam MI. Stress-related primary intracerebral hemorrhage. *Stroke*. 2000;31:1426–1428.

Marinkovic I, Strbian D, Pedrono EM, et al. Decompressive cranietomy for intracerebral hemorrhage. *Neurosurgery*. 2009;65(4):780–786.

Martin-Schild S, Albright KC, Hallevi H, et al. Intracerebral hemorrhage in cocaine users. *Stroke*. 2010;41:680–684.

Mayer SA, Brun NC, Broderick J, et al. Recombinant activated factor VII for acute intracerebral hemorrhage *US phase IIa* trial. *Neurocrit Care*. 2006;4(3):206–214.

Mehta RH, Cox M, Smith EE, et al. Race/Ethic differences in the risk of hemorrhagic complications among patients with ischemic stroke receiving thrombolytic therapy. *Stroke*. 2014;45(8):2263–2269.

Morgenstern LD, Viscoli CM, Kernan WN, et al. Use of *Ephedra*-containing products and risk for hemorrhagic stroke. *Neurology*. 2003;60(1):123–135.

Phan TG, Koh M, Wijdicks EF. Safety of discontinuation of anticoagulation in patients with intracranial hemorrhage at high thromboembolic risk. *Arch Neurol*. 2000;57(12):1710–1713.

Piepgras DG, Morgan MK, Sundt TM, Yanigihara T, Mussman LM. Intracerebral hemorrhage after carotid endarterectomy. *J Neurosurg*. 1988;68(4):532–536.

Russell D, VorderBruegge M, Burns SM. Effect of an outcomes-managed approach to care of neuroscience patients by acute care nurse practitioners. *Am J Crit Care*. 2002;11(4):353–362.

Zavier AR, Qureshi AL, Kirmani JF, Yahia AM, Bakshi R. Neuroimaging of stroke: a review. *South Med J*. 2003;96(4):367–379.

34

SUBARACHNOID HEMORRHAGE

Joli Vavao, Teresa Bell-Stephens, J.J. Baumann, and Gary K. Steinberg

Case vignette

Mrs. K is a 42-year-old Caucasian female who presented to an outside hospital 18 hours ago when she developed a sudden headache, nausea, and vomiting. Initially thought to be a migraine, after a long, stressful day at the office, she was treated with IV Dilaudid and Phenergan and released but presented 2 hours later with somnolence and profuse vomiting. A head computed tomography (CT) scan demonstrated evidence of an acute subarachnoid hemorrhage (SAH) (Figure 34.1) with early signs of hydrocephalus. She was then transferred to your facility for a higher level of care. Mrs. K's husband is at the bedside, and his demeanor can best be described as a combination of fear, anxiety, and guilt. He is frantically asking staff for updates as she has continued to become more difficult to arouse in transport.

Upon arrival to the intensive care unit (ICU), the patient is noted to have increased somnolence. The decision is made to insert an external ventricular drain (EVD). Bloody cerebral spinal fluid begins to drain into the collection chamber, and Mrs. K becomes more arousable and able to say her name, while complaining of a terrible headache and neck pain. She is moving all extremities. Vital signs: 170/90, pulse 90 with regular rate and normal sinus rhythm, temperature 98.1 F. Laboratory results: Na 136; K 3.8; creatinine 1.0; glucose 105; white blood cells 11,000; hemoglobin 11.6; hematocrit 35.8; platelets 300,000. She is started on IV nicardipine to lower her blood pressure to a systolic blood pressure <160. A CT angiogram is performed and shows a 7 mm right middle cerebral artery (MCA) aneurysm with a wide neck (Figure 34.2), and she is felt to be a candidate for surgical clipping of her ruptured aneurysm. She tolerates the procedure well and continues to be monitored for vasospasm, receiving daily transcranial Dopplers (TCDs). On post-bleed day 5 she starts to experience intermittent left arm drift and TCDs are elevated in the right MCA. A cerebral angiogram demonstrates moderate vasospasm in the proximal right MCA. Intraarterial nicardipine is administered by the interventional neuroradiologist in the catheterization (cath) lab with good results (Figure 34.3). Her blood pressure is augmented with Neo-Synephrine, and mean arterial pressure (MAP) goals are kept in the range of 110–120. She continues to improve neurologically over the next 3 days and shows no further clinical or TCD signs of cerebral vasospasm. Her blood pressure is relaxed, and her EVD is weaned and able to be removed postbleed day 8. Physical, occupational, and speech therapy have been involved in her care and recommend that she go home with outpatient physical therapy (PT) and speech therapy for deconditioning and cognitive rehabilitation. She is discharged on oral analgesia, a bowel regimen, nimodipine, and an H2 blocker. She is able to return to work in 4 months.

This typical progression for a patient with an acute SAH highlights several situations in which advanced practice provider (APP) interventions influenced Mrs. K's clinical course and outcome. Each situation must be prioritized, investigated, and either prevented or treated. Some factors are present at the initial time of hemorrhage, while others can have a delayed onset of hours or weeks. The APP has an active role in stabilizing the patient and requesting admission orders, labs, and tests, as well as communicating the plan to the family. So where do you begin with the clinical care of Mrs. K, and how do you communicate the complexity of her acute situation to the family, preparing them for the next hours, days, weeks, or months?

Overview

The incidence of nontraumatic SAH in the United States is estimated to be 9.7 per 100,000 (Labovitz et al., 2006) and accounts for 5% of strokes. Patients have a significant mortality rate despite current management and available resources. A quarter of patients with SAH die, and 15% of those deaths occur prior to hospitalization (Shea et al., 2007). Close to 50% of survivors are left with persistent neurologic deficits (Connolly et al., 2012). It is estimated that as many as 46% of survivors of SAH have long-term cognitive impairment that affects functional status and quality of life (Qureshi et al., 2007). One-third of SAH survivors require long-term care. Thus, SAH patients also cause a substantial burden on health-care resources in the acute and long term. The mean acute hospital care charge for a single patient is $65,900, and the cost per survivor of SAH is $978,054 (Qureshi et al., 2007).

Biologic and physiologic process and anatomy

The leading cause of spontaneous SAH is rupture of an intracranial aneurysm. Aneurysms most commonly are located at branch points in the circle of Willis at the base of the brain (Figure 34.1). There are known risk factors contributing to the formation of cerebral aneurysms, which are listed in Table 34.1 (Caranci et al., 2013).

At the time of hemorrhage, there is extravasation of blood into the subarachnoid spaces covering the central nervous system, which contains cerebrospinal fluid (Figure 34.2). Most deaths after SAH occur rapidly after the initial bleed. The sudden volume of blood in the subarachnoid space causes a profound

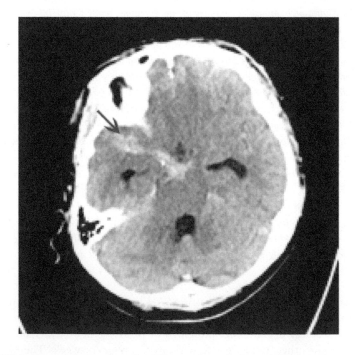

Figure 34.1 Axial CT head scan: Dense subarachnoid hemorrhage (Fisher CT Grade 3) in suprasellar cistern and right Sylvian fissure (arrow).

Table 34.1 Risk Factors for Cerebral Aneurysm Formation and Hemorrhage

- Smoking
- High blood pressure or hypertension
- Congenital resulting from inborn abnormality in artery wall
- Family history of brain aneurysms
- Age over 40
- Gender, women compared with men have an increased incidence of aneurysms at a ratio of 3:2
- Other disorders affecting the connective tissues: Ehlers-Danlos syndrome, polycystic kidney disease, Marfan syndrome, and fibromuscular dysplasia (FMD)
- Presence of an arteriovenous malformation (AVM)
- Drug use, particularly cocaine
- Infection
- Tumors
- Traumatic head injury

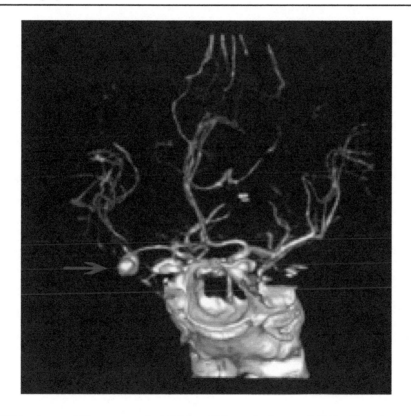

Figure 34.2 CT Angiogram (3D reconstruction): Right middle cerebral artery (MCA) trifurcation ruptured aneurysm (arrow). The aneurysm is multilobulated, irregularly shaped, and points inferiorly and laterally, measuring approximately 7 mm in largest diameter with a 3 mm neck.

reduction in cerebral blood flow, reduced cerebral autoregulation, and acute cerebral ischemia (Broderick et al., 2009). This results in increased intracranial pressure, decreased cerebral perfusion, acute vasoconstriction, and increased microvascular permeability. In addition to the insult to the brain at the time of initial hemorrhage, if the patient survives, there is a 70% chance of re-bleed within the first 24 hours, with a high fatality rate. Therefore, the main focus in the first 24 hours after an SAH is to stabilize the patient, identify the source of hemorrhage, and reduce the chance of re-bleeding.

Physical findings

The hallmark presentation of an SAH is a headache that is extremely sudden and immediately reaches maximal intensity, often described as the "worst headache of his or her life" or a "thunderclap headache."

Other clinical signs and symptoms of an SAH are listed in order from most to least common in Table 34.2 (Cohen-Gadol and Bohnstedt, 2013).

Diagnostic tests

There are four main foci of diagnostic studies for SAH: (1) identify subarachnoid blood; (2) identify aneurysm size, location, and morphology; (3) identify cerebral vasospasm and infarct; and (4) identify hydrocephalus. When an SAH is suspected, the priority should be to obtain a rapid noncontrast CT scan to detect the presence of subarachnoid blood. A CT scan has a sensitivity of 98% or better to detect SAH (Provenzale and Hacein-Bey, 2009). If the head CT scan is negative, but SAH is still highly suspected, a lumbar puncture should be performed to look for the presence of elevated red blood cells (Czuczman et al., 2013). If an SAH is present, the patient should undergo either a CT angiogram or a formal digital subtraction cerebral angiogram (DSA) to define the architecture of the aneurysm and plan treatment (Nagai and Watanabe, 2010). If a CT angiogram is negative, but there is a diffuse aneurysm pattern of SAH, a DSA should be performed (Agid et al., 2010).

Other studies for patients with an SAH are included in Table 34.3.

Classifications

The severity of clinical presentation is the strongest prognostic indicator in SAH. Initial clinical severity is measured by the Hunt and Hess grading system (Table 34.4) (Hunt and Hess, 1968). Higher scores correlate to poorer outcomes. Other factors predictive of poor prognosis include the following:

Table 34.2 Clinical Signs and Symptoms of SAH

- Meningismus
- Recent atypical "warning" headaches that have lasted for days or weeks prior to the hemorrhage
- Nausea and vomiting
- Focal neurologic deficit, especially cranial nerve deficits
- Seizure
- Back or neck pain
- Lightheadedness or dizziness
- Dysphasia
- Syncope
- Ataxia
- Vision changes

Table 34.3 Other Diagnostic Tests to Consider for SAH Patients

---

- Serum chemistry panel
- Complete blood count
- Prothrombin time (PT) and activated partial thromboplastin time (aPTT)—assess for coagulopathy
- Blood typing/screening—preparation for intraoperative transfusions, if necessary
- Cardiac enzymes—assess for myocardial ischemia
- Arterial blood gas (ABG)—patients with respiratory compromise
- Baseline electrocardiogram
- Baseline chest x-ray, particularly if aspiration is suspected

---

- Older age
- Preexisting severe medical illness
- Global cerebral edema on CT scan
- Intraventricular and intracerebral hemorrhage
- Symptomatic vasospasm
- Delayed cerebral infarction (especially if multiple)
- Hyperglycemia
- Fever
- Anemia
- Pneumonia and sepsis

The Fisher Grading System, which measures the amount of blood seen on the initial CT scan, is also useful in the prediction of cerebral vasospasm (Table 34.5) (Fisher et al., 1980).

Interventional procedures

If a CT scan reveals an SAH and the CT or cerebral angiogram shows the presence of an aneurysm, a decision is made whether an aneurysm is amenable to coiling or whether to expedite microsurgery to prevent risk of re-bleeding. According to current American Heart Association guidelines, microsurgical clipping may receive increased consideration in patients presenting with large (>50 mL) intraparenchymal hematomas and middle cerebral artery aneurysms. Endovascular coiling may be preferable in the elderly (>70 years of age), in those presenting with poor-grade SAH, and in those with aneurysms of the basilar apex (Connolly et al., 2012). Due to the complexity of care required by an SAH patient, several factors need to be considered during treatment planning, such as the health-care environment, the existing equipment, the availability of relevant neurosurgical and endovascular skills, the anatomy and location of the aneurysm, the

Table 34.4 Hunt and Hess Grading for SAH Severity

Clinical grade	Mortality (%)
Grade 0: Unruptured aneurysm without symptoms	0
Grade I: Asymptomatic, or minimal headache and slight nuchal rigidity	1
Grade II: Moderate to severe headache, nuchal rigidity, no neurologic deficit other than cranial nerve palsy	5
Grade III: Drowsiness, confusion, or mild focal deficit	19
Grade IV: Stupor, moderate to severe hemiparesis, possibly early decerebrate rigidity and vegetative disturbances	42
Grade V: Deep coma, decerebrate rigidity, moribund appearance	77

Note: The *Hunt and Hess Score* is based on the clinical presentation of a patient with subarachnoid hemorrhage, with the higher score correlating to poorer outcome.

Table 34.5 Fisher CT Grading System for Aneurysmal SAH

1 = No hemorrhage evident
2 = Subarachnoid hemorrhage <1 mm thick
3 = Subarachnoid hemorrhage >1 mm thick
4 = Intraventricular hemorrhage (IVH) or intraparenchymal hemorrhage, without subarachnoid hemorrhage

Note: The *Fisher Grading System* is based on the location of blood on the CT scan (Fisher et al., 1980). Grades 1–3 are ranked less to most severe and predict increasing risk of vasospasm after subarachnoid hemorrhage. Grade 4 has a low risk of developing vasospasm.

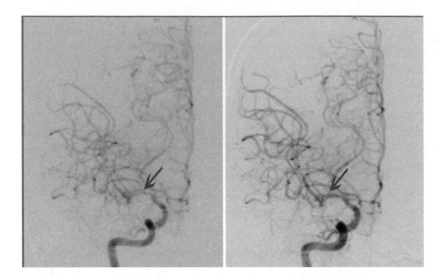

Figure 34.3 Left internal carotid artery angiograms. AP views: Pretreatment angiogram (left) shows moderate left M1 MCA vasospasm (arrow); postnicardipine angiogram (right) shows successful dilation of M1 MCA segment following intraarterial nicardipine treatment (arrow).

relative difficulties for the endovascular or surgical approach in the specific case, and the age and clinical state of the patient. These are all factors that could affect the final recommendation and should be discussed with the patients and/or their relatives (Molyneux et al., 2009).

- *Surgical clipping*—For most anterior circulation aneurysms, a skin incision is made and a small portion of skull removed. After the dura is opened, the temporal lobe can be separated from the parietal and frontal lobe along the Sylvian fissure. Separation of the lobes provides a window through which the aneurysm is visualized. When the aneurysm can be clearly seen, a surgical clip is attached at the base of the aneurysm. Application of the surgical clip prevents blood from entering the aneurysm and re-bleeding. When the surgical clip is in place, the dome of the aneurysm is punctured, and the aneurysm is inspected to assure no more blood is filling it (Figure 34.4). Systemic mild hypothermia (33°C –34°C) has also been used for this type of surgery, as well as in several other clinical settings, including head injury, ischemic stroke, and circulatory arrest, to protect the brain against ischemic injury (Nguyen et al., 2010).
- *Coiling embolization*—Cerebral angiographic techniques are used to guide a catheter to the location of the aneurysm. Platinum coils are attached to the end of a guide wire and advanced through a microcatheter into the dome of the aneurysm, where they are detached. Coils are packed into the aneurysm until it is filled, after which blood can no longer enter the aneurysm, and it is considered secure. The blood in the aneurysm where the coils are placed will clot and solidify, but there is no additional blood entering the aneurysm, and there is no further risk of re-bleed (Figure 34.5).

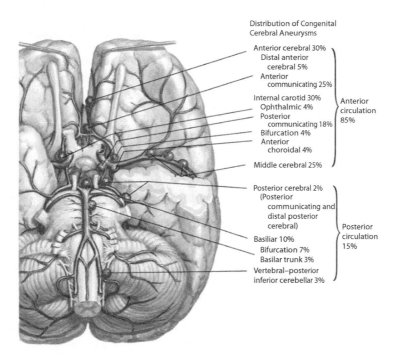

Distribution of Congenital
Cerebral Aneurysms

Anterior cerebral 30%
Distal anterior
cerebral 5%
Anterior
communicating 25%

Internal carotid 30%
Ophthalmic 4%
Posterior
communicating 18%
Bifurcation 4%
Anterior
choroidal 4%

Middle cerebral 25%

Anterior
circulation
85%

Posterior cerebral 2%
(Posterior
communicating and
distal posterior
cerebral)

Basiliar 10%
Bifurcation 7%
Basilar trunk 3%

Vertebral–posterior
inferior cerebellar 3%

Posterior
circulation
15%

Figure 34.4   Circle of Willis. (Published from *Cerebral Vascular Anatomy, Illustrating Common Sites and Approximate Distribution of Congenital Aneurysm Formation*, 2011, Elsevier Inc., Netter Image Collection. With permission.)

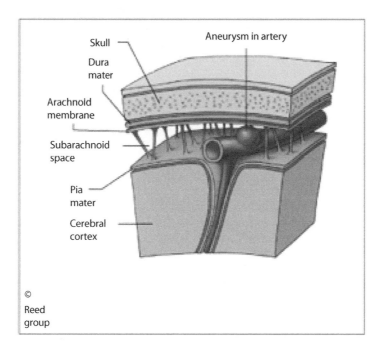

Skull
Dura
mater
Arachnoid
membrane
Subarachnoid
space
Pia
mater
Cerebral
cortex

Aneurysm in artery

©
Reed
group

Figure 34.5   Anatomy of the subarachnoid space with an aneurysm on a subarachnoid artery. (Published from Reed Group Westminster, CO. With permission.)

Table 34.6 Critical Care Management of the SAH Patent

Airway	• Intubation should be performed on patients with altered mental status who cannot protect their airway, have suspected aspiration, or have pulmonary edema.
	• Mechanical ventilation settings should not compromise intracranial pressure or cerebral perfusion pressure.
Circulatory	• Acute hypertension should be controlled after SAH and until aneurysm obliteration with IV titratable vasoactive medication (systolic BP 90–140 mm Hg or MAP 60–80 mm Hg).
	• Post securing of the aneurysm, the blood pressure should be managed at higher levels to prevent cerebral vasospasm.
Neurologic	• Full neurologic exam should be performed hourly in the ICU.
Vasospasm	• Narrowing of the cerebral arteries after SAH is common, occurring most frequently 7–10 days after aneurysm rupture and resolving spontaneously after 21 days. Prevention of vasospasm includes:
	• Oral nimodipine administration (Dorhout Mees et al., 2007).
	• Maintenance of euvolemia, as well as treatment with induced hypertension (monitored by arterial line) and volume expansion (monitored by central venous line) for symptomatic vasospasm.
	• Daily transcranial Doppler to monitor for the development of arterial vasospasm.
	• Endovascular therapy with vasodilators and angioplasty balloons.
Hydrocephalus	• Acute hydrocephalus occurs in 15%–87% of patients with SAH (Chan et al., 2009).
	• EVD placement indicated for cerebrospinal fluid diversion in symptomatic patients.
	• Attempted weaning of the EVD should take place.
	• Patients with chronic symptomatic hydrocephalus after SAH should undergo placement of a ventriculoperitoneal shunt.
Seizure	• Continuous EEG can be beneficial in a patient with fluctuating neurologic exam but negative workup for vasospasm.
Endocrine	• Hyponatremia—incidence of hyponatremia in this disease ranges from 10% to 30%. Hyponatremia has been associated with the onset of elevated TCD and clinical signs of vasospasm (Nakagawa et al., 2009).
	• Cerebral salt wasting (CSW)—excessive secretion of natriuretic peptides and causes hyponatremia from excessive natriuresis.
	• CSW is corrected by administration of hypertonic saline IV (Al-Rawi et al., 2010).
	• Hyperglycemia—associated with poor outcomes and should be corrected with aggressive insulin sliding scale.
Fever	• Associated with worse cognitive outcome in survivors of SAH (Zhang et al., 2011).
	• Antipyretics or cooling blanket to maintain normothermia.
Laboratory	• Assess cardiac and pulmonary function.
	• Fluid/electrolyte balance.
Deep vein thrombosis (DVT)	• Frequent occurrence after SAH, due to immobility and poor mental status.
	• Prophylactic subcutaneous low molecular weight heparin after treatment of an aneurysm.
	• Ultrasound screening of lower extremity.
	• If DVT occurs, consider placement of an inferior vena cava filter in postoperative patients, if anticoagulation contraindicated; consider anticoagulation in endovascularly treated patients.

(Continued)

Nutrition	• Enteral feeding should be started on patients with altered mental status.
	• A bedside swallow exam should be performed prior to any oral intake to avoid aspiration.
Medications	• Vasopressors (IV or oral).
	• Pain management.
	• Bowel regimen.
	• GI protectant.
	• Nimodipine.
Rehabilitation	• Early assessment by physical, occupational, and speech therapy should be performed in the ICU (Olkowski et al., 2013).
	• Referral to inpatient or outpatient therapy at discharge including neuropsychological/cognitive therapy.
Psychosocial	• Screening for depression prior to discharge and referral to psychiatry or primary care physician for ongoing management during recovery (Kreiter et al., 2013).
	• Social services referral for family members to provide housing during hospitalization and any disability or insurance issues due to acute nature of event.
	• Case manager referral for assessment of discharge needs.

Critical care management in SAH

The priority and focus of the management of the acute SAH patient are listed in Table 34.6.

Family counseling

- ICU management goals
    - Explanation of vasospasm and hydrocephalus (acute and delayed)
    - EVD, arterial lines, endotracheal tube, feeding tube, or other monitoring equipment
    - Radiological testing and results
    - Return to the cath angiography suite with or without intervention
- Preparation of the family of a an SAH patient for a prolonged recovery and the setting of realistic expectations
- Early rehabilitation
- Discharge planning

Common questions

- *Are certain activities more likely to cause a subarachnoid hemorrhage?* The highest incidence of rupture occurs while patients are engaged in their daily routines, in the absence of strenuous physical activity (Matsuda et al., 2007). Many family members feel a sense of guilt or anger if a patient has been going through a stressful time in his or her life prior to the hemorrhage or if the patient was with the family member when the hemorrhage occurred.
- *Will the patient regain a good quality of life?* Cognitive impairment, behavioral changes, social readjustment, and low energy may substantially affect surviving patients' function and quality of life. Multiple studies using diverse designs have consistently demonstrated that intellectual impairment is very prevalent after an SAH. Although cognitive function tends to improve over the first year, global cognitive impairment is still present in approximately 20% of SAH patients and is associated with poorer functional recovery and lower quality of life (Samra et al., 2007). Therefore, after discharge, it is reasonable to refer patients with SAH for a comprehensive evaluation, including cognitive, behavioral, and psychosocial assessments (Connolly et al., 2012).

- Should family members be screened for aneurysms? Noninvasive screening of people with familial (at least a first-degree relative) SAH and/or a history of SAH is recommended to evaluate for aneurysms or late regrowth of a treated aneurysm (Broderick et al., 2009).

Common pitfalls and medicolegal concerns

- Misdiagnosis of SAH—Recent data suggest an SAH misdiagnosis rate of 12% (Kowalski et al., 2004). Reasons for misdiagnosis are listed in Table 34.7 (Cohen-Gadol and Bohnstedt, 2013).
- Nonrecognition of vasospasm—It is common for SAH patients in the acute care setting to have fluctuating neurologic exams. Diagnosis requires appropriate evaluation of other potential conditions that could also produce neurologic deterioration, as shown in Table 34.8.
- Clear documentation of symptoms, assessment, and interventions, as well as patient and family consent and education.

APP Role in the care of SAH Patients

The APP ensures the highest-quality patient outcomes for the SAH patient. Competencies within the domains of professional practice include the following:

- Incorporate pathophysiology, evidence-based practice, and clinical guidelines with critical thinking to guide clinical decision making.
- Apply advanced skills such as EVD or neuromonitoring placement to help treat and guide care.

Table 34.7 Misdiagnosis of Subarachnoid Hemorrhage

- Failure to obtain CT of the head at first contact with the patient
- Failure to perform a lumbar puncture with a negative CT scan
- Misinterpretation of diagnostic test results
- Misinterpretation of CT results
- Patient's inability to recognize serious symptoms and seek immediate medical care

---

Table 34.8 Diagnosis of Vasospasm

- Delayed onset or persisting neurologic deficit
- Onset timing (4–20 days posthemorrhage, maximal at 7–10 days)
- Deficit is appropriate to involved arteries
- Other causes of deterioration ruled out
  - Hydrocephalus
  - Cerebral edema
  - Seizure
  - Hyponatremia
  - Hypoxia
  - Sepsis
- Diagnostic testing
  - Transcranial Doppler
  - Angiogram
  - CT or MRI scan
  - Labs (electrolytes, complete blood count, arterial blood gasses)
  - Electroencephalogram

- Provide education regarding the care and management of the SAH patient to a variety of recipients. Information on diagnosis, interventions, treatment options, risk factors, and expectations are provided to the patient and family.
- Give instructions on care to various health-care providers within the APP's own organization, as well as to referring institutions and transport providers on initial management of the SAH patient, and at discharge, to facilitate communication and clinical handoff to the patient's primary care provider and ongoing management and follow-up recommendations.
- Collect and analyze data that can lead to quality improvement projects and practice change.
- Incorporate new technology, test new equipment, become an expert user, and ensure its safety and feasibility.
- Incorporate the latest research into practice, conduct independent research projects, be actively involved in a professional organization, and write or edit peer-reviewed articles.

Common communication requests (Elliott and Walden, 2014)

- Blood pressure parameters
  - Pretreatment—Systolic 90–140 mm Hg
  - Posttreatment
    - Assess neurologic function at each MAP to determine if a higher target is appropriate.
    - Nimodipine—Adjust dosing to more frequent smaller doses if hypotension results after administration.
- Fluctuating neurologic exam
  - Determine if likely vasospasm, especially if focal neurologic deficit is referable to affected vascular distribution; TCD elevation over the last 24 hours or >200 cm/s is suggestive of vasospasm; if clinical symptoms/signs do not respond to medical therapy (induced hypertension and volume expansion), consider DSA for diagnosis and treatment.
  - Exclude hydrocephalus with CT scan.
  - Continuous electroencephalogram (EEG) monitoring to exclude seizures should be considered in patients with neurologic deterioration of undetermined etiology (Diringer et al., 2011).
  - Check for abnormal serum electrolytes and other blood parameters, poor systemic oxygenation, and rule out infection as causes of neurologic deterioration.
- Patient and family questions regarding care and prognosis
  - Provide early, frequent, and consistent multidisciplinary communication regarding the patient's condition.
  - Clinicians provide clear information regarding condition and prognosis and include a discussion of prognostic uncertainty, if appropriate.
  - Consider using a family support specialist or social worker to improve ongoing education and support.
  - Encourage proximity and involvement in care when desired by the family (Souter et al., 2015).

Acknowledgments

We thank Cindy H. Samos for assistance with the manuscript. This work was supported in part from funding provided by Bernard and Ronni Lacroute, the William Randolph Hearst Foundation, and Russell and Elizabeth Siegelman.

References

Agid R, Andersson T, Almqvist H, et al. Negative CT angiography findings in patients with spontaneous subarachnoid hemorrhage: when is digital subtraction angiography still needed? *AJNR Am J Neuroradiol.* 2010;31:696–705.

Al-Rawi PG, Tseng MY, Richards HK, et al. Hypertonic saline in patients with poor-grade subarachnoid hemorrhage improves cerebral blood flow, brain tissue oxygen, and pH. *Stroke.* 2010;41:122–128.

Broderick JP, Brown RD Jr, Sauerbeck L, et al. Greater rupture risk for familial as compared to sporadic unruptured intracranial aneurysms. *Stroke.* 2009;40:1952–1957.

Caranci F, Briganti F, Cirillo L, Leonardi M, Muto M. Epidemiology and genetics of intracranial aneurysms. *Eur J Radiol.* 2013;82:1598–1605.

Chan M, Alaraj A, Calderon M, et al. Prediction of ventriculoperitoneal shunt dependency in patients with aneurysmal subarachnoid hemorrhage. *J Neurosurg.* 2009;110:44–49.

Cohen-Gadol AA, Bohnstedt BN. Recognition and evaluation of nontraumatic subarachnoid hemorrhage and ruptured cerebral aneurysm. *Am Fam Physician.* 2013;88:451–456.

Connolly ES Jr, Rabinstein AA, Carhuapoma JR, et al. Guidelines for the management of aneurysmal subarachnoid hemorrhage: a guideline for healthcare professionals from the American Heart Association/american Stroke Association. *Stroke.* 2012;43:1711–1737.

Czuczman AD, Thomas LE, Boulanger AB, et al. Interpreting red blood cells in lumbar puncture: distinguishing true subarachnoid hemorrhage from traumatic tap. *Acad Emerg Med.* 2013;20:247–256.

Diringer MN, Bleck TP, Claude Hemphill J 3rd, et al. Critical care management of patients following aneurysmal subarachnoid hemorrhage: recommendations from the Neurocritical Care Society's Multidisciplinary Consensus Conference. *Neurocrit Care.* 2011;15:211–240.

Dorhout Mees SM, Rinkel GJ, Feigin VL, et al. Calcium antagonists for aneurysmal subarachnoid haemorrhage. *Cochrane Database Syst Rev.* 2007:CD000277.

Elliott EC, Walden M. Development of the transformational advanced professional practice model. *J Am Assoc Nurse Pract.* 2014;27(9):479–487.

Fisher CM, Kistler JP, Davis JM. Relation of cerebral vasospasm to subarachnoid hemorrhage visualized by computerized tomographic scanning. *Neurosurgery.* 1980;6:1–9.

Hunt WE, Hess RM. Surgical risk as related to time of intervention in the repair of intracranial aneurysms. *J Neurosurg.* 1968;28:14–20.

Kowalski RG, Claassen J, Kreiter KT, et al. Initial misdiagnosis and outcome after subarachnoid hemorrhage. *JAMA.* 2004;291:866–869.

Kreiter KT, Rosengart AJ, Claassen J, et al. Depressed mood and quality of life after subarachnoid hemorrhage. *J Neurol Sci.* 2013;335:64–71.

Labovitz DL, Halim AX, Brent B, Boden-Albala B, Hauser WA, Sacco RL. Subarachnoid hemorrhage incidence among Whites, Blacks and Caribbean Hispanics: the Northern Manhattan study. *Neuroepidemiology.* 2006;26:147–150.

Matsuda M, Watanabe K, Saito A, Matsumura K, Ichikawa M. Circumstances, activities, and events precipitating aneurysmal subarachnoid hemorrhage. *J Stroke Cerebrovasc Dis.* 2007;16:25–29.

Molyneux AJ, Kerr RS, Birks J, et al. Risk of recurrent subarachnoid haemorrhage, death, or dependence and standardised mortality ratios after clipping or coiling of an intracranial aneurysm in the International Subarachnoid Aneurysm Trial (ISAT): long-term follow-up. *Lancet Neurol.* 2009;8:427–433.

Nagai M, Watanabe E. Benefits of clipping surgery based on three-dimensional computed tomography angiography. *Neurol Med Chir.* 2010;50:630–637.

Nakagawa I, Kurokawa S, Takayama K, Wada T, Nakase H. [Increased urinary sodium excretion in the early phase of aneurysmal subarachnoid hemorrhage as a predictor of cerebral salt wasting syndrome]. *Brain Nerve.* 2009;61:1419–1423.

Nguyen HP, Zaroff JG, Bayman EO, Gelb AW, Todd MM, Hindman BJ. Perioperative hypothermia (33 degrees C) does not increase the occurrence of cardiovascular events in patients undergoing cerebral aneurysm surgery: findings from the Intraoperative Hypothermia for Aneurysm Surgery Trial. *Anesthesiology.* 2010;113:327–342.

Olkowski BF, Devine MA, Slotnick LE, et al. Safety and feasibility of an early mobilization program for patients with aneurysmal subarachnoid hemorrhage. *Phys Ther.* 2013;93:208–215.

Provenzale JM, Hacein-Bey L. CT evaluation of subarachnoid hemorrhage: a practical review for the radiologist interpreting emergency room studies. *Emerg Radiol.* 2009;16:441–451.

Qureshi AI, Suri MF, Nasar A, et al. Changes in cost and outcome among U.S. patients with stroke hospitalized in 1990 to 1991 and those hospitalized in 2000 to 2001. *Stroke.* 2007;38:2180–2184.

Samra SK, Giordani B, Caveney AF, et al. Recovery of cognitive function after surgery for aneurysmal subarachnoid hemorrhage. *Stroke.* 2007;38:1864–1872.

Shea AM, Reed SD, Curtis LH, Alexander MJ, Villani JJ, Schulman KA. Characteristics of nontraumatic subarachnoid hemorrhage in the United States in 2003. *Neurosurgery.* 2007;61:1131–1137; discussion 1137-1138.

Souter MJ, Blissitt PA, Blosser S, et al. Recommendations for the critical care management of devastating brain injury: prognostication, psychosocial, and ethical management: a position statement for healthcare professionals from the Neurocritical Care Society. *Neurocrit Care.* 2015;23:4–13.

Zhang G, Zhang JH, Qin X. Fever increased in-hospital mortality after subarachnoid hemorrhage. *Acta Neurochir Suppl.* 2011;110:239–243.

35

HYDROCEPHALUS

Nadine Bradley, Jimmi Amick, and Brandon G. Rocque

Case vignette: Hydrocephalus and ventriculoperitoneal shunt failure

A 10-year-old boy presents to the emergency department with several days of headache, 2 days of vomiting, and new onset of increasing sleepiness. His medical history is significant for premature birth, intraventricular hemorrhage with hydrocephalus, treated by ventriculoperitoneal (VP) shunting. He has not had a shunt malfunction in many years. Neurologic examination reveals a well-nourished child, tired but easily aroused, with no focal neurologic deficits.

A computed tomography (CT) scan is performed (Figure 35.1a). Comparison of the CT to his baseline magnetic resonance imaging (MRI) (Figure 35.1b) shows a marked increase in ventricular size. The clinical scenario and imaging findings are consistent with VP shunt failure.

The patient underwent VP shunt revision. Intraoperative assessment of the shunt revealed an occluded ventricular catheter and normal function of the valve and distal catheter. The ventricular catheter was replaced and connected to the existing valve. The patient returned to his neurologic baseline upon emergence from anesthesia. He had no further headaches. At 9 months follow-up, he continued to do well.

Overview

Epidemiology

According to the National Institutes of Health, 1–2 out of every 1000 live births results in hydrocephalus. Another 6000 children develop hydrocephalus within the first two years of life (NHFOnline, 2015). Although more than 50% of hydrocephalus cases are congenital, traumatic brain injuries or cerebral hemorrhage can also lead to hydrocephalus. A related condition, normal pressure hydrocephalus, develops later in life and can be a cause of dementia and movement difficulties in older adults.

Societal significance

Placement of a ventricular shunt for treatment of hydrocephalus is one of the most common procedures performed by neurosurgeons. According to the National Hydrocephalus Foundation, there are approximately 75,000 discharges from American hospitals each year with the diagnosis of hydrocephalus. Based on a study of hospital admissions, treatment of hydrocephalus may result in over $1 billion of health-care expenditures per year (Simon et al., 2008).

The impact of hydrocephalus on the individual is highly variable. A child with hydrocephalus, if adequately treated, may develop normally without any outward signs of neurologic dysfunction. However, if severely affected, a patient with hydrocephalus may be totally dependent on others for care throughout life.

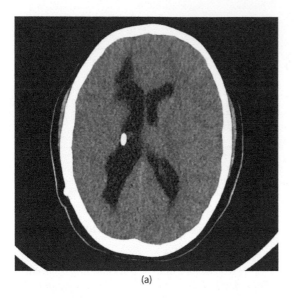 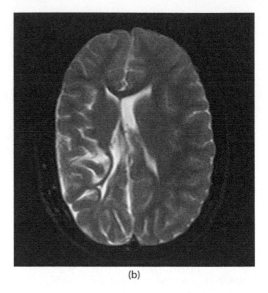

(a)   (b)

Figure 35.1   (a) CT scan performed to evaluate a patient with suspected shunt malfunction. (b) MRI of the same patient performed at baseline. Note the change in ventricle size in the CT performed during a period of shunt failure.

Basic biologic and physiologic processes

The traditional theory of cerebrospinal fluid (CSF) circulation posits that CSF is produced by the choroid plexus within the ventricles. CSF then passes through the ventricles, ultimately exiting the ventricular system through the outlets of the fourth ventricle. Reabsorption of CSF is thought to occur in the subarachnoid space, particularly via arachnoid granulations into the cerebral venous sinuses. However, this classic theory is not supported by modern evidence and does not explain the ventricular dilation observed in most cases of hydrocephalus.

A complete explanation for the physiology of CSF circulation and the pathophysiology of hydrocephalus is beyond the scope of this text. We address this topic briefly: The majority of CSF is produced by the choroid plexus, though CSF production also occurs throughout the brain. CSF "circulation" includes flow in both directions in the interventricular foramina (i.e., foramen of Monro and cerebral aqueduct). Absorption occurs largely at the level of the cerebral capillaries both from the subarachnoid space and from the ventricles. The ventriculomegaly seen in hydrocephalus is likely the result of a combination of increased intraventricular pulsations, decreased capillary CSF absorption, and increased venous pressure (Warf, 2013; Greitz, 2004).

The consequence of these processes in infants with open cranial sutures is expansion of the ventricles leading to increasing head size and thinning of the cortical mantle. Untreated, this process can lead to grotesque head enlargement and fatal failure of brain function. In older children and adults, new-onset hydrocephalus may be caused by obstruction or inflammation that leads to derangement of the CSF physiology described above. This in turn leads to increased ventricular size and increased intracranial pressure, the symptoms of which are well known (headache, nausea, vomiting, lethargy, etc.).

Treatment is directed at normalizing intracranial pressure, normalizing ventricular size, and preventing the consequences of prolonged ventricular dilation.

Figure 35.2 is an example of hydrocephalus due to focal obstruction of the cerebral aqueduct by a tectal tumor of the midbrain.

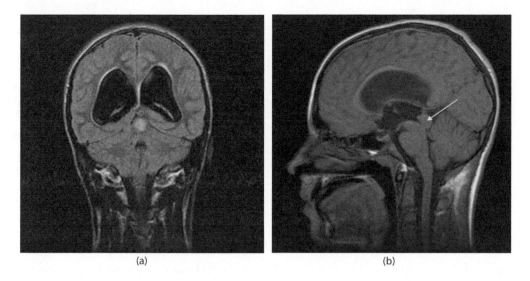

Figure 35.2 (a) Coronal MRI showing dilated lateral ventricles. (b) Sagittal MRI showing dilated third ventricle and normal-size fourth ventricle. Note the presence of a dilated midbrain tectum indicating the presence of a tectal tumor (arrow).

Common physical exam findings

Infants:

- Increasing head circumference—Crossing percentiles on growth chart
- Prominent scalp veins
- Bulging fontanel
- Irritability
- Vomiting
- Increased sleepiness
- Impaired upgaze: "sun-setting" eyes

Toddlers and young children:

- Headaches or head banging
- Nausea/vomiting
- Increased sleepiness
- Increased irritability
- Visual changes
- Regression in motor and cognitive abilities
- Large head circumference

Teens and adults:

- Headaches (especially that wake you up from sleep or first thing upon waking)
- Nausea/vomiting
- Irritability
- Increased sleepiness
- Visual changes

- Regression in motor or cognitive abilities
- Decline in school performance

Relevant diagnostic tests

- Head ultrasound: This is used for preemies and infants while a fontanel is still present (Figure 35.3).
- Head CT: Able to visualize the ventricles but hard to assess the other structures of the brain. It is used less in children due to the radiation exposure.
- MRI: It provides a more detailed study of the brain and can be used to determine the reason behind the cause of the hydrocephalus (i.e., tumor, hemorrhage). Recently, a rapid-protocol MRI has been advocated to evaluate the ventricle size and configuration of children with hydrocephalus while avoiding sedation and radiation exposure.
- Shunt series: Anteroposterior (AP) and lateral x-rays of the head, and AP views of the chest and abdomen that allow assessment of shunt hardware to evaluate for breakage or discontinuity (Figure 35.4).

Surgical treatments

There are two main approaches to surgical treatment of hydrocephalus: CSF shunting and endoscopic CSF diversion. In both cases, the goal of treatment is to normalize intracranial pressure and ventricular size and allow for normal brain function.

CSF shunting

The mainstay of hydrocephalus treatment for decades has been VP shunting. A cranial incision is made at the site for ventricular catheter insertion, either frontal or posterior depending on surgeon preference. A burr hole is made. In infants, the anterior fontanelle may be used as a site to enter the cranium without bony removal. A second incision is made in the abdomen, and the peritoneum is opened. A tunneling device is used to pass the distal catheter subcutaneously from the head to the abdomen. In the case of coronal placement, a small intervening incision is often required to complete the pass. Once the valve and distal catheter are in position, the dura is opened, and the ventricular catheter is passed into the ventricle.

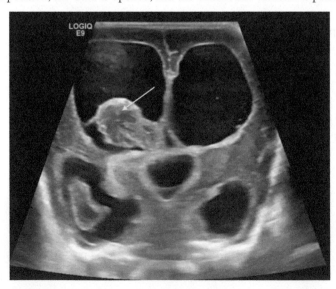

Figure 35.3 Ultrasound of an infant with hydrocephalus. Note the dilated lateral and third ventricles and the presence of hemorrhage (arrow) within the ventricle.

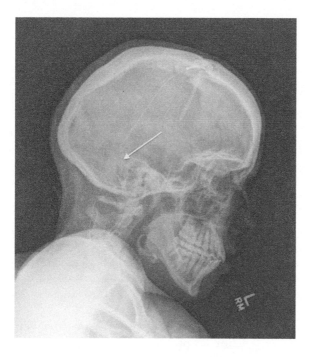

Figure 35.4 Example of one component of the shunt series, a lateral skull x-ray, showing a discontinuity in the distal shunt catheter.

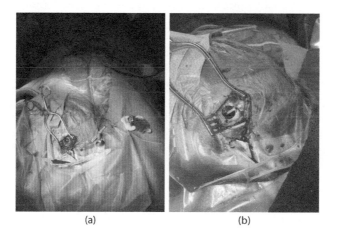

(a)   (b)

Figure 35.5 Both images show a VP shunt placement in the operating room.

Endoscopy, ultrasound, and stereotactic techniques have all been used to guide placement of the ventricular catheter. Once the ventricular catheter is connected to the distal shunt system, the distal tubing is placed into the open peritoneum. All incisions are closed (Figure 35.5).

In cases where the peritoneum is not a viable shunt target (e.g., infants with history of necrotizing enterocolitis or patients with history of insufficient peritoneal absorption of CSF), alternate locations for the distal shunt catheter are the atrium of the heart (ventriculoatrial [VA] shunt), the plural cavity (ventriculopleural [VPL] shunt), as well as other less common locations.

As with any implanted foreign body, shunts are prone to infection. Shunt infection rates vary from 2% to 15%. The most common organisms are skin flora, suggesting contamination at the time of surgical implantation or revision. Careful adherence to a shunt placement protocol has been shown to decrease shunt infection rates (Kestle et al., 2011). At most centers, the protocol for treatment of a shunt infection involves complete removal of all shunt hardware along with a period of external ventricular drainage and antibiotics. After completion of the course of antibiotics and documentation of clearance of bacteria from the CSF, a new shunt system is placed.

The other major risk of shunting is that of shunt failure or obstruction (like that described in the case vignette). In children, the rate of shunt failure is as high as 40% in the first year and 50% by the end of the second year after shunt placement (Kestle et al., 2000). Typical symptoms of shunt failure are headache, nausea/vomiting, and lethargy, as noted above. Greater than 80% of shunt failures are a result of occlusion of the ventricular catheter.

The revision procedure typically involves opening of the cranial incision; disconnection of the ventricular catheter from the valve; and assessment of flow through the valve and distal catheter using a manometer. If good distal runoff is seen, than the ventricular catheter is removed, a new catheter placed, and the new catheter connected to the existing distal system. In the rare event that the distal runoff through the manometer is poor, the valve or distal catheter must be replaced. Some surgeons will advocate replacing the ventricular catheter in these cases, as well (i.e., replace the entire shunt), given the high likelihood of ventricular catheter occlusion.

Endoscopic third ventriculostomy and endoscopic third ventriculostomy/ Choroid plexus cauterization

An alternative to shunting is endoscopic third ventriculostomy (ETV). This procedure is particularly well suited to treatment of hydrocephalus due to obstruction of CSF pathways within the ventricles or at the outlet of the fourth ventricle (e.g., aqueductal stenosis or posterior fossa tumor). The procedure involves introduction of an endoscope into the lateral ventricle, navigation of the endoscope through the foramen of Monro, and creation of an ostomy in the floor of the third ventricle. The ETV Success Score (ETVSS) is a model designed to predict the probability of successful ETV based on preoperative factors (Kulkarni et al., 2010) (Table 35.1).

In children under 2 years of age, ETV alone has not had a high level of success. However, the addition of choroid plexus cauterization (ETV/CPC), a technique pioneered by Dr. Ben Warf in Uganda and now gaining popularity in the United States as well, substantially increases the likelihood of successful hydrocephalus treatment without a shunt (Warf, 2005). Depending on the etiology of hydrocephalus, 50%–80% of children with hydrocephalus are successfully treated with ETV/CPC and do not require subsequent shunting.

Because of the lack of implanted hardware, ETV/CPC does not carry the same infection risk as shunting. However, the site of the ETV is in close proximity to the infundibulum, and there is a small risk of

Table 35.1 Endoscopic Third Ventriculostomy Success Score (ETVSS)

Score	Age	Etiology	Previous shunt
0	<1 month	Postinfectious	Previous shunt
10	1 month to <6 months		No previous shunt
20		Myelomeningocele, intraventricular hemorrhage, nontectal brain tumor	
30	6 months to <1 year	Aqueductal stenosis, tectal tumor, other	
40	1 year to <10 years		
50	≥10 years		

Note: The ETVSS is calculated as Age Score + Etiology Score + Previous Shunt Score.

inducing diabetes insipidus. There is also a small risk of damage to the basilar artery. Both of these complications have the potential to result in severe, lifelong consequences.

Family counseling

Prognosis

The diagnosis of hydrocephalus can be overwhelming and frightening, but with early diagnosis and timely treatment, the prognosis can be greatly improved. Many patients with hydrocephalus as their primary condition go on to lead productive lives with few restrictions. Patients who suffer from other medical conditions along with hydrocephalus may experience more complications related to hydrocephalus than patients without comorbidities. The key to having a positive prognosis with hydrocephalus is establishing a plan of care in a timely manner, under the direction of a neurosurgeon, and maintaining the care plan with the help of other team members, such as the advanced practice health professional.

Common questions

- *What caused it?*
  - There are two types of hydrocephalus, congenital or acquired. Congenital hydrocephalus is present at birth from genetic abnormalities or deviation from normal events during fetal development. Acquired hydrocephalus occurs either at the time of birth or sometime after. It can be caused by an injury or disease and can happen at any age.
- *What are the treatment options?*
  - There are a few different surgical options available. These options are outlined previously in the chapter. There is no effective nonsurgical treatment for hydrocephalus.
- *Are multiple surgeries required?*
  - Multiple surgeries are a possibility. Shunts often require revisions for infection, malfunction, or a break in the catheter.
- *Can I hurt the shunt once it is in place?*
  - Typically, shunts are not affected by everyday activities. Patients can lie on the side in which the shunt is placed without concern. Children with shunts can be held by parents without concern.
- *When are revisions necessary?*
  - Revisions are necessary when an infection is detected, the shunt is malfunctioning, or there is a break in the catheter system. Revisions may also be necessary if the patient is symptomatic or shows increased ventricular size on imaging.
- *What should I look for to know if the shunt is malfunctioning?*
  - Common symptoms of shunt malfunction include headache, nausea, vomiting, change in personality, and sun-setting eyes. Other signs of malfunction are palpable fluid collections around the catheter or an obvious break in the catheter (usually seen in the neck).

Pitfalls

- Multiple surgeries
- Lifelong dependency on shunt
- Lifelong requirement for neurosurgical care

Relevance to the advanced practice health professional

The advanced practice health professional plays a vital role in the lives of patients with hydrocephalus and their families. They are the direct link from home to the care team. It is important that they are familiar with the disease process, have knowledge of treatment options, and provide support for the families. The advanced practice health professional should be able to answer questions concerning the disease process, including treatment options, with the support of the care team. They should be familiar with signs and symptoms of malfunction or infection so that they can recognize a problem in a timely manner. Most importantly, the advanced practice health professional must develop relationships with the families to provide necessary support and to develop trust. Through these, the patient's care plan will flow seamlessly across disciplines to provide optimum care.

Common phone calls, pages, and requests with answers

- A patient with a shunt has been complaining of a headache for 2 days. The patient vomited this morning after breakfast. No fever, diarrhea, or vision changes were reported.
  - The patient should come to the hospital to be evaluated, including images, to see if the shunt is malfunctioning.
    - Fast-sequence MRI and shunt series
    - Possible shunt tap
- Two days after discharge from a shunt revision, the surgical incision is red, warm to touch, and draining clear fluid.
  - The patient should come to the hospital for the care team to evaluate the incision.
    - CSF studies should be sent to evaluate for possible shunt infection.
- Can a 10-year-old patient with a shunt play sports?
  - Contact or collision sports are not advised.
    - Suggest swimming, tennis, dance, golf, etc.
- A patient with a shunt revision 6 months ago complains of abdominal pain.
  - The patient should come to the hospital for evaluation of pseudocyst
    - Abdominal ultrasound
    - CSF studies

References

Greitz D. Radiological assessment of hydrocephalus: new theories and implications for therapy. *Neurosurg Rev.* 2004;27(3):145-165–discussion166-167. doi:10.1007/s10143-004-0326-9.

Kestle J, Drake J, Milner R, Sainte-Rose C. Long-term follow-up data from the shunt design trial. *Pediatric.* 2000;33(5):230–236. doi:10.1159/000055960.

Kestle JR, Riva-Cambrin J, Wellons JC 3rd, et al. A standardized protocol to reduce cerebrospinal fluid shunt infection: the hydrocephalus clinical research network quality improvement initiative. *J Neurosurg Pediatr.* 2011;8(1):22–29. doi:10.3171/2011.4.PEDS10551.

Kulkarni AV, Drake JM, Kestle JR, Mallucci CL, Sgouros S, Constantini S. Predicting who will benefit from endoscopic third ventriculostomy compared with shunt insertion in childhood hydrocephalus using the ETV success score. *J Neurosurg Pediatr.* 2010;6(4):310–315. doi:10.3171/2010.8.PEDS103.

NHFOnline. Facts about hydrocephalus | Hydrocephalus statistics | NHFOnline.org. http://nhfonline.org/facts-about-hydrocephalus.html., 2015 (Accessed August 26, 2017).

Simon TD, Riva-Cambrin J, Srivastava R, Bratton SL, Dean JM, Kestle JR. Hospital care for children with hydrocephalus in the United States: utilization, charges, comorbidities, and deaths. *J Neurosurg Pediatr.* 2008;1(2):131–137. doi:10.3171/PED/2008/1/2/131.

Warf BC. Comparison of endoscopic third ventriculostomy alone and combined with choroid plexus cauterization in infants younger than 1 year of age: a prospective study in 550 African children. *J Neurosurg.* 2005;103(suppl 6):475–481. doi:10.3171/ped.2005.103.6.0475.

Warf BC. Congenital idiopathic hydrocephalus of infancy: the results of treatment by endoscopic third ventriculostomy with or without choroid plexus cauterization and suggestions for how it works. *Child's Nerv Syst.* 2013; 29(6):935–940.

36

MALIGNANT BRAIN NEOPLASMS AND BRAIN METASTASIS

Cathy M. Rosenberg, Simon Buttrick, and Ricardo Komotar

Case vignette

The patient is a previously healthy, right-handed, 30-year-old male. He presents with a 2–3 week history of dizziness, nausea, and intermittent vomiting. He initially attributed his symptoms to an upper respiratory infection but sought care in the emergency room when his symptoms progressed.

Imaging studies revealed a lesion within the right cerebellar peduncle, slightly indenting the brainstem. The lesion was hyperintense on T2 weighted magnetic resonance imaging (MRI), and did not enhance with contrast.

He was subsequently scheduled for a stereotactic needle biopsy to obtain a tissue diagnosis, to further guide treatment. Unfortunately, the patient deteriorated suddenly the day prior to surgery with increased headache and increased nausea and vomiting. Shortly thereafter, he became unresponsive.

An emergency computed tomography (CT) was performed and revealed a large right cerebellar hemorrhage with extension into, and compression of the brainstem.

An extraventricular drain (EVD) was placed at the bedside, and the patient was taken emergently to the operating room for evacuation of the hematoma and partial tumor resection.

Postoperatively, the patient never regained consciousness. Brain death protocol was initiated and confirmed by two physicians. Testing revealed absent pupillary reactions to light, absent oculocephalic reflexes, absent corneal reflexes, and mild preservation of the gag reflex.

Extensive counseling was held with the family regarding the patient's condition and the significance of the clinical findings. Eventually, family members elected to proceed with organ procurement after cardiac death. Pathology revealed World Health Organization (WHO) grade 4 glioma with hemorrhagic components.

Introduction

The purpose of this chapter is to introduce and discuss the most common malignant adult brain tumors, their clinical presentation, relevant diagnostic imaging, treatment options, and clinical points or patient education pertinent to the nurse or midlevel provider.

The vast majority of intracranial neoplasms are either gliomas, arising from glial cells, the support network of the central nervous system (CNS) (Batchelor, 2015), or metastases from extracranial malignancies (Wong and Wu, 2015). Management of intracranial neoplasms is complex, often requiring a combination of surgery, chemotherapy, and radiation. We consider the clinical and diagnostic features of both gliomas and metastases together, and then separately discuss the management of each. Nurses and midlevel

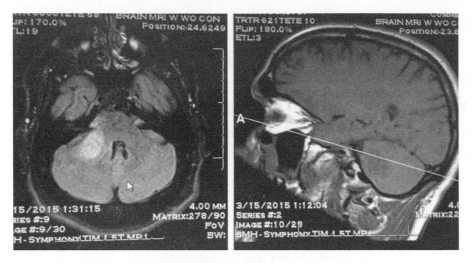

Figure 36.1   (a) Right cerebellar mass and (b) nonenhancing with contrast.

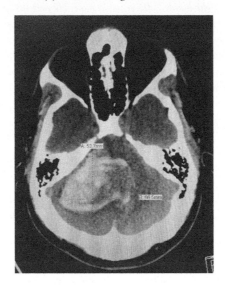

Figure 36.2   Hemorrhage, right cerebellar with brainstem compression.

providers should ensure that the patient and family understand the overall goals of care and the roles of various providers along the continuum.

Clinical presentation

Signs and symptoms of brain tumors can be localized, related to the anatomic location of the lesion, or generalized, as a result of increased intracranial pressure, hydrocephalus, or meningeal irritation. Common localizing signs and symptoms include the following:

Frontal lobe: Contralateral weakness, motor seizures, impaired cognition/higher-level functioning, changes in personality, impaired fluency of speech, dysphasia

Parietal lobe: Contralateral cortical sensory deficit, impaired spatial relations, agnosia, apraxia

Temporal lobe: Visual field deficits, impaired memory, impaired speech and comprehension, impaired emotional responses, psychomotor seizures

Occipital lobe: Homonymous hemianopsia, visual hallucinations/seizures

Cerebellum: Ipsilateral limb ataxia or truncal ataxia, nystagmus

Brainstem: Cranial nerve deficits and long tract findings

Generalized symptoms include headache, seizure, cognitive or behavioral change, fatigue, decreased responsiveness, lethargy, apathy, and confusion. Signs and symptoms related to elevated intracranial pressure include papilledema, headache, nausea, and vomiting (Wong and Wu, 2015).

Headache is the most common initial presenting symptom of a brain tumor; however, only a very small percentage of patients with headaches end up harboring a tumor. Therefore, it is essential to elicit the specific features of the headaches. Brain tumors often present with headaches that are progressive over several months. Classically, the headache is worse in the morning, as intracranial vessels are dilated from hypoventilation during sleep, which further contributes to intracranial pressure. This feature is not found in every patient with a brain tumor, but if present, should raise suspicion for an intracranial lesion. Other features warranting further evaluation for brain tumor are the presence of headache associated with nausea and vomiting or a headache that worsens with changes in body position or maneuvers that increase intrathoracic pressure (Wong and Wu, 2015).

Workup

Contrast-enhanced MRI is the most useful diagnostic study in the workup of a suspected intracranial neoplasm. Gliomas appear as T2 hyperintense, diffuse lesions. Although there are rare exceptions, higher-grade neoplasms (grades III and IV) are usually contrast enhancing, while lower-grade neoplasms are not. Metastases tend to be more sharply demarcated, are often found at the gray–white junction, and generally have more peritumoral edema than primary intracranial neoplasms. Crucially, metastases often come in multiples, which is rare for gliomas. Nevertheless, it is impossible to definitively distinguish between gliomas and metastases based purely on MRI. Several novel imaging techniques have somewhat improved our ability to noninvasively diagnose intracranial lesions, but histopathologic analysis remains the gold standard. In the absence of significant past medical history, further workup often includes an HIV test, as there is a wide differential diagnosis for intracranial lesions in HIV-positive patients, and a basic metastatic workup consisting of a CT of the chest, abdomen, and pelvis with intravenous contrast. If this reveals a likely primary malignancy, it should be biopsied to obtain tissue for diagnosis, as the type of cancer can significantly impact the management of the intracranial metastases. Even if this metastatic workup does not reveal any primary malignancy, intracranial metastases cannot be ruled out.

Initial management is highly dependent on the specific clinical situation. The rare patient with a large mass lesion, who is rapidly deteriorating, should be taken to the operating room immediately to relieve the mass effect. Patients who are clinically stable but symptomatic from mass effect and edema can be treated with steroids, which usually results in significant improvement of symptoms. It is important to keep in mind, however, that steroids rapidly shrink primary CNS lymphomas. If this diagnosis is considered likely, steroids should be used sparingly to avoid losing a target to biopsy (AANN, 2014). Patients are usually started on antiepileptic medications to decrease the risk of seizures, although there is still significant debate as to the benefit of this practice.

Gliomas

Classification

Gliomas are classified in the WHO system according to the specific glial cell they originate from, and their malignancy potential. Astrocytomas arise from astrocytes, while oligodendrogliomas arise from oligodendrocytes and portend a somewhat better prognosis. Malignancy potential is graded on a scale from

I to IV. Grade IV astrocytomas are termed *glioblastoma* (previously *glioblastoma multiforme* [GBM]). They are the most common primary intracranial malignancy and have the worst prognosis, with median survival between 12 and 18 months with optimal therapy. Grade III astrocytomas, or anaplastic astrocytomas, are less common, and median survival is generally between 2 and 3 years. Grade II astrocytomas, also known as low-grade gliomas, have a better prognosis, but despite being considered benign lesions, they frequently transform into higher-grade gliomas over time. Grade I astrocytomas, which comprise several rarer tumors, are of a more benign nature and are often cured completely with surgical resection. Oligodendrogliomas occur in grades II and III, each with somewhat improved survival compared to their astrocytoma counterparts. With the use of advanced histochemistry and genetic analysis, we are learning that specific gene mutations found in tumor cells can have profound effects on survival, allowing for more accurate prognostication than by using the WHO grading system alone.

Management

When a high-grade glioma is suspected based on imaging characteristics, the tumor is resected if in a surgically accessible area. In addition to providing ample tissue for histopathologic diagnosis, aggressive resection has been shown to improve survival. Extent of resection has been found to correlate with survival; however, if less than 80% of the tumor is resected, it likely offers no benefit over biopsy alone. The principal goal of glioma surgery is therefore achieving maximal resection without creating a neurologic deficit. Intraoperative monitoring, including somatosensory evoked potentials (SSEPs) and motor evoked potentials (MEPs), which allows for real-time assessment of neural pathways, has made surgery on eloquent region tumors safer. Awake craniotomies are also becoming more commonplace and are especially useful for tumors close to language and motor areas. In awake craniotomies, electrical stimulation is used to "stun" a small area of brain tissue. If no changes occur in the patient's neurologic exam, the stimulated area can likely be resected safely.

It is important for patients and families to understand that gliomas are highly infiltrative lesions. Complete resection of the enhancing tumor, referred to as "gross total resection," does not imply removal of all tumor cells. Patients and families often misinterpret this statement and need reinforcement to understand the pathology and need for continued treatment. Especially with high-grade gliomas, tumor cells can be found at sites quite distant from the enhancing tumor. Therefore, gliomas can never be cured surgically. If the lesion is deep or in an eloquent area of the brain, and aggressive resection is deemed to be associated with a high risk of neurologic injury, the tumor should be biopsied instead to provide a definitive tissue diagnosis to guide treatment (Recht, 2015). Postoperatively, MRI is usually done to evaluate the extent of resection.

Patients are kept on steroids, commonly dexamethasone, to reduce swelling close to the surgical cavity, and antiepileptic medications. Steroids are tapered according to the patient's clinical exam, the presence of edema and neurologic symptoms (AANN, 2014). Providing clear written instructions regarding the details of the steroid weaning process to include dates and dosages reduces phone calls related to mistakes in dosing or confusion regarding the correct scheduling of medications. Patients are continued on low-dose steroids throughout radiation and may require tapering during treatment under the direction of the radiation oncology or neurology team. Patients are placed on proton pump inhibitors or H2 blockers while taking steroids to minimize gastrointestinal (GI) side effects such as gastritis and ulceration. Patients should be instructed to monitor for and report GI side effects. They should also receive education as to the increased risk of infection while on steroids related to impaired immunity, alterations in blood sugar management if diabetic, possible worsening of hypertension, and the possibility of mood swings, agitation, and anxiety. Psychological side effects can be significant enough to warrant referral to a psychiatrist to assist with symptom management or be cause for referral to the emergency room if the patient has a crisis. Patients on long-term steroids should also receive protection against osteoporosis. Long-term use of corticosteroids can suppress the hypothalamic-pituitary-adrenal axis and cause secondary adrenal insufficiency (Roth et al., 2010).

Prophylactic antiepileptic medications remain controversial in the postoperative period. Treatment should be individualized to the patient's need. If a patient presented preoperatively with a seizure, or if tumor was resected from a more epileptogenic region, then medications are often continued and eventually weaned off under the direction of a neurologist if the patient remains seizure free. Patients presenting with seizures need to be counseled regarding driving restrictions according to individual state laws and counseled regarding safety precautions. Seizures and subsequent safety precautions can create multiple changes in personal and family dynamics related to role alterations within the family unit, challenges or inability to earn income, and new or increased dependence on others, and may serve as a significant source of distress related to lost independence. Patients may also experience depression or suicidal thoughts and should be counseled to report any thoughts of hurting themselves or others when taking antiepileptic medications. Stevens-Johnson syndrome is a rare but serious skin disorder that causes fever, severe rash, and blistering and may be life threatening. Patients should be counseled to monitor for and report any rash immediately (Schachter, 2015).

The current mainstay of therapy for high-grade gliomas is radiation and chemotherapy since Stupp et al. demonstrated in 2005 that the addition of temozolomide to standard radiation therapy significantly improves survival in newly diagnosed glioblastoma. The benefit is modest, prolonging mean survival from 12.1 months with radiation therapy alone to 14.6 months. Strikingly, temozolomide appears to have a robust effect on the tail end of the survival curve, improving 2-year survival rates from 10% to 25%. Temozolomide is taken orally and is generally well tolerated. The efficiency of temozolomide has been found to be dependent on the methylation stats of the *MGMT* gene. *MGMT* encodes a DNA repair enzyme, which helps tumor cells repair damage created by temozolomide. Tumors that have the *MGMT* gene inactivated by methylation therefore portend a better prognosis. Radiation tends to be given in daily fractions of 2 Gy, 5 days a week for 6 weeks. Regimens may require adjustment to make treatment more tolerable for patients. Both chemotherapy and radiation impair wound healing; therefore, it is imperative to wait at least 2 weeks after surgery before initiating therapy.

Patients with gliomas require close observation with frequent imaging to assess for recurrence or progression of disease. At our institution, we routinely obtain MRI imaging every 3 months for glioblastoma and less frequently for lower-grade gliomas. Radiotherapy causes radiation necrosis in some patients. This often results in worsening symptoms and is hard to distinguish from tumor recurrence based on MRI. Novel imaging techniques, such as magnetic resonance spectroscopy, perfusion imaging, and positron emission tomography are often utilized in an attempt to differentiate between radiation necrosis and recurrence, but their benefit is unproven.

For focal recurrences, repeat craniotomy has been shown to increase survival. A small subset of patients, who maintain good functional status, may benefit from additional surgeries, although the risks of wound infection and wound breakdown increase with every intervention. Bevacizumab is a monoclonal antibody that inhibits angiogenesis, which offers a modest survival benefit in patients with recurrent glioblastoma. Providers prescribing bevacizumab need to inform patients that this agent carries a black box warning about impaired wound healing and wound dehiscence as well as severe and occasionally fatal hemorrhage.

Additional clinical trials are underway to assess the efficacy of novel treatment strategies, including stem cells, tumor vaccines, and targeted molecular therapies. Many of these therapies are in their infancy and are years away from being integrated into mainstream clinical practice. Smaller community facilities may not offer these options, and referral to larger academic institutions should be considered to improve the patient's access to care when feasible. Clinicaltrials.gov offers information about currently approved research studies that patients may be eligible to pursue within the continental United States and 189 countries.

Brain metastasis

Metastatic brain tumors originate outside of the CNS and then spread to the CNS, creating a common neurologic complication of cancer. Metastatic brain tumors are the most common intracranial tumors in adults and are at least twice as likely to occur as gliomas (AANN, 2014). Metastatic brain tumors occur in up to 30% of adults with systemic cancer, at least three-fourths of these occur within the first year of diagnosis (Ahluwalia et al., 2014). The incidence of metastasis appears to be increasing secondary to several factors: enhanced imaging techniques; more frequent utilization of intracranial imaging in the staging of asymptomatic patients; more effective, life-prolonging systemic treatment options; the inability of many chemotherapeutic agents to cross the blood-brain barrier (BBB), creating a haven for intracranial tumor deposition; and transient weakening of the BBB by certain chemotherapeutic agents allowing for seeding of CNS malignancies (Ahluwahlia et al., 2014).

Common systemic malignancies that metastasize to the brain in descending order include lung, breast, melanoma, renal, and colon. Gastrointestinal malignancies and prostate cancer rarely metastasize to the brain, although prostate cancer has a propensity to spread along the meninges. Brain metastases tend to spread hematogenously and are usually found at the gray-white junction.

Management of brain metastases involves four basic treatment modalities: surgery, chemotherapy, stereotactic radiosurgery, and whole brain radiation. Planning treatment takes into account several factors: the history of the patient's cancer, the current status of the cancer, overall patient health, number and size of metastatic tumors, and finally the location of the tumor(s) within the brain (ABTA, 2012). Surgery provides the most definitive method for treating metastases but may carry the greatest risk. It is generally reserved for large metastases in patients with otherwise well-controlled disease and good functional status. Stereotactic radiosurgery, such as linear accelerator (LINAC) radiosurgery, CyberKnife, or Gamma Knife, delivers radiation to a specific area of the brain, with rapid drop off of tissue damage to surrounding structures. This is usually delivered in a single session, but patients may return for additional metastases. It is generally accepted that stereotactic radiosurgery is effective for lesions up to 3 cm in size, and several targets can be treated simultaneously. Furthermore, it is often used to treat the resection cavity after surgical removal of metastases in order to destroy any remaining tumor cells. Whole brain radiation involves radiotherapy evenly distributed over the entre brain. Some cancers, such as small cell lung carcinoma, are exquisitely sensitive to radiation, while others, such as melanoma or renal cell carcinoma, are not. Whole brain radiation is used for patients with multiple, diffuse brain metastases, or patients with poor functional status. Due to their radiosensitivity and poor prognosis, small cell cancer metastases are unique in that they are almost never treated surgically. Finally, in rare instances, intrathecal chemotherapy is used. This method allows direct contact between the chemotherapy agent and the cancer cells. The drug can be delivered via repeated lumbar punctures, or through an Ommaya reservoir, a surgically implanted device.

Patients and families need to be informed that evidence of results may take a few months to become evident on follow-up imaging. Posttreatment imaging is obtained at short intervals, usually every 2–3 months, to evaluate the patient's response to treatment and to monitor for recurrence. It is important for cancer patients to continue to maintain their regularly scheduled visits even when their cancer is under control.

Many patients and families require assistance while living with cancer. Various forms of support are available through support groups to help connect patients with others in similar situations. Social workers can help connect patients to these resources, as well as financial, transportation, home care, palliative care, or hospice services. TrialConnect is the American Brain Tumor Association's Clinical Trial Matching Service and is available at www.abtatrialconnect.org.

End-of-life care

Metastatic disease and high-grade gliomas are often incurable, and determining when to stop treatment can be a very difficult decision for the patient and family. However, the decision to stop treating does not mean to stop providing care to the patient. Patients and families want to know what to expect during the dying process as well as have their emotional and spiritual needs met. Palliative care and hospice services should be considered when the patient is unlikely to survive greater than 6 months.

Hospice services may also provide additional levels of support for the patient and family, which may not be otherwise available compared to traditional medical services, such as respite care (Batchelor, 2015). Research demonstrates that patients enrolled in hospice were hospitalized less frequently at the end of life, received less intensive care, underwent fewer invasive procedures, and were less likely to die in a hospital or skilled nursing setting. Most patients when surveyed do not demonstrate these preferences. Therefore, it is important to have frank but sensitive discussions between providers and patients about end-of-life care (Obermeyer et al., 2014).

Common phone calls, relevant information, and recommendations for nurses and midlevel providers

Midlevel providers and nurses should avoid the misconception that preoperative patients are more stable clinically than postoperative patients as demonstrated in the clinical vignette. Patients awaiting surgery are often symptomatically controlled with steroids. New symptoms and worsening of the neurologic exam, especially alterations in consciousness, warrant a repeat detailed neurologic examination, possible reimaging, emergency measures to decrease cerebral edema, and possibly earlier neurosurgical intervention.

Family members have the primary responsibility of supporting a person with a brain tumor. It is essential that the midlevel provider and nurse anticipate and prepare the family for the physical, behavioral, cognitive, and emotional effects of the disease process and treatment. Shorter hospital stays and overwhelming amounts of information need to be delivered in manageable amounts. Providing information frequently, verbally and in writing or by video, may help improve retention.

Patients or family members often call with alterations in the neurologic status during the steroid weaning process. This is frequently related to tapering the steroid more rapidly than the patient can tolerate and resultant cerebral edema. Instruct the patient to resume the previously effective dosage for 24–48 hours. If improved, reattempt weaning and monitor for symptom recurrence. If steroids have been used for a prolonged period of time, consider suppression of the hypothalamic-pituitary-adrenal axis and secondary renal insufficiency during the weaning process, especially if associated with headache, nausea, myalgias, and hypotension (AANN, 2014).

Table 36.1 is a combination of the Kernohan grading scale, which divides tumors into four grades, and a tiered grading system that helps to distinguish histopathologic characteristics between tumor grades (Greenberg, 2006). Understanding the cellular characteristics and WHO grading scales allows providers to anticipate and plan options for treatment.

Determine if the midlevel provider will be sharing pathology results. Discuss the approach with the collaborating physician. Consistent language regarding pathology is important in maintaining trust between providers. Shared information regarding pathology needs to be delivered in a culturally sensitive manner that is suitable to the patient's preferences. Inconsistencies in delivering difficult information can create misunderstanding and dissatisfaction with caregivers and may cause patients to inappropriately seek care from others.

Table 36.1 Astrocytoma Grading and Characteristics

Kernohan grade	WHO designation	Hypercellularity	Pleomorphism	Vascular proliferation	Necrosis
I	Low-grade astrocytoma	Slight	Slight	None	None
II	Low-grade astrocytoma	Low	Minimal	None	None
III	Anaplastic astrocytoma	Moderate	Moderate	Permitted	None
IV	Glioblastoma multiforme	Hypercellular	Moderate and marked	Common	Required

Conclusion

Diagnosis and management of primary and metastatic intracranial neoplasms are complex. In many cases, a combination of surgery, radiation, and chemotherapy is required. The field is rapidly evolving with advances in molecular biology and immunotherapy offering hope that the dismal prognosis of these disease processes may improve in the near future.

References

Ahluwalia MS, Vogelbaum MV, Chao ST, Mehta MM. Brain Metastasis and Treatment. *F1000 Prime Reports.* Chicago, IL: AANN; 2014.

American Association of Neuroscience Nurses. *Care of the Adult Patient with a Brain Tumor. AANN Clinical Practice Guideline Series.* Chicago, IL: AANN; 2014.

American Brain Tumor Association. Metastatic brain tumors. www.abta.org (accessed 26 August, 2017). 2012.

Batchelor T. Patient information: High grade glioma in adults (Beyond the basics). Up to Date. www.uptodate.com (accessed 26 August, 2017). 2015.

Obermeyer Z, Makar M, Abujabe S, Dominii F, Block S, Cutler DM. Association between the medicare hospice benefit and health care utilization for patients with poor prognosis cancer. *JAMA.* 2014;312(18):1888–1896.

Roth P, Wick W, Weller M. Steroids in neurooncology: Actions, indications and side effects. *Curr Opin Neurol.* 2010;23(6):597–602.

Recht LD. Patient information: Primary low grade glioma in adults (beyond the basics). Up to Date. www.uptodate.com (accessed 26 August, 2017). 2015.

Schachter SC. Seizures in adults (Beyond the basics). Up to Date. www.uptodate.com (accessed 26 August, 2017). 2015.

Stupp R, Mason WP. van den Bent MJ et al. Radiotherapy plus concomitant and adjuvant temozolomide for glioblastoma. *N Engl J Med.* 2005;352:987–996.

Wong ET, Wu JK. Clinical presentation and diagnosis of brain tumors. Up to Date. www.uptodate.com (accessed 26 August, 2017). 2015.

37

PITUITARY SURGERY

Valentina Pennacchietti and Nelson M. Oyesiku

Case vignette

A 59-year-old male patient was admitted with a history of headaches, nausea, vomiting, and generalized weakness. He was severly hyponatremic and hypopituitaric. Magnetic resonance imaging (MRI) showed a large enhancing sellar mass (Figure 37.1). Hydrocortisone, testosterone, and levothyroxine replacements were started after an endocrinologic evaluation. The patient underwent a bilateral three-dimensional (3D) endoscopic transsphenoidal resection of the tumor, a pituitary nonfunctioning macroadenoma. At day 4 after surgery, the patient was discharged with hormonal replacement therapy. A 3-month follow-up, MRI showed total resection of the tumor (Figure 37.2); the patient went back to his usual activities, still on replacement therapy.

Epidemiology

The most common lesions affecting the sellar region are pituitary nonsecreting or secreting adenomas (10% of intracranial neoplasms). They occur in 10%–15% of the general population and are sometimes diagnosed incidentally. They typically occur in the third to fourth decades of life and in both sexes equally (Kopczak et al., 2014).

Clinically significant pituitary tumors are associated with high morbidity and decreased quality of life. Morbidity comprises visual impairment, endocrine disturbances, and neurologic deficit related to mass effect.

Pathogenesis

In 95% of cases, pituitary tumors occur sporadically, with both genetic and epigenetic abnormalities (Kopczak et al., 2014). Several pituitary selective oncogenes, tumor suppressor genes, and mediators of the pituitary cell cycle are involved in pituitary tumorigenesis (Rogers et al., 2014). About 5% have a familial genetic background (e.g., as part of multiple endocrine neoplasia [MEN] type 1, Carney complex (CNC), or familial isolated pituitary adenomas (FIPAs) (Kopczak et al., 2014). MEN type 1 is an autosomal dominant disorder due to mutations in the tumor suppressor gene *MEN1* and is characterized by the occurrence of tumors in the parathyroid glands, pancreatic islets, and anterior pituitary (2.7% of all pituitary tumors). MEN type 4, due to mutations in *CDN1B*, occurs in 3% of patients with a *MEN1*-like syndrome without mutations of *MEN1* (Rogers et al., 2014).

Anatomy of the sellar region

The sellar region is at the center of the cranial base and hosts the pituitary gland. Its boundaries are the optic nerves, chiasm, and circle of Willis, above; the cavernous sinuses and internal carotid arteries, laterally; and the brainstem and basilar artery, behind (Figure 37.3).

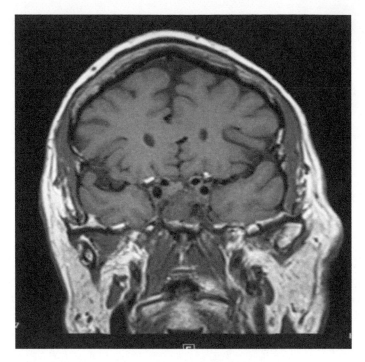

Figure 37.1 Preoperative MRI showing an enhancing hyperintense sellar mass.

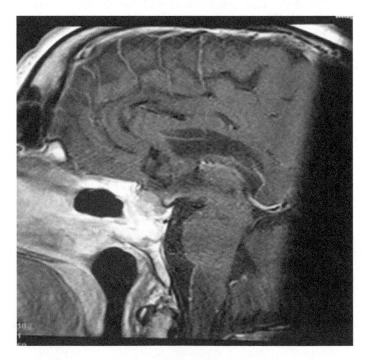

Figure 37.2 Three months follow-up postoperative MRI.

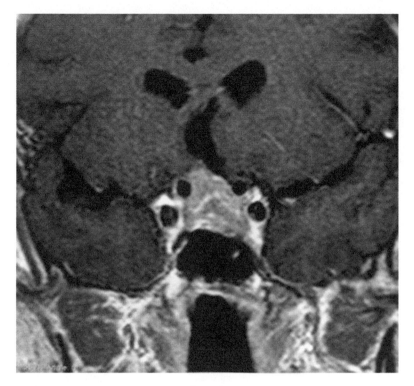

Figure 37.3 Anterior view of the pituitary gland, in relationship with optic chiasm, above, and intracavernous segments of internal carotid arteries, laterally (1: pituitary gland, 2: cavernous segment of the internal carotid artery, 3: internal carotid artery, 4: pituitary stalk, 5: optic chiasm, 6: superior hypophyseal artery).

The nasal cavity provides access to this space, because the sphenoid bone connects it to the pituitary gland above. The carotid arteries are in close relationship to the sphenoid bone, creating an impression in the lateral wall of the sphenoid sinus. Also, both cavernous sinuses lie laterally to the sphenoid bone. The pituitary gland rests in the center of the bone, the sella turcica, limited anteriorly by the tuberculum sellae and posteriorly by the dorsum sellae. The sphenoid sinus is an air cavity inside the sphenoid body. It separates the cavernous sinuses, the cavernous segments of the carotid arteries, the optic, extraocular, and trigeminal nerves, and the pituitary gland from the nasal cavity (Figure 37.4). The sella turcica is separated from the rest of the brain by the diaphragma sellae, a membrane that covers the pituitary gland, except for a small opening in its center for the pituitary stalk.

The cavernous sinus is a venous space that lies in the space between the superior orbital fissure and the petrous apex, hosts the horizontal part of the internal carotid artery, and forms the lateral wall of the sella. The carotid artery enters the cavernous sinus after the foramen lacerum, it reaches the anterior clinoid process and penetrates the roof of the cavernous sinus, bending anteriorly. The cavernous sinus hosts, from rostral to caudal, the oculomotor, trochlear, ophthalmic, and abducens nerves. The oculomotor, trochlear, and ophthalmic nerves are in the lateral sinus wall, between two dural leaves. The abducens nerve lies lateral to the carotid artery, within the sinus.

The suprasellar area is the region above the sella turcica. It extends from the ventral surface of the midbrain, around the optic chiasm, to the subcallosal area. The cerebral peduncles form its posterior wall. The infundibulum of the pituitary gland passes through this region to go in the diaphragma sellae. The suprasellar region also hosts the optic nerves and chiasm. Above the optic chiasm lie the anterior cerebral and anterior communicating arteries, the lamina terminalis, and the third ventricle (Rhoton, 2002).

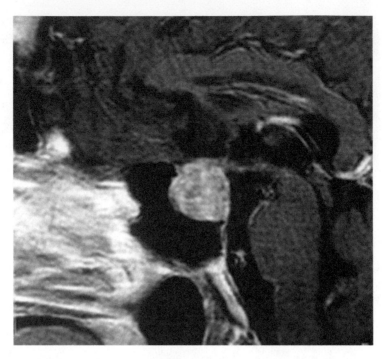

Figure 37.4 Lateral wall of the nasal cavity, showing the concha (1: frontal sinus, 2: superior meatus, 3: sphenoid ostia, 4: sphenoid sinus, 5: superior nasal concha, 6: middle concha, 7: middle meatus, 8: eustachian tube, 9: inferior meatus).

Clinical features

Pituitary adenomas can present with signs and symptoms related to a derangement in hormone production (overproduction or underproduction) or mass effect, or both. In general, patients with visual symptoms should be referred urgently for investigation. Prolactinomas more frequently occur in women, while in men they are diagnosed later because of symptoms of libido and erectile dysfunction. Women develop menstrual irregularities, galactorrhea, or infertility. Cerebrospinal fluid (CSF) rhinorrea may be seen with macroprolactinomas, resulting from erosion of the sphenoid bone.

Nonfunctioning adenomas usually cause clinical manifestations from mass effect to surrounding structures: compression of the pituitary stalk can cause headache, optic chiasm involvement results in unitemporal or bitemporal visual field defects, and extension laterally into the cavernous sinus may rarely cause ophthalmoparesis.

Pituitary apoplexy (hemorrhage into or infarction of the pituitary gland) is uncommon (0.2 per 100 patient-years) and is characterized by severe headache, sudden onset of visual disturbance, meningism, and hypotension. It can be fatal as a result of sudden hypopituitarism and cortisol deficiency (Rogers et al., 2014). Factors that may predispose patients to apoplexy are rarely identified and include acute blood pressure changes (hypotension or hypertension), dynamic stimulatory tests of the pituitary gland, and anticoagulation (Miller et al., 2014).

Diagnosis

Laboratory tests

Preoperative endocrine evaluation should investigate pituitary hormone deficiencies (frequent in cases of large pituitary masses) and hypersecretion. The evaluation includes measurement of anterior pituitary hormones (prolactin, thyroid-stimulating hormone, adrenocorticotropic hormone [ACTH], growth hormone [GH], luteinizing hormone, follicle-stimulating hormone, α-subunit) as well as target hormones (free thyroxine, cortisol, insulin-like growth factor-I; testosterone in men; estradiol in women). An ACTH-secreting tumor causes Cushing disease, a complex of signs and symptoms related to hypercortisolism (hypertension, diabetes mellitus, obesity, osteoporosis), whereas a GH-secreting tumor causes acromegaly, a clinical syndrome characterized by cardiomyopathy, hypertension, diabetes, musculoskeletal abnormalities, sleep apnea, and increased incidence of colon cancer.

Patients with suspected Cushing disease should undergo a comprehensive battery of tests, including nighttime salivary and 24-hour urinary cortisol determinations, low-dose and high-dose dexamethasone suppression tests, and, in equivocal cases, inferior petrosal sinus sampling. In cases of clinical or biochemical suspicion for acromegaly, GH suppression during oral glucose tolerance is indicated (Miller et al., 2014).

Visual evaluation

In patients with lesions in close proximity of the optic chiasm, visual acuity, formal assessment of visual fields using Goldman or Humphrey perimetry, optic disc examination, eye movements, and pupillary responses are necessary (Rogers et al., 2014; Miller et al., 2014).

Neuroradiologic imaging

Patients should be investigated with MRI with and without contrast agent. Dedicated vascular imaging may be indicated in cases of lesions with cavernous sinus involvement, and computed tomography may be performed to obtain clearer delineation of bony anatomy (Miller et al., 2014).

The differential diagnosis of a sellar mass lesion is long and mainly includes pituitary adenoma, craniopharyngioma, Rathke cleft cyst, epidermoid cyst, chordoma, meningioma, metastatic tumor, lymphoma, aneurysm, lymphocytic hypophysitis, arachnoid cyst, mucocele, pituitary abscess, or sarcoidosis (Rogers et al., 2014).

Treatment options

Before surgery, other surgical and nonsurgical options must be properly considered. An appropriate endocrine workup must be completed because certain pituitary tumors may be amenable to medical therapy.

Medical treatment with a dopamine agonist, such as cabergoline, bromocriptine, or quinagolide, is the preferred treatment for prolactinomas. Normoprolactinemia is achieved in 85%–90% of patients using cabergoline and 75% using bromocriptine. Side effects include headache, postural hypotension, nausea, and sedation, and 3.5% of patients stop treatment because of intolerance to cabergoline. Occasionally, dopamine agonist treatment of an invasive prolactinoma that is eroding the skull base can result in leakage of cerebrospinal fluid, manifesting as cerebrospinal rhinorrhea. The indications for pituitary surgery in prolactinoma include pituitary apoplexy with neurologic signs, failure of medical treatment, and increasing tumor size associated with neurologic deficits.

At the present time, a transsphenoidal approach is the method of choice for resection of pituitary adenomas. Indications for a transsphenoidal approach have expanded with the development of extended transsphenoidal approaches that involve removal of additional bone to widen the surgical corridor, allowing access to skull base lesions. Although microscopic techniques are used, the endoscopic technique is gaining favor as the preferred approach in experienced hands. New 3D endoscopes are gaining popularity as a solution to the limitations of the 2D view provided by traditional endoscopes. Intraoperatively, manipulation of CSF volume via a lumbar drain can help bring the tumor into the operative field or help unload the prolapsed diaphragma sellae and arachnoid after tumor removal. CSF drainage is also therapeutic in case of an intraoperative CSF leak, allowing drainage of CSF while the site of the leak heals.

Limitations to the endoscopic approach may be vascular, such as carotid arteries that critically constrict the sellar corridor, or anatomic variants of the skull base (e.g., conchal sinus). Intracavernous extension of tumor lateral to the carotid arteries may be a challenge for transsphenoidal resection.

With the availability of postoperative radiosurgery, it is quite reasonable to treat residual tumor in the lateral cavernous sinus after an endoscopic approach rather than use a transcranial approach purely for the resection of cavernous sinus disease, as long as residual disease is minimal. Several studies of radiosurgery for pituitary adenomas have shown good results. The most common reason to perform a craniotomy for pituitary adenoma is that the extent of residual disease after transsphenoidal operation is not amenable to radiotherapy (Rogers et al., 2014; Miller et al., 2014).

Grading systems

Traditionally, pituitary tumors were classified based on their tinctorial properties with histology reagents and were associated with a clinical disease in eosinophilic or acidophilic (acromegaly), basophilic (Cushing disease), and chromophobic adenomas.

Pituitary adenomas are also classified depending on their size into microadenomas (<1 cm) and macroadenomas (>1 cm).

A common grading system is the Knosp classification, based on the invasion of the intracavernous segment of the internal carotid artery by the tumor: a grade from 0 to 4 is assigned, detecting the lateral extent of the lesion on coronal MRI sections. Tumors with grades 0–2 are contained within the lateral carotid artery tangential, while tumors that extend beyond the carotid artery tangential are grades 3–4 (Micko et al., 2015).

According to the 2004 WHO classification, pituitary tumors arising from adenohypophyseal cells are clinically divided into functioning (mainly GH, prolactin, and ACTH) and nonfunctioning (mainly follicle-stimulating and luteinizing hormones [FSH–LH]) tumors, which constitute half to one-third of all pituitary adenomas.

The 2004 WHO classification also classifies all benign tumors as typical adenomas, while atypical adenomas included all tumors showing "borderline or uncertain behavior." Such tumors were classified as having atypical morphologic features suggestive of aggressive behavior such as invasive growth. Other features include an elevated mitotic index and a Ki-67 labeling index >3% and extensive nuclear staining for p53 immunoreactivity (Raverot et al., 2014; Kopczak et al., 2014; Dallapiazza et al., 2014).

Family counseling

Prognosis

Survival rates after surgical treatment are high (91%–98%), and usually gross total resection is achieved in 80% of cases. For the follow-up and treatment, a pituitary multidisciplinary team should comprise endocrinologists, neurosurgeons, neuroradiologists, neuropathologists, and oncologists (Kopczak et al., 2014; Rogers et al., 2014).

Common questions

After pituitary surgery, common concerns are the rate of remission of the endocrinologic symptoms and signs and the rate of recurrence of these tumors. Cushing disease has a high success rate of surgical cure with transsphenoidal surgery. Short-term remission supported by normalization of serum or urine cortisol levels is >80%, with a higher rate of success in microadenomas than in macroadenomas. The recurrence rate is 17%.

Biochemical remission of acromegaly is based on normal GH and insulin-like growth hormone levels as well as GH suppression test. In cases of persistent disease after surgery, repeat transsphenoidal operation may be successful in 60% of patients, although this percentage is much lower if the tumor is invasive or difficult to visualize on MRI.

In prolactinomas, normalization of prolactin postoperatively has been reported to be 80%–90% for microadenomas and 40% for macroadenomas.

Early surgery in a patient with pituitary apoplexy is associated with a good outcome, with vision preservation in most cases and resolution of blindness in some cases. Adenomas manifesting with apoplexy have been shown to recur more often; for this reason, close follow-up and eventual postoperative radiation therapy after surgery are warranted.

Macroadenomas have been shown to recur even more than 10 years after initial surgery with a mean time to recurrence of 5–7 years (Miller et al., 2014).

Pitfalls

Mortality associated with endoscopic endonasal transsphenoidal pituitary surgery performed by an experienced pituitary neurosurgeon is low (<1%), and complications such as CSF leak and meningitis are rare (3%–5% and about 1%, respectively) (Rogers et al., 2014). Injury to the internal carotid arteries is an uncommon event (less than 1%). Partial or complete pituitary insufficiency occurs in about 5%–15% of all cases (Sauer et al., 2014).

Endonasal endoscopic techniques are associated with lower complication rates and lower health-care costs when compared with transcranial techniques (Villwock et al., 2015).

Relevance to the advanced practice health professional

Patients should be monitored postoperatively for water metabolism (diabetes insipidus or hyponatremia), hypopituitarism, and neurosurgical complications such as CSF leak (rhinorrea) or meningitis. Water metabolism perturbations are transient in most cases, and new permanent hypopituitarism is rare.

At the time of discharge, patients should be warned of the risk of late CSF leak, avoiding efforts, such as coughing, sneezing, or bending forward, almost for the first 30 days after surgery. An endocrine evaluation should be performed at 6–12 weeks postoperatively. Postoperative imaging (MRI with and without gadolinium) should be obtained after 12 weeks because early postoperative changes can obscure residual tumor or underestimate the resection (Miller et al., 2014).

Common phone calls, pages, and requests with answers

Q: *Which are the most common complaints after transsphenoidal surgery?*

A: Headache is the most frequent postoperative complaint. If used, nasal packing is removed on the second or third postoperative day, and this may be uncomfortable for the patient. The patient should be taught not to blow the nose, cough, or sneeze through the nose due to risk of injury to the surgical cavity. Dressings placed under the nose can be changed as needed. The patient can get out of bed to walk on postoperative day 1 and may be discharged on the third day after surgery if no complications occurred.

Q: *Which blood tests are useful in the early postoperative management of a patient with a pituitary lesion?*

A: Morning serum cortisol levels on days 2 and 3 after surgery verify hypothalamic-pituitary-adrenal (HPA) axis integrity and indicate if oral hydrocortisone replacement is necessary after discharge. If the cortisol level is less than 10 mcg/dL, patients are discharged with low-dose oral hydrocortisone. The cortisol levels need to be rechecked 1 week after discharge. Patients not in cortisol replacement have to recognize and report flu-like symptoms, which may indicate eventual hypocortisolemia or hyponatremia.

Q: *Which exams are necessary to assess a postoperative diabetes insipidus?*

A: Polydipsia, polyuria, hypovolemia, excessive thirst, hypotension, altered mental status, and fever are common signs of diabetes insipidus. Urinary output is high, even up to 4–18 L/day; urine-specific gravity, sodium, and osmolality are low; and serum sodium and osmolality are high.

References

Dallapiazza R, Bond AE, Grober Y et al. Retrospective analysis of a concurrent series of microscopic versus endoscopic transsphenoidal surgeries for Knosp grades 0-2 nonfunctioning pituitary macroadenomas at a single institution. *J Neurosurg.* 2014;121(3):511–517.

Kopczak A, Renner U, Stalla GK. Advances in understanding pituitary tumors. *F1000Prime Rep.* 2014;6:5.

Micko AS, Wohrer A, Wolfsberger S, Knosp E. Invasion of the cavernous sinus space in pituitary adenomas: endoscopic verification and its correlation with an MRI-based classification. *J Neurosurg.* 2015;122(4):803–811.

Miller BA, Ioachimescu AG, Oyesiku NM. Contemporary indications for transsphenoidal pituitary surgery. *World Neurosurg.* 2014;82(suppl 6):S147–151.

Raverot G, Jouanneau E, Trouillas J. Management of endocrine disease: clinicopathological classification and molecular markers of pituitary tumours for personalized therapeutic strategies. *Eur J Endocrinol.* 2014;170(4):R121–32.

Rhoton AL Jr. The sellar region. *Neurosurgery.* 2002;51(suppl 4):S335–374.

Rogers A, Karavitaki N, Wass JA. Diagnosis and management of prolactinomas and non-functioning pituitary adenomas. *BMJ.* 2014;349:g5390.

Sauer N, Flitsch J, Doeing I, Dannheim V, Burkhardt T, Aberle J. Non-functioning pituitary macroadenomas: benefit from early growth hormone substitution after surgery. *Growth Horm IGF Res.* 2014;24(2–3):71–75.

Villwock JA, Villwock MR, Goyal P, Deshaies EM. Current trends in surgical approach and outcomes following pituitary tumor resection. *Laryngoscope.* 2015;125(6):1307–1312.

38

SKULL BASE TUMORS

Angela Richardson, Cathy M. Rosenberg, and Jacques Morcos

Case vignette

This patient is a 16-year-old female who presented with amenorrhea. On initial evaluation, her pediatrician attributed her symptoms to aggressive athletic training with her track and field team since the age of 15. Evaluation by a pediatric endocrinologist did not reveal any abnormalities in her hormonal levels. These hormone levels were evaluated again 6 months later and remained unremarkable. Due to ongoing symptoms, her family requested additional testing. A magnetic resonance imaging (MRI) scan of the brain was performed. These images revealed a suprasellar enhancing mass with both solid and cystic components compressing the optic chiasm and hypothalamus (Figure 38.1a and b). Several areas of calcification were seen on a computed tomography (CT) scan (Figure 38.1c). Due to the calcifications and the heterogeneous appearance, this mass was believed to be most consistent with a craniopharyngioma.

Once this intracranial mass was diagnosed, she was referred for neurosurgical evaluation. Her neurologic exam was grossly normal, but because of the proximity of the lesion to the optic chiasm, she was referred for formal visual field testing. Ophthalmologic evaluation demonstrated visual acuity 20/20 bilaterally with full extraocular movements without diplopia. Formal visual field testing demonstrated a left homonymous hemianopsia (Figure 38.2). A repeat endocrine panel performed at this time remained normal.

The initial neurosurgical consultant offered a limited resection. Another consultant deemed the tumor inoperable and suggested no intervention. Several radiation options were also discussed: intratumoral seed radiation, cystic aspiration, or radiation alone. The family sought a third opinion from a neurosurgeon specializing in skull base surgery. This surgeon offered an attempt at gross total resection, which would be the most likely approach to result in a cure. Since craniopharyngiomas have a high recurrence rate, many experts believe the first attempt at surgery offers the best hope for a cure (Cheng et al., 2016). Ultimately, the patient and her parents opted for maximal safe resection with the hope for a cure, or if not possible, for a delay in recurrence.

The attending physician performed the informed consent process. He described resection of the craniopharyngioma via a right cranio-orbital and transsylvian approach. He also discussed the possible complications including coma, death, and paralysis, as well as the risk of development of diabetes insipidus (DI) or other transient or permanent endocrine abnormalities (Tan et al., 2017). The pituitary stalk was sectioned at the time of surgery to allow for maximal resection. There were no obvious intraoperative complications.

The patient was at her neurologic baseline postoperatively, but she was diagnosed with DI when she developed increased urine output and increased serum sodium. She was treated with desmopressin acetate (DDAVP), resulting in normalization of her electrolytes and urine output. She then developed the syndrome of inappropriate antidiuretic hormone (SIADH) with serum sodium levels as low as 119. Her hyponatremia required treatment with fluid restriction,

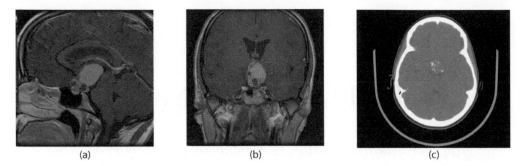

(a) (b) (c)

Figure 38.1 (a) Sagittal MRI T1 sequence with gadolinium contrast demonstrating midline enhancing mass with cystic components. (b) Coronal MRI T1 sequence with gadolinium contrast showing an enhancing mass with solid and cystic components at the level of the foramen of Monroe. (c) Axial CT scan without contrast with calcifications at the periphery of the lesion.

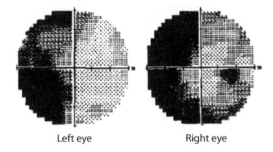

Left eye Right eye

Figure 38.2 Patient's visual fields demonstrating a left homonymous hemianopsia.

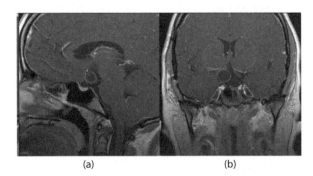

(a) (b)

Figure 38.3 MRI T1 sequence with gadolinium preformed 1 year after surgery. (a) Sagittal image demonstrating a suprasellar peripherally enhancing cystic lesion. (b) Coronal image showing the same mass eccentric to the right side.

close monitoring of her serum sodium, and sodium replacement as clinically indicated. Her SIADH resolved, and she again developed DI. She was discharged home on postop day 19 with oral DDAVP.

She underwent routine postoperative follow-up including an interval MRI at 1 year after surgery. This imaging study (Figure 38.3) demonstrated a peripherally enhancing suprasellar cystic structure to the right of midline elevating the right optic tract. She was diagnosed with recurrent disease. Her neurologic exam remained stable with a persistent left lower quadrantanopsia improved from her preoperative homonymous hemianopsia. As the risks of further surgery were thought to outweigh the possible clinical benefit, she was referred to a radiation oncologist. This physician recommended external beam radiation over 6 weeks as an adjunctive treatment; she completed this without complication. Her MRI at the completion of radiation was stable, and 1 year after radiation treatment, imaging demonstrated shrinkage of the cystic mass. She has been followed for 10 years after completing this treatment and has remained neurologically stable with stable findings on interval MRIs, and persistent endocrine dysfunction is managed satisfactorily with medication.

Introduction

In contrast to the convexity of the cranium, the base of the skull has a more complicated anatomy. The bones of this region contain foraminae (openings) that allow the cranial nerves and major blood vessels to enter and exit the skull. Due to the bony anatomy and these exiting blood vessels and nerves, retraction of the nervous system tissue can be difficult, and specialized surgical approaches may be required. These approaches may be performed using the microscope or can be performed using an endoscope. Due to the difficult anatomy and the rarity of these approaches in clinical practice, neurosurgeons may elect to undergo specialized fellowship training in either open or endoscopic skull base surgery. An additional aspect of skull base surgery is the proximity of other structures such as the orbit, the nasopharynx, the external and middle ear, and the facial sinuses. Understanding the anatomic relationship of these structures to the skull base is crucial, as some approaches to lesions at the base of the skull require traversing these extracranial areas (Patel et al., 2016; Slattery, 2015). Skull base surgery thus often requires a team of neurosurgeons; ear, nose throat (ENT) specialists; and/or oculoplastic and orbital surgeons to obtain optimal patient outcomes.

Some lesions encountered at the skull base also occur elsewhere (i.e., meningiomas), and other lesions are only seen at the skull base. For a list of pathologies commonly encountered by skull base surgeons, see Table 38.1. Although these tumors may not be the most common brain tumors, they are responsible for significant morbidity in patients who have them. The close proximity to the cranial nerves can frequently result in cranial neuropathies. The surgical approaches to these tumors are complex, and there can be significant risks associated with these surgeries of either temporary or permanent cranial neuropathies.

Clinical presentation

Patients with lesions of the skull base can present in a variety of ways—their presentation in combination with clinical exam and imaging findings will determine the course of treatment. With the increased imaging, some patients may be referred with an incidentally found tumor. More commonly they will have symptoms referable to the tumor. These symptoms can be general or related to tumor location. General symptoms are often due to increased intracranial pressure (ICP). This set of symptoms would include headaches (characteristically worse in the morning), vision changes (blurry vision, diplopia), and nausea/vomiting.

In contrast to these general symptoms, another subset of symptoms is specific to tumor location; if cranial nerve deficits are present, they can help localize the tumor. (Refer to Chapter 9 for a review of the cranial nerve exam.) Lesions of the anterior skull base such as olfactory groove meningiomas can present with anosmia, or lack of a sense of smell. Involvement in the orbit or along the optic nerves, chiasm, or tract can produce specific visual field defects depending on the location. Tumors of the orbital apex or cavernous sinus may result in diplopia due to compromise of the nerves controlling the extraocular movements (CN III, IV, VI). Involvement of the cavernous sinus is more likely if facial sensation is impaired. Facial sensation (CN V) can be altered by lesions interrupting any or all of the three branches (V_1, V_2, V_3) of the trigeminal nerve. Lesions of the cerebellopontine angle (CPA) can alter facial sensation, abduction

Table 38.1 Common Skull Base Tumors

Lesion	Common symptoms	Location	Cranial nerves involved
Acoustic neuroma (vestibular schwannoma)	Hearing loss, tinnitus, dysequilibrium	Posterior fossa	VIII, VII, V, VI
Meningiomas	Location specific, as meningiomas may occur anywhere in the skull base	Nonspecific	Any possible
Pituitary adenoma	Cushing disease, acromegaly, bitemporal hemianopsia, see Chapter 37 for more information	Midline in sella with sella expanded	II, VI, III
Craniopharyngioma	Headache, hydrocephalus, bitemporal hemianopsia, loss of visual acuity, DI	Sella and suprasellar	II, VI, III, V
Paraganglioma— Tympanicum, jugulare, or caroticum (aka glomus)	Location specific, may vary depending on which location	Middle ear, neck	Varies with location
Chordoma	Diplopia, headache (retro-orbital or occipital)	Midline	VI most commonly
Chondrosarcoma	Pain, diplopia	Parasagittal	VI most commonly
Esthesioneuroblastoma	Nasal obstruction, epistaxis, anosmia, diplopia	Anterior skull base/paranasal sinuses	I
Sinonasal carcinoma	Nasal obstruction, epistaxis, anosmia, diplopia	Anterior skull base	I

Note: The tumor types in this table are those most frequently encountered by skull base specialists. Some tumor types (i.e., meningiomas) may occur in any location, while others, such as acoustic neuromas, occur in one particular location. Cranial nerve deficits will vary depending on the location of the tumor.

of the eye, hearing, vestibular function, and/or facial movement. More extensive lesions of this region, or lesions arising closer to the jugular foramen and hypoglossal canal, can cause significant difficulties swallowing or with vocal cord function or tongue movement due to compression of the lower cranial nerves (CN IX, X, XI, XII).

Endocrinopathies can also occur with tumors of the skull base. The abnormal over- or underproduction of hormones can cause significant morbidity and mortality; thus, vigilance is important for early detection and treatment. These endocrine abnormalities can occur early in the course of the tumor (preoperative), intra- or perioperatively, as a delayed response to radiation/surgery, or as a result of tumor progression/recurrence (Tan et al., 2017). As discussed in Chapter 37, these tumors, as well as craniopharyngiomas, are the most likely to be associated with endocrine abnormalities. In these patients, particularly in the immediate postoperative period, urine output and serum sodium level must be carefully monitored to detect DI. This requires aggressive fluid replacement and, potentially, treatment with vasopressin. Patients may also develop the syndrome of SIADH, which is treated with fluid restriction. One of the most severe hormone abnormalities that may be seen is a low cortisol state. This can result in profound hypotension refractory to treatment and electrolyte abnormalities; this can even be fatal. Patient symptoms are nonspecific and usually include malaise, fatigue, and nausea/vomiting. Prompt administration of stress dose steroids can result in a rapid reversal of symptoms.

Patients may also present with cerebrospinal fluid (CSF) leak. These patients will often complain of clear water-like fluid dripping or flowing from the nose or ear. More fluid may leak with a Valsalva maneuver, any straining, or bending over. Even if a CSF leak is not present before surgery, it may occur after surgery—through the nose (rhinorrhea) or ear (otorrhea), or at the incision site.

Lesions of the skull base can occur sporadically or may be associated with other diseases or genetic syndromes. A full discussion of all the possible syndromes and genetic diseases is beyond the scope of this chapter; however, one disease of note is neurofibromatosis type 2 (NF2). This disease can occur sporadically or be inherited in an autosomal dominant fashion. The clinical features are caused by a mutation on chromosome 22 resulting in absent or defective merlin protein. Patients with bilateral vestibular schwannomas, by definition, have NF2 (Slattery, 2015). Special consideration must be given to the goal of hearing preservation in these patients. Patients with unilateral vestibular schwannoma or other lesions characteristically associated with NF2 and/or a positive family history should be referred for a genetics consultation.

Workup

Usually a patient will be referred with imaging studies demonstrating an intracranial lesion. Most surgeons will require MRI with and without contrast for surgical planning; additional sequences may be requested depending on tumor type and location. For bony lesions or to better define bony anatomy, a CT scan may be warranted. Depending on the location and type of tumor, as well as specific patient complaints, other specialists may be consulted. Ophthalmologic evaluation includes formal visual fields, visual acuity, and funduscopic exam for the assessment of papilledema. Evaluation by an otolaryngologist is useful for lesions of the anterior skull base where an endoscopic endonasal approach is considered. For acoustic neuromas, neurootologists can perform vestibular and audiometric evaluations. Endocrinologists will typically be involved in the care of patients with preoperative endocrinopathies. Additional specialists may be consulted as needed.

Management

Management is nearly always based on a multidisciplinary approach, to include neurosurgery, ophthalmology, oculoplastics, ENT, endocrinology, radiation oncology, physical therapy, occupational therapy, nutritionists, and speech therapy. Where feasible without undue risk, surgical resection is often considered. For lesions less than 3 cm in a difficult to access location, where tissue diagnosis is not needed, stereotactic radiosurgery may be considered. Patients undergoing surgery need to be warned of the risks. Depending on tumor location and surgical approach, specific postoperative deficits, whether permanent or temporary, may be predicted. Surgeries of this type are frequently long, and where appropriate, patients and families should be warned that they might remain intubated following the procedure. Specifically in cases where the lower cranial nerves are at risk, patients may suffer from vocal cord paralysis or dysphagia, either of which can lead to compromised respiratory function. Evaluation of vocal cord function can be completed by ENT prior to extubation, if necessary. In some cases, tracheostomy or feeding tube placement may be required in the perioperative period. In patients where the facial nerve is at risk, postoperative assessment should include documentation of facial nerve function. Particular attention should be given to whether the patient is able to completely close his or her eye. If they are unable to do so, artificial tears and Lacri-Lube, along with taping the eye closed at night, are necessary to protect the cornea.

Adjuncts to treatment

One common adjunct to treatment following surgeries of skull base lesions, or as a conservative measure for the treatment of CSF leaks, is a lumbar drain (Stokken et al., 2015). A lumbar drainage device is a closed, sterile system allowing for continuous drainage of CSF from the subarachnoid space. These devices are often placed for diversion of CSF to promote healing of dura and to decrease tension at the surgical site. Insertion is performed under sterile conditions, most frequently at the L3-L4 or L4-L5 interspace or, occasionally, at the C1-C2 interspace (Farhat et al., 2011). The proximal catheter is advanced to approximately the level of T12-L1, and the distal end is attached to a sterile, closed CSF collection system. Dependent on provider preference, drainage may be set to a specific level, a specific volume (such as 10–15 cc/hr), or to a specific pressure. Documentation and assessment should include color, clarity, and volume drained hourly. Patient assessment should be performed every 1–4 hours and include level of consciousness, neurologic exam, insertion site appearance, presence or absence of headache, photophobia, nuchal rigidity, Kernig sign, and so on. While photophobia, nuchal rigidity, and Kernig sign would suggest meningeal irritation, the presence of headache is nonspecific and can be caused by meningeal irritation or potentially overdrainage of CSF (Attia et al., 1999). System maintenance includes an occlusive dressing over the site and tubing, and maintenance of the tubing without kinking. If the insertion site or system leaks, contact the provider for immediate system repair or replacement, as this can lead to overdrainage and tension pneumocephalus or increase the risk of CSF infection and meningitis through microbial spread. Connections, ports, and stopcocks should be observed to ensure they are intact. Aseptic technique is maintained to obtain samples and change drainage bags. Dressing changes and catheter care should be performed according to institutional protocols. Occlusion of the tubing may occur from blood products. The provider may flush the system with preservative-free sterile saline per institutional protocol (Slazinski et al., 2012).

Other critical components of patient care involve movement and positioning, which should be undertaken with care in these patients. The head of bed should be maintained at the ordered level, usually 30°–45°. Neutral positioning should be implemented when possible, to avoid hyperflexion or rotation of the hips. Clamping the lumbar drain (LD) is essential when the head of bed is changed significantly or the patient changes from lying to sitting or standing to avoid overdraining CSF. Consider placing a sign over the bed to increase awareness of the lumbar drain and assist in maintaining the appropriate precautions (Nestler, 1992).

Removal of the LD occurs when the patient's condition warrants. Timing of catheter removal should be clearly communicated by the surgeon. Often the drain is clamped, patient activity is increased, and the patient is observed for CSF leakage prior to discontinuing the LD. Drainage usually lasts 3–5 days as the dura heals and can withstand increased hydrostatic pressure at that time. Therapy longer than 5 days may be associated with an increased risk of infectious complications such as meningitis (Coplin et al., 1999).

Placement of the LD or CSF drainage can result in additional complications. Radicular pain can occur from nerve root irritation by the catheter. This may be treated with position changes, withdrawing the catheter slightly, analgesics, or complete removal of the catheter. Tension pneumocephalus (the presence of air within the cranial vault causing mass effect on the brain) can occur from a siphoning effect and may manifest by a sudden change in mental status or neurologic deficit. This can be treated by shutting off the drainage system and placing the patient supine or in slight Trendelenburg. An urgent call to the surgeon is warranted for this complication as it can lead to brain herniation (Pepper et al., 2011). High-flow oxygen and a nonrebreather may be used to promote resolution of pneumocephalus. Other complications may include herniation in the presence of high ICP. Signs and symptoms may include altered mental status, irritability, weakness, paresis, posturing, abnormal breathing, and/or pupillary changes. Should this occur, the provider would close the drain and institute measures for herniation. Overdrainage can also result in the development of subdural hematomas. This would be treated acutely with drain closure and treatment of elevated ICP, followed by CT scan. Surgery may be required depending on the results of imaging studies. Intradural hematoma may occur at the drain site after removal of the drain. Manifestations may include lower extremity paresis, changes in tone, and reflexes. Should this occur, notify the surgeon immediately and anticipate surgical decompression and correction of any possible coagulopathies.

Patient and family education

Patient and family education is essential for optimal outcomes. They should be informed that maintaining the head of bed at the prescribed level facilitates healing of the surgical site and minimizes the risk of CSF leakage. Patients and family members should be instructed to request nursing assistance prior to activity to prevent dislodging or disconnecting the catheter or overdraining CSF. Patients should also be instructed to avoid Valsalva maneuvers, heavy lifting, or bending with the head below the heart to reduce the risk of CSF leak.

Advanced-level providers should proactively treat discomfort and evaluate the efficacy of treatments. The patient should remain free of complications, and safety will be maintained. The patient and family will understand the rationale for placement as well as the risks and benefits of treatment modalities.

Common phone calls, relevant information, and recommendations for nurses and advanced practice providers

Nursing considerations include ensuring patients understand the following: goals of pain management; nausea and vomiting; nutrition, especially if the patient has required a feeding tube; bowel regimen; and deep vein thrombosis prophylaxis. Advanced practice providers should expect to write and enforce orders regarding bowel regimens and early prophylaxis for nausea and vomiting to avoid straining and increasing the risk of CSF leak.

One of the most common phone calls to the advance practice provider includes leaking drainage systems or insufficient drainage from the lumbar drain. Blood or CSF at the insertion site warrants immediate bedside evaluation to ensure the integrity of the system and to avoid more devastating complications such as herniation. The risk-benefit analysis of chemical DVT prophylaxis with an indwelling catheter present must be considered. Some providers recommend holding chemical prophylaxis when the LD is to be discontinued to minimize the risk of hematoma formation at the site, although most published studies demonstrate the safety of prophylactic subcutaneous heparin, with no increase in bleeding risk.

Patients complaining of diplopia may be treated with a variety of options. The simplest is patching the eye or taping one side of their glasses to occlude vision. Prism glasses may be prescribed after consultation with ophthalmology. Diplopia may also manifest as or exacerbate nausea and/or headache, and these symptoms may respond to treatment of the diplopia. Eliminating or reducing diplopia also improves patient safety by reducing the risk of falls.

Patients and families often inquire about typical follow-up. Postoperative routines vary, but in general, patients are seen at 2 weeks after surgery for suture removal and wound assessment. Patients with persistent vertigo may benefit from vestibular rehabilitation. Additional follow-up is at the discretion of the surgeon but includes interval imaging to follow tumor growth and/or recurrence. Adjunctive treatment such as radiation and chemotherapy is dependent on tumor pathology and grade, residual tumor, and progression.

Endocrine dysfunction can cause significant morbidity and even mortality, so vigilance in monitoring urine output, sodium levels, and patient's mental status is essential. In patients susceptible to endocrine dysfunction postoperatively with unexplained hypotension refractory to treatment with fluids, along with malaise, nausea, and/or vomiting may signal a hypocortisol state. Treatment is with prompt administration of steroids. As seen in the clinical vignette, increased urine output with decreased urine specific gravity and a rising serum sodium can signal the development of DI. This needs to be treated promptly to prevent volume depletion and electrolyte abnormalities. This process described in the vignette (DI followed by SIADH and then again by DI) is termed the triphasic response. Patients at risk require close monitoring of their urine output (UOP) and sodium levels and awareness that excess excretion of free water may be followed by excess retention with the development of hyponatremia and possible cerebral edema.

Conclusion

Tumors of the base of the skull often present with hormonal and cranial neuropathies due to the proximity of the brainstem, pituitary gland, and hypothalamus. Treatment is complex and often requires the care of multiple specialists to achieve optimal outcomes. The role of the advanced practice provider is to understand and coordinate the care of the multidisciplinary team. Helping the patient and family to understand the goals of care and the roles of the different providers in this complex scenario can be challenging. The advanced practice provider can assist in making this daunting process more understandable and comfortable.

As demonstrated by the clinical case vignette, this patient has been seen at her 10-year follow-up. She had hypopituitarism and is maintained on estrogen, progesterone, thyroid replacement, and prednisone. She has been able to discontinue her DDAVP despite the pituitary stalk resection. She follows up with her endocrinologist every 6–12 months to assess her lab values and to ensure she is on the minimum amount of medications to be physiologically stable. She is also followed by the ophthalmologist and neurosurgeon annually for formal visual field testing and cranial imaging with contrast-enhanced MRI to ensure she remains clinically and radiographically stable without progression.

References

Attia J, Hatala R, Cook DJ, Wong JG. The rational clinical examination. Does this adult patient have acute meningitis? *JAMA*. 1999;282(2):175–181.

Cheng J, Shao Q, Pan Z, You J. Analysis and long-term follow-up of the surgical treatment of children with craniopharyngioma. *J Craniofac Surg*. 2016;27(8):e763–e766. doi:10.1097/SCS.0000000000003176.

Coplin WM, Avellino AM, Kim DK, Winn HR, Grady MS. Bacterial meningitis associated with lumbar drains: a retrospective cohort study. *J Neurol Neurosurg Psychiatry*. 1999;67(4):468–473.

Farhat HI, Elhammady MS, Levi AD, Aziz-Sultan MA. Cervical subarachnoid catheter placement for continuous cerebrospinal fluid drainage: a safe and efficacious alternative to the classic lumbar cistern drain. *Neurosurgery*. 2011;68(1 Suppl Operative):52–56; discussion 56. doi:10.1227/NEU.0b013e318207b20a.

Nestler AP. Integral nursing interventions for cranial base surgical patients. *Otolaryngol Head Neck Surg*. 1992;10(1):7.

Patel CR, Fernandez-Miranda JC, Wang WH, Wang EW. Skull base anatomy. *Otolaryngol Clin North Am*. 2016;49(1):9–20. doi:10.1016/j.otc.2015.09.001.

Pepper JP, Lin EM, Sullivan SE, Marentette LJ. Perioperative lumbar drain placement: an independent predictor of tension pneumocephalus and intracranial complications following anterior skull base surgery. *Laryngoscope*. 2011;121(3):468–473. doi:10.1002/lary.21409.

Slattery WH. Neurofibromatosis type 2. *Otolaryngol Clin North Am*. 2015;48(3):443–460. doi:10.1016/j.otc.2015.02.005

Slazinski T, Anderson TA, Cattell E et al. Care of the Patient Undergoing Intracranial Pressure Monitoring/External Ventricular Drainage or Lumbar Drainage. *AANN Clinical Practice Guidelines*. Chicago, IL: AANN; 2012.

Stokken J, Recinos PF, Woodard T, Sindwani R. The utility of lumbar drains in modern endoscopic skull base surgery. *Curr Opin Otolaryngol Head Neck Surg*. 2015;23(1):78–82. doi:10.1097/MOO.0000000000000119.

Tan TS, Patel L, Gopal-Kothandapani et al. The neuroendocrine sequelae of paediatric craniopharyngioma: a 40 year meta-data analysis of 185 cases from three UK centres. *Eur J Endocrinol*. 2017;176(3):359–369. doi:10.1530/EJE-16-0812.

39

POSTERIOR FOSSA SURGERY

Solomon Ondoma, Yiping Li, and Mustafa Baskaya

Case vignette

We present the case of a 62-year-old female who for the past month has been having unsteadiness while walking. She reports being unsteady on her feet only, without weakness of the lower extremities or upper extremities. She also notes that she has been having visual symptoms such as intermittent blurriness when staring at objects. This has also been going on for a month. She denies any nausea or vomiting. She also denies any headaches that have been going on for the last few months. Past medical history is otherwise unremarkable. She has no prior history of malignancy but has a 20 pack-year history of smoking.

On examination she is neurologically intact except for slight dysmetria on finger-to-nose testing and is obviously unsteady on her feet with poor lower extremity coordination and a positive Romberg sign (Figures 39.1 and 39.2).

The patient went to the operating room where a posterior fossa craniotomy was performed, and gross total resection of the tumor was achieved.

Postoperatively the patient did well but did have some nausea and vomiting that resolved over a few hours. She recovered in the neurointensive care unit (Neuro-ICU) on postoperative day 1 and transitioned to general care by postoperative day 2. By the third day, the patient was medically stable and discharged to rehabilitation for further improvement in her balance and coordination.

Overview

The posterior fossa is an intracranial cavity that contains the brainstem, cerebellum, and cranial nerves. Because of its relatively small size and the vital structures housed within the posterior fossa, mass effect is poorly tolerated in this location (Figure 39.3). Common complications from mass effect include brainstem compression leading to paralysis or cardiopulmonary dysfunction, cerebellum compression resulting in ataxia or dysmetria, obstruction of cerebrospinal fluid (CSF) flow leading to hydrocephalus, and lower cranial nerve dysfunction causing dysarthria or dysphagia.

Posterior fossa surgery is commonly performed to remove infratentorial tumors and vascular malformations. Posterior fossa tumors are more common in children than adults and account for up to 70% of all childhood brain tumors and up to 20% of all adult brain tumors. Besides tumor resection, posterior fossa surgery is also indicated in cases of malignant cerebellar strokes, Chiari malformations, or posterior fossa hemorrhages where neurologic deficits can arise from mass effect.

Posterior fossa surgery can be a lifesaving procedure aimed at reducing mass effect on the vital neurologic structures and clearance of obstruction for normal flow of cerebrospinal fluid. Overall posterior fossa surgery is extremely common and should be part of the armamentarium of every neurosurgeon. It is the workhorse surgical approach to all traumatic, infections, neoplastic, vascular,

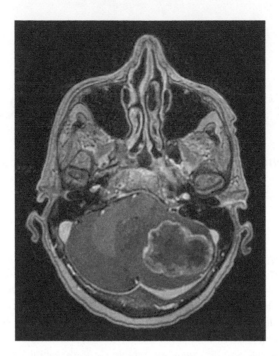

Figure 39.1 Magnetic resonance imaging of the head shows a large heterogenously enhancing lesion in the left cerebellar hemisphere with significant edema and mass effect upon the fourth ventricle.

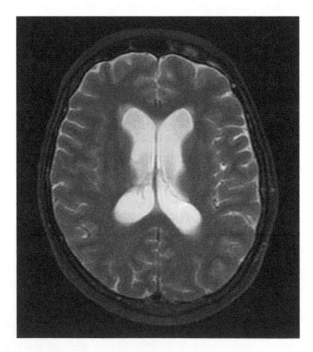

Figure 39.2 T2 sequence shows ventricular enlargement with evidence of hydrocephalus manifested by transependymal lucency.

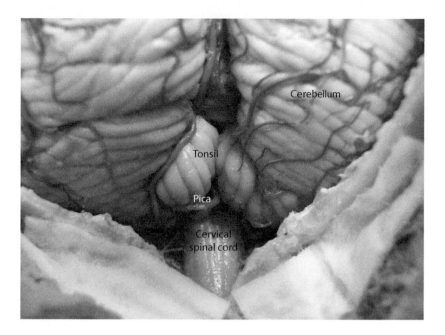

Figure 39.3 Cadaveric/intraoperative photo of a posterior fossa craniotomy. (© Mustafa Baskaya, MD, Department of Neurological Surgery, University of Wisconsin School of Medicine and Public Health.)

or congenital lesions within the infratentorial intracranial cavity. Knowledge of the posterior fossa and the potential surgical complications are vital to intensive care nurses and advanced practice health professionals.

Common physical examination findings

- *Headache*—The most common symptom. Typically more severe in the morning due to increased intracranial pressure from hypoventilation and recumbence during sleep. May be exacerbated by coughing, bearing down, or maneuvers that increase intrathoracic pressure.
- *Nausea and vomiting*—Due to increased intracranial pressure, vestibular dysfunction, or pressure on the area postrema of the fourth ventricle.
- *Cranial neuropathies*—Include opthalmoplegia, dysarthria, dysphagia, or hearing loss.
- *Hydrocephalus*—Resulting in papilledema, blurry vision, and headache.
- *Ataxia and dysmetria*—Due to dysfunction of the cerebellar vermis or hemisphere.

Relevant diagnostic tests

For more information, see Conolly et al. (2010) and Greenberg (2010).

Laboratory

- Complete blood count (CBC) with differential
- Basic metabolic profile, magnesium, and phosphate
- Type and screen

- International normalized ratio/partial thromboplastin (INR/PTT)
- Erythrocyte sedimentation rate (ESR) and C-reactive protein (CRP)

* The hematocrit may be markedly elevated in some patients with hemangioblastoma of the posterior fossa.

Vascular/Electrophysiologic

- ECG
- Computed tomography angiography (CTA)—Presence of an occipital sinus, the vertebral arteries, and the bony anatomy
- CT venogram (CTV)—Evaluate the patency of the venous sinuses in some CPA masses such as tentorial meningiomas
- Magnetic resonance angiography (MRA)
- Diagnostic angiogram
- Transcranial Doppler for evaluation of vasospasm
- Cranial nerve monitoring for acoustic neuromas or tumors of the fourth ventricle
- Indocyanine green (ICG) during aneurysm surgery

Radiologic

- Chest x-ray (CXR) as part of general preoperative workup
- Flexion and extension x-rays to evaluate instability at the craniocervical junction
- CT of the head and cervical spine
- MRI of the brain, cervical spine, and thoracic spine—important in evaluating for drop metastases to the spinal cord or spine, evaluation for syrinxes associated with Chiari I, as well as associated spinal tumors in cases of hemangioblastoma in patients with Von Hippel-Lindau
- CSF flow studies in case of Chiari type I malformations
- Ultrasound as an intraoperative adjunct
- Stealth navigation

Review of relevant interventional procedures and surgeries

Procedures for the posterior fossa are usually open surgical procedures. Endovascular procedures address cerebrovascular disorders as well as preoperative tumor embolization.

The open surgical approaches are discussed in the next sections (Greenberg, 2010).

Midline subocciptal craniotomy

Indications include the following:

1. Midline posterior fossa lesions
   a. Cerebellar vermian and paravermian lesions, including vermian arteriovenous malformation (AVM), cerebellar astrocytoma near the midline
   b. Tumors of the fourth ventricle
   c. Pineal region tumors
   d. Brainstem lesions
2. Decompressive craniectomy for trauma or Chiari malformation
3. Cerebellar hemispheric tumors

Paramedian subocciptal craniotomy

Indications include the following:

1. Access to the CPA for either CPA tumors or for microvascular decompression for trigeminal neuralgia
2. Tumors of the cerebellar hemisphere
3. Access to the vertebral artery for treatment of vertebrobasilar junction anomalies

Far-lateral transcondylar approach

Indication:

Access to the anterolateral intrinsic brainstem tumors or extraaxial craniocervical junction tumors such as foramen magnum tumors

Family counseling

Counseling begins in the office or the emergency room.

Discussions address the nature of the lesion or disease and its relationship to the vital structures of the posterior fossa.

The natural history of the disease, the treatment alternatives, and the risks and complications associated with the treatment alternatives are also discussed.

With this information clearly presented, the patient and his or her family then make an informed decision.

If surgery is to be performed, the precise goals of the surgery are addressed. Again these are dependent on the disease being treated. It is important to know whether an open biopsy, a gross total resection, or a subtotal resection will be performed in case of tumors. Relieving hydrocephalus and obtaining tissue for definitive pathological diagnosis are additional important goals.

Palliation may be the goal for metastatic lesions to the posterior fossa.

Risks and complications (Conolly et al., 2010; Albright et al., 2014)

Infection:

Bleeding—both introperatively or postoperative hematoma

Injury to important brain structures to cause temporary or permanent deficit, coma, vegetative state, or death

The specific related neurological deficits may include:

*   Ataxia
*   Injury to lower cranial nerves causing balance, hearing, and swallowing difficulties and facial weakness

CSF leak that may lead to meningitis.

Air embolism, especially in cases performed in the sitting position.

The risks of general anesthetic medications and the state of being under general anesthesia with endotracheal intubation are often addressed by the anesthesia team. These include:

*   Anaphylactic reactions to the drugs
*   Nausea, vomiting
*   DVT

- Atelectasis, aspiration pneumonia
- Malignant hyperthermia

Surgery

This is performed under general anesthesia with endotracheal intubation. The patient is either prone or in the sitting position depending on the precise nature of the lesion and/or surgeon preference. A preoperative antibiotic is given to prevent infection. Compressive stockings and sequential compression devices (SCDs) are applied for DVT prophylaxis. Chemical DVT prophylaxis is not given for intracranial surgery for concerns of postoperative hematoma. An indwelling bladder catheter is placed to closely monitor urine output (Conolly et al., 2010; Albright et al., 2014).

It is common for an external ventricular drain to be placed before posterior fossa surgery to temporize hydrocephalus.

The hair at the back of the head is often clipped. A midline or paramedian incision is made depending on the pathology.

The length of the surgery is dependent on the lesion size, location, vascularity, and intraoperative complications.

At the end of surgery, the patient is usually extubated in the operating room, if the patient met criteria, and allowed to recover in the postanesthesia care unit. When stable, the patient is then taken to the Neuro-ICU for close monitoring, typically for 1–2 nights. If the patient has an external ventricular drain (EVD), he or she may stay longer until weaned from it or converted to a permanent CSF shunt. Blood pressure is kept strictly within a normal range. Pain is treated expectantly and as needed.

That night, if the patient feels up to it, he or she may eat, drink, and dangle his or her feet at the bedside.

When transitioned to general care, the patient is evaluated by the physical and occupational therapists to determine safety for return to home. Sometimes a short stay in an acute or subacute rehabilitation facility may be needed.

Criteria for discharge home, other than physical and occupational therapists' clearances, are as follows:

- Tolerating a diet with adequate caloric intake.
- Voiding—Some patients may need to go home with a bladder catheter.
- Passing flatus or having bowel movements.
- Having well-controlled pain on oral medications.
- Being ambulatory with little or no assistance.
- Having no outstanding medical issues.

Prognosis

Usually, the patient returns to the clinic in 2 weeks from surgery for a wound check and removal of stiches or staples. At that point, definitive pathology results, the prognosis, and/or the need for adjuvant therapies are discussed.

A cure is established with resection of

- AVMs in the adult patient; pediatric patients have to be followed into adulthood
- Clipped aneurysms
- Benign tumors such as hemangioblastoma and pilocytic astrocytoma

For high-grade gliomas, adjuvant chemotherapy and radiation are needed. Unfortunately, for grade 4 astrocytomas, even with the standard therapies, the median survival is less than 18 months.

There is no cure or effective chemotherapy for diffuse pontine glioma in children. Death occurs.

The prognosis for metastatic tumors is dependent on the primary tumor behavior, efficacy of the available adjuvant therapies, and involvement of other organs. When tumors metastasize to the brain, they usually are, by definition, stage 4.

In acute presentations of trauma or aneurysmal subarachnoid hemorrhage, recovery can be very protracted, with outcomes dependent on the patent's age, premorbid state, and the aggressiveness of physical and occupational therapy.

Common questions

- What are the risks and possible complications associated with surgery?
- How will the surgery be performed?
- Will residents be involved in the surgery?
- Have you performed similar surgeries before?
- Is this a common problem?
- Is it familial or genetic?
- How long will the surgery take?
- What is the recovery period from surgery like?
- When can I return to work?
- How should I care for the wound/incision?

Pitfalls

Perioperative complications include:

- Venous air embolism, which is classic for the sitting position.
- Inadequate subocciptal craniotomy for removal of the lesion.
- Failure to achieve meticulous hemostasis, leading to postoperative hematoma.
- Splitting the vermis can cause permanent truncal ataxia and has been associated with a higher incidence of cerebellar mutism, a part of the posterior fossa syndrome.
- CSF leak from lack of watertight closure.
- Acute hydrocephalus with no EVD in place. This necessitates immediate intervention and can cause rapid deterioration leading to death.

Common pitfalls and medicolegal concerns

Complications are due to the nature of the complexity of posterior fossa surgery and the vital structures involved.

It is important for the consenting process to be thorough, and it must be an informed written consent. The majority of patients tend to be children, on whose behalf parents act. It is said that the well-informed patient is the surgeon's best ally. Most of the potential medicolegal aspects will be obviated by the up-front detailed and honest discussion about the goals, outcomes, and potential risks and complications of the surgery.

Relevance to the advanced practice health professional

The posterior fossa is small, crowded, and occupied by the brain structures that control or regulate the vital functions of breathing, cardiac function, balance, and coordination, as well as cranial nerves mediation of special sensory functions. Obstructive lesions progressively or acutely lead to hydrocephalus. The surgery is complex and is performed, usually, in a prone position. The potential risks and complications are myriad and unforgiving. The patients are usually young. All of these factors call for a proper understanding of the anatomy; well-coordinated teamwork between the surgeons, anesthetists, and nursing team in the peri- and postoperative periods; as well as a family-centered care approach.

Common phone calls, pages, and requests with answers

These can be from the unit or home:

- Pain medication increases
- Concerns regarding postoperative nausea and vomiting
- Elevations in blood pressure requiring continuous infusions of antihypertensive medications
- Problems with functioning of EVDs
- Elevations in intracranial pressure
- Postoperative pseudomeningocele with or without CSF leak
- Wound care

References

Greenberg MS. *Handbook of Neurosurgery.* New York, NY: Thieme; 2010.

Conolly ES, McKhann G II, Huang J, Chouhru TF, Komotar RJ, Mocco, J. *Fundamentals of Operative Techniques in Neurosurgery.* New York, NY: Thieme; 2010.

Albright AL, Pollack LF, Adelson PD. *Principles and Practices of Pediatirc Neurosurgery.* New York, NY: Thieme; 2014.

40

EPILEPSY SURGERY

Wendell Lake and Kyle Swanson

Case vignette

JZ is a 30-year-old man who suffers from epilepsy. He experiences approximately one seizure per month. His epilepsy prevents him from driving and limits his activities. During a seizure, JZ is unresponsive; he stares and turns his head to the right while repetitively grasping his clothes. After the seizure, he is confused and sleepy for 30 minutes to an hour. Prior to having a seizure, he often hallucinates that he smells an indescribable bad odor.

JZ has been on multiple antiepileptic medications. He is currently on three medications but continues to have seizures. He has previously discontinued other medications due to side effects. The dosages of his current antiepileptics are at the maximum level. Electroencephalogram (EEG) demonstrates that seizures localize to the left temporal lobe. Magnetic resonance imaging (MRI) shows that the medial part of the left temporal lobe is shrunken and appears abnormal.

Diagnosis: Mesial temporal sclerosis resulting in medically refractory epilepsy with predominantly complex partial seizures.

Treatment: Left-sided temporal lobectomy followed by slow tapering of antiepileptic medications after the patient is seizure-free for 2 years postoperatively. Figure 40.1 demonstrates the patient's axial and coronal postoperative MRI scan.

Overview

Epilepsy is a common medical problem with 1% of the U.S. population suffering from the illness. Although the mechanisms of epilepsy are not completely understood, it is thought to be due to a population of neurons firing in a synchronized, unregulated fashion that disrupts normal brain function. Causes of epilepsy are various but include idiopathic, genetic, traumatic, and damage due to infection (Duncan et al., 2006; Avoli et al., 2005).

Approximately one-third of epilepsy patients are refractory to medical therapy. Failure of medical therapy is defined as the inability to control seizures with two or more drugs given at therapeutic doses. Currently, only 0.2% of patients with medically refractory epilepsy undergo surgery. If a patient cannot be successfully managed with medications alone, then referral to an epilepsy center that offers surgical therapy is warranted to determine whether the patient is a surgical candidate. Surgical therapy for epilepsy is significantly underutilized, and efforts are underway to increase awareness and access (Duncan et al., 2006; Brodie et al., 2009).

The majority of drug-resistant epilepsy patients that undergo surgery have temporal lobe epilepsy. Patients with temporal lobe epilepsy often have mesial temporal sclerosis. In this condition, the hippocampus and medial temporal lobe are dysfunctional and act as a seizure focus. Microscopic examination of the hippocampus reveals loss of neurons and scarring of the structure, called gliosis. For these cases, the goal of surgery is to remove the damaged hippocampus and, to various degrees, other portions of the temporal lobe, including the amygdala or lateral temporal cortex. This can be accomplished by craniotomy, but some

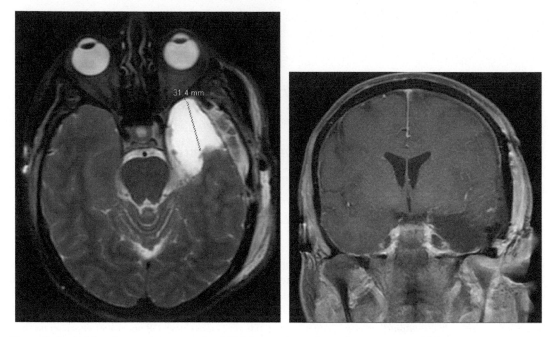

Figure 40.1   Axial and coronal postoperative MRI for a patient who underwent temporal lobectomy.

centers now offer percutaneous laser ablation of the medial temporal lobe in select patients (Engel et al., 1982).

Randomized controlled trials have shown that epilepsy surgery is superior to medical therapy in achieving seizure freedom (Jobst and Cascino, 2015; Téllez-Zenteno et al., 2005). In one trial, only 8% of patients treated with only medications were free of awareness-impairing seizures as opposed to the surgical arm in which 58% of patients were free of awareness-impairing seizures. If patients become seizure free, the risk of sudden death due to epilepsy significantly declines. Data from randomized trials also indicate that epilepsy surgery significantly improves quality of life (Fiest et al., 2014). Other studies have demonstrated that epilepsy surgery is cost-effective when compared to long-term medical therapy (King et al., 1997).

Anatomical review

The anatomy relevant to epilepsy surgery depends on the origin of the epileptic activity. Since the goal of epilepsy surgery is generally to resect the origin of epileptic activity or to modulate the activity of the brain either by disconnection or stimulation, the anatomy relevant to the procedure varies. Disconnection procedures focus on severing white matter connections, such as the corpus callosum (the connection between the cerebral hemispheres), to prevent seizure generalization and loss of consciousness. Stimulation procedures attempt to prevent seizures by altering electrical activity with stimulation of the epileptic focus, as is the case with the Neuropace responsive neurostimulation (RNS) system, or with stimulation of the anterior thalamus, in the case of deep brain stimulation (DBS) for epilepsy, or by stimulation of the vagus nerve. When reviewing the anatomy relevant to epilepsy surgery, temporal lobe anatomy deserves special mention, since approximately 75% of epilepsy surgery cases involve resection of the anterior temporal lobe or some portion of the medial temporal lobe.

Often epilepsy surgery is performed to treat mesial temporal sclerosis. In these cases, the medial structures of the temporal lobe, the hippocampus, and to some degree the amygdala, are thought to be epileptogenic. In some cases, the lateral temporal cortex may also be a focus of epilepsy. When the temporal lobe is viewed laterally, the superior, middle, and inferior temporal gyri are evident. Viewed medially, the uncus and parahippocampal gyrus are evident (Figure 40.2 and 40.3). A coronal section of the anterior temporal lobe demonstrates the hippocampus, temporal horn, optic tract, and parahippocampal gyrus (Figure 40.4). Traditionally, a portion of the lateral temporal cortex is removed with the hippocampus and amygdala (anterior temporal lobectomy); however, there are procedures that preserve the lateral temporal cortex and only remove the medial temporal lobe structures (selective amygdalohippocampectomy). On the dominant side, the left brain for most people, the surgeon may choose to limit the posterior extent of resection of the temporal lobe to avoid creating language deficits (taking the resection back to only 3.5–4 cm from the temporal pole on the dominant side as opposed to 5–5.5 cm from the temporal pole on the nondominant side) (Van Hoesen, 1995).

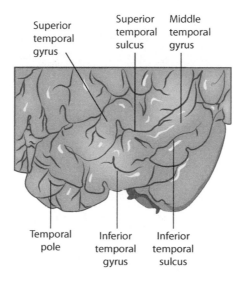

Figure 40.2   An anatomical specimen demonstrating the lateral temporal lobe.

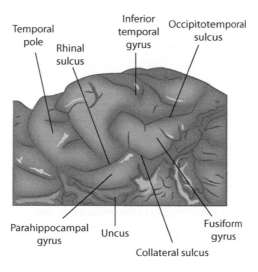

Figure 40.3   An anatomical specimen demonstrating the inferior surface of the temporal lobe.

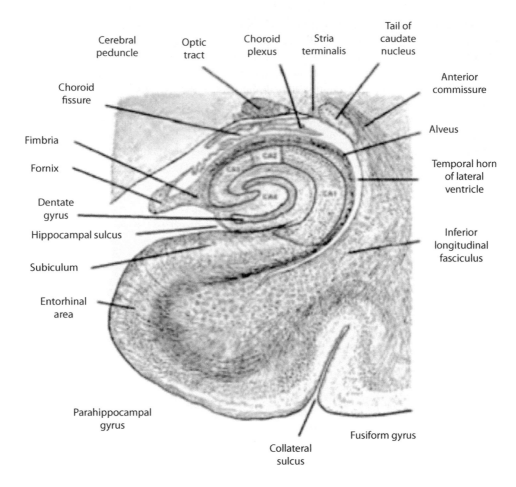

Figure 40.4 An anatomical drawing of a coronal section through the anterior temporal lobe at the level of the hippocampus. (Copyright © 2012 J. A. Kiernan.)

Since working memory is an integral function of the hippocampus, the patient may undergo specialized memory testing preoperatively (Wada testing or functional MRI) to determine how much memory function resides in the hippocampus that is to be resected. Some patients may experience transient or mild permanent memory deficits after temporal lobe surgery, so the risks of this must be weighed against the benefits of seizure control. Visual fibers also transit through the temporal lobe carrying visual information from the contralateral upper visual quadrant in both eyes. Following temporal lobe surgery, many patients may have a reduction of vision in the contralateral upper quadrant, often called a "pie in the sky" deficit. However, this rarely results in any decreased function or subjective complaints and is often only noted on more detailed confrontational or formal visual field testing (Blumer et al., 1998; Katz et al., 1989; Salanova et al., 2002).

Common physical examination findings

- Physical exam findings for epilepsy surgery patients vary depending on the type of epilepsy they have and the presence of any structural abnormalities of the brain.
- Many epilepsy surgery patients suffer from memory problems preoperatively and/or postoperatively. This is more common in patients with temporal lobe epilepsy.

- The patient's behavior during a seizure often depends on the location of the epileptic focus. In patients with temporal lobe epilepsy, behavior during a seizure often consists of both simple and complex partial seizures. In a simple partial seizure, the patient may have the sensation of a bad smell or taste coupled with feelings of fear or other emotion. In simple partial seizures, they do not lose awareness. In complex partial seizures, awareness is impaired, and the patient may participate in automatisms including lip smacking, picking at clothing, and staring (Marks and Laxer, 1998).
- In some patients, seizures may generalize and become tonic-clonic in nature.

Diagnostic tests

- In epilepsy surgery patients, it is important to preoperatively localize the epileptic focus in the brain and determine if it can be resected. A variety of imaging and electrophysiologic tests are used for this end.
- All epilepsy patients undergo preoperative monitoring in an epilepsy unit with scalp EEG. In this environment, antiepileptics may be withdrawn in a controlled fashion to elicit seizures and better localize the seizure focus.
- Some epilepsy surgery patients require further localization and undergo invasive EEG monitoring. In this group of patients, EEG grids or wires are placed intracranially via surgery in selected areas of the brain to help exactly localize the origin of epileptic activity.
- Imaging studies are employed to find structural brain abnormalities, which may be serving as epileptic foci and can be considered for resection or stimulation. Methods employed include MRI, functional MRI, positron emission tomography (PET), and single photon emission computerized tomography (SPECT).
- Postoperatively, epilepsy surgery patients may undergo an additional MRI to verify complete resection of a structural abnormality and to rule out significant hemorrhage or stroke.

Types of epilepsy surgery

Epilepsy surgery may be categorized as diagnostic or therapeutic. In some patients, invasive monitoring is used diagnostically to better localize the seizure focus. In these patients, EEG grids or electrodes are placed in the brain, and the patient is monitored in an epilepsy unit for the course of several days to weeks. Anticonvulsants are withdrawn in a controlled fashion to increase the likelihood of capturing seizures. Information from this episode may then be used to make further therapeutic decisions. Most patients who have invasive monitoring will eventually go on to have a therapeutic surgery, but some patients are found to have multiple sources of their seizures, and surgical resection is not an option.

Therapeutic epilepsy surgery may be classified as resective surgery or stimulation surgery. The majority of resective epilepsy surgeries will involve removal of a portion of the temporal lobe, but resective surgery may also be performed to remove extratemporal seizure foci from the frontal, parietal, or occipital lobes. The success rate of extratemporal epilepsy surgery is generally lower. Another form of resective epilepsy surgery is often called *disconnection surgery*. This surgery is usually palliative, with a goal of decreasing the frequency or severity of seizures, as opposed to eliminating seizures. Examples of disconnection surgery include corpus callosotomy and functional hemispherotomy. In these surgeries, the white matter connections for various brain regions are severed to prevent seizure propagation and generalization.

With advancing technology, stimulation devices are now commercially available that reduce seizure frequency. Of these technologies, vagal nerve stimulation (VNS) is the most long-established technology. In VNS a coiled electrode is wrapped around the vagal nerve (usually on the left side) and connected to a battery placed subcutaneously on the chest. This technology stimulates the vagus nerve and reduces seizure frequency for some patients. A newer technology, Neuropace RNS, allows for the treatment of seizures arising from eloquent areas of the brain that cannot be resected due to functional importance. Intracranial wire or paddle electrodes are implanted at a seizure focus and are then connected to a small battery/computer that is recessed into the skull. This device records brain activity looking for epileptic activity and then, under the supervision of a clinician, is iteratively programmed to provide brain stimulation that reduces seizure frequency (Rolston et al., 2012).

There are certain universal tenets for epilepsy surgery. If a patient has had an intracranial procedure, his or her neurologic status needs to be monitored closely. For patients undergoing invasive monitoring, the nursing care team must work with the EEG technicians to ensure that the grids and electrodes are properly connected. Extra care must be taken with epilepsy surgery patients to correctly record their home antiepileptic drugs (AEDs) and develop an appropriate plan for inpatient AED administration. If the patient is undergoing invasive monitoring, the neurology and surgical teams will prescribe a controlled withdrawal of AEDs in order to capture epileptic activity for surgical planning. In the case of patients who have undergone a respective surgery, the neurology and surgery teams will generally maintain the patient on his or her home AEDs and taper them as an outpatient at some later date. Patients who are receiving palliative stimulation therapy, such as Neuropace RNS or VNS, will usually continue on their baseline home AEDs. In these patients, the neurology or surgical team should communicate to the nursing team whether or not the stimulator has been activated and whether the device limits future MRI imaging.

Common grading scheme

The Engel system and International League Against Epilepsy (ILAE) system are the most common classifications for outcome following epilepsy surgery. The Engel system is presented here because it is the scale most commonly used and has been shown to have good interrater reliability (Durnford et al., 2011).

Engel 1: Free from disabling seizures
Engel 2: Rare disabling seizures
Engel 3: Worthwhile improvement of seizures following epilepsy surgery
Engel 4: No worthwhile improvement following epilepsy surgery

Family counseling

As with any chronic illness, family counseling is a very important part of caring for epilepsy surgery patients. Some patients undergoing epilepsy surgery may have cognitive or education limitations. Patients also may have difficulty obtaining transportation since they cannot drive.

Prognosis is one of the common points of discussion regarding epilepsy surgery. The chance of seizure freedom following epilepsy surgery depends on the type of epilepsy and the anatomical location of the seizure focus. Patients undergoing temporal resective surgery have the best rates of seizure freedom, with 66% of patients achieving long-term seizure freedom (Engel class 1). The rates of seizure freedom are significantly lower for patients with extratemporal seizure foci, with a 46% rate of seizure freedom after occipital or parietal lobe epilepsy surgery and a 27% rate of seizure freedom after frontal lobe epilepsy surgery. Palliative procedures, such as callosotomy, VNS, or Neuropace RNS placement, are meant to decrease the frequency of seizures and only rarely result in complete freedom from disabling seizures (Téllez-Zenteno et al., 2005). Possible complications following epilepsy surgery also depend on location of the epileptic focus and the type of surgical intervention (stimulation therapy versus resection). The complication rates in one large series of patients treated surgically for temporal lobe epilepsy were as follows: 0% mortality, 0.9% hemiparesis, 3.7% transient language deficits, and 3.2% transient cranial nerve deficits. For this group, 69% became seizure free (Salanova et al., 2002). Other important potential complications include surgical site infection, vision deficits, and changes in mood, memory, or speech.

Postoperative questions related to epilepsy surgery may be general concerns such as wound care, but others are specific to epilepsy surgery. Many questions relate to driving or activity restrictions, and others are related to medication weaning. With regard to driving, laws vary depending on region, but generally patients should not consider driving until they are seizure free for at least 6 months. If the patient has never driven before, he or she may need to be referred to occupational health for testing in a driving simulator to see if he or she is neurologically appropriate for driving. The issues related to driving generally will be addressed during outpatient follow-up. There is no general consensus on how to wean anti-pileptic drugs following epilepsy surgery. Many neurologists only begin weaning medications following 2 years of postoperative seizure freedom, but often this decision is individualized to the patient by the neurologist and neurosurgeon (Berg et al., 2007).

Common pitfalls and medicolegal concerns

- Epilepsy surgery patients are susceptible to seizures and should have seizure precautions, including appropriately padded beds.
- Work closely with the neurology/neurosurgery team to determine when seizures should be treated for patients undergoing invasive EEG monitoring. (The goal is to capture seizures to localize the lesion.) In some cases, it may be necessary to administer IV lorazepam or another benzodiazepine if a seizure persists too long.
- The lifting of driving restrictions for patients with epilepsy varies depending on the local governmental authority.
- Memory and neuropsychologic changes may occur following epilepsy surgery, and patients, as well as their families, must be counseled accordingly. Generally, any negative changes resulting from surgery are more than offset by improved epilepsy control, particularly if the patient becomes seizure free.

Relevance to the advanced practice health provider

Advanced practice health providers (APHPs) continue to increase in number and the services they offer. Many APHPs are now an integral part of neurosurgical care teams. Epilepsy surgery is an exciting field with the potential to provide a significant positive impact for carefully selected patients. As the field of epilepsy surgery expands, APHPs will continue to have an important role in patient care and research.

Common phone calls, pages, and requests with answers

Q: *What action should be taken when an epilepsy patient, undergoing invasive monitoring, has a seizure?*

A: Press the event recorder button. Note the start time of the seizure. Note the symptoms, and talk to the patient to see if he or she is conscious or can remember the event (e.g., say, "remember the color red" to the patient).

Q: *When should seizures be treated for patients undergoing monitoring?*

A: The neurology and neurosurgery teams will assist with this decision, and you should ask for ground rules prior to each patient's admission to the unit. Seizures persisting longer than 2–3 minutes or successive seizures occurring prior to the patient's return to his or her baseline neurologic status may require treatment urgently with lorazepam or another benzodiazepine.

Q: *Does resective temporal lobe epilepsy surgery lead to memory impairment?*

A: Many temporal lobe epilepsy patients suffer from memory problems preoperatively. These deficits can be due to structural problems with one of the temporal lobes or due to the AEDs that they take. The epilepsy surgery team makes every effort to ensure that the surgical procedure does not lead to increased memory deficits. This may include invasive monitoring or other testing such as functional MRI or Wada testing. Memory is generally stable following resective surgery for temporal lobe epilepsy and may even improve if the patient stops having seizures or is able to be weaned off of AEDs.

References

Avoli M, Louvel J, Pumain R, Köhling R. Cellular and molecular mechanisms of epilepsy in the human brain. *Prog Neurobiol.* 2005;77(3):166–200.

Berg AT, Langfitt JT, Spencer MD, Vickrey MD. Stopping antiepileptic drugs after epilepsy surgery: a survey of U.S. epilepsy center neurologists. *Epilepsy Behav.* 2007;10(2):219–222.

Blumer D, Wakhlu S, Davies K, Hermann B. Psychiatric outcome of temporal lobectomy for epilepsy: incidence and treatment of psychiatric complications. *Epilepsia.* 1998;39(5):478–486.

Brodie MJ, Elder AT, Kwan P. Epilepsy in later life. *The Lancet Neurol.* 2009;8(11):1019–1030. http://dx.doi.org/10.1016/S1474-4422(09)70240-6.

Duncan JS, Sander JW, Sisodiya SM, Walker MC. Adult epilepsy. *Lancet.* 2006;367(9516):1087–1100.

Durnford AJ, Rodgers W, Kirkham FJ et al. Very good inter-rater reliability of Engel and ILAE epilepsy surgery outcome classifications in a series of 76 patients. *Seizure.* 2011;20(10):809–812. http://dx.doi.org/10.1016/j.seizure.2011.08.004.

Engel J, Brown WJ, Kuhl DE, Phelps ME, Mazziotta JC, Crandall PH. Pathological findings underlying focal temporal lobe hypometabolism in partial epilepsy. *Ann Neurol.* 1982;12(6):518–528.

Fiest KM, Sajobi TT, Wiebe S. Epilepsy surgery and meaningful improvements in quality of life: results from a randomized controlled trial. *Epilepsia.* 2014;55(6):886–892.

Van Hoesen GW. Anatomy of the medial temporal lobe. *Mag Reson Imaging.* 1995;13(8):1047–1055.

Jobst BC, Cascino GD. Resective epilepsy surgery for drug-resistant focal epilepsy. *JAMA.* 2015. 313(3):285. http://jama.jamanetwork.com/article.aspx?doi=10.1001/jama.2014.17426.

Katz A, Awad IA, Kong AK et al. Extent of resection in temporal lobectomy for epilepsy. II. Memory changes and neurologic complications. *Epilepsia.* 1989;30(6):763–771.

King JT, Sperling MR, Justice AC, O'Connor MJ. A cost-effectiveness analysis of anterior temporal lobectomy for intractable temporal lobe epilepsy. *J Neurosurg.* 1997;87(1):20–28.

Marks WJ, Laxer KD. Semiology of temporal lobe seizures: value in lateralizing the seizure focus. *Epilepsia.* 1998;39(7):721–726.

Rolston JD, Englot DJ, Wang DD, Shih T, Chang EF. Comparison of seizure control outcomes and the safety of vagus nerve, thalamic deep brain, and responsive neurostimulation: evidence from randomized controlled trials. *Neurosurg Focus.* 2012;32(3):E14.

Salanova V, Markand O, Worth R. Temporal lobe epilepsy urgery: outcome, complications, and late mortality rate in 215 patients. *Epilepsia.* 2002;43(2):170–174.

Téllez-Zenteno JF, Dhar R, Wiebe S. Long-term seizure outcomes following epilepsy surgery: a systematic review and meta-analysis. *Brain.* 2005;128(5):1188–1198.

41

BRAIN ABSCESS

Andrea L. Strayer and Wendell B. Lake

Case vignette

A 51-year-old male presented to the emergency department (ED) following a seizure. Prehospital personnel treated his seizure with midazolam and lorazepam. Prior to this witnessed generalized tonic-clonic seizure, the patient had no history of epilepsy, but he did complain of recent frontal headaches, worse at night. The patient, who immigrated to the Midwest from Mexico, had no major health problems other than tobacco use. Additionally, he had no known history of tuberculosis. Computed tomography (CT) scan of the head revealed a right frontal lobe lesion. Magnetic resonance imaging (MRI) of the brain with gadolinium demonstrated a multiloculated ring-enhancing lesion, centered in the right middle frontal gyrus, 2.0 × 2.3 × 2.3 cm with restricted diffusion and associated vasogenic edema (Figure 41.1).

The patient underwent a right frontal craniotomy for abscess resection. An encapsulated area of pus was noted and resected. After the abscess was removed, the resection cavity was irrigated. Broad-spectrum antimicrobial coverage was started with ceftriaxone, metronidazole, and vancomycin. Infectious disease (ID) was consulted and provided recommendations for antibiotic therapy and follow-up testing.

Evaluation included dental x-rays, transthoracic echocardiogram (TTE), laboratory studies, and blood and intraoperative cultures.

Intraoperative cultures from the resected brain abscess demonstrated a polymicrobial infection with Fusobacterium, Staphylococcus aureus, Parvimonas, and coagulase-negative staphylococci. These cultures were consistent with a dental

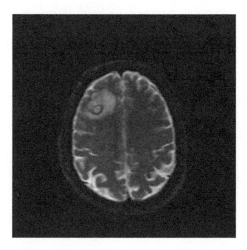

Figure 41.1 Multiloculated rim-enhancing lesion centered on the right middle frontal gyrus, measuring 2 × 2.3 × 2.3 cm. This scan demonstrates areas of restriction centrally with adjacent vasogenic edema.

source, and the patient's dental x-rays demonstrated dental abscesses. An oral surgeon performed multiple tooth extractions to control the source of his intracranial infection.

He was discharged to home on long-term antibiotic therapy consisting of vancomycin, ceftriaxone, and metronidazole.

Epidemiology and social significance

The most common microorganisms associated with brain abscess are *Streptococcus* spp and *Staphylococcus* spp, comprising 34% and 18%, respectively (Brouwer et al., 2014, p. 809) Table 41.1. Geographical distribution is similar across the world, with the average age 34 years and males affected 2.4 times more often than females. Brouwer notes only 20% presented with fever, headache, and focal neurologic deficits. Additionally, over the past 50 years, fatality has decreased from 40% to 20%, and full recovery increased from 33% to 70% (Brouwer et al., 2014, p. 809).

Pathophysiology

Initially, a brain abscess begins as a focal area of cerebritis, evolving to a pus-filled encapsulated mass lesion with associated vasogenic edema. A brain abscess often has an associated predisposing condition (86%). Conditions associated with brain abscess include otitis, mastoiditis, sinusitis, meningitis, dental abscess, pneumonia, endocarditis, prior brain surgery, and head injury. Brain abscess can occur secondary to either hematogenous spread (endocarditis or other remote infection source) or direct contiguous spread (sinusitis or mastoiditis) (Brouwer et al., 2014, p. 808; Slazinski, 2013, p. 382). Immunocompromised patients are at higher risk of developing fungal infections. Additionally, those who live in or have visited tropical countries are at risk of amebic and typhoid brain abscesses (Wiwanitkit, 2012, p. 247).

Moazzam et al. evaluated previously published case reports via systematic review of the literature of intracranial abscesses of odontogenic origin. In this review of the literature, men comprised 82% of the cases. Periodontitis and caries with periapical abscess were the most common oral sources of brain abscess. The most common procedure prior to brain abscess discovery was wisdom tooth extraction. The authors' review found 47% of those infected reflected polymicrobial growth (Moazzam, 2015, p. 801).

Presenting signs and symptoms

Seizure is not an uncommon presenting symptom for brain abscess, occurring in 25%–34% of patients (Muzumdar, 2011, p. 137). Other presentations of brain abscess include focal neurologic deficit, headache, fever, nausea, and/or vomiting. Please refer to Table 41.2 for a list of presenting signs and symptoms as noted by Brouwer et al. (2014, p. 809).

Table 41.1 Culture Results and Major Groups of Causative Microorganisms

Characteristic	All patients	Children
Positive culture	4543/6663 (68)	631/1093 (63)
Monomicrobial	3067 (77)	325 (73)
Polymicrobial	902 (23)	117 (27)
Cultured microorganisms	5894	724
Streptococcus spp.	2000 (34)	260 (36)
Viridans streptococci	755 (13)	58 (6)
S. pneumoniae	139 (2)	27 (4)
Enterococcus	49 (0.8)	2 (0.3)

Table 41.1 (Continued) Culture Results and Major Groups of Causative Microorganisms

Characteristic	All patients	Children
Other/not specified	1057 (18)	173 (24)
Staphylococcus spp.	1076 (18)	128 (18)
S. aureus	782 (13)	80 (11)
S. epidermidis	148 (3)	31 (4)
Not specified	146 (2)	16 (2)
Gram-negative enteric	861 (15)	114 (16)
Proteus spp.	417 (7)	60 (8)
Klebsiella pneumoniae	135 (2)	11 (2)
Escherichia coli	126 (2)	18 (2)
Enterobacteriaceae	101 (2)	9 (1)
Pseudomonas spp.	122 (2)	13 (2)
Actinomycetales	148 (3)	16 (2)
Nocardia	57 (1)	0
Corynebacterium	49 (0.8)	7 (1)
Actinomyces	48 (0.8)	8 (1)
Mycobacterium tuberculosis	41 (0.7)	1 (0.2)
Haemophilus spp.	124 (2)	41 (6)
Peptostreptococcus spp.	165 (3)	45 (6)
Bacteroides spp.	370 (6)	33 (5)
Fusobacterium spp.	119 (2)	17 (2)
Parasites	5 (0.1)	0
Fungi	83 (1)	8 (1)
Other	821 (13)	49 (7)

Source: Brouwer MC et al., *Neurology.*, 82, 807, 2014.
Data are *n* (%).

Table 41.2 Clinical Characteristics and Laboratory and CSF Examinations in Patients with Brain Abscess

Characteristic	n/N (%)[a]
Age, y, mean[b]	33.6
Sex, male	5,333/7,585 (70)
Predisposing conditions[c]	
Otitis/mastoiditis	2,754/8,727 (32)
Sinusitis	660/6,499 (10)
Heart disease[d]	911/6,841 (13)
Posttraumatic	950/6,858 (14)
Hematogenous[e]	384/3,025 (13)
Pulmonary disease	403/4,909 (8)
Postoperative	469/5,421 (9)
Odontogenic	178/3,721 (5)
Immunocompromise	172/1,957 (9)
Meningitis	216/3,883 (6)
Unknown	1,350/7,198 (19)
Other	230/4,361 (5)

(Continued)

Table 41.2 (Continued) Clinical Characteristics and Laboratory and CSF Examinations in Patients with Brain Abscess

Characteristic	n/N (%)[a]
Symptoms and signs	
Headache	4,526/6,575 (69)
Nausea/vomiting	1,993/4,286 (47)
Fever	3,718/6,970 (53)
Altered consciousness	3,207/7,479 (43)
Neurologic deficits	2,996/6,241 (48)
Seizures	1,647/6,581 (25)
Nuchal rigidity	1,465/4,629 (32)
Papilloedema	845/2,428 (35)
Mean duration of symptoms[f]	8.3 d
Triad of fever, headache, focal neurologic deficits	131/668 (20)
Blood investigation	
Leukocytosis	1,366/2,273 (60)
Elevated CRP	196/316 (60)
Elevated ESR	311/434 (72)
Positive blood culture	135/484 (28)
CSF investigation	1,392/3,955 (35)
LP	1,286/1,298 (99)
Normal CSF	96/588 (16)
Pleocytosis	758/1,063 (71)
Elevated CSF protein	222/381 (58)
Culture positive	263/1,108 (24)
Clinical deterioration attributed to LP	76/1,030 (7)

Source: Brouwer MC et al., *Neurology.*, 82, 809, 2014.
Abbreviations: CRP = C-reactive protein; ESR = erythrocyte sedimentation rate; LP = lumbar puncture.
[a] All data are presented with the total number of patients included in studies that presented the specific patient characteristic.
[b] The mean age was recalculated from averages presented in 85 studies including 5,391 patients.
[c] Numbers do not add up to 100% because multiple predisposing conditions could be present in 1 patient.
[d] Heart disease includes congenital heart defects and endocarditis.
[e] Source not specified.
[f] Recalculated from averages presented in 15 studies including 989 patients.

Diagnostic tests

Acutely, CT scan of the head is often obtained if a mass, such as a brain abscess, is suspected. It is further characterized with an MRI of the brain. If a cerebral abscess is present, it usually demonstrates ring enhancement with gadolinium. Diffusion restriction on MRI sequences is characteristic of brain abscess.

Laboratory data

    Complete blood count with differential (CBC with diff)
    Erythrocyte sedimentation rate (ESR)
    C-reactive protein (CRP)
    Blood cultures from two sites
    Basic metabolic panel (BMP)
    Intraoperative abscess fluid Gram stain, culture, sensitivities
    Transthoracic echocardiogram
    Chest x-ray
    Dental x-rays (if indicated)

Treatment

Goals of treatment include the following:

- Accurate identification of the causative pathogen.
- Appropriate antimicrobial therapy with complete treatment of the primary infection foci.
- Support and rehabilitation of the neurologic sequela of the brain abscess.

Surgical therapy

Both needle aspiration and resection are surgical options for brain abscess treatment. A literature review between 1990 and 2008 revealed a lower mortality rate with aspiration (6.6%) versus excision (12.7%) (Ratnaike, 2011, p. 433). Although the specific surgical approach depends on the abscess location and characteristics, the goals of surgical treatment are the same. One goal is to decrease the volume of the abscess. This has two benefits: one is decreasing intracranial pressure, and another is decreasing the total amount of infected material. Another goal is to obtain cultures such that specific antimicrobial therapy can be initiated. Finally, surgical drainage and débridement breaks down the fibrous rind surrounding the brain abscess. This allows antimicrobials and the patient's immunological system to better access the infectious nidus and thereby more rapidly clear the infection.

Brain abscess is a neurosurgical emergency, requiring emergent attention and a team-based approach. Medical, nonsurgical treatment may be an option if the source is known and the abscess is small (Arlotti, 2010, p. S88). While outcomes have improved, pyogenic intraparenchymal abscess can be life threatening. Brouwer and colleagues conducted a literature review and found that 84% of patients underwent a neurosurgical procedure, including abscess stereotactic aspiration alone or craniotomy with débridement and aspiration (Brouwer et al., 2014, p. 809–810).

Antimicrobial therapy

Immediately following abscess aspiration, broad-spectrum antibiotics are started at central nervous system/cerebrospinal fluid penetrating doses. These may include vancomycin, ceftriaxone, metronidazole, and others. Infectious disease specialists are crucial in the initiation and monitoring of antimicrobials.

Once final speciation is identified, antibiotic therapy is tailored. A long-term intravenous access catheter is placed. Appropriate surveillance laboratory studies occur at recommended intervals. For instance, vancomycin will require appropriate trough levels and dosing adjustments.

Anticonvulsant therapy

Antiepileptic therapy may include levetiracetam or an equivalent medication. In some patients, even if the patient did not present with seizures, antiepileptics are started for seizure prophylaxis. Once the abscess is treated, tapering of the antiepileptic medications can be considered.

Counseling and education

Key points to consider include:

Initial evaluation: Severity of illness; treatment goals as above in conjunction with patient-centered goals
Acute care: Rehabilitation needs; long-term antibiotic therapy

Pitfalls

Long-term antibiotics will be required. Providers will coordinate management responsibility of the antibiotics. Discharge case managers/social services can assist with discharge planning. Variables include the following:

- Insurance coverage
- The patient or family's ability to learn and provide long-term antibiotics
- The patient's neurologic status

Long-term antibiotics require surveillance laboratory studies to assess antibiotic effectiveness and to evaluate for complications (such as kidney injury). Discharge planning requires arranging these surveillance labs and how the studies will be communicated to the infectious disease team.

Relevance to the advanced health practice provider

Advanced practice providers are pivotal members of the team and are involved throughout the continuum of care. All aspects of the care of the patient with a brain abscess are pertinent for the advanced practice provider.

Common phone calls, pages, and requests with answers

Q: My patient would like oral antibiotics for discharge. Is this an option?

A: Oral antibiotics are rarely sufficient for treatment of brain abscess. The patient should contact the ID specialist to determine what their antibiotic options are.

Q: My patient is going to discharge on long-term antibiotics. What adjuvant medications can assist in this therapy?

A: Probiotics may help prevent gastrointestinal upset. Antibiotic therapy can place the patient at risk for developing other complications such as Clostridium difficile colitis.

Q: The provider thinks my patient's brain abscess came from his dental abscess, but the dentist would prefer not to pull his tooth/teeth while he is inpatient. He would like him to see his local dentist. Is this OK?

A: No. The treatment of the causative foci, in this case tooth abscess, requires treatment as soon as identified.

References

Arlotti M, Grossi P, Pea F et al. Consensus document on controversial issues for the treatment of infections of the central nervous system: Bacterial brain abscesses. *Int J Infect Dis.* 2010;14(suppl 4):S79–S92.

Brouwer MC, Coutinho JM, van de Beek D. Clinical characteristics an outcome of brain abscess: systematic review and meta-analysis. *Neurology.* 2014;82:806–813.

Moazzam AA, Rajagopal SM, Sedghizadeh PP, Zada G, Habibian M. Intracranial bacterial infections of oral origin. *J Clin Neurosci.* 2015;22:800–805.

Muzumdar D, Jhawar J, Goel A. Brain abscess: An overview. *Int J Surg.* 2011;9:136–144.

Ratnaike TE, Das S, Gregson BA, Mendolow AD. A review of brain abscess surgical treatment-78 years: Aspiration versus excision. *World Neurosurg.* 2011;76:431–436.

Slazinski T. Brain abscess. *Crit Care Nurs Clin North Am.* 2013;25:381–388.

Wiwanitkit S, Wiwanitkit V. Pyogenic brain abscess in Thailand. *N Am J Med Sci.* 2012;4:245–248.

42

TYPE I CHIARI MALFORMATIONS

George M. Ghobrial, Karthik Madhavan, and S. Shelby Burks

Case vignette

A 24-year-old female presents to your office seeking neurosurgical consultation after referral from her primary care physician. The patient describes a 4-year history of worsening headaches localizing toward the posterior aspect of her head. These headaches are exacerbated whenever she coughs and with any activities associated with abdominal straining, such as weight lifting. Additionally, when she coughs, she experiences pain radiating into her arms, and sometimes into her shoulders and scapula. The pain frequently manifests as a pins and needles sensation, or less frequently, as a burning sensation. Lately, the patient describes intermittent blurry vision or double vision, which seems to be increasing in frequency over the last 6 months. When she saw her primary care physician, she had described intermittent numbness, tingling, and clumsiness in her hands. Upon directed questioning, she has felt clumsy on her feet. Her primary physician obtained magnetic resonance imaging (MRI) of her brain (Figure 42.1) and cervical spine (Figure 42.2), as well as a cerebrospinal fluid (CSF) flow study (Figure 42.3) in lieu of her history and clinical findings, ultimately followed by a neurosurgical referral.

Overview

1. *Epidemiology:* Given the MRI finding of tonsillar descent in tandem with a common constellation of symptoms encountered, the diagnosis is consistent with a Chiari type I malformation. The true incidence is not known. However, increased usage of MRI and CT have made it clear that the incidental finding of tonsillar descent that defines a Chiari type I malformation is as high as 0.77% on imaging studies (Bejjani, 2001).

2. *Societal significance:* The most commonly encountered symptom in type I Chiari malformations is pain, occurring in up to 90% of patients (Todor, Mu, Milhorat, 2000). Due to the high rate of tonsillar descent observed on cranial imaging and the wide spectrum of symptoms that have been reported to occur with Chiari malformations, a large population of patients will seek further diagnostic workup , pursue disease-specific therapies, and even undergo neurosurgical treatment for symptomatic relief (Todor, Mu, Milhorat, 2000). Given the wide spectrum of clinical presentation, the diagnosis, management, and surgical decision-making process can be challenging.

3. *Basic biologic and physiologic processes:* A Chiari malformation is a condition defined by cerebellar tonsillar descent with disruption of physiologic CSF flow, with or without the presence of gross syrinx formation in the cervical cord. Several overlapping theories have been proposed. One theoretical inciting event is the incomplete development or lack of formation of one or more fourth ventricular foramina, resulting in the gradual buildup of pressure in the posterior fossa, resulting in cerebellar tonsillar elongation and descent. Furthermore, as the tonsils descend, CSF flow can be obstructed at

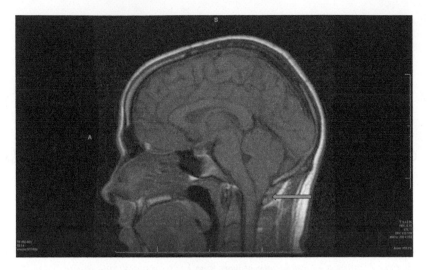

Figure 42.1   T1 noncontrasted MRI, sagittal projection, of the brain demonstrating tonsillar descent to the level of the C1 vertebrae (arrow).

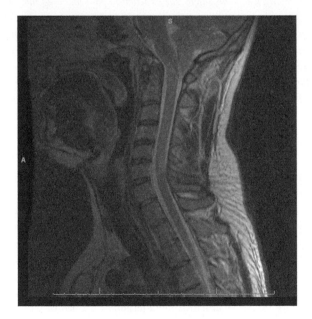

Figure 42.2   T2-weighted MRI of the cervical spine, sagittal projection, demonstrating tonsillar descent. This study demonstrates the lack of CSF space around the upper cervical cord, which is abnormal. In some patients a syrinx is present in the cervical spine, and this would appear as T2 hyperintensity within the spinal cord (not present here). Medullary kinking of the cervical spine is also present, a finding commonly encountered in congenital Chiari malformation.

the cervicomedullary junction (Figure 42.4). This may lead to pressured flow of CSF into the central canal of the spinal cord and syrinx formation through the obex (superior foramen of the central canal). Syrinx progression occurs gradually through pressure waves created by cardiac systole. One proposal is that systole can direct the flow of CSF within the spinal canal from outside-to-inside, directly through spinal cord tissue, by pressure-mediated diffusion of water through the interstitium. These mechanisms explain that disruption of the natural flow of CSF can result in arachnoid cysts,

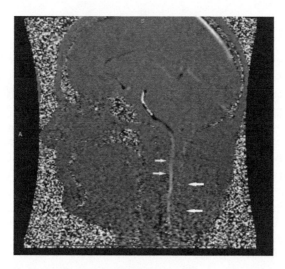

Figure 42.3   MRI of the brain, sagittal projection, CINE study (cardiac-gated synchronization). The cardiac cycle causes pulsatile changes in venous pressure that directly affect the flow of CSF in the subarachnoid space. By timing signal acquisition with the cardiac cycle, higher-resolution imaging of the subarachnoid space can be obtained and is therefore helpful in demonstrating normal flow of CSF in the cervical spine (gray arrows) as well as severely diminished or absent CSF flow (white arrows).

spinal cord cysts, and expansion of the central canal into a syrinx causing cord compression, atrophy of the parenchyma (myelomalacia), and symptomatic expansion of the central canal into syringomyelia (Bejjani, 2001; Alden et al., 2001; Calliauw and Dehaene, 1977; Dyste et al., 1989).

Anatomical review

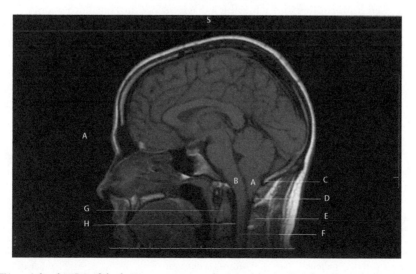

Figure 42.4   T1-weighted MRI of the brain, noncontrasted, sagittal projection demonstrating type I Chiari malformation in a 30-year-old male. (A) Cerebellar tonsil; (B) medulla, with cervicomedullary kinking; (C) opisthion, posterior aspect foramen magnum; (D) posterior arch of C1; (E) spinous process of C2; (F) cervical spinal cord, level of C3; (G) dens of C2; and (H) cervical subarachnoid space.

Common physical examination findings

Pain is the most common complaint of type I Chiari malformation in adults and can often precede significant clinical exam findings. Often, a radiographic diagnosis precedes any physical exam finding. In the event of progressive tonsillar descent and compression of the cervical spinal cord, and/or cervicomedullary kinking, cervical myelopathy may manifest first as hyperreflexia in the upper followed by lower extremities. A routine examination of motor strength of the upper and lower extremities will commonly demonstrate weakness affecting the arms more often than the legs. Atrophy is also a common finding, even in younger patients. Tandem gait assessment is critical in detecting early myelopathy. The formation of a cervical syrinx can cause dissociative cervical sensory and motor deficits in the upper extremities and hands. Therefore, sensory modalities including pain, coarse and light touch, and proprioception may likely provide useful clinical findings.

Further tonsillar herniation and syrinx formation can cause upper cervical spine and brainstem findings termed *syringobulbia*. These cranial neuropathies may manifest through diplopia, dysconjugate gaze, and downbeat nystagmus to the more onerous findings of sleep apnea and arrhythmia. Horner syndrome may be evident as well. Coordination, gaze, and balance should be examined to assess as a clinical correlate to cerebellar and tonsillar deformation in the posterior fossa. In a review of 50 patients with Chiari malformation, Dyste et al. found weakness to be by far the most common exam finding followed by sensory loss ($n = 17$). Pain was by far the most common chief complaint in 60% of patients ($n = 30$), with headache the most specific pain-type complaint ($n = 12$), followed by neck ($n = 9$), arm ($n = 6$), and chest/upper back ($n = 5$) pain. Glossopharyngeal and vagal nerve function can be tested, via cough and gag reflexes, which are surprisingly abnormal in a significant number of patients. However, in the absence of a relevant clinical history, routine testing of cough and gag can unnecessarily provide significant discomfort for young patients (Table 42.1).

Relevant diagnostic tests

- *MRI Brain:* MRI of the brain, particularly sagittal-projection imaging encompassing the upper cervical spine in the caudal-most extent, is critical for capturing the extent of tonsillar herniation and providing useful information and achieving a diagnosis of Chiari malformation.
- *MRI Cervical spine:* T2-weighted sagittal sequences are helpful in assessing the extent of cervical canal stenosis caused by tonsillar herniation, as well as determining the lowermost extent of descent. It is important in the author's opinion to always include T1-weighted postgadolinium sequences to exclude intramedullary neoplasms as the causative pathology of any cyst in the spinal cord, which can occur in adults with ependymomas, hemangioblastomas, metastatic disease, and even low-grade astrocytomas of the pilocytic subtype, which are rarely encountered in the spinal cord. As such, views of the remaining neuroaxis must be obtained if the caudal-most aspect of the syrinx is not visualized on a cervical spine MRI.
- *CINE-flow MRI:* CINE (from *cinema*) is a method of acquiring short-duration MRI sequences over a few seconds to evaluate the flow of CSF around the posterior fossa into the spinal canal and

Table 42.1 Chiari Malformation: Anatomic Differences among the General Subtypes

Type I	Type II	Type III
• Tonsillar descent with or without syringomyelia (50%–76%)	• Tonsillar descent • Vermis descent • Myelomeningocele • Syringomyelia	• Tonsillar descent • Posterior cerebellar descent • Cervical meningocele

subarachnoid spaces (Figure 42.3). This study is often regarded as an adjunctive test in surgical decision making and is technically difficult to administer well, requiring a skilled MR technician and neuroradiologist, an obstacle to being available everywhere.

Review of relevant interventional procedures and surgeries

The surgical management of Chiari I malformation is chiefly a decompressive operation, directed at the foramen magnum and upper cervical spine, where the underlying cerebellar tonsils are impacting the lower brainstem and cervical spine.

The standard decompression has been addressed through a midline posterior cervical, suboccipital approach. A lower portion of the occipital bone surrounding the foramen magnum is resected along with the C1 posterior ring. Uncommonly, if the tonsillar descent is below the C1 ring, additional portions of the C2 lamina may need to be resected, increasing the risk of postoperative neck pain via disarticulating supporting paraspinal muscles, and placing the patient at increased risk for postlaminectomy cervical kyphosis. Posterior cervical midline dissections are relatively more painful for the patient postoperatively, regardless of how well the surgeon maintains a strict plane in the midline avascular ligamentum nuchae, avoiding muscles and bleeding laterally. Intraoperative ultrasound of the dura to evaluate the impact of bony and ligamentous decompression on the tonsils as well as their rostrocaudal height is a useful tool.

Otherwise, after exposure, some surgeons open the dura and shrink the tonsils via bipolar coagulation for added decompression and CSF flow restoration. This can also allow the surgeon to visualize and dissect any adhesions potentially obstructing CSF flow in and out of the fourth ventricle. A duraplasty is then performed to allow for additional space for CSF flow in the subarachnoid space. A watertight closure is vital in preventing a persistent CSF leak or pseudomeningocele.

Arguably, maintenance of a bloodless exposure and strict hemostasis will prevent bone dust and blood from entering the intradural space, which can be a source of aseptic chemical meningitis, and increased postoperative pain. Physiologic flow restoration via CSF flow diversion is reserved for pediatric populations with cranial abnormalities thought to be resulting in syrinx formation. It has also been repeatedly published that obliteration of the obex with compressed muscle, and hence obstruction of flow to the central canal, can be preventative of syrinx progression.

Common grading schemes

Family counseling

1. *Prognosis:* The discussion of the management of Chiari malformations with the patient and family is often tenuous, given the relatively young age of onset, and could potentially lead to neurosurgical treatment.
2. *Common questions:* The family and patient will most often ask the risks and benefits of the surgical procedure, the expected postoperative course of stay, and how long after surgery before they can return to various activities. These answers should all be predetermined with the primary surgeon and vary based on his or her comfort level and experience.
3. *Pitfalls:* One very common pitfall surrounding the management of Chiari malformation is significant pain with a reduction in quality of life. Therefore, it is important that the family understands this so that their expectations of surgery match the surgeon's expectations. Young patients will commonly have unrealistic expectations about the natural course of recovery after treatment. One prevalent issue is the challenge of effectively communicating to a young patient that recovery from significant myelopathy, atrophy, and weakness, as well as lower cranial nerve palsies may take months, and it may not lead to a total return to all activities of daily living.

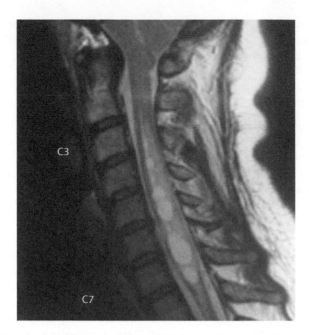

Figure 42.5 Syringomyelia seen as the low-intensity signal pockets of fluid within the cervical spinal cord as a result of the CSF flow abnormalities in a Chiari I malformation.

Common pitfalls and medicolegal concerns

Syringomyelia is encountered most commonly in adult patients and is a condition of symptomatic cord compression by intramedullary cyst formation and expansion. Syringomyelia can occur in the setting of a Chiari malformation, and it is most often the disordered CSF flow that is the underlying pathophysiologic basis of disease. The treatment of syringomyelia in adults most often is due to posttraumatic arachnolysis, and tonsillar herniation is not routinely encountered. Therefore, the management will differ and usually entails either duraplasty and arachnolysis alone, or duraplasty and shunting of the cyst cavity. There is a high rate of syrinx recurrence regardless of treatment modality; reoperations are unfortunately encountered periodically throughout the life of a patient with syringomyelia.

Relevance to the advanced practice health professional

This disease process is highly complex and commonly encountered in the neurosurgical community. This patient population is young, and the families that accompany them are often apprehensive due to the looming possibility of an upcoming neurosurgical procedure. Therefore, it is important to understand the disease process, its clinical manifestations, how to care for these patients, as well as the patient's full medical history and surgical plans. In either the clinic or the postoperative care setting, how well pain is managed will dictate how the patient and/or family defines a successful operation. To say the least, these patients and social aspects of care are among the most challenging in neurosurgery.

Common phone calls, pages, and requests with answers

1. *Pain management:* The most common phone call, page, or request will be regarding the escalation of pain. A clear plan with the patient, family, nursing staff, and adjunctive care staff must be made regarding pain management in order to limit complications from analgesics.

2. *Aseptic meningitis:* The duraplasty procedure can result in aseptic or chemical meningitis occurring postoperatively, presumably due to residual blood and other inflammatory particulate matter retained within the subarachnoid cisterns. Fever, neck pain, photophobia, nausea, vomiting, and mild lethargy can all occur but will occur early within the first 24–48 hours postoperatively and therefore will be highly unlikely related to bacterial meningitis. Routine workup for bacterial meningitis is most often unnecessary. Glucocorticoids, such as dexamethasone, are effective at limiting the meningitis and treating the pain, and aseptic meningitis has a self-limited course.

3. *Due to the likely extensive dural openings,* a patient with Chiari I malformation is exposed to a high rate of potential CSF leakage through the dural repair.

References

Alden TD, Ojemann JG, Park TS. Surgical treatment of Chiari I malformation: Indications and approaches. *Neurosurg Focus.* 2001;11:E2.

Bejjani GK. Definition of the adult Chiari malformation: A brief historical overview. *Neurosurg Focus.* 2001;11:E1.

Calliauw L, Dehaene I. The surgical risk in the treatment of Arnold Chiari malformations. *Acta Neurochir (Wien).* 1977;39:173–179.

Dyste GN, Menezes AH, VanGilder JC. Symptomatic Chiari malformations. An analysis of presentation, management, and long-term outcome. *J Neurosurg.* 1989;71:159–168.

Todor DR, Mu HT, Milhorat TH. Pain and syringomyelia: A review. *Neurosurg Focus.* 2000;8:E11.

43

BRAIN DEATH AND ORGAN DONATION

Arun Paul Amar

Key points

- Brain death is the irreversible cessation of all brain function.
- From a legal standpoint, brain death is tantamount to circulatory arrest and is recognized as a valid determination of death.
- The principal elements of brain death are a known mechanism of injury, absence of response to verbal and noxious stimulation, absence of brainstem reflexes, absence of respiratory drive (apnea) on formal testing, and exclusion of all possible confounders.
- Federal, state, and institutional policies about brain death declaration vary. Compliance with these statutes and appropriate documentation are essential.
- Use of a checklist can improve the accuracy and reliability of diagnosis as well as satisfy local requirements for certifying brain death.
- Brain dead patients represent a significant potential source of organ donation.
- Organ donation after designated cardiac death is an option for patients who do not meet criteria for brain death but have catastrophic neurologic injury that will not likely improve with medical or surgical intervention.

Brain death

The concept of brain death lives at the intersection of science, religion, medicine, ethics, and law. Though the term is commonly used in clinical parlance, "brain death" is one of the most poorly understood notions among laypeople, and explaining the nuances of this subject to patients' families can be one of the most daunting tasks faced by health-care professionals. A widely accepted definition is that brain death is the condition of irreversible cessation of all brain function (Wijdics, 2013, p. 191; Sawicki et al., 2014, p. 417; Wang et al., 2002, p. 732; Youn and Greer, 2014, p. 813).

Physiology of brain death

Although catastrophic neurologic injury has been recognized since antiquity, the challenges pertaining to brain death are the by-product of modern resuscitation techniques and intensive care measures that defy previously nonsurvivable brain damage (Wijdicks, 2013, p. 191; Wang et al., 2002, p. 731). A person declared brain dead can still have a beating heart (at least temporarily) as a result of "artificial life support" that sustains cardiopulmonary function, such as mechanical ventilation and vasopressor medication. This can cause considerable consternation or confusion among the patients' family and impede their acceptance of death. However, from a legal standpoint, the declaration of brain death is tantamount to circulatory arrest and is recognized as a valid determination of death throughout much of the world. This includes the United States, under the Uniform Determination of Death Act (UDDA) (Wijdicks, 2013, p. 193; Wang et al., 2002, p. 732). Therefore, because of these implications, it is imperative to differentiate true brain death from other conditions of devastating coma in which the loss of brain function is either incomplete or reversible. Furthermore, determination of brain death should not be undertaken if a therapeutic intervention (medical or surgical) may plausibly reverse the underlying malady.

It is now recognized that cessation of brainstem function underlies brain death and is its *sine qua non* (Wijdicks, 2013, p. 192). As a result, clinical assessment of brain death emphasizes the examination of brainstem function.

Although there has been extensive debate about the criteria that define brain death, current guidelines specify that the following conditions be fulfilled (Wijdics 2013, 195–196; Sawicki et al., 2014, p. 417; Wang et al., 2002, p. 731):

A known mechanism of acute catastrophic brain injury, typically corroborated by appropriate neuro-imaging findings.

Absence of response to verbal and noxious stimulation (coma), including eye opening, grimacing, or other motor activity. However, some reflexive "spinal" movements such as the triple flexion response are compatible with brain death.

Absence of brainstem reflexes (pupillary, corneal, oculocephalic/vestibuloocular, cough, and gag reflexes).

Absence of respiratory drive (apnea) on formal testing with hypercarbic challenge.

The exclusion of all possible confounders, such as drugs (sedatives, hypnotics, narcotics, neuromuscular blocking agents, etc.), severe electrolyte or metabolic imbalances, or other neurologic conditions that could mimic brain death, such as high cervical cord injury, Guillain-Barré syndrome, etc. The patient should also be normothermic and normotensive.

As explained in the section pertaining to organ donation, brain death is accompanied by cardiovascular repercussions (hypotension due to loss of vascular tone and invariant heart rate), but these are not brain death criteria, per se.

Despite the seeming simplicity of this schema, declaration of brain death is far from straightforward, and many omissions of documentation occur. In one study conducted at a major urban trauma center, audit of brain death notes from the medical record revealed that the majority were deficient in documenting one or more elements, such as specific brainstem reflexes or the absence of confounding factors (Wang et al., 2002, p. 731). Implementation of a checklist can help ensure the accuracy and reliability of diagnosis as well as satisfy local requirements for certifying brain death (Wang et al., 2002, p. 735). It enumerates the systematic assessments that establish the diagnosis and documentation of brain death.

Apnea test

Particular attention must be paid to the apnea test. Properly performed, the apnea test produces acute hypercarbia, resulting in cerebrospinal fluid acidosis that stimulates respiratory centers of the brainstem. Thus, the absence of respirations confirms brainstem dysfunction. If improperly performed, however, validity of the test is questioned. Also, in unstable patients the test may precipitate cardiac arrest. Therefore, it should only be performed after clinical assessment suggests that the patient is brain dead and the apnea test is needed for confirmation.

Patients should be preoxygenated with 100% oxygen for 10 minutes. A baseline arterial blood gas (ABG) should be drawn, verifying that the patient is normocarbic. If hypocarbia is present (e.g., due to deliberate hyperventilation used to mitigate elevated intracranial pressure), it will take longer to achieve the target value of hypercarbia. After 10 minutes of disconnection from the ventilator, the ABG is repeated. A partial pressure of carbon dioxide (pCO_2) ≥ 60 mm Hg is necessary to establish the validity of the apnea test.

Confirmatory tests

Centers vary in terms of the requirements for ancillary studies that confirm cessation of blood flow to the brain and/or the absence of cerebral electrical activity (on electroencephalography or evoked potentials) as diagnostic criteria of brain death. Sometimes these studies are employed when the clinical assessment suggests brain death but a confirmatory apnea test cannot be performed, or when uncertainty exists about the reliability of the clinical exam due to confounding conditions (Sawicki et al., 2014, p. 417; Youn and Greer, 2014, p. 821). However, these tests are notoriously inaccurate due to false-positive and false-negative results, and their interpretation in the context of brain death can be misleading (Wijdicks, 2013, p. 196). Nonetheless, even though the necessity and utility of these tests remain the subject of controversy, it is always necessary to comply with the policies of the individual institution in obtaining them.

Brain death declaration

In many jurisdictions, the declaration of brain death requires assessment by more than one physician and/ or more than one examination, separated by a variable time interval. Criteria for adults and children, such as the need for confirmatory tests, may also differ (Wijdicks, 2013, p. 197). Many facilities restrict declaration to physicians who have certain backgrounds (e.g., neurology and neurosurgery) or have passed a test that certifies proficiency in brain death examination. Again, adherence to local institutional policy is mandatory.

In communicating the diagnosis of brain death, it is important to be unequivocal in expressing the fact that the patient has died, despite the presence of a beating heart. Patients' families often get confused at this time about whether they need to make decisions to "pull the plug" and withdraw life support. However, unlike conditions of coma in which the loss of brain function is either incomplete or reversible, brain death declaration enables the physician to remove the body from life support without any assent from family or other legally authorized representative (LAR) under the UDDA, except in New York and New Jersey, where physicians are required to honor religious objections (Wijdicks, 2013, p. 193).

Understandably, receiving the news of brain death can be quite upsetting for families, and some may react with threatening comments. It is often helpful to allow them a reasonable period of time to process this information or to summon other relatives to observe the body before it is disconnected from the ventilator. Engagement of a religious figure from the family's faith as well as the hospital's ethics council and risk management team can also help diffuse tension during these difficult moments.

Organ donation

Brain dead patients represent an important source of organ transplantation, as more than three–fourths of them become donors (Wijdicks, 2013, p. 201). However, the success of this process requires the synchronized efforts of a large team to address the physiological needs of the donor body as well as the psychological needs of the donor's family. Typically, these endeavors are managed by the local organ procurement organization (OPO), a federally regulated agency that coordinates arrangements between the brain dead patient, transplant surgeons, and other entities.

Approaching the donor's family

Because of the considerable preparation that must occur prior to transplantation, early identification of patients with irreversible devastating brain injury is essential to maintain the pool of potential donors. At most centers, it is obligatory to notify the regional OPO of patients who meet criteria of catastrophic brain damage and might progress to brain death.

However, the issue of organ donation should not be discussed with the patient's family or other LAR until the brain death declaration has been first explained to them. Furthermore, in order to avoid the appearance of conflict of interest or ulterior motives, the clinicians who cared for the brain dead patient are discouraged from initiating conversations about organ donation with the family. Instead, such discussions are best had with the regional OPO agent acting as mediator. But if the family of a patient in whom brain death is imminent requests withdrawal of care, it may be appropriate for the clinicians to bring up the potential of organ donation at that time.

Preservation of organs

As a result of the central role of the brainstem in maintaining homeostasis, brain dead patients suffer many systemic problems, including poikilothermia, diabetes insipidus, and marked hypotension due to loss of vascular tone and an invariant heart rate (Wijdicks, 2013, p. 192; Youn and Greer, 2014, p. 823; Westphal et al., 2012, p. 2260–2266). Maintenance of the body's organs for potential transplantation requires aggressive hemodynamic support and other intensive care unit measures that maximize tissue perfusion; but once consent for organ donation is signed, the treating team often cedes such management to the OPO.

Specific management protocols are beyond the scope of this chapter but can be found elsewhere (Youn and Greer, 2014, p. 823–825; Westphal et al., 2012, p. 2260–2266). The goals include ensuring hemodynamic stability, correcting oxygen deficits, treating bacterial infections, reversing hypothermia, and correcting metabolic disorders (Westphal et al., 2012, p. 2261). Adoption of these aggressive protocols can improve the yield of organ donation by up to 80% or more (Westphal et al., 2012, p. 2261).

Donation after cardiac (circulatory) death

In patients with devastating brain injury who do not meet criteria of brain death, the donation after cardiac death (DCD) protocol allows for the potential of organ donation. If family members wish to withdraw care due to medical futility, terminal extubation is performed in the operating room with the transplant team on standby. The patient is then monitored for circulatory arrest, and once this occurs, organ procurement is initiated immediately. However, as a result of the inherent delay during which organs are not perfused, ischemic injury may preclude their subsequent use for donation (Neyrinck et al., 2013, p. 1–9). The DCD protocol is a relatively recent program and is associated with unique ethical considerations and resource strains. As such, it is not available at all centers.

Conclusions

Brain death represents a challenging situation for all involved parties, including health-care providers and patients' families. Sensitivity to cultural or religious issues is paramount, and clear communication is essential. Adherence to local policies for documentation helps minimize error and facilitate successful management.

References

Neyrinck A, Raemdonck DV, Monbaliu D. Donation after circulatory death: current status. *Curr Opin Anesthesiol.* 2013;26:1–9.

Sawicki M, Bohatyrewicz R, Walecka A, Sotek-Pastuszka J, Rowinski O, Walecki J. CT angiography in the diagnosis of brain death. *Pol J Radiol.* 2014;79:417–421.

Wang MY, Wallace P, Gruen PJ. Brain death documentation: Analysis and issues. *Neurosurgery.* 2002;51:731–736.

Westphal GA, Caldeira Filho M, Fiorelli A et al. Guidelines for maintenance of adult patients with brain death and potential for multiple organ donations: The Task Force of the Brazilian Association of Intensive Medicine the Brazilian Association of Organs Transplantation, and the Transplantation Center of Santa Catarina. *Transplant Proc.* 2012;44:2260–2267.

Wijdicks E. 2013. Brain death. In: Bernat JL, Beresford R, eds. *Handbook of Clinical Neurology, Volume 118. Ethical and Legal Issues in Neurology.* New York, NY: Elsevier; 2013:191–203.

Youn TS, Greer DM. Brain death and management of a potential organ donor in the intensive care unit. *Crit Care Clin.* 2014;30:813–831.

PART VI

Clinical Pathologies and Scenarios: Spine

44

SPINAL CORD INJURIES AND FRACTURES

Laura Sweeney, George M. Ghobrial, and James S. Harrop

Case vignette

A 47-year-old female is transferred to a regional trauma center for evaluation following an unfortunate diving accident. Witnesses describe that the patient dove into shallow water, sustaining a blunt force trauma to the head and neck followed by an immediate loss of consciousness. Cardiopulmonary resuscitation was initiated for a few minutes until emergency medical services arrived. An airway was established, and the cervical spine was secured. The patient was brought to the emergency department of the regional spinal cord injury center. After a primary evaluation for cardiopulmonary injuries, the patient was examined neurologically and was found to be awake and responsive. Greatly diminished strength in the bilateral upper and lower extremities was observed along with decreased rectal tone.

Urgent computed tomography (CT) scan demonstrated bilateral facet dislocation at the C5-C6 level (Figure 44.1). Sagittal T2-weighted magnetic resonance imaging (MRI) shows spinal cord compression and edema, along with disruption of the posterior ligamentous complex (Figure 44.2). The patient was cleared for additional injuries. Her mean arterial pressures are elevated to 85, and the patient is taken to the operative suite for posterior decompression and stabilization (Figure 44.3). Postoperatively, the patient exhibits markedly improved strength in the upper and lower extremities.

Overview

Epidemiology

The incidence of spinal cord injury (SCI) is approximately 12,500 new cases annually in the United States. The average age of injury is steadily rising in accordance with an aging general population. Eighty percent of SCIs involve males. Motor vehicle collisions (MVCs) are the leading cause of SCI, followed by falls, violence/gunshot wounds, and sports. Due to the use of seat belts, sport regulations, and other preventative measures, the incidence of complete SCI is decreasing, while the relative proportion of cervical SCI is increasing.

Societal significance

The proportion of SCI in the elderly is increasing, with low-velocity injuries, such as falls, a leading cause. Consequently, preventative measures should be incorporated at assisted living centers wherever possible in an attempt to reduce these injuries.

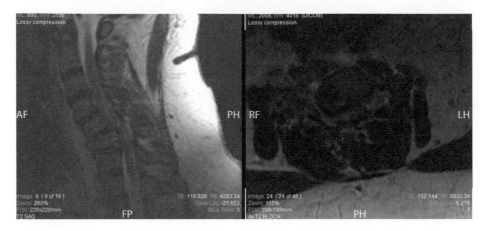

Figure 44.1 Sagittal (*left*) and axial (*right*) CT scan demonstrating traumatic subluxation of C5 and C6, with approximately 50% narrowing of the spinal canal.

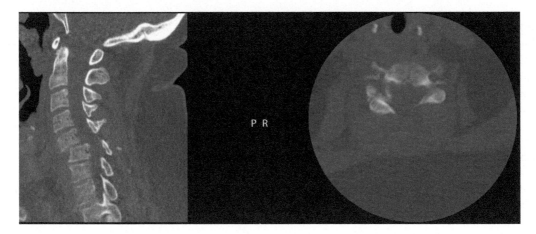

Figure 44.2 Sagittal (*left*) and axial (*right*) T2-weighted MRI demonstrating a C5-C6 subluxation with disruption of the posterior ligamentous complex, spinal cord compression, with spinal cord edema.

Basic biologic and physiologic processes

Traumatic SCI involves a transfer of kinetic injury to the spinal cord parenchyma, resulting in disruption of ascending and descending axonal tracts, which carry sensory and motor information, respectively. Also occurring is the initial destruction of supporting cellular architecture, including Schwann cells, neurons, and astrocytes. This initial destruction is referred to as the primary injury and is thought to be largely irreparable. Following the initial injury, cellular death triggers spinal cord inflammation through the migration of inflammatory mediators. The inflammatory environment is acidic and is replete with prostaglandins and free radicals, which are toxic to injured neurons, Schwann cells, and astrocytes. The destruction of spinal cord architecture after the initial injury by way of cell-mediated means (i.e., inflammation) is referred to as the secondary injury. Secondary injury is also exacerbated by hypoperfusion or anoxia of the spinal cord.

The primary injury is preventable through means that lower an individual's risk for SCI (e.g., protective gear in high-risk sports, seat belts), whereas the secondary injury historically has been the main focus of scientific and clinical research for SCI. In the past few decades, investigations have been underway that

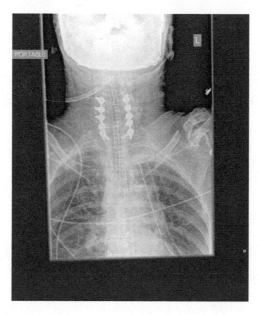

Figure 44.3   Anteroposterior plain film radiograph demonstrating posterior cervical instrumented fusion from C3 to C7.

implicate cellular-based therapies (i.e., stem cell transplants) as a means to replenish lost cellular architecture and treat the primary injury. These are presently the available pathways to limit any further destruction of the spinal cord, and to maximize future recovery.

Anatomical review

Tetraplegia, previously referred to as quadriplegia, occurs when there is loss of motor strength and tone in all four extremities, due to traumatic injury of the spinal cord. Injuries involving the thoracic, lumbar, or sacral regions can cause paraplegia. Throughout the years, the rates of complete tetraplegia and complete paraplegia have decreased, while incomplete tetraplegia has increased.

In order to classify the level of injury, health-care providers use the functional American Spinal Injury Association (ASIA or AIS) Impairment Scale, which is discussed later in the chapter.

Common physical examination findings

The neurologic examination is essential for early surgical decision making in the face of SCI and spinal fractures. Patients with neurologic deficits such as decreased strength in the setting of acute SCI have shown relatively better improvement with immediate surgery when compared to delayed surgery (>24 hours). As a result, the neurologic exam carries significant importance in the early care setting.

Prognosis

The neurologic exam in the spinal cord injured patient is also paramount in determining patient prognosis with regard to extent of improvement. However, clinical research indicates that a detailed SCI examination by a certified examiner 2 weeks beyond the initial injury is relatively more useful when compared to an examination of a patient in the early stage to estimate the extent of recovery.

Neurologic examination

The neurologic examination on a patient with a suspected spinal injury is well described, and an emphasis is placed on understanding the level of injury and the presence of radiculopathy or myelopathy, which is suggestive of nerve root or spinal cord compression, respectively.

1. Lower motor neuron (LMN) injury
    LMN findings are indicated most commonly by nerve root compression and can present with unilateral radicular pain and paresthesias in a classic dermatomal distribution, weakness, and decreased reflexes.
2. Upper motor neuron (UMN) injury
    UMN findings are suggestive of spinal cord involvement above the level of the trauma, and can manifest with bilateral weakness and paresthesias, hyperreflexia and clonus, ataxia, bowel and bladder incontinence, and priapism denoting severe SCI.

The neurologic evaluation is made up of a six-point scale of the 10 major muscle groups. The six-point scale consists of five (full strength), four (movement against resistance), three (movement against gravity), two (movement without gravity), one (trace movement), and zero (no movement). The major muscle groups include C5 deltoids/biceps, C6 wrist/extensors, C7 triceps, C8 middle finger flexors, T1 small finger flexors, L2 hip flexion/quads, L3 knee extension, L4 ankle dorsiflexion, L5 foot/big toe dorsiflexion, S1 gastrocnemius/foot plantar flexion. In addition to the previously stated evaluation, sensory examination is important to test. Health-care providers test sensation with light touch and pinprick for normal (two), impaired (one), and absent (zero). The human body has 28 dermatomes to test for sensation.

Relevant diagnostic tests

Laboratory

Patients with SCI are at an elevated risk of gastrointestinal ulcers. As such, routine evaluation of a patient with SCI with or without multisystem trauma requires periodic evaluation of

*   Complete blood count (CBC)—This is recommended for routine monitoring of anemia related to surgical procedures and occult bleeding.
*   Albumin/prealbumin—Labs are useful for weekly monitoring of nutrition often with conditions preventing normal oral feeding (e.g., traumatic brain injury [TBI], tracheotomies, prolonged endotracheal intubation, cervical spine surgery).
*   International normalized ratio/prothrombin time/partial thromboplastin (INR/PT/PTT)—This should be followed periprocedurally and coagulopathies treated. More frequent monitoring is recommended in the setting of epidural hematoma or intracranial hemorrhage.

Vascular/Electrophysiologic

*   Ultrasound of the bilateral lower extremity veins is recommended on a weekly basis due to the increased risk of deep vein thrombosis (DVT) in the SCI patient. With patients at increased risk (e.g., ventilated patient, para-/tetraplegic patient), more frequent screening may be considered.

Radiologic

- Consider the following imaging in the acute traumatic SCI patient:
  - Cervical/thoracic/lumbar spine CT: In a patient with a spine fracture, the risk of concomitant fracture is 10%–15%; therefore, it is warranted to obtain CT imaging of the complete spine.
  - Chest/abdomen/pelvis CT: This should be routinely obtained in the unresponsive trauma patient with suspected injuries. In this case, the radiologist can reconstruct CT thoracic and lumbar spine imaging to lower the overall radiation exposure.
  - Head CT: In longitudinal studies of TBI and SCI, the risk of co-occurring TBI and SCI is as high as 60%.
  - MRI: Axial and sagittal view T2- and T1-weighted imaging as well as short T1 inversion recovery (STIR) sequence imaging should be localized to the level of injury suspected by a neurologic examination. In the case of unresponsive patients, it is prudent to begin with an MRI assessment of trauma identified on CT (e.g., fracture, soft tissue swelling), and scout imaging of the adjacent spinal regions when suspicion of additional injury arises.

Review of relevant interventional procedures and surgeries

Spinal decompression and arthrodesis

As previously mentioned, patient functional outcomes have been shown in prospectively designed clinical research to show greater improvements when the spine is decompressed and stabilized within the first 24 hours in the case of more severe SCI involving greater motor deficits (e.g., no motor or sensory function below, or within three anatomic levels of injury; ASIA grade A [referred to as "ASIA A"]).

Ventriculostomy/Intraparenchymal tissue monitor

In the setting of co-occurrent severe TBI (Glasgow Coma Scale ≤8) and SCI, intracranial pressure (ICP) monitoring is warranted with either intraparenchymal tissue monitor or external ventricular drain (EVD/ventriculostomy), as the patient lacks sufficient neurologic status for adequate monitoring. In the case of intracranial hemorrhage with a GCS >8 (moderate or mild TBI), consider ICP monitor placement if a patient requires prolonged surgical intervention. This will allow the surgeon to continue to monitor for changes in ICP or intracranial hemorrhage size during a long surgery, which can be deadly if left untreated.

Common grading schemes

The American Spinal Injury Association Impairment Scale (AIS): International Standards for Neurological Classification of Spinal Cord Injury (ISNCSCI) is the most widely used to date. Numerous studies have validated AIS, with a high correlation coefficient. Ten muscle groups bilaterally are scaled from 1 to 5 for a total strength score of 100. Twenty-eight dermatomes are assessed bilaterally using pinprick and light touch in addition to assessment of anal sensory and motor sensation. Scoring is based on an A–E grade:

- A (complete injury): No sensory or motor function below the level of injury including sacral levels S4–S5.
- B (sensory incomplete): Loss of motor function three levels below injury level but preserved sensory function.
- C (partial motor loss): More than half of all muscle groups below the level of injury are less than a grade 3 (able to contract muscle group against gravity).

- D (partial motor loss): More than half of all muscle groups above the level of injury are greater than a grade 3.
- E (normal): A transient neurologic deficit must be noted, but the patient must have returned to normal in all motor and sensory areas tested.

Family counseling

- **Prognosis**

  As mentioned above, prognosis is often difficult to gauge appropriately in the acute setting, as factors such as multisystem trauma, medication, ventilation, and TBI are all confounders limiting an accurate AIS determination. Family counseling is a multidisciplinary approach and should include the expertise of rehabilitation medicine specialists in regard to specific recovery plans of care and realistic goals for recovery. Patients and family members need time to accept this life-changing adjustment. However, each individual goes through this process differently. Some remain optimistic, whereas others quickly start the grieving process.

- **Common questions**

  Will I ever walk again?

  Will I be able to go back to work? More than half of the individuals that have a SCI were working before injury. About one-third of SCI patients go back to work after injury.

  How long will I be in the hospital? The average length of stay in the acute care hospital is about 11 days. The average stay in rehabilitation is about 36 days. Both of these numbers have decreased significantly over the years.

  What are common complications after SCI? Blood clots (VTE), pneumonia, septicemia, pressure ulcers, spasticity, depression, pain, and renal stones. Pneumonia and septicemia are the leading cause of death in SCI patients. Autonomic dysreflexia is a medical emergency that patients with SCI can develop due to noxious stimuli leading to hypertension, bradycardia, diaphoresis, and flushing.

  Will I be able to have sex again? Yes, although it may be different prior to injury. There are many different techniques, medications, and assistive devices that can be used.

- **Pitfalls**

  Comorbidities and the patient's general health can be detrimental in recovery and early ambulation. A patient may not be able to fully participate in rehabilitation due to his or her preinjury health and mobility status.

Common pitfalls and medicolegal concerns

SCI patients typically have a prolonged hospital stay, which necessitates daily attention to detail in a medically fragile patient population. As a result, the most common pitfalls and medicolegal concerns are often avoidable.

Decubitus ulcers

SCI patients are prone to decubitus ulcers due to prolonged hospitalization in an immobilized state. Patients unable to ambulate should still work with physical therapy (e.g., range of motion, strengthening of intact muscle groups, positioning), not only to maximize recovery and prevent contractures, but also because it lowers patient morbidity for a number of reasons. Through therapy, patients can develop a number of pressure relief methods, ranging from rolling to a variety of specialized seating systems. Importantly, pressure redistribution via a tilt in space wheelchair reduces pressure from the buttocks, posterior thighs, and posterior trunk. If a patient is unable to be mobilized or complete rolling independently, a schedule should be implemented for pressure redistribution, to aid in reperfusion of the skin.

Skin barrier cream, spray, or skin prep should be applied to pressure points, such as the sacrum and under cervical collars, to prevent breakdown. At times, cervical collars and thoracic or lumbar spine braces can cause skin breakdown, so these areas should also have frequent skin assessments. Also, attention to detail is needed for patients with fragile skin, as this raises the risk of ulcer, as well as nutritionally depleted patients, who have the highest relative risk for decubitus ulcer.

Thromboembolism

The risk of DVT is higher in patients with SCI and can precipitate life-threatening pulmonary embolism (PE) if not dealt with promptly. DVT prophylaxis must be instituted upon admission, and it is even more important in patients with multisystem traumatic injuries due to the raised risk. Two noninvasive ways to prevent DVTs are by applying pneumatic compression stockings and T.E.D. antiembolism stockings. In addition, unfractionated heparin is one of several anticoagulant medications used as DVT prophylaxis. Many times patients are sent to rehab on either unfractionated heparin or low molecular weight heparin (e.g., enoxaparin). Inferior vena cava (IVC) filters should be used in patients who cannot be anticoagulated and/or failed anticoagulation.

Urinary tract infection

Patients with acute trauma and subsequent surgery most commonly have a Foley catheter for careful monitoring of fluid balance. However, daily attention should be paid to evaluating the medical necessity of the Foley, and it should be removed as soon as possible. Furthermore, the sterile placement of a Foley as well as sterile straight catheters, bladder training, and suprapubic catheters are important with patients with SCIs. Bladder training normally begins when the patient is transferred to rehabilitation.

Bowel Regimen

Bowel dysfunction is devastating in patients with SCI because it does not only affect skin integrity but also quality of life. Patients can develop many gastrointestinal complications, such as ileus, ulcers, reflux, autonomic dysreflexia, constipation, distention, and so on. It is important to establish a bowel regimen early on in the injury. These regimens normally include a stool softener three times a day, a gentle laxative (such as Senokot), and an enema once a day. The patient can administer these medications whenever he or she desires. Some individuals like to do it at the start of their day, and others before bedtime. In addition, a patient should have a nutritious, high-residue diet, with plenty of fluids.

Autonomic dysreflexia

Autonomic dysreflexia (AD) is considered a medical emergency. AD occurs in patients with SCI above the T6 region, although it has been reported to occur with injury as low as T10. Noxious stimuli, such as kinked Foley catheter, bowel obstruction, and undetected urinary tract infection, below the level of injury trigger AD. Some of the symptoms of AD include hypertension, bradycardia, diaphoresis, flushing above the level of injury, anxiety, and headaches. The treatment for AD is removal of the noxious stimuli (unkink the Foley, perform manual disimpaction, treat the UTI). At times, patients might need antihypertensives to control the rise of blood pressure.

Relevance to the advanced practice health professional

SCI can be a devastating, life-changing injury not only to the patient but also to family members. Health-care professionals need to be able to inform patients about the level of injury using an appropriate, good bedside manner. Patients and family members need time to absorb this information. However, health-care providers should be ready to answer any questions that patients and their family members might have regarding SCI. Education about the injury and what to expect in the future is key. In order to start the disposition process, which should begin upon admission to the hospital, case management (CM) and social work (SW) should be consulted. Case managers know which rehabilitation facilities specialize in SCI and what health care insurances will require. Social workers can provide health care insurance applications for uninsured patients and provide resource and support groups for not only the patient, but also family members.

The need for surgery should be assessed first in order to provide spinal stability for the patient. After surgery, management of the body systems is important. Respiratory management includes early ventilator weaning, aggressive chest therapy, and determination of the need for tracheostomy or diaphragmatic pacemaker. Cardiovascular management is important in the early injury state. As health-care providers, we aim to have adequate spinal cord perfusion with elevated blood pressures (mean arterial pressure >85 mm Hg) for our patients. We also attempt to prevent autonomic dysreflexia. Other interventions we implement are skin protection, bowel and bladder regimens, pain control, and DVT prophylaxis.

Early therapy and rehabilitation are critical in the acute phase of injury. Range of motion (ROM), early mobilization, and physical medicine and rehabilitation (PMR) are all essential interventions that should be implemented early. Patients with SCI will need management of long-term issues, such as bowel/bladder incontinence, chronic pain, and mobility limitations. There are many new advances to assist patients with SCI when they finish their rehabilitation and are discharged home.

SCI is an injury that requires a multidisciplinary approach. In the acute injury phase, patients will be followed by their surgeon (normally neurosurgery or orthopedic), PMR, physical and occupational therapists, nutritionist, social worker, and case manager. After the acute phase, appropriate follow-up is necessary. Patients will require follow-up with their surgeons, where they will be examined and postoperative films, such as x-rays of their spines, will be reviewed. In addition, due to the spasticity that patients with SCI frequently encounter, a PMR doctor is important. These physicians can help control spasms with different medications (baclofen, Valium, Zanaflex) and modalities (intrathecal baclofen pumps).

Common phone calls, pages, and requests

After spinal surgery or SCI there are common medications, nursing alerts, and activity sets that are ordered automatically. However, it is common for certain orders to be overlooked or missing. Some things that we get called about are bowel medications, such as enemas or oral laxatives per PMR. Due to the side effects and dosage choices, pain medications or antispasmodics are other medications that need to be adjusted during the acute phase. A patient should not have uncontrolled pain or spasms; however, the patient needs to be alert enough to participate in therapy. Although some patients cannot feel below their umbilicus, they often experience pain above their injury level. Other times, spasms are not properly controlled, which may necessitate a medication increase or dose adjustment. In addition, some patients may develop anxiety following the injury and its resultant prognosis.

After spinal surgery, spine stability is important. Patients may need to wear cervical collars (i.e., Philadelphia, Miami J, Aspen collars), cervical-thoracic orthoses (CTOs), or thoracic or lumbar braces (custom clamshell, lumbosacral orthosis [LSO], thoracolumbosacral orthosis [TLSO]). Physical and occupational therapy work with these patients daily and sometimes even twice a day. In order to safely participate in therapy, patients need to have clear spine stability orders in place, including which collar or brace to wear, and when to don the brace (supine or sitting). If these orders are not prepared, we get contacted in order to clarify such specifications. This causes a delay in therapy, as the therapist will not be able to work with the patient until the orders are complete.

Another role we play is to educate and communicate with caregivers. Patients and caregivers are typically overwhelmed in the acute phase of injury. Therefore, it is important to discuss not only the current plan, but also the future with both the patient and the family (with the patient's consent). As previously mentioned, rehabilitation is vital to a patient's recovery. While the patient is in the acute hospital, family members can tour rehabilitation facilities and assist in choosing the proper rehabilitation setting. Once stable for discharge to rehab, as health-care providers, we provide the appropriate follow-up needed for the patient. We make sure the patient has the appropriate collar or brace and prescription for x-ray prior to follow-up appointment. We answer any questions that the patient, family members, or rehab facilities may have. In addition, we make sure that when the patient is discharged to rehab, he or she has a DVT prophylaxis (unfractionated heparin, Lovenox, or T.E.D.s) prescribed.

References

Benevento BT, Sipski ML. Neurogenic bladder, neurogenic bowel, and sexual dysfunction in people with spinal cord injury. *Phys Ther.* 2002;82(6):601–612.

Masri WS, Kumar N. Traumatic spinal cord injuries. *Lancet.* 2011;377(9770):972–974. doi: 10.1016/S0140-6736(11)60248-1.

National Spinal Cord Injury Statistical Center. Spinal cord injury facts and figures at a glance. J Spinal Cord Med. 2012;35(6):480–481.

National Spinal Cord Injury Statistical Center. Facts and figures at a glance. Birmingham, AL: University of Alabama at Birmingham. Accessed February 2014. https://www.nscisc.uab.edu/PublicDocuments/fact_figures_docs/Facts%202014.pdf.

45

CAUDA EQUINA SYNDROME

Jasmin Stefani and Luis M. Tumialán

Case vignette

History

A 24-year-old man who works at a hardware store presented to the emergency department after he lifted a 50-pound bag of cement and felt a "pop" in his back. He reported debilitating axial back pain without radiculopathy. His physical examination was limited by his pain, and a test of his motor skills against confrontation was likewise difficult to perform. The patient reported no bowel or bladder issues. Plain radiographs were negative for abnormal findings, and the patient was discharged with narcotic pain medication and was instructed to follow up with his primary care provider. On two subsequent occasions, he returned to the emergency department, but his assessments were unremarkable and he was discharged. The treating physician noted a concern about potential drug-seeking behavior.

The patient returned to the emergency department a fourth time, complaining of urinary retention. A catheter was placed, and 1.5 L of urine were drained from his bladder. A neurosurgical consultation was then requested.

Neurosurgical examination

The patient was nonambulatory because of his high level of pain. Evaluation of muscle group strength by confrontation resulted in scores of 3/5 bilateral quadriceps strength and 3/5 plantar flexion and dorsiflexion function. Sensory examination demonstrated unequivocal saddle anesthesia along with nondermatomal sensory loss in the lower extremities. Reflex examination demonstrated complete areflexia on the left patellar and Achilles tendons, and hyporeflexia in the right leg.

Radiographic studies and surgical intervention

Magnetic resonance imaging (MRI) revealed a large disc herniation at L1-L2 and severe compression of the cauda equina (Figure 45.1). A minimally invasive approach was used to access the L1-L2 segment of the spine. A generous hemilaminectomy and a medial facetectomy were performed, allowing safe mobilization of the thecal sac and removal of the disc herniation (Figure 45.2).

Postoperative course

The patient had resolution of urinary retention after the Foley catheter was removed on postoperative day 1. He experienced gradual strengthening in the quadriceps over the ensuing weeks and returned to work without limitations 3 months postoperatively.

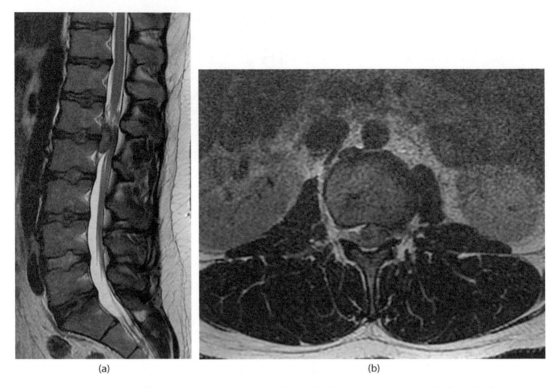

(a)　　　　　　　　　　　　　　　(b)

Figure 45.1　(a) T2-weighted sagittal MRI demonstrates a large disc herniation at L1-L2, which resulted in severe compression of the cauda equina. Note that the conus medullaris is rostral to the disc herniation. (b) T2-weighted axial MRI demonstrates complete obliteration of the cerebrospinal fluid signal secondary to the large disc herniation. (From Barrow Neurological Institute, Phoenix, Arizona. With permission.)

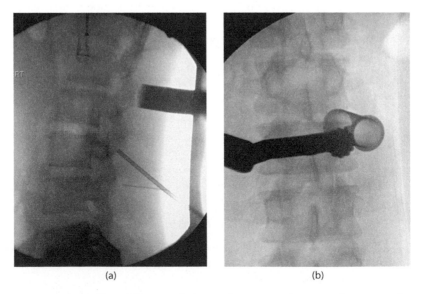

(a)　　　　　　　　　　　　　　　(b)

Figure 45.2　Anteroposterior and lateral fluoroscopic images demonstrate the minimal access port in position for the decompression. (From Barrow Neurological Institute, Phoenix, Arizona. With permission.)

Overview of cauda equina syndrome
Epidemiology

Although rare, cauda equina syndrome (CES) may be a neurosurgical emergency. The incidence of CES has been estimated to be between 1 per 33,000 cases (Fuso et al., 2013) and 7 per 100,000 inhabitants (Schoenfeld and Bader, 2012). The most common cause of CES is prolapse of a lumbar intervertebral disc, which compresses the spinal nerve roots at the cauda equina (Fuso et al., 2013). CES accounts for 2%–3% of all lumbar disc herniation surgeries, in which approximately 70% of patients had a reported history of chronic back pain (Gleave et al., 2002; Sun et al., 2014). Although the majority of CES cases may be secondary to lumbar disc herniation, it is important to bear in mind that other disorders can contribute to CES, including malignancy, vascular or infectious lesions, iatrogenic causes such as lumbar anesthesia or spinal manipulation, trauma, structural anomalies, or an occupying lesion compressing the nerve roots within the cauda equina (Ahn et al., 2000; Allorent et al., 2013; Amini et al., 2006; Ampil et al., 2001; Bartels and de Vries, 1996; Fayeye et al., 2010; Neuman et al., 2012; Paolini et al., 2002; Sales et al., 2013; Solheim et al., 2007; Shapiro, 1993). Men in their fourth and fifth decades of life have a higher prevalence of disc herniations; therefore, those in this demographic group are more likely than others to present with CES. The most common levels of injury are L4, L5, and S1 (Gleave et al., 2002).

Societal significance

CES can cause significant physical and mental disabilities and may result in considerable social and financial costs (McCarthy et al., 2007). Undiagnosed CES can lead to lifelong devastating medical morbidities, such as sexual dysfunction or loss of bladder and bowel function (Fuso et al., 2013; Arrigo et al., 2011; DeLong et al., 2008). Neurologic deficits may also include temporary or permanent foot drop or flail foot (absence of plantar flexion and dorsiflexion) (Hamilton et al., 2011).

Basic biologic and physiologic processes

The cauda equina comprises the lumbar, sacral, and coccygeal nerve roots in the lumbar spine distal to the conus medullaris (Gitelman et al., 2008). Nerve roots in the cauda equina are made up of a dorsal root, which consists of afferent fibers for transmission of sensation, and a ventral root, which consists of the efferent pathway and allows transmission of motor and sympathetic fibers (Gitelman et al., 2008; Hamilton et al., 2011; Sun et al., 2014). CES is caused by the compression of the cauda equina nerve roots, which in turn causes obstruction of axoplasmic flow, venous congestion, and ischemia (Figure 45.3) (Gleave et al., 2002). Diagnosis is made based on symptoms that include lower back pain with unilateral or bilateral radicular pain, in combination with secondary neurologic deficits (specifically, the loss of visceral functions) (Kostuik, 2004; McCarthy et al., 2007; DeLong et al., 2008).

Anatomical review

MRI showed a large disc herniation at L1–L2 causing severe compression of the cauda equina (Figure 45.1a) and complete obliteration of the cerebrospinal fluid signal (Figure 45.1b). Anteroposterior and lateral fluoroscopic imaging showed the minimal access port positioned for decompression (Figure 45.2).

Common physical examination findings

CES is usually diagnosed after a thorough clinical examination that includes both a physical component and a comprehensive patient history (Gitelman et al., 2008). Symptom onset may be sudden, within

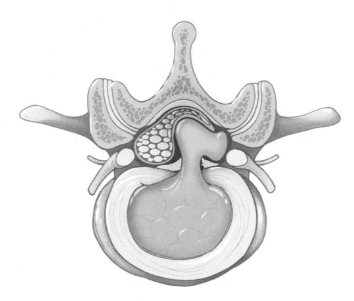

Figure 45.3   A central disc herniation causing severe central canal stenosis. Central disc extrusions of this size have the capacity to cause severe compression of the neural elements that can lead to cauda equine syndrome. (From Barrow Neurological Institute, Phoenix, Arizona. With permission.)

24 hours, or symptoms may occur gradually over several weeks (Shapiro, 2000). A complete neurologic examination should be completed before addressing the red flag symptoms mentioned below.

The most common CES findings are as follows:

- Severe lower back pain in the form of unilateral or bilateral sciatica (96%–100%) (Shapiro, 2000)
- Saddle anesthesia (81%); check using light touch and pinprick (Tarulli, 2015)
- Neurogenic bowel and bladder dysfunction, and diminished urinary function (93%) (Shapiro, 1993) and anal sphincter tone (47%) (Tarulli, 2015); check anal sphincter tone and "wink" reflex; test trigone sensation by pulling gently on catheter
- Bilaterally absent Achilles reflexes (Gitelman et al., 2008)
- Unilateral or bilateral calf muscle weakness; monitor for deterioration (Gitelman et al., 2008)
- Sexual dysfunction (<5%) (Gitelman et al., 2008)

Patients with higher lesions may present with

- Foot drop, toe drop, or both
- Reduced or complete loss of knee-jerk reflexes
- Unilateral or bilateral quadriceps weakness; monitor for deterioration (Shapiro, 2000)

Relevant diagnostic tests

Imaging of the lumbosacral spine can identify conus or root compression that may cause CES. The most common cause of CES is intervertebral disc herniation (Shapiro, 1993; Tarulli, 2015; Ahn et al., 2000; Gardner et al., 2011).

- MRI of the lumbar spine is the gold standard of imaging for CES. It accurately displays soft tissue pathology, allowing for evaluation of stenosis, compression, and etiology (Tarulli, 2015).

- Computed tomography (CT) with myelography is often recommended for patients who cannot undergo MRI. A CT with or without contrast of the lumbar spine may also reveal stenosis and intervertebral disc degeneration and herniation.
- A lumbar myelogram may reveal obstruction of the spinal canal.
- Plain radiographs of the spine are not recommended as a first-line imaging modality when CES is suspected, but they may have value for evaluation of spinal trauma, listhesis, scoliosis, and disc degeneration.

Review of relevant interventional procedures and surgeries

CES is often a neurosurgical emergency. Delay in treatment may cause irreversible progression of symptoms, resulting in permanent neurologic deficits (Tarulli, 2015). Selection of a treatment modality depends largely on the underlying cause of CES. Previously published reports (Kostuik, 2004; Gleave et al., 2002; Shapiro, 2000; Shapiro, 1993; Gardner et al., 2011) indicate that prompt diagnosis and urgent or emergent surgery may improve patient outcome.

Decompression should be conducted within 48 hours (or, ideally, within 24 hours) of symptom onset or syndrome diagnosis to relieve mechanical or chemical pressure and to prevent further progression of neurologic deficits (Tarulli, 2015; Shapiro, 2000; Gitelman et al., 2008). The opportune time to perform surgical intervention is at the onset of urinary or bowel dysfunction (Olivero et al., 2009; Gleave et al., 2002; Gitelman et al., 2008; Domen et al., 2009; DeLong et al., 2008; Bell et al., 2007).

Laminectomy (with discectomy) with complete decompression of the neural elements is the surgical intervention of choice for CES (Ahn et al., 2000; Gardner et al., 2011; Gitelman et al., 2008). This procedure is focused on eliminating stenosis and relieving the pressure from the compressed nerves in the cauda equina region. For CES caused by compressive lesions such as malignancies, hematomas, or abscesses, surgery to remove the compressing lesion is the preferred treatment modality.

Common grading schemes

Two systems are commonly used to evaluate CES. One such system differentiates between incomplete or complete CES (Table 45.1); the second grades the degree of CES by the timing of symptoms (Gleave et al., 2002; Gardner et al., 2011).

CES caused by lumbar disc prolapse can be divided into three different groups. These groups and common presenting symptoms of CES are described in Table 45.2.

Family counseling

Prognosis

Rehabilitation therapy is a critical component of the healing process. The prognosis of patients with CES is variable, but some researchers have suggested that those with incomplete CES (CES-I) have better

Table 45.1 Types of Cauda Equina Syndrome (CES) and Symptoms

CES type	Prevalence	Management	Symptoms
Incomplete CES (CES-I)	30%–50%	Surgical decompression	Perianal saddle anesthesia with altered urinary sensation, loss of desire to void, poor urinary stream, strain to micturate
CES with retention (CES-R)	50%–70%	Surgical decompression	Perianal saddle anesthesia with painless urinary retention and overflow incontinence

Table 45.2 Common Presenting Symptoms of Cauda Equina Syndrome (CES)

Group	History	Symptoms
1	No previous history of low back pain	Rapid onset with severe neurologic deficit
2	History of lower back pain and sciatica	Exacerbation leads to severe neurologic deficit such as acute bladder dysfunction
3	History of chronic back pain and sciatica	Gradual progression of CES symptoms with canal stenosis

prognoses than patients who suffer from CES with retention (CES-R) (Gardner et al., 2011; Tarulli, 2015). Most (79%) patients with CES will have an acceptable return of urological function, with 44% returning to normal function; 28% of patients will continue to have residual back pain and motor and/or sensory deficits in the perineum and lower extremities (Gleave et al., 2002; Shapiro, 2000; Gardner et al., 2011). Unfortunately, approximately 20%–28% of all CES patients will have poor outcomes and will require ongoing treatment such as physical therapy, Foley catheters, or straight catheterization (Shapiro, 2000). The most common benefit of surgical intervention is pain relief, but long-term problems with sexual dysfunction (44%), micturition (48%), and defecation (50%) may persist (Tarulli, 2015). The recovery process may continue for several years after decompression (Tarulli, 2015).

Common questions

Patients experiencing CES often have similar concerns regarding their diagnosis. Below are some common patient concerns and possible responses to these questions.

Q: Will I be able to urinate on my own?
A: Bladder function may take up to 5 years to recover (Gleave et al., 2002). Straight catheterization may be required initially, but bladder training can be learned with rehabilitation.
Q: Will my pain get better?
A: Severe pain should be relieved postoperatively, but as with any surgical intervention, there will be some postoperative pain. This should improve over time. If you have a history of chronic back pain, surgery may not completely eradicate the pain (Shapiro, 2000).
Q: Will I be able to walk?
A: Complete motor recovery may take up to a year (Gleave et al., 2002).
Q: Will I be able to have sex again?
A: Some patients (30%–47%) may experience some form of erectile dysfunction or long-term sexual dysfunction despite receiving timely treatment (McCarthy et al., 2007).

Even if surgical decompression is performed in a timely manner, neurologic deficits may persist. An important component of preoperative counseling should be the establishment of realistic patient expectations. It is critical to emphasize that although decompression is the only surgical option to possibly restore neurologic function, it is impossible to predict the extent of recovery for each patient.

Common pitfalls and medicolegal concerns

CES has a high medicolegal profile (Arrigo et al., 2011; Daniels et al., 2012; Gardner et al., 2011; Kostuik, 2004). The rarity of the syndrome can cause misdiagnosis and delay in treatment (Gardner et al., 2011; Arrigo et al., 2011). Treatment delays can be multifactorial, but common causes of delayed treatment include postponement in seeking medical attention, failure by outpatient providers to recommend immediate hospitalization, failure by medical providers to recognize the symptoms in an emergent or clinic setting, miscommunication between medical personnel, failure by a nurse to examine and report neurologic deficits, or unavailability of MRI (Kostuik, 2004). These breakdowns in the system may ultimately lead to delayed treatment for CES and increase the potential for malpractice claims. Of the 95 CES cases reported to the Medical Defence Union in the United Kingdom in 2003, 65% progressed to claims and 48% resulted in an average settlement of £336,000 (US$549,427). Just under one-half of these 95 cases were reported by general providers and involved incorrect and delayed diagnosis (Markham, 2004). Negligence allegations appear to be the main cause of substantial damages awarded to plaintiffs. An omission in the medical record—timing of events, undocumented neurologic deficits, or unreported changes in bowel and bladder function—may constitute negligence (Kostuik, 2004).

The practitioner's ultimate goal is to relieve compression within 24–48 hours of CES onset, specifically when the patient presents with CES-I and has signs of progression. Decompression during CES-I has been documented to have favorable patient outcomes; however, CES-R has been associated with poor patient outcomes, and reversal of neurologic deficits is unlikely (Gardner et al., 2011).

Relevance to the advanced practice health professional

Any patient who reports acute onset low back pain should be evaluated for CES. Practitioners should perform a thorough neurologic assessment, including a detailed sensory assessment of the patient and documentation of all findings. Any increase in low back pain should be followed up with an examination of functional status, including function of the bowel and bladder. Bladder functional assessment should include postvoid residual evaluation. Suspicion of saddle anesthesia must be urgently reported to the surgeon. It is equally important to counsel patients with back pain to immediately contact a medical provider if they experience symptoms such as increased pain, radicular pain, bilateral weakness, or incontinence (Kostuik, 2004).

References

Ahn UM, Ahn NU, Buchowski JM, Garrett ES, Sieber AN, Kostuik JP. Cauda equina syndrome secondary to lumbar disc herniation: a meta-analysis of surgical outcomes. *Spine(Phila Pa 1976)*. 2000;25(12):1515–1522.

Allorent J, Cozic C, Guimard T, Tanguy G, Cormier G. Sciatica with motor loss and hemi-cauda equina syndrome due to varicella-zoster virus meningoradiculitis. *Joint Bone Spine*. 2013;80(4):436–437.

Amini A, Liu JK, Kan P, Brockmeyer DL. Cerebrospinal fluid dissecting into spinal epidural space after lumbar puncture causing cauda equina syndrome: review of literature and illustrative case. *Childs Nerv Syst*. 2006;22(12):1639–1641.

Ampil FL, Burton GV, Mills GM, Jawahar A, Pelser R, Nanda A. Cauda equina compression in breast cancer—incidence and treatment outcome. *Eur J Gynaecol Oncol*. 2001;22(4):257–259.

Arrigo RT, Kalanithi P, Boakye M. Is cauda equina syndrome being treated within the recommended time frame? *Neurosurgery*. 2011;68(6):1520–1526; discussion 1526.

Bartels RH, de Vries J. Hemi-cauda equina syndrome from herniated lumbar disc: a neurosurgical emergency? *Can J Neurol Sci*. 1996;23(4):296–299.

Bell DA, Collie D, Statham PF. Cauda equina syndrome: what is the correlation between clinical assessment and MRI scanning? *Br J Neurosurg*. 2007;21(2):201–203.

Daniels EW, Gordon Z, French K, Ahn UM, Ahn NU. Review of medicolegal cases for cauda equina syndrome: what factors lead to an adverse outcome for the provider? *Orthopedics*. 2012;35(3):e414–419.

DeLong WB, Polissar N, Neradilek B. Timing of surgery in cauda equina syndrome with urinary retention: meta-analysis of observational studies. *J Neurosurg Spine*. 2008;8(4):305–320.

Domen PM, Hofman PA, van Santbrink H, Weber WE. Predictive value of clinical characteristics in patients with suspected cauda equina syndrome. *Eur J Neurol*. 2009;16(3):416–419.

Fayeye O, Sankaran V, Sherlala K, Choksey M. Oligodendroglioma presenting with intradural spinal metastases: an unusual cause of cauda equina syndrome. *J Clin Neurosci*. 2010;17(2):265–267.

Fuso FA, Dias AL, Letaif OB, Cristante AF, Marcon RM, de Barros TE. Epidemiological study of cauda equina syndrome. *Acta Ortop Bras*. 2013;21(3):159–162.

Gardner AE. Gardner E, Morley T. Cauda equina syndrome: a review of the current clinical and medico-legal position. *Eur Spine J.* 2011;20(5):690–697.

Gitelman A, Hishmeh S, Morelli BN et al. Cauda equina syndrome: a comprehensive review. *Am J Orthop (Belle Mead NJ).* 2008;37(11):556–562.

Gleave JR, Macfarlane R. Cauda equina syndrome: what is the relationship between timing of surgery and outcome? *Br J Neurosurg.* 2002;16(4):325–328.

Hamilton DK, Smith JS, Sansur CA et al. Rates of new neurological deficit associated with spine surgery based on 108,419 procedures: a report of the scoliosis research society morbidity and mortality committee. *Spine.* 2011;36(15):1218–1228.

Kostuik JP. Medicolegal consequences of cauda equina syndrome: an overview. *Neurosurg Focus.* 2004;16(6):e8.

Markham DE. Cauda equina syndrome: diagnosis, delay and litigation risk. *Curr Orthop.* 2004;18(1):58–62.

McCarthy MJ, Aylott CE, Grevitt MP, Hegarty J. Cauda equina syndrome: factors affecting long-term functional and sphincteric outcome. *Spine.* 2007;32(2):207–216.

Neuman BJ, Radcliff K, Rihn J. Cauda equina syndrome after a TLIF resulting from postoperative expansion of a hydrogel dural sealant. *Clin Orthop Relat Res.* 2012;470(6):1640–1645.

Olivero WC, Wang H, Hanigan WC et al. Cauda equina syndrome (CES) from lumbar disc herniations. *J Spinal Disord Tech.* 2009;22(3):202–206.

Paolini S, Ciappetta P, Santoro A, Ramieri A. Rapid, symptomatic enlargement of a lumbar juxtafacet cyst: case report. *Spine.* 2002;27(11):E281–283.

Sales JG, Tabrizi A, Elmi A, Soleimanpour J, Gavidel E. Adolescence spinal epidural abscess with neurological symptoms: case report, a lesson to be re-learnt. *Med J Islam Repub Iran.* 2013;27(1):38–41.

Schoenfeld AJ, Bader JO. Cauda equina syndrome: an analysis of incidence rates and risk factors among a closed North American military population. *Clin Neurol Neurosurg.* 2012;114(7):947–950.

Shapiro S. Cauda equina syndrome secondary to lumbar disc herniation. *Neurosurgery.* 1993;32(5):743–746;discussion 46-47.

Shapiro S. Medical realities of cauda equina syndrome secondary to lumbar disc herniation. *Spine.* 2000;25(3):348–351; discussion 52.

Solheim O, Jorgensen JV, Nygaard OP. Lumbar epidural hematoma after chiropractic manipulation for lower-back pain: case report. *Neurosurgery.* 2007;61(1):E170–171;discussion E71.

Sun JC, Xu T, Chen KF et al. Assessment of cauda equina syndrome progression pattern to improve diagnosis. *Spine (Phila Pa 1976).* 2014;39(7):596–602.

Tarulli AW. Disorders of the cauda equina. *Continuum (Minneap Minn).* 2015;21(1):146–158.

46

ACUTE LOW BACK PAIN

Laura Ellen Prado and David Benglis

Case vignette

A patient picked up his 4-year-old son, and he immediately felt a sharp pain in his lower back that worsened over the course of the day. He took an ibuprofen, tried icing the lower back, but experienced no relief.

The patient awoke the next morning with worsened pain and spasms, and he could not mobilize from the bed. He took some more ibuprofen and rested the remainder of the weekend. He cancelled work on Monday.

Over the course of the day, the patient's condition progressed to involve his back and his left leg (along the outside to the top of the foot). The nature of the pain was throbbing and caused produced diaphoresis (sweating). He called his primary care provider and spoke to his advanced practice registered nurse (APRN) who evaluated him and recommended initial treatment with a short course of oral steroids and nonsteroidal anti-inflammatory drugs (NSAIDS).

The patient gave a typical initial presentation of acute low back pain brought about by a minor trauma. The most common cause of acute low back pain is musculoskeletal trauma causing a lumbar muscle spasm, and it usually resolves with conservative treatment (rest, ice, heat, NSAIDs, oral steroids, physical therapy, stronger pain medication, and steroid injections). Other reasons for back pain include degenerated discs or discogenic back pain, facet/joint mediated back pain, or spondylolisthesis (congenital reasons, traumatic, or degenerative).

The patient failed conservative treatment and magnetic resonance imaging (MRI) was done. He had a moderate left-sided herniated disc at L4-L5 causing his pain.

Overview

Low back pain ranks as one of the primary causes of disability around the world, accounts for the most frequent diagnosed musculoskeletal disorders affecting persons annually, and is a leading cause of global disability (The Global Burden of Disease Collaborators, 2015, p. 23; Manchikanti, 2000, p. 169). Approximately 65%–80% of Americans will be affected by low back pain in their lifetime. Many of those people will go on to develop lifelong debilitating chronic back pain (Manchikanti, 2000, p. 183).

Forty percent of all lost workdays are attributed to acute low back pain annually (Manchikanti, 2000, p. 169). In the United States, the cost associated with this condition is upward of $50 billion annually (Shaheed et al., 2014, p. 2).

Low back pain is localized to the lumbosacral region. There may be a radicular component if there is compression on an exiting nerve root. Typically, there are five lumbar vertebrae and five respective intervertebral discs between those vertebrae. (The bottom lumbar vertebra is connected via a disc to the sacrum.) The posterior aspect of the spine consists of the spinous process, lamina, transverse process, pars interarticularis, and facet joint. The intervertebral disc has a tough annulus fibrosus surrounding the softer nucleus pulposus. The nerve root exits the intervertebral foramen (where it lies close to the disc) and innervates a specific dermatome.

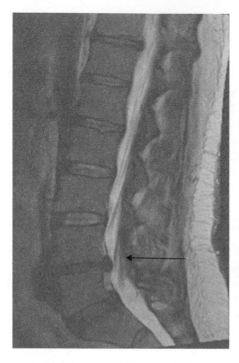

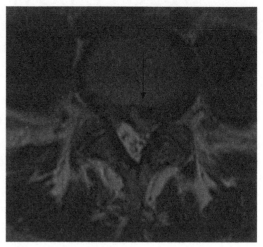

MRI, sagittal view of the lumbar spine demonstrating an L4-5 herniated disc.

MRI, axial view demonstrating an L4-5 herniated disc, eccentric to the left.

The most common cause for acute low back pain is musculoskeletal or lumbar muscular strain. Another common cause may be from degenerative disc disease or spondylosis as the disc itself is innervated by nerves. More rare conditions may cause back pain, such as spondylolisthesis (loose spine) resulting from trauma, certain boney defects (i.e., pars), aging (degenerative), or congenital. Keep infectious origins of back pain in the differential in a patient with fevers, elevated white blood cell count, and poorly controlled diabetes (Greenberg, 2010, p. 428). Tumors should be considered in patients with prior history of cancer.

Most acute low back pain episodes will improve within 2 weeks (Deyo and Weinstein, 2001, p. 366), and for 80%–90% of people they will resolve in 6 weeks (Manchikanti, 2000, p. 167). Common initial treatment involves NSAIDS, steroids, muscle relaxer medications, and physical therapy. Injections such as an epidural steroid injection, facet joint injection, or transforaminal injection (which targets a particular exiting nerve root) may provide some benefit. If pain persists longer than 6 weeks despite conservative treatment, further diagnostic imaging should be pursued.

Relevant diagnostic tests

Imaging

1. X-rays: Typical initial screening test to evaluate for spondylosis (degenerated disc and facet joints), fractures, spondylolisthesis/instability (with flexion and extension views), deformities/scoliosis, and infections (erosions of the disc space).
2. MRI: Best to evaluate soft tissues including herniated discs, nerve compression, tumors, infectious process.

3. Computed tomography (CT) scan: Best to evaluate for boney osteophytes causing compression on nerves, fractures, and pars defects.
4. CT/myelogram: Invasive test that demonstrates compression of nerves, osteophytes; good for patients with prior surgery/spine hardware preventing adequate imaging on MRI, or patients with devices that are not MRI compatible (i.e., pacemakers).
5. Bone scan: Helpful to evaluate for occult fractures, arthritic conditions, infections, or tumor (metastases).
6. Electromyogram (EMG)/nerve conduction study (NCS): Test that provides information on which nerves are irritated in a patient with radicular pain (help hone in on a particular nerve in a patient who has multiple nerves compressed on imaging); can be used to rule out nerve irritation due to compression of a peripheral nerve (nerve outside the spine), or neuropathy (a condition that is intrinsic to the nerve); can indicate acute, chronic changes, and show if a nerve is regenerating.

Labs

1. Fever, elevated white blood count (WBC), sedimentation rate, and C-reactive protein (CRP) would be concerning for infectious or autoimmune pathology

Common physical exam findings

Primary back pain

1. Tenderness with palpation of the lumbar spine; be aware of sacroiliac joint pain (the great mimicker)
2. Extension of lumbar spine elicits pain that could be due to facet joint pathology

Primary back pain with a radicular component

1. Perform a motor exam in the lower extremities to evaluate for weakness:
   a. Weakness of dorsiflexion, would indicate compression of the L5 nerve root.
   b. Weakness of plantar flexion would indicate compression of the S1 nerve root.
2. Hypoactive reflexes may reflect nerve root compression:
   a. Diminished knee reflex may reflect L3 compression.
   b. Diminished Achilles reflex may reflect S1 compression.
3. A straight leg raise and a crossed straight leg raise may indicate a herniated disc causing compression on the nerve root.
4. A pain diagram represents classic dermatomal distribution of respective nerve root compressive pathologies.

Relevant surgeries

If the cause of acute back pain is a herniated disc, with associated radiculopathy, and conservative treatment failed, then the patient may be referred to a surgeon. The surgeon may consider a microdiscectomy, laminectomy, and/or foraminotomy. This would involve removing the lamina, which would provide access to remove the herniated disc material, as well as provide adequate space in the foramen for the exiting nerve root.

If the acute back pain has an underlying structural issue and has failed conservative therapy and progressed to becoming a chronic condition, a lumbar fusion may sometimes be indicated. There are various ways to perform a fusion that are related to the approach a surgeon takes, the material used for the fusion, and the devices used to stabilize the spine (Resnick et al, 2008).

Prognosis

Prognosis is typically good with time. Ideal body weight, activity modification, rest, and physical therapy are the gold standard treatments. As listed in the above section, most acute back pain is musculoskeletal, and episodes resolve within 6 weeks.

Patients having surgery to relieve a painful radiculopathy may take 2 weeks to 6 months to recover on average. Patients with more than one acute back pain episode may progress into a chronic stage, which is one of the most difficult entities to treat. Rarely is back pain alone a surgical problem.

Common pitfalls and medicolegal concerns

1. Neoplasm or cancer
   a. If past medical history is pertinent for cancer, there could be metastatic disease to the spine.
   b. Pain may be nocturnal and unrelenting, and there is little ability to obtain relief.
   c. Unexplained weight loss is common.

2. Cauda equina syndrome—significant disc herniation that compromises the entire spinal canal
   a. Bowel incontinence or urinary dysfunction.
   b. Back and leg pain, paresthesia.
   c. Saddle anesthesia.
   d. Loss of sphincter tone.

3. Infection
   a. Past medical history is pertinent for immunosuppression (HIV, prolonged steroid use, etc.), diabetes, infectious exposure (e.g., tuberculosis) (Greenberg, 2010, p. 431).
4. Visceral nonspine etiology—aortic aneurysm, pyelonephritis, renal calculi, or pancreatitis (Deyo, 2001, p. 365).

Relevance to the advanced practice health professional

A nurse practitioner or physician assistant is likely to encounter a patient with acute back pain in his or her career multiple times. The provider should be aware of how to treat the patient initially, know when further diagnostic testing should be ordered, and know when a surgical consult is appropriate.

When should imaging be done?

X-rays are always a good start with recommended views being anteroposterior/lateral (AP/LAT) and flexion/extension to evaluate for fractures or instability (spondylolisthesis). One may order oblique views to evaluate for foraminal compression. If pain persists more than 6 weeks, consider obtaining a MRI. A CT may identify boney deformities such as occult fractures (those not noticed on x-rays). If there is a contraindication to having a MRI or there is extensive instrumentation from previous surgeries, then a CT/myelogram is a good alternative test.

Diagnostic imaging should be done immediately if motor weakness is found on examination or there is bowel and/or urinary dysfunction. While pain per se is not typically an emergency, urgent detailed MRI imaging may be warranted in the patient with significant unrelenting back or leg pain affecting quality of life.

When to refer to a surgeon?

Once conservative therapy has been completed and pain persists, referral to a surgeon may be warrented. Pathologic processes that warrant a referral to a surgeon are as follows:

1. Herniated lumbar disc
2. Spondylolisthesis (including anterolisthesis [forward displacement of vertebrae] and retrolisthesis [backward displacement of vertebrae])
3. Pars defects
4. Tumors
5. Stenosis (pressure on nerves from arthritis)

Always consider motor weakness or bowel or urinary dysfunction an urgent issue until proven otherwise.

Conclusions

Acute low back pain is a debilitating condition causing loss of work hours and productivity. It is one of the most common conditions that leads patients to a primary care provider and the emergency room in the United States. The first line of treatment includes NSAIDs, oral steroids, muscle relaxers, and gabapentin. Rest, heat and ice, and physiotherapy concurrently may also provide benefit. Opioids may be required to help a patient control severe pain; however, they should be utilized on a limited basis. Steroid injections may temporize and reduce severe pain involving the back and legs. Surgery is typically the last resort except in certain emergent circumstances.

References

Abdel Shaheed C, Maher CG, Williams KA, McLachlan AJ. Interventions available over the counter and adice for acute low back pain: Systematic review and meta-analysis. *J Pain.* 2014;15:2–15.

Deyo RA, Weinstein JN. Low back pain. *N Engl J Med.* 2001;344:363–370.

Global Burden of Disease Collaborators. Global, regional, and national incidence, prevalence, and years lived with disability for 301 acute and chronic diseases and injuries in 188 countries, 1990-2013: a systematic analysis for the Global Burden of Disease Study 2013. *Lancet.* 2015;386:743–800. http://dx.doi.org/10.1016/S0140-6736(15)60692-4

Greenberg MS. *Handbook of Neurosurgery.* New York, NY: Theime Medical Publishers; 2010.

Manchikanti L. Epidemiology of low back pain. *Pain Physician.* 2000;3:167–192.

Resnick DK, Haid RW Jr, Wang JC. *Surgical Management of Low Back Pain.* New York, NY: Theime Medical Publishers; 2008.

47

ACUTE NECK PAIN AND WHIPLASH

Kelly Walters, John Lee, and Honglian Huang

Case vignette

A 35-year-old, previously healthy, male grocery store stocker presented to the urgent care clinic 3 days after a motor vehicle accident in which he was a passenger in a stationary car rear-ended by a vehicle traveling at approximately 25 mph. He felt well immediately after the accident, without pain, but over the next few days developed neck and upper back pain and stiffness that progressively worsened (7/10 on visual analog scale [VAS]). The pain worsened with movement of the neck and shoulders and was better with rest. He also had intermittent headaches emanating from the occipital to frontal regions of the head. He does not have any numbness, tingling, dizziness, visual disturbances, speech difficulties, or difficulty walking. He has tried to rest as much as possible and has taken ibuprofen with limited effectiveness. He presented to urgent care because he was anxious about the persistent symptoms and does not feel he can return to work in this state.

On exam, he had a rigid stance with guarding of the neck. There was significant soreness to palpation at the paravertebral and shoulder muscles and at the cervical spinous and transverse processes. Active range of motion at the cervical spine was limited by pain in all directions. There was no radiation of pain in the arms on exam. Shoulder exam demonstrated limited shoulder abduction and flexion due to soreness of the neck and shoulder muscles but otherwise unremarkable. Neurologic exam was within normal motor, sensation, and reflexes. X-ray of the cervical spine obtained demonstrated flattening of cervical lordosis without subluxation or fractures.

Overview

Epidemiology

Whiplash has recently been defined by the Quebec Task Force as "an acceleration-deceleration mechanism of energy transfer to the neck. It may result from rear-end or side-impact motor vehicle collisions, but can also occur during diving or other mishaps" (Spitzer et al., 1995). The term *whiplash* describes both a mechanism of injury and the symptoms resulting from it (NAAS, 2003-2009). The impact may result in bony or soft-tissue injuries, which in turn may lead to a variety of clinical manifestations called whiplash-associated disorders (WADs) (Spitzer et al., 1995). The worldwide annual incidence of WAD ranges widely from 70 to 598 cases per 100,000 people (Spitzer et al., 1995; Quinlan et al., 2004; Cassidy et al., 2000; Otremski et al., 1989). WAD is the most common complaint after a motor vehicle accident (Versteegen et al., 2000). While most people recover quickly from whiplash injury, 4%–42% may describe symptoms years later (Eck et al., 2001). Whiplash symptoms that persist more than 6 months postinjury are considered chronic WAD (persistent symptoms) or late whiplash syndrome (persistent symptoms plus psychological emotional sequelae) (Kasch et al., 2001). Fully defining and treating whiplash can be a challenge as symptoms can vary to a large degree, and imaging is often normal.

Societal significance

Whiplash injuries generally are not life-threatening and in most cases, symptoms are transient and possibly go unreported. When symptoms persist, chronic WAD can lead to a decrease in quality of life and can have significant economic costs with up to $3.9 billion in the United States due to medical cares and the loss of work time (Eck et al., 2001).

Biologic and physiologic processes

The most common cause of WAD is rear-end collisions. In a rear-end collision, the chest is thrust forward causing rapid hyperextension and tension of the lower cervical spine with flexion of the upper cervical spine causing an "S" shape of the spine. The trauma force may be lateral as well, with the trunk being forced left or right with lateral hyperextension of the neck. The consequence of this rapid and forceful movement causes strain and injury to the tissues and bony structures of the cervical spine including discs, joint capsules, ligaments, facet joints, muscles, and nerves (Magnusson et al., 2014).

Whiplash process

Clinical symptoms and physical exam findings

Clinical symptoms may include (Erk et al., 2001) the following:
- Pain or stiffness in the neck, shoulders, arms, and back
- Weakness/paresthesias
- Headache, dizziness, vertigo
- Fatigue
- Visual disturbance
- Tinnitus/hearing loss
- Dysphasia
- Temporomandibular joint symptoms
- Difficulties with concentration and memory
- Psychological symptoms
  - Depression/anxiety, anger, frustration
  - Family or occupational stress, posttraumatic stress disorder (PTSD)
  - Sleep disturbances
  - Social isolation
  - Hypochondriasis
  - Drug dependency

Exam findings may include the following:
- Altered posture with guarding of the neck region
- Neck pain, stiffness, and tenderness to palpation
- Limited range of motion of the neck
- Normal neurological exam in most cases; may have impairments in sensory, motor, and reflex testing

Grading schemes

A Quebec Task Force (QTF) was assembled by request of the Quebec Automobile Insurance Society to analyze the impact of whiplash on individuals and on society. The Task Force reviewed over 10,000 publications and released the findings in April 1995 (Spitzer et al., 1995). In that report, a grading and classification

Table 47.1 Quebec Task Force (QTF) WAD Grades

WAD grade	Classification
0	No complaint about the neck; no physical signs
I	Neck complaint of pain, stiffness, or tenderness only; no physical signs
II	Neck complaint and musculoskeletal signs; musculoskeletal signs include decreased range of motion and point tenderness
III	Neck complaint and neurological signs; neurological signs include decreased or absent deep tendon reflexes, weakness, and sensory deficits
IV	Neck complaint and fracture or dislocation

Source: Spitzer W.O., *Spine* (Phila PA 1976), 20, 1-73, 1995.

scheme (Table 47.1) was generated based on the type and severity of signs and symptoms shortly after the whiplash injury. Now this scheme is used widely in many clinical evaluations related to whiplash injuries.

Diagnostic tests

The diagnosis of WAD is primarily clinical. In the acute, posttrauma setting, ruling out fracture or spinal cord compression is important. The following tests may be useful for QTF grades II–IV or in the subacute phase when symptoms are persisting or even worse:

- X-ray: Cervical and upper thoracic spine x-ray (anteroposterior, lateral, open-mouth, and oblique views) should be obtained if there are neurological signs (Daffner, 2010). In acute whiplash patients who are alert and stable, the decision to obtain x-rays is dependent on history, clinical exam, and judgement. Clinical tools such as the Canadian C-Spine Rule can help aid in deciding whether to obtain x-rays (Stiell et al., 2003) When there are no fractures or dislocations, the most common radiographic findings include preexisting degenerative changes or a slight flattening of the normal lordotic curvature of the cervical spine (Erk et al., 2001).
- Specialized imaging studies (computed tomography [CT], magnetic resonance imaging [MRI]) should be considered in QTF WAD grades III and IV. In general, specialized imaging studies are not necessary in QTF WAD grades I and II, but can be obtained depending on clinical judgement.
- CT: Allows good views of calcified tissues such as bone.
- MRI: Useful for viewing interspinous, anterior and posterior longitudinal ligament tears, intervertebral discs, nerve roots, spinal cord, soft tissue and muscle injury, edema, and hemorrhage (Grenier et al., 1991).

Treatment

The goal is pain relief and return to normal function and activities of daily living as soon as possible. Appropriate management of acute pain reduces risk of chronic pain. The following consensus recommendations are based on appropriate whiplash therapies from widely varying studies.

Follow-ups postinjury should take place in 1 week, 3 weeks, 6 weeks, and 3 months. Typically, whiplash symptoms have resolved in 50% of cases by 3 months. Follow-ups can be provided by the patient's primary care provider.

Patient/Family counseling

Maintaining good posture while returning to usual activities as soon as possible will expedite recovery, because activity restrictions can lengthen the healing process. Care providers should educate patients

Table 47.2 Treatment of WAD at Different Phases

Phase	Treatment options
Acute phase	Ice/heat therapy
Up to 3 days	Pain medications: Alternate acetaminophen and NSAIDs. Narcotic pain medications for a short course in severe cases.
Local reaction and inflammation	Muscle relaxants.
	No heavy lifting, excessive bending, or twisting of cervical spine.
	Depending on activity required at the patient's job, no work until first follow-up appointment in 1 week.
	Encourage good posture.
Subacute phase	Continue acute phase treatment as appropriate.
Greater than 3 days to 3 months	Physical therapy.
Repair and remodeling	Massage therapy, joint mobilization, relaxation techniques.
	Serotonin/norepinephrine reuptake inhibitors (SNRIs) can help with pain and dizziness.
	Some patients have found pain relief with transcutaneous electrical nerve stimulation (TENS) and acupuncture.
Chronic phase	Continued physical therapy with functional, range of motion, strengthening exercises.
Greater than 3 months	Consider referrals to neurologist, psychologist.
Modified movement strategies for normal daily activities	Consider multidisciplinary cognitive behavioral approach to treatment.

Source: Croft AC, *Palmer J Res.*, 1, 10-21,1994; TRACsa, *Trauma and Injury Recovery. Clinical Guidelines for Best Practice Management of Acute and Chronic Whiplash-Associated Disorders—Evidence Report*, Adelaide: TRACsa; 2008.

and their families on signs of neurologic decline (changes in motor, sensory, bowel or bladder functions). Patients with neurologic signs or changes in clinical status should seek medical attention immediately.

Prognosis

The whiplash prognosis depends on the severity of the injuries. Mild whiplash injuries can resolve within 1–2 weeks; moderate injuries with muscle spasm or ligament strains may take 4–8 weeks; and severe injuries with nerve, ligament, and/or spinal disc damage may result in chronic or permanent disability. Factors associated with prolonged recovery and likely need for more intensive treatment or earlier referrals include severity of neck symptoms and radicular irritation, presence of specific symptoms such as headache; muscle pain; pain or numbness radiating from neck to arms, hands, or shoulders; more initial subjective complaints and concern regarding long-term prognosis; multiple initial symptoms; older age; female gender; not in full-time employment; having dependents; and presence of osteoarthritis on x-ray (2001).

Common questions

1. *When can I return to work?*
    Typically after the first follow-up appointment, 1 week after injury, depending on the type of job. Mild exercise is encouraged, but heavy lifting should be avoided until the symptoms have improved.

2. *When can I return to driving?*

No driving while taking medications is recommended because medications such as narcotics or muscle relaxants can impair driving ability.

3. *Why am I in pain when my tests are normal?*

Pain after whiplash injuries is often soft tissue related and may not be readily evident on imaging studies. In addition, emotional and psychological factors associated with whiplash injuries may contribute to heightened pain perception.

4. *How long will it take to heal?*

This varies depending on your age, previous neck injury, and degree of whiplash. You may have symptoms for a few weeks to over 12 months.

Pitfalls

- Narcotic pain-seeking behaviors or addiction
- Failing to diagnosis more serious injuries such as spine fracture or cord injury
- Association of WAD with lawsuits

Medicolegal concerns

WAD is the most common complaint after automobile accidents. Attorneys and insurance companies may be involved. Thorough history taking, physical examination, appropriate and timely choice of studies, treatment, follow-ups, and appropriate documentation on the part of the health care provider are essential.

Relevance to the advanced practice health professional

Whiplash is a relatively common occurrence but is easily overlooked or mistreated due to the lack of objective findings. It is critical for advanced practice health professionals to understand the mechanism of the injury and apply appropriate assessment, diagnosis, and therapeutic strategies at different phases to maximize the clinical outcomes.

Common phone calls, pages, and requests

- What are the next steps with new neurological symptoms?
- When should a patient be referred to a specialist?
- Change or refill pain management medication.
- Provide documentation for Family and Medical Leave Act (FMLA) or other work/school/insurance needs.

Acknowledgments

The authors would like to extend their sincere appreciation to Dr. Vernon Lin for giving them an opportunity to work on this chapter and for providing them advice, support, and guidance. The author is also very grateful for Dr. Xiaoming Zhang's suggestions and editing of this manuscript.

References

Cassidy JD, Carroll LJ, Côté P, Lemstra M, Berglund A, Nygren A. Effect of eliminating compensation for pain and suffering on the outcome of insurance claims for whiplash injury. *N. Engl. J.Med.* 2000;342:1179–1186.

Croft AC. A proposed classification of cervical acceleration/deceleration injuries with a review of prognostic research. *Palmer J Res.* 1994;1(1):10–21.

Daffner RH. Radiologic evaluation of chronic neck pain. *Am Fam Physician.* 2010;82(8):959–964.

Eck JC, Hodges SD, Humphreys SC. Whiplash: a review of a commonly misunderstood injury. *Am J Med.* 2001;110:651–656.

Elliott JM, Noteboom JT, Flynn TW, Sterling M. Characterization of acute and chronic whiplash-associated disorders. *J Orthop Sports Phys Ther.* 2009;39(5):312–323.

Fleming B. Whiplash: the role of imaging—to X-ray or not? *BCMJ.* 2002;44(5):248–251.

Grenier N, Halini PH, Frija G, Sigal R. Traumatismes. In: Sigal R, Grenier N, Doyon D, Garcia-Torres E, eds. *IRM de la Moelle et du Rachis.* Paris/Milan: Masson; 1991.

Kasch H, Stengaard-Pedersen K, Arendt-Nielsen L, Staehelin Jensen T. Headache, neck pain, and neck mobility after acute whiplash injury: a prospective study. *Spine(Phila Pa 1976).* 2001;26:1246–1251.

Magnusson M, Karlberg M, Mariconda C, Bucalossi A, Dalmazzo G. Pathophysiology of whiplash-associated disorders: theories and controversies. In: Alpini DC, Brugnoni G, Cesarani A, eds. *Whiplash Injuries, Diagnosis and Treatment* (2nd ed.). Milan, Italy: Springer-Verlag Italia. 2014;89–94.

Motor Accidents Authority. Guidelines for the management of whiplash-associated disorders. Sydney, Australia: Motor Accident Authority; 2001.

North American Spine Society (NAAS). 2003-2009. North American Spine Society Public Education Series. http://www.knowyourback.org/Documents/whiplash.pdf.

Otremski I, Marsh JL, Wilde BR, McLardy Smith PD, Newman RJ. Soft tissue cervical spinal injuries in motor vehicle accidents. *Injury.* 1989;20:349–351.

Quinlan KP, Annest JL, Myers B, Ryan G, Hill H. Neck strains and sprains among motor vehicle occupants – United States, 2000. *Accid Anal Prev.* 2004;36:21–27.

Spitzer WO, Skovron ML, Salmi LR et al. Scientific monograph of Quebec Task Force on Whiplash-Associated Disorders: redefining "whiplash" and its management. *Spine (Phila Pa 1976).* 1995;20(suppl 8):1–73.

Stiell IG, Clement CM, McKnight RD. The Canadian C-spine rule versus the NEXUS low-risk criteria in patients with trauma. *N Engl J Med.* 2003;349:2510–2518.

TRACsa. Trauma and Injury Recovery. Clinical guidelines for best practice management of acute and chronic whiplash-associated disorders—Evidence Report. Adelaide, SA: TRACsa; 2008.

Versteegen GJ, Kingma J, Meijler WJ, ten Duis HJ. Neck sprain after motor vehicle accidents indrivers and passengers. *Eur Spine J.* 2000;9:547–552.

Yadla S, Ratliff JK, Harrop JS. Whiplash: diagnosis, treatment, and associated injuries. *Curr Rev Musculoskelet Med.* 2008;1(1):65–68.

48

ANTERIOR CERVICAL SURGERY

Álvaro Martín Gallego, Chelsie McCarthy, and Roger Härtl

Case vignette

A 78-year-old male with a history of atrial fibrillation and gout presents with subjective bilateral lower extremity weakness and difficulty walking for many years. The patient reports that these symptoms are becoming progressively worse, especially over the past year. On examination, he is noted to have mild bilateral ankle plantar flexion weakness (4/5) and patellar reflex hyperreflexia.

Magnetic resonance imaging (MRI) revealed C5-C6 disc herniation with anterior medullary and bilateral foraminal compression, C4-C5-C6 spondylosis with anterior and posterior osteophytes, and C3-C5 kyphosis.

A C5-C6 anterior cervical discectomy and fusion (ACDF) with placement of a polyetheretherketone (PEEK) interbody cage and ventral screws was decided to be the best treatment for this patient.

A 45-year-old female patient with no significant past medical history (PMH) or past surgical history (PSH) presents with neck pain, right shoulder and arm pain with intermittent numbness and pain radiating to the right middle two fingers for the past 7 years. The patient reports the pain is severely limiting daily activity. Pain is worse with exercise, lifting, and computer work; the pain is improved with topical anesthetic creams and rest. Previously attempted nonoperative treatments provided no relief of symptoms; they include cervical epidural steroid injection, physical therapy, acupuncture, chiropractics, and nonsteroidal anti-inflammatory drugs (NSAIDs).

Exam revealed no myelopathy or weakness; pain worsened with movement. Cervical MRI revealed a C6-C7 disc herniation on the right; there was no spondylosis or subluxation. Other levels appear unaffected.

Based on the patient's symptoms, radiologic findings, and persistent symptoms despite nonoperative treatments, surgical options were discussed. It was decided that the patient would undergo a C6-C7 discectomy and placement of artificial disc through an anterior approach under general anesthesia.

Basic concepts

- **Disc herniation:** The intervertebral disc is composed of a ligamentous outer fibrous annulus and a gelatinous inner nucleus pulposus. The combination of intervertebral pressure and degeneration of the ligamentous fibers can lead to a tear in the annulus, allowing the nucleus pulposus to prolapse, which can compress the spinal cord and/or the cervical nerve roots.
- **Radiculopathy**: Symptoms are caused by conditions that affect the nerve roots. Cervical nerve roots provide innervation to a specific region of upper extremities. The nerve root is irritated (by compression) at its exit from the cervical spinal cord. This irritation can result in pain, weakness,

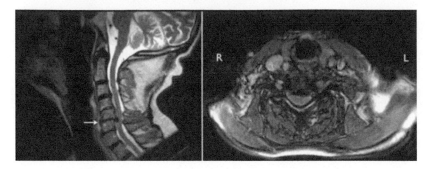

Figure 48.1 Preoperative cervical MRI showing C5-C6 central disc herniation with ventral cord compression and bilateral foraminal stenosis.

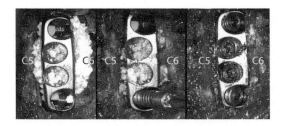

Figure 48.2 Placement of a PEEK interbody cage with ventral titanium screws. A synthetic bone substitute is added to facilitate bone fusion.

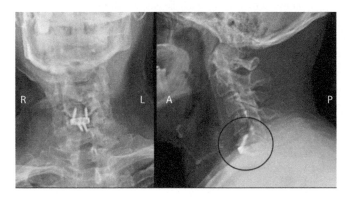

Figure 48.3 Immediate postoperative x-rays following a C5-C6 ACDF (AP and lateral projection).

numbness, or hyperpathia in the neck or upper extremities. Cervical disc herniation is one of the most frequent causes of cervical radiculopathy. Disc herniations are responsible for only 20%–25% of radiculopathy cases, and approximately 70%–75% are from spondylosis.

- **Spondylosis**: Degenerative changes in vertebral discs, ligaments, joints, and vertebral bodies. Gradually there is bone formation in these areas, called *hard disc* or *osteophyte*. These structures can compress the spinal cord and nerve root, as well as cause instability.
- **Myelopathy**: This term refers to any damage or functional disturbance, acute or chronic, in the spinal cord. Compression of the cervical spinal cord may yield symptoms of spinal cord dysfunction known as cervical spondylotic myelopathy. The normal transmission of the neural signals to the

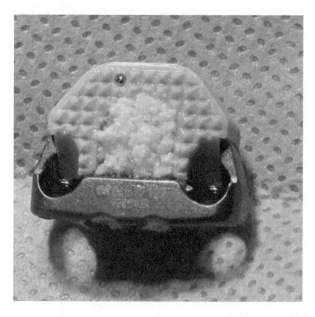

Figure 48.4 (a) Interbody cage. (b) "In situ" PEEK and titanium interbody cage used for ACDF.

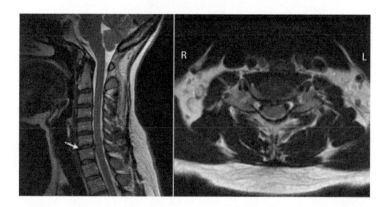

Figure 48.5 Preoperative MRI showing a C6–C7 right disc herniation with right foraminal stenosis.

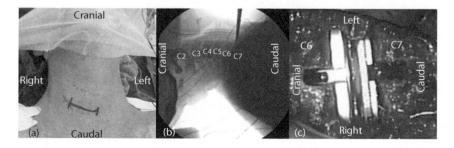

Figure 48.6 (a) Neck incision. (b) Confirmatory localization with x-ray (lateral projection), a radiopaque instrument is used. (c) Arthroplasty is placed between C6 and C7.

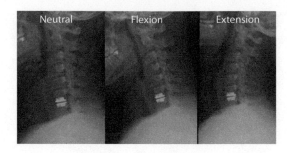

Figure 48.7   Postoperative dynamic x-rays following a C6–C7 arthroplasty.

upper and lower limbs is disrupted. This syndrome occurs in 5%–10% of patients with symptomatic cervical spondylosis and may be exhibited as

- Arm and hand weakness
- Leg stiffness
- Hyperreflexia
- Loss of balance with falling episodes
- Poor coordination or lack of fine motor dexterity
- Bowel or bladder changes

Epidemiology

- Incidence of cervical radiculopathy: 83.2 per 100,000 population
- Mean age: 50 years old
- Male-to-female ratio: 1:7
- Between 180,000 and 200,000 cervical procedures are performed in the United States per year
- Anterior cervical fusion represents 80% of all cervical surgeries

Common physical examination findings

- Painful limitation of neck motion occurs with almost all herniated cervical discs.
- Motor weakness, numbness, paresthesias, and hyperesthesia may be present.
- Upper extremities' reflexes may be diminished in patients with radiculopathy who do not have myelopathy.
- Neck extension and lateral bending usually aggravate pain.
- Neck pain predominantly suggests cervical instability.
- Radiculopathy suggests cervical and foraminal stenosis.
- Neck flexion may cause an "electrical shock-like sensation radiating down the spine" (Lhermitte sign).

Diagnosis

- **Imaging studies:**
  - MRI: Best assessment of spinal canal/cord
  - Computed tomography (CT): Best assessment of bone

Table 48.1 Cervical Syndromes

	C4-C5	C5-C6	C6-C7	C7-T1
%	2%	20%	70%	8%
Compressed root	C5	C6	C7	C8
Reflex affected	Deltoid and pectoralis	Biceps and brachioradialis	Triceps	Finger jerk
Main motor weakness	Arm abduction	Forearm flexion	Wrist flexion	Finger extension
Paresthesia and hyperesthesia	Neck, shoulder, scapula	Lateral arm, and forearm, thumb and index finger	Fingers 2 and 3, palm	Fingers 4 and 5

- Myelogram: If MRI is inconclusive; more accurate but more invasive
- Flexion/extension (Dynamic) x-rays: Evaluate possible instability

- **Electrodiagnostic studies:** Help to confirm the diagnosis of radiculopathy

  - Upper extremities electromyography (EMG): Show dysfunction of the nerve conduction (radiculopathies)
  - Nerve conduction study (NCS): Excludes distal neuropathies (carpal tunnel syndrome and others)

Treatment

Most patients with acute cervical radiculopathy due to cervical disc herniation may improve without surgery. Conservative therapy, consisting of anti-inflammatory medications, pain medications, and resting, should be utilized before making the surgical decision.

If surgical treatment is indicated, an anterior cervical discectomy with fusion or arthroplasty is the gold standard approach. This allows for decompression of the spinal canal in cervical disc herniations and/or spinal and foraminal stenosis through a small cervical skin incision with the help of a microscope. After discectomy and decompression of the neural structures, a cervical implant is placed into the intervertebral space. If the aim of the implant is to provide cervical fusion and stability, a cage or a bone graft should be placed; if it is to maintain a segment's motion, an arthroplasty may be used instead.

Surgical management
Indications

- Persistent symptoms that do not resolve within 4–6 weeks of conservative therapy
- Significant and progressive neurologic findings or localizing symptoms (motor weakness or disabling pain)

Anesthetic issues

- Some patients require special intubation techniques (fiberoptic) to minimize neck manipulation (i.e., cervical myelopathy patients).

- Prophylactic intravenous antibiotics (cefazolin 1–2 g for adults) 30 minutes prior to incision
- Foley catheter for prolonged surgery
- Consider arterial line for patients who require enhanced monitoring of blood pressure
- Special anesthetic regimens may be needed if spinal neurophysiologic monitoring used
- Bite block when using motor evoked potentials

Surgical procedure

Positioning

- The patient is positioned in a supine and neutral posture.
- Appropriate padding for extremities is provided to prevent compression neuropathies.
- Gentle extension and traction are given to the neck.
- Shoulder traction is given to help radiographically image lower cervical levels, and arms are tucked at sides.
- A shoulder roll is used to create cervical lordosis.

Sterile preparation

- Minimal shave if needed
- Meticulous sterilization of cervical area in standard fashion
- Sterile towel to dry

Marking the incision

- Initial localization is made using anatomic landmarks.
- Final localization is confirmed with x-ray (lateral projection).

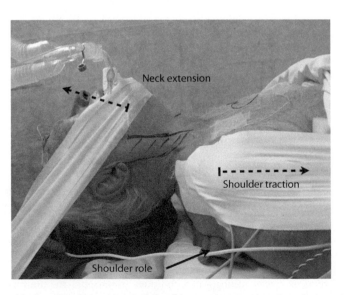

Figure 48.8 Patient positioning: Head extension and shoulder traction are given in order to gain cervical exposure. A shoulder roll is used to enhance cervical lordosis.

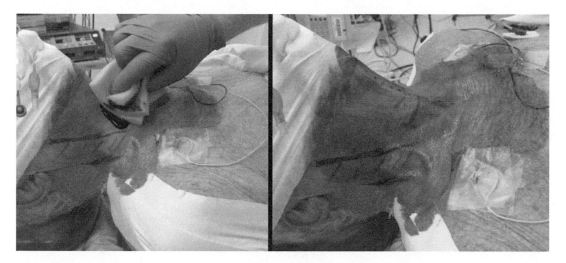

Figure 48.9   Cervical area should be widely sterilized. In this photograph a brush with Betadine gel was used.

- Side: The majority of surgeons prefer right-side neck exposure because it is more comfortable for right-handed surgeons. An approach through the left side may, theoretically, decrease the possibility of injuring the recurrent laryngeal nerve (but recent studies do not prove this).
- Transverse incision is used for most cases for cosmetically favorable results (along cervical skin lines). It is marked from the midline to 3 cm lateral. Alternatively, a longitudinal incision along the medial sternocleidomastoid muscle can be used (multilevel discectomies and obese patients).
- To obtain an iliac bone autograft, an 8 cm oblique line is marked 6 cm lateral to the anterior superior iliac spine (optional).

Surgical approach

- A skin incision is made.
- Platysma is dissected and split.
- Dissection is made along the medial border of the sternocleidomastoid.
- Identify the carotid sheath structures and work medially.
- Use blunt dissection to reach the prevertebral space—longus colli muscles, prevertebral fascia, underlying disc spaces, and vertebral bodies.
- Verify levels with x-ray—a needle is inserted into the disc space of interest.
- Insert a self-retaining anterior cervical retractor system.

Microdiscectomy

- Interbody pins may be screwed into the middle of the adjacent vertebrae under x-ray control. Pin distraction provides gentle distraction to open the disc space.
- The anterior longitudinal ligament and the fibrous ring of the disc are incised.
- The disc is removed, and disc space cartilage is cleared with curettes.
- The posterior longitudinal ligament is resected with 1- to 2-mm Kerrison rongeurs.
- A blunt nerve hook may be gently inserted into the neural foramen and canal to ensure adequate decompression.
- Epidural bleeding is managed with bipolar electrocautery and thrombin-soaked Gelfoam.

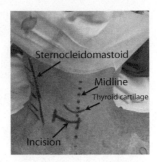

Figure 48.10 Incision for a C5–C6 approach is marked from the midline to 3–4 cm lateral, next to the medial border of the sternocleidomastoid. Thyroid cartilage points to the C4–C5 level.

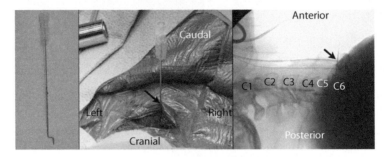

Figure 48.11 A bent needle is used to point the right level under intraoperative x-rays (lateral projection).

- The endplates are drilled to remove all disc material and osteophytes and to decorticate the bone.
- Either an interbody graft/cage or an arthroplasty is placed. These may be secured with anterior screws or a plate.

Closure

- Meticulous hemostasis
- Irrigation of wound with sterile saline
- Verification of integrity of important regional structures (e.g., esophagus, carotid, jugular)
- Use of transient submuscular drainage in multilevel surgery, corpectomy, or with persistent bleeding
- Layered closure
- Vicryl interrupted sutures for platysma
- Continuous absorbable intradermal suture for skin

Postoperative

- If soft-tissue drainage is used, remove after 24 hours.
- Antibiotics are given for 24 hours postoperatively.
- A soft collar may be offered depending on preference.
- Early ambulation is encouraged.
- If dysphagia, a liquid diet is ordered and advanced as tolerated. Consider speech/swallowing and ear, nose, throat (ENT) consult if problematic.

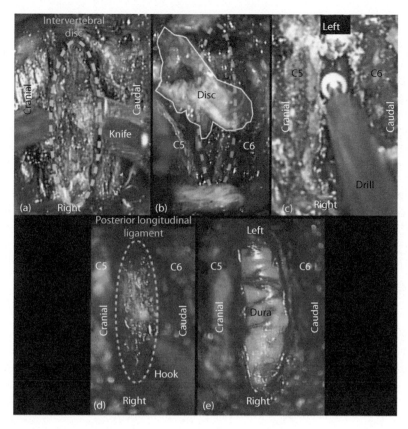

Figure 48.12 (a) Opening the fibrous ring with a knife; (b) extracting the disc; (c) drilling the vertebral plates to decorticate the vertebral bodies and widen the intervertebral space; (d) exposing the posterior longitudinal ligament; and (e) widely exposing the dura.

- An oral narcotic and muscular relaxant are prescribed with intravenous breakthrough medication if needed.
- The patient is typically discharged the day following surgery.
- Postoperative radiographs are taken before discharge.
- The patient should be instructed to inspect the incision regularly for signs of wound infection.

Complications of approach

- Postoperative cervical wound hematoma (typically within the first 12 hours): May require emergent return to operating room.
  - Respiratory distress
  - Extreme difficulty swallowing
  - Tracheal deviation in anteroposterior cervical spine x-ray

- Recurrent laryngeal palsy: Hoarseness
  - Temporary dysfunction (11%) with recovery within 3–6 months
  - Permanent dysfunction less common (4%)

- Swallowing difficulty
  - Transient: 50%
  - Delayed (5% at 6 months): May result from anterior plate or screw dislodgment, causing esophageal obstruction; if surgical conditions ruled out and persists >2 weeks, may refer patient to ENT for further evaluation

- Wound infection (1%)
- Weakness of nerve root of level operated
- Postoperative fluid collection possibly indicating cerebrospinal fluid leak or esophageal injury
- Injuries of the visceral (esophagus or trachea) or vascular structures (carotid, jugular, or vertebral)
- Injuries to the spinal cord and cervical roots (0.1%–3.3%)
- Horner syndrome: Sympathetic plexus injury
- Stroke, possibly resulting from carotid retraction in susceptible patients with carotid stenosis
- Delayed neurologic deterioration possibly indicating epidural abscess, graft dislocation, or subluxation

Anterior cervical fusion

Overview

Cervical spondylosis and disc degeneration can lead to radiculopathy and myelopathy from progressive foraminal and central stenosis. Decompression of a degenerative spine can yield cervical instability. In order to prevent instability and neck pain, once a decompression of the intervertebral disc and neural foramen is performed, an intervertebral graft is inserted to maintain disc space height and enhance fusion. The choice of graft material will be dictated by surgeon preference. Autograft (iliac crest and other autologous bones) or allograft/cage (PEEK, titanium filled with bone graft) can be used.

Advantages

- Provides multilevel stability

Indications

- Intractable or progressive cervical radiculopathy or myelopathy refractory to conservative management with evidence of spondylosis or disc herniation causing foraminal or central stenosis
- Cervical discitis or epidural abscess causing neurologic symptoms
- Anterior cervical tumor
- Degenerative or traumatic cervical subluxation
- Traumatic cervical instability

Contraindications

- No absolute contraindications
- Predominant posterior pathology (hypertrophied ligamentum flavum)
- Severe osteoporosis
- Ossification of the posterior longitudinal ligament (OPLL) (if there is no ventral dura in continuous OPLL cases)

Surgical procedure

- Anterior cervical approach
- Implantation of interbody graft
  - Autograft: Iliac crest
  - Allograft: Structural or with a cage (PEEK, titanium)

- Plating and screws (common)
- Placement of local bone or synthetic substitutes as filler over the grafts to fill gaps and facilitate bone fusion

Anterior cervical arthroplasty

Overview

Cervical arthroplasty has gained attention as an alternative to traditional arthrodesis, as artificial discs can maintain the motion of the cervical disc.

Advantages

- Maintenance of range of motion and maneuverability
- Avoidance of adjacent-segment degeneration
- Reconstitution of disc height and spinal alignment
- Earlier return to previous functional state

Indications

- Single-level or two disc herniations between C3 and C7 with radiculopathy, myelopathy, or both with minimal spondylosis and no adjacent-level degeneration
- Typically recommended in patients under 60 years old

Contraindications

- Infection or inflammatory disease
- Neck pain related to facet arthropathy
- Myelopathy caused by posterior compression, deformity, and/or instability
- Inadequate endplate integrity (osteoporosis or metabolic bone disease)
- Intervertebral disc collapse (more than 50% of normal height)

Surgical procedure

- Anterior cervical approach plus discectomy as previously described
- Implantation of cervical arthroplasty:

  - A trial is inserted to assess with fluoroscopy the appropriate implant size and position.
  - The arthroplasty is selected and implanted.
  - The surgeon should ensure that the optimal size of the artificial disc is selected. If too small, the artificial disc may migrate, and if too big, it may inhibit the range of motion.

Patient and family counseling

Preoperative counseling regarding surgical risks

- Swallowing dysfunction: Common, usually very transient
- Hoarseness: Less common. Also typically transient but there is a very small risk of permanent vocal cord paresis; important to discuss with patients, especially those who rely on their voice in their profession (i.e., singers, broadcasters)
- Blood loss: Very low risk due to microsurgical approach
- Infection: Very low risk, decreased further with antibiotics in the operating room and for 24 hours following surgery
- Damage to the dura causing cerebrospinal fluid leak: Very low risk
- Spinal cord injury resulting in para- or quadriplegia: Very infrequent but the most feared complication
- Loss of range of motion: Some loss of range of motion at the levels fused
- Pseudarthrosis (2%–20%): Failure of bone to fuse after ACDF surgery—patients should be counseled on smoking cessation prior to surgery as smoking can interfere with bony fusion

Prognosis

The primary goal of this procedure is to prevent any progression or worsening of neurologic symptoms (weakness, paralysis, etc.) by decompressing the spinal cord and/or nerves and stabilizing the spine. Most patients experience varying degrees of relief of their previous symptoms and have great improvement in functionality, which is often further improved with physical and occupational therapy after recovery. While this procedure addresses the currently diseased levels, there is some risk for adjacent-level disease in the future following this surgery.

Common questions from patients and families

- *What are the restrictions after surgery?*
  - For 6 weeks after surgery, patients are advised to avoid lifting more than 10 pounds and to avoid any repetitive turning or bending of the neck. Patients are also advised to avoid NSAIDs for 6 weeks after surgery to avoid any interference or delay of the bony fusion (if an ACDF was performed, not for arthroplasty). Patients are encouraged to walk daily after surgery. For multiple-level fusions, patients may be required to wear a hard cervical collar for 6 weeks after surgery.
- *Will there be a stay in the hospital?*
  - After most cervical spine surgeries, patients are usually up and able to walk within a few hours. Often there is a very short stay (1 night) in the hospital (especially after a one-level surgery) to ensure pain is well controlled. There is typically no need for a prolonged hospital stay or to stay in bed during the recovery period.
- *What will the pain be like?*
  - It is imperative to ensure that the patient's expectations are appropriately managed preoperatively. Counseling patients that some pain is expected but medications will be provided to control it is key. The most common source of pain is muscle spasms, which usually respond very well to muscle relaxers. Pain medications are taken as needed and weaned as tolerated. If narcotic pain medication is used, a bowel regimen is key to prevent constipation.

- *What care will the incision need?*
  - The incision is most commonly closed with intradermal absorbable sutures and Steri-Strips. It is important to keep the incision dry for 3–5 days after surgery; after that, patients may shower. There is usually no need for any dressing changes; ointments should be avoided during the postoperative period.
- *Will there be loss of range of motion after surgery?*
  - There can be some loss of range of motion after an ACDF, which usually goes unnoticed with normal activities of daily living. If multiple levels are fused, the decreased range of motion will be more noticeable. Arthroplasty will typically preserve the range of motion.
- *Will my symptoms resolve?*
  - There is no guarantee that symptoms will resolve. The main goal of the surgery is to prevent any neurologic worsening. Patients often have relief of their previous symptoms, but this can take time as nerve recovery is a gradual process and is not guaranteed.
- *Will the patient need rehab services?*

  - Depending on the baseline functional status of the patient and the patient's support system, some patients may benefit from rehabilitation services after surgery. Based on a postoperative evaluation, necessary services may be identified and arranged. If patients have imbalance or gait disturbance prior to surgery, for example, they would benefit from physical therapy immediately postop for gait training. Most patients are recommended to start outpatient physical therapy for further strengthening and range of motion at 6 weeks postop.

Common pitfalls and medicolegal concerns

- **Wrong indication:** It is very important to evaluate the cases thoroughly with an optimal neurologic examination and radiologic exam visualization. The radiographic and clinical evaluations should be correlated. A wrong indication of surgery can lead the patient to additional chronic pain and more surgeries.
- **Wrong-level surgery:** A nonoptimal preoperative preparation can lead the surgeon to perform the surgery in a wrong cervical level. This is one of the most important medicolegal issues that can occur. This confusion is greater in lower-level surgeries (C6-C7) because of the difficulties in localization of these levels with the intraoperative x-rays. There are shoulder traction devices available that provide continuous traction to the shoulders and can decrease the rate of wrong-level errors. This mistake can be decreased with routine x-rays before incision and intraoperatively, when the vertebral body is reached.
- Use caution to widely open cervical tissue planes to maximize exposure and minimize retraction force on tracheoesophageal structures.
- For difficult anatomy (reoperations, cervical infection, irradiated fields, etc.), it is helpful to have ENT specialists for routine assistance with the exposure.

Relevance to the advanced practice health professional

Advanced practice health professionals play an important role in guiding patients and families through the surgical process. It is imperative to ensure that patients' expectations are appropriately managed in discussing surgical treatment. Providing patients and their families with accurate information and education regarding the procedure, goals, risks, and recovery can help decrease stress and anxiety and ensure a positive experience. Having a strong grasp of the pathophysiology, procedure, and recovery is critical in serving as a resource and support for patients.

Common phone calls, pages, and requests

- *Difficulty swallowing:* Patients may call with difficulty swallowing after surgery. This is usually mild and temporary—resolving within a few weeks. It is important to evaluate patients for aspiration risk. If symptoms are persistent, worsening, or do not improve, it may be necessary to arrange for a speech and swallow evaluation.
- *Muscle spasms:* Patients may call with muscle spasm pain in the neck and often radiating to the shoulder blades during the first few weeks. This is usually alleviated with consistent muscle relaxers; application of a heating pad can also be beneficial.
- *Driving:* While patients are taking narcotic pain medications or muscle relaxers, patients should be restricted from operating any vehicles. The activity restrictions during the acute postoperative period usually prohibit patients from driving.
- *Collar questions:* With multilevel fusions, patients may need to wear a hard collar for the first 6 weeks. Collars should be properly fitted and worn when a patient is up and out of bed. Patients may use a soft collar as needed for comfort if a hard collar is not indicated (i.e., one-level surgery).
- *Wound care:* Five to seven days after surgery, patients may get the incisional area wet during a quick shower. After showering, the area should be patted dry with a clean towel. Steri-Strips usually fall off on their own or will be removed during the postoperative visit. There is usually no need for any additional dressing. Patients should avoid applying any ointments or oils to the incision during the first few weeks after surgery.

49

POSTERIOR CERVICAL SURGERY

Dennis T. Lockney, Angela Wolfe, and Daniel J. Hoh

Case vignette

History

A 60-year-old male with a history of hypertension and 15-year history of diabetes mellitus presents with a 1-year history of neck pain radiating into the shoulders, as well as numbness in bilateral arms, right greater than left. He also has a 30 pack-year history of smoking but quit 12 years ago. He has occasional paresthesias in both arms and some difficulty using his cell phone. Symptoms are worsened with neck flexion and have been nonresponsive to physical therapy.

Physical examination

Motor	Right	Left
Deltoid	5	5
Biceps	5	5
Wrist extension	5	5
Triceps	5	5
Hand grip	5	5
Iliopsoas	5	5
Quadriceps	5	5
Tibialis anterior	5	5
Extensor hallucis longus	5	5

Sensory: Diminished to pinprick testing in right greater than left C5 distributions.

Reflexes	Right	Left
Biceps	2+	2+
Triceps	2+	2+
Brachioradialis	3+	3+
Patellar	3+	3+
Ankle jerk	3+	3+
Hoffman	Present	Absent

Gait: Spastic.

Magnetic resonance imaging (MRI) is shown in Figures 49.1 and 49.2.

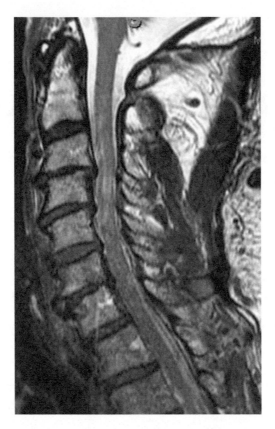

Figure 49.1　Sagittal T2 MRI of the cervical spine revealing multilevel cervical stenosis with spinal cord compression.

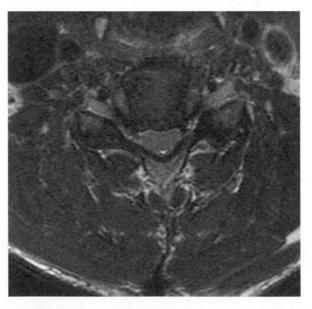

Figure 49.2　T2-weighted axial MRI of the cervical spine demonstrating absence of CSF signal surrounding the spinal cord and spinal cord compression.

Diagnosis

Cervical spondylotic myelopathy secondary to cervical stenosis, C3–C7

Management

Surgical treatment, C3–C7 laminectomy and decompression, C3–T1 posterior instrumented fusion

Overview

Epidemiology

Cervical spondylosis is the most common cause of myelopathy and spinal cord dysfunction in patients older than 55 years of age (Steinmetz et al., 2012, p. 1801). In the United States, the estimated incidence is four new cases annually per 100,000 and prevalence of 60 per 100,000 (Nouri et al., 2015, p. E675).

Societal significance

Clinical presentation of cervical spondylotic myelopathy (CSM) is highly variable with some presenting with mild symptoms, whereas others may have severe disability. Those with severe disabling CSM often are dependent and require significant health-care and societal resources. Given the increasing elderly population, the potential societal impact of untreated CSM may become increasingly more relevant.

Pathobiology

CSM is caused by progressive compression of the spinal cord and/or nerve roots secondary most commonly to degenerative processes of the vertebral column. Specifically, neural compression can occur from various degenerative etiologies including acute or chronic disc herniation/protrusion, hypertrophy of the ligamentum flavum, facet joint degeneration and hypertrophy, and progressive osteophyte formation. Individuals with a congenitally narrow cervical spinal canal may be more susceptible to clinically significant CSM. With even minor progressive degenerative changes, those with a congenitally smaller spinal canal may have diminished capacity to tolerate discoligamentous hypertrophy.

As the spinal cord and nerve roots undergo acute and/or chronic compression, symptoms result from progressive neurologic dysfunction of these neural structures. This may manifest as pain, numbness, paresthesias, weakness, and potentially long spinal cord tract signs such as gait instability, incoordination, and bowel or bladder dysfunction.

Common physical exam findings

Gross physical exam

- Loss of range of motion
- Painful range of motion
- Muscle spasm

Neurologic exam

- Radiculopathy:
    - Pain, paresthesias, or numbness in a dermatome of an affected nerve root; weakness of muscles innervated by an affected nerve root

- Diminished reflex (cervical root dysfunction)
  - Spurling maneuver—reproduction of radicular pain with neck extension when patient's head is turned toward the affected side and examiner applies downward pressure on the forehead
- Myelopathy
  - Extremity paresthesias across multiple dermatomes or below a spinal cord level
  - Weakness and loss of hand dexterity (e.g., difficulty with buttoning shirts, writing, opening jars, dropping objects)
  - Gait instability—broad based, use of ambulatory assistance, feeling unsteady, trouble ascending or descending stairs
  - Urinary or bowel incontinence—less common and generally represents long-standing severe myelopathy
    - Lhermitte sign—electrical shock–like sensation down the back with neck extension or flexion
- Motor
  - Weakness of extremities—may or may not be present.
  - Grip-and-release test—inability to rapidly flex and fully extend digits greater than 20 times in 10 seconds
    - Increased tone or spasticity of major muscle groups leading to "spastic gait"
- Sensory
  - Proprioceptive dysfunction
  - Positive Romberg sign
    - Diminished pinprick testing
  - Pathologic reflexes
  - Brisk deep tendon reflexes (>2+)—may be absent with concomitant peripheral neuropathy (e.g., chronic diabetic neuropathy)
  - Present Hoffman sign—flexion of fingers when middle digit distal phalanx flicked
  - Present inverted radial sign—flexion of fingers while testing brachioradialis deep tendon reflex (DTR)
  - Present Babinski sign—extension of great toe and fanning of other toes when mildly noxious stimulus applied from lateral sole of foot to medial ball of foot
    - Sustained clonus at ankle joint

Relevant diagnostic tests

Magnetic resonance imaging

MRI is the gold standard for evaluation of the spinal cord, nerve roots, and vertebral column in suspected cervical spondylotic myelopathy. Multiplanar visualization (sagittal and axial views) allows for evaluation of potential compressive pathology with specific localization. Additionally, MRI may reveal "T2 signal abnormality" within the spinal cord, a finding that suggests more severe spinal cord dysfunction in the setting of severe compression.

Degree of spinal cord compression can be quantified by measuring the overall space available for the spinal cord (SAC). Myelopathy is rarely present with a SAC > 14 mm. On the contrary, a SAC < 6 mm is nearly always associated with myelopathy. A SAC between 6 and 14 mm can present with variable degrees of dysfunction (Matsunaga et al., 2002, p. 168).

Computed tomography (CT) imaging

CT imaging is useful for fine detail evaluation of bony and potentially calcified structures. For example, patients with significant osteophyte formation may be better evaluated on CT. CT may also be better for distinguishing other types of calcified compressive lesions such as ossification of the posterior longitudinal ligament (OPLL). The presence of a calcified anterior longitudinal ligament or diffuse idiopathic skeletal hyperostosis may impact surgical approach (particularly ventral approaches) and may be more apparent on CT. Last, for those patients in whom MRI is contraindicated (e.g., pacemaker), CT myelography can provide visualization of the neural elements and assessment for SAC.

Plain film x-ray

Routine anteroposterior (AP) and lateral x-rays assess overall alignment, show the presence of osteophytes, and evaluate any existing instrumentation in the setting of prior surgery. Lateral flexion and extension plain films may be used to evaluate for dynamic instability.

Posterior cervical surgical techniques

The goal of posterior cervical surgery is to decompress the neural elements and to fuse the vertebral column when indicated.

Advantages of posterior approaches

- Facile treatment of multilevel disease
- Ability to directly address dorsal pathology to the spinal cord/nerve roots
- Avoidance of risk to anterior neck soft tissue structures such as the esophagus, trachea, carotid sheath, and other potential nerve injuries (e.g., recurrent laryngeal nerve, sympathetic chain) with resultant dysphagia, dysphonia, or Horner syndrome

Disadvantages/Contraindications

- It is contraindicated in patients with cervical kyphosis. Posterior decompression in the setting of kyphosis does not allow the spinal cord to posteriorly migrate away from ventral compression in patients with cervical kyphosis.
- It does not directly address anterior focal pathology (e.g., a large central disc herniation).
- Postoperative C5 root palsy with shoulder abduction weakness is more common after posterior surgery. More extensive posterior muscle dissection likely results in increased postoperative pain, lengthier recovery, increased blood loss, and higher infection rate.

Cervical spine surgery can be divided into anterior versus posterior approaches. Three common posterior cervical operations include laminectomy, laminoplasty, and laminectomy with instrumented fusion. There is a paucity of literature that demonstrates superiority of one technique over another. In general, surgical series have demonstrated successful improvement in neurologic function with each of these approaches. Further study is necessary to determine the potential advantages of specific techniques for a given patient population.

1. **Laminectomy**—Cervical laminectomy involves removal of the lamina at the levels of spinal cord and/or nerve root compression. Decompression is achieved either by direct removal of any posterior compression (e.g., hypertrophied ligamentum flavum) or by indirect decompression, allowing the spinal cord to passively migrate posteriorly away from any ventral compression. Careful preservation of the facet joints maintains alignment and stability. Laminectomy alone (without instrumentation and fusion), however, has been shown in some cases to result in delayed kyphosis.

2. **Laminoplasty**—Laminoplasty is a procedure in which the spinal canal is expanded while preserving aspects of the posterior elements. There are historically a number of described techniques. A common approach, the expansile "open-door" technique, involves partial-thickness drilling on one side at the lamino-facet junction, and a full-thickness drilling on the contralateral side. This allows the lamina to be expanded by gently opening the full-thickness side, while "hinging" on the partial-thickness cut. Small metal plates are then applied to maintain the surgically expanded canal. A potential advantage of laminoplasty is that it is a nonfusion approach; therefore, there is relative preservation of cervical range of motion and the risk of pseudarthrosis (e.g., high-risk patients such as those with tobacco history) is obviated. The laminoplasty literature, however, reports a variable rate of postoperative neck and shoulder girdle pain.

3. **Laminectomy with posterior instrumentation and fusion**—The addition of instrumentation and fusion after laminectomy may prevent delayed kyphosis progression. Screw placement in the lateral masses with connecting rods allows for internal fixation and stabilization. Preparation of the posterolateral bony margins with implanting of bone graft material allows for eventual bony arthrodesis. In addition to preventing delayed kyphosis, successful fusion may improve preoperative symptoms of axial neck pain. Fusion, however, reduces range of motion. This may impact risk of degeneration at nonfused levels. Pseudarthrosis is a potential risk after fusion surgery and may result in the need for additional treatment. Common risk factors for pseudarthrosis include tobacco history and steroid or nonsteroidal anti-inflammatory use.

Common grading schemes

Family counseling

Prognosis

Cervical spondylotic myelopathy is a condition of progressive neurologic decline. Natural history suggests that 75% of patients have a step-wise worsening of their disease, with intervening periods of stable function. Twenty percent have a gradual, progressive decline, and 5% suffer more rapid deterioration. Surgical outcomes depend largely on severity and duration of preoperative symptoms and function. In general, longer duration and worse deficits are associated with poorer prognosis. Therefore, intervening early before severe chronic disability may be advised.

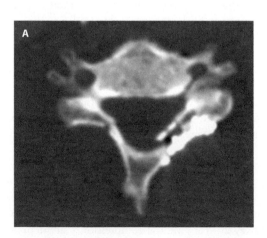
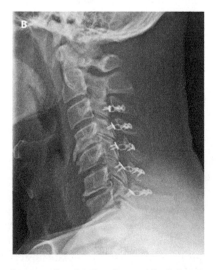

Figure 49.3 (a) Postoperative axial CT scan demonstrating expansile open-door laminoplasty with plating system. (b) Lateral x-ray after laminoplasty demonstrating increased spinal canal from C3-C7.

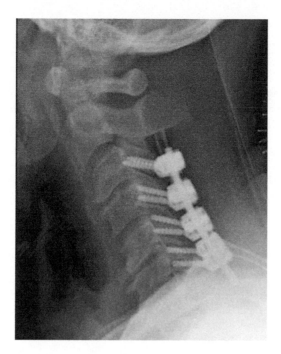

Figure 49.4 Postoperative lateral plain film demonstrating laminectomy and instrumented fusion using lateral mass screws.

Table 49.1 Nurick Classification of Disability

Grade 0	Nerve root signs and symptoms only or normal
Grade 1	Signs of cord compression, normal gait
Grade 2	Mild gait involvement, fully employed
Grade 3	Gait difficulties prevent employment, walks unassisted
Grade 4	Unable to walk without assistance
Grade 5	Wheelchair or bedbound

Common questions from patients

Q: How Do I Care for My Incision at Home?

A: In general, keep your incision clean and dry, no ointments or lotions applied to the incision and no submersion of the incision under water (e.g. swimming pool, bathtub) until it is well healed. Shower daily and wear clean, loose fitting clothing. Avoid pets (e.g. sleeping with cats and dogs) while sutures and/or staples are in place.

Q: How Will I Manage Postoperative Pain When I Get Home?

A: Surgeons will provide prescriptions when you leave the hospital for pain medication that will generally include an opiate and possibly muscle relaxant. Non-medication measures to control postoperative pain include changing positions and ice packs applied to areas surrounding the incision intermittently. If pain is poorly controlled at home, contact your surgeon's office.

Table 49.2 Modified Japanese Orthopedic Association (mJOA) Score

I. Motor dysfunction score of the upper extremities	
Inability to move hands	0
Inability to eat with a spoon but able to move hands	1
Inability to button shirt but able to eat with a spoon	2
Able to button shirt with great difficulty	3
Able to button shirt with slight difficulty	4
No dysfunction	5
II. Motor dysfunction score of the lower extremities	
Complete loss of motor and sensory function	0
Sensory preservation without ability to move legs	1
Able to move legs but unable to walk	2
Able to walk on flat floor with a walking aid (i.e., cane or crutch)	3
Able to walk up and/or down stairs with handrail	4
Moderate to significant lack of stability but able to walk up and/or down stairs without handrail	5
Mild lack of stability but walk unaided with smooth reciprocation	6
No dysfunction	7
III. Sensation	
Complete loss of hand sensation	0
Severe sensory loss or pain	1
Mild sensory loss	2
No sensory loss	3
IV. Sphincter dysfunction	
Inability to urinate voluntarily	0
Marked difficulty with micturition	1
Mild to moderate difficulty with micturition	2
Normal micturition	3

Source: Adapted from Japanese Orthopaedic Association (mJOA) Score (from Nurick S, *Brain*, 95, 87–100, 1972).

Q: When Will I Return to See My Surgeon?

A: Generally, you will return to see your surgeon within 3-6 weeks after surgery. Staples and/ or sutures should be removed approximately two weeks postoperatively.

Q: Will I Need to Wear a Neck Brace/Collar after Surgery?

A: Postoperative cervical collar use depends on various individual factors, as well as surgeon recommendation. If a collar is used, the skin under the collar should be inspected for pressure sores (e.g., redness, skin breakdown) at least daily. At home, patients will need assistance with skin inspection and removal of the collar and replacement of pads. The collar should fit snugly to maintain neutral position of the cervical spine but also allow eating. If there is concern regarding collar use or pressure sores, the patient should call the surgeon's office.

Q: What Activities Should Be Avoided after Surgery?

A: In general, early after surgery, avoid activities that cause excessive pain. If numbness, tingling, electrical shock pain, or weakness develop with any activity, stop the activity and notify your surgeon's office. Excessive bending or twisting of the neck should be avoided. Riding in a car is generally safe. Driving, however, should be avoided if you are wearing a collar (i.e., unable to look over your shoulder for other vehicles) or taking opiate or sedating medications.

Common pitfalls and medicolegal concerns

- Wrong level surgery
- Nerve or spinal cord injury
- Failure to relieve symptoms
- Failure of fusion
- Instrumentation failure
- Wound infection
- Postoperative hematoma

Relevance to the advanced practice health professional

Cervical spondylotic myelopathy is the most common cause of spinal cord dysfunction in adults older than 55 years (Steinmetz et al., 2012, p. 1801). As life expectancy of the population increases, diagnosis and management of cervical spine disorders will become increasingly important for health-care professionals. As up to 80% of patients have improved functional outcomes with surgery, surgical intervention represents one of the most effective treatments for this common, disabling condition.

Common phone calls, pages, and requests

Postoperative pain

During the patient's hospitalization, nurses may page regarding inadequate pain control. Pain is a common problem after surgery, and there may be times when the patient receives too much (e.g., excessive sedation) or too little pain medication (e.g., severe discomfort). One should review any pain medications the patient may have been using before surgery and compare to inpatient medications. Usually patients experience more pain postoperatively and, therefore, will likely require a higher dose, frequency, or additional pain medications than their pre-op regimen.

Opiates and muscle relaxants are commonly used postoperatively. Prior history of opiate use, patient weight, and allergies should always be considered when initiating analgesics. Consultation with the hospital pharmacist may be helpful for patients who require complex dosing regimens. Overmedicating with opiates and some muscle relaxants can lead to confusion, lethargy, respiratory depression, or hypotension. If these occur, the medication should be held, with subsequent close clinical evaluation before resuming pain medication. If the patient is clinically unstable (e.g., hypoxemic, unarousable), then a physician should be called emergently for evaluation.

Nonsteroidal anti-inflammatory medications (NSAIDS) should be avoided after spinal fusion as they may inhibit bone fusion.

In general, postoperative pain is normal and expected. You should always keep in mind that some complications, however, might present as pain (e.g., postoperative hematoma with spinal cord or nerve compression, infection). A careful history and physical exam should be performed if the patient experiences an unexpected increase in pain, or pain associated with other abnormal exam findings like weakness, numbness, or wound breakdown.

Superficial wound infection

If there is concern for a wound infection, it is important to both visually assess the wound and inquire if the patient has any associated symptoms such as pain or neurologic deficit. This initial assessment can be performed at bedside, a review of a photo sent from home, or an office visit. You should know the general practice of the surgeon and how the surgeon prefers to manage superficial wound infections. This may include serologic tests, vital signs (particularly temperature), neurologic assessment, and potentially imaging.

When evaluating a patient for a wound infection, perform a focused exam of the surgical area for redness, tenderness, fluctuance, drainage, dehiscence, and for any exposed muscle, bone, or instrumentation. Discuss your findings with the surgeon, and formulate a treatment plan. This should include clear communication with the patient and family regarding wound care, any antibiotics, and subsequent follow-up assessment.

Postoperative urinary retention

Postoperative urinary retention is common after surgery with general anesthesia. Patients, particularly older men, should be educated preoperatively about this possibility as it frequently occurs in patients with a history of benign prostatic hypertrophy (BPH). Home medications should be reviewed for those that may be used to treat other chronic urinary problems including BPH. If urinary retention is associated with fever, dysuria, or hematuria, you should evaluate for possible urinary tract infection.

Return to work

Timing for return to work is generally related to the type of work they perform, the physical activity required (e.g., desk job versus manual labor), and when their postoperative pain is adequately managed without significant opiate pain medications. Most patients after posterior cervical surgery can expect to be out of work for 3–6 weeks. For those who engage in strenuous physical labor, you may advise not resuming work until after the first postoperative outpatient visit, and/or after adequate time for tissue healing (e.g., successful bony fusion).

References

Gray H. *Anatomy of the Human Body.* Philadelphia, PA: Lea & Febiger; 1918.

Matsunaga S, Kukita M, Hayashi K, Shinkura R, Koriyama C, Sakou T, Komiya S. Pathogenesis of myelopathy in patients with ossification of the posterior longitudinal ligament. *J Neurosurg.* 2002;96:168–172.

Nouri A, Tetreault L, Singh A, Karadimas SK, Fehlings MG. Degenerative cervical myelopathy: epidemiology, genetics, and pathogenesis. *Spine.* 2015:40:E675–E693.

Nurick S. The pathogenesis of spinal cord disorder associated with cervical spondylosis. *Brain.* 1972;95:87–100.

Steinmetz M, Placide R, Benzel E, Krishnaney A. Management of cervical spondylotic myelopathy. In: Alfredo Quinones-Hinojosa, ed. *Schmidek & Sweet Operative Neurosurgical Techniques. Indications, Methods, and Results.* 6th ed. Philadelphia, PA: Elsevier; 2012:1801–1813.

50

SPINAL DECOMPRESSIVE SURGERIES AND LUMBAR MICRODISCECTOMY

Gabriel Duhancioglu, Rahul Kamath, Junyoung Ahn, and Kern Singh

Case vignette

A 51-year-old male presents with 7/10 pain radiating down the anterior aspect of his right thigh with a slight "pulling" sensation in the lower back that occurred following lifting a 50-pound weight. The patient describes the pain as intermittent and sharp that worsens with prolonged sitting and standing. The patient's magnetic resonance imaging (MRI) demonstrates a right-sided lumbar disc herniation at the L5-S1 level (Figure 50.1a and b).

Initially, the patient's symptoms responded well to physical therapy and nonsteroidal anti-inflammatory drugs (NSAIDS). However, the patient's radiculopathy continued to worsen. Following 8 months of conservative management, surgical intervention was recommended for the patient's persistent pain. Following a right-sided, hemi-laminectomy and microdiscectomy at the L5-S1 level, the patient demonstrated significant improvement in pain and strength that was maximized during postoperative physical therapy.

Overview

Approximately 70%–80% of the population will experience low back pain at some point in their lives (van Tulder et al., 2002; National Institute of Neurological Disorders and Stroke [NINDS], 2004). Low back pain has been described as the most common reason for missed workdays and occupational-related disability (NINDS, 2004). In addition, the annual costs associated with the treatment and disability secondary to low back pain have been estimated to be approximately $50 billion (Besen et al., 2015). As such, the societal consequence of low back pain is substantial and wide reaching.

The discs between the vertebral bodies are susceptible to wear and tear from injuries and/or normal aging. These intervertebral discs may rupture or bulge and result in a condition known as a disc herniation. A disc herniation in the lumbar spine can contribute to low back and leg pain if the surrounding neural structures are compressed. While previous studies have demonstrated that a herniated disc may be treated nonoperatively, the efficacy of the surgical removal of the herniated disc has also been demonstrated (Weinstein et al., 2006; Tullberg et al., 1993).

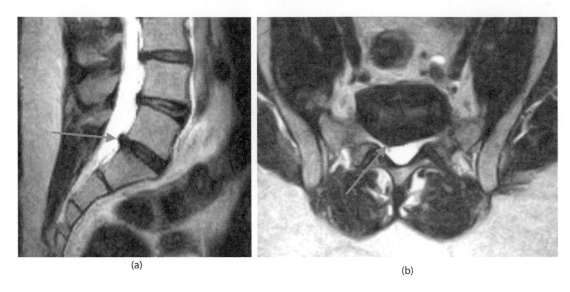

(a)

(b)

Figure 50.1 (a) Preoperative parasagittal T2-weighted MRI demonstrating a herniated disc bulge at the L5–S1 level. (b) Preoperative axial T2-weighted MRI demonstrating the same herniated disc bulge on the right side at the L5–S1 level causing traversing S1 nerve root compression.

Review of the anatomy

Lumbar disc herniations most often occur at the L4–L5 and L5–S1 disc levels (Moore and Agur, 2007). Terminology to describe disc herniation according to morphology and the relationship of the disc material to the annulus fibrosus (surrounding the nucleus pulposus) are described in Table 50.1.

Common physical examination findings

Typical presentation of a lumbar disc herniation is as follows:

- Patients have leg pain (radiculopathy) accompanied by lower back pain or a sensation of numbness or tingling in the legs and/or feet.
- Patients may also present with walking difficulties.
- Bending forward or sitting down may ease the symptoms for some patients.

Relevant diagnostic tests

History and physical examination

- Examination is essential for the purposes of diagnosis before any diagnostic imaging or laboratory tests are obtained.
- Radiographic evidence should corroborate the clinical presentation if surgical intervention is necessary.

Table 50.1 Nomenclature for Lumbar Disc Herniation Based on Morphology of Displaced Disc Material

Nomenclature	Description
Protrusion	The width of the displaced disc material is greater than the distance between the outermost point of disc material to the base.
Extrusion	The distance of the disc material beyond the edge of the disc space is greater than the width of the disc material (as measured on any plane).
Sequestration	This describes cases of extrusion in which the disc material is no longer in continuity with the intervertebral disc.
Schmorl nodes	Disc material displacement in the head-to-toe direction is through an opening in the vertebral body endplates.
Contained	Displaced disc material is covered by the fibers of the outer annulus fibrosus and/or the posterior longitudinal ligament.

Source: Data from Fardon D.F. et al., *Spine J.*, 14, 2525–2545, 2014.

Imaging

Plain radiograph

- Appropriate initial imaging modality to detect misalignment of vertebrae (spondylolisthesis)
- May provide information regarding degeneration, instability, or fracture, but limited in detecting soft tissue injury (Deyo and Weinstein, 2001: Finch, 2006)

Computed tomography (CT)

- It may be utilized to characterize the morphology of the spinal canal and the surrounding structures.
- It may not be adequate to confirm the diagnosis of a disc herniation.
- For lumbar disc herniation, the reported sensitivity is 80%–95% and specificity is 68%–88% (Greenberg and Greenberg, 2010).
- It is typically used in situations in which prior instrumentation has been placed. Ideally, a CT myelogram is used in these scenarios when an MRI cannot be obtained.

Magnetic resonance imaging (MRI)

- Offers high-resolution visualization of the spinal cord, nerve roots, surrounding soft tissue, degenerative processes, or spinal masses (Humphreys et al., 2002).
- MRI is currently the gold standard for confirming the diagnosis of disc herniation as well as evaluating the surrounding soft tissue and neural structures.
- MRI offers the highest sensitivity and specificity for detection of lumbar disc herniation (Lotke et al., 2008).

Review of relevant interventional procedures and surgeries

The surgical approach for the microdiscectomy may influence the postoperative course. Specifically, the minimally invasive microdiscectomy technique has been associated with a shorter length of hospitalization, lower postoperative narcotic medication use, and lower risk of surgical site infections when compared to the traditional open technique (Harrington and French, 2008; Rasouli et al., 2014). However, complications and reported improvements in clinical outcomes have been similar between the microscopic and open techniques (Harrington and French, 2008; Dasenbrock et al., 2012: Rasouli et al., 2014).

Common grading schemes

Recently, the combined task forces of the North American Spine Society, the American Society of Spine Radiology, and the American Society of Neuroradiology reported on their recommendations regarding the nomenclature for describing pathology of the lumbar disc (Fardon et al., 2014). Herniation was defined as a localized displacement of the disc material (nucleus pulposus, cartilage, fragments of apophyseal bone, and/or annular tissue) beyond the border of the disc space. Descriptive terms for the morphology of lumbar disc herniations are listed in Table 50.1.

In addition, disc herniation may be classified according to the anatomical position (far lateral, paracentral, center) in relation to the vertebral body. This terminology may be useful in determining the appropriate surgical approach (posterior, lateral) based on the location of the herniation.

Family counseling

Prognosis

Pain and depressive mood symptoms secondary to chronic low back pain are often significantly improved in the majority of patients immediately following a microdiscectomy (Harrington and French, 2008; Dasenbrock et al., 2012; Lau et al., 2011). However, appropriate postoperative management may expedite recovery. Engagement in rehabilitative activities (patient education, therapist-led exercise regimens) has been associated with significant improvements in postoperative functional status (McGregor et al., 2014). In addition, smoking cessation is recommended for all patients, as smoking has been identified as an independent risk factor for reoperation following a single or multilevel lumbar decompression (Bydon et al., 2015).

Common questions

- What are some common complications during the operation?
- Nerve root injury, incidental dural tears, and recurrent disc herniation are possible complications of a discectomy (Harrington and French, 2008; Rasouli et al., 2014).
- Is the patient at risk of paralysis or death following surgery?

Paralysis is not a relevant complication with this procedure, as the spinal cord terminates in the lower thoracic–upper lumbar level (T12-L1). Complications such as death are rare and are not typically encountered during this outpatient procedure.

- How long does it typically take for the patient to recover from the surgery and be released from the hospital?

Recovery following surgery may vary based on the extent of the surgery, patient comorbidities, and any intraoperative or perioperative complications. Typically, lumbar microdiscectomies are outpatient procedures that may require 23-hour hospitalization.

- How long does it typically take for symptoms to be resolved?

Symptom resolution may vary between patients based on the chronicity of preoperative pain complaints. In general, symptoms resolve within hours after the procedure. However, maximal improvement may not be observed until 6 months following the intervention (Porchet et al., 2009).

- What does the rehabilitation process entail?

Patients who receive postoperative rehabilitation education along with participation in a therapist-led exercise program experience improved functional outcomes in both the short term and long term (McGregor et al., 2014).

Pitfalls

Approximately 7%–10% of patients experience recurrent herniation within 6 months of the primary operation, making the first few months following the operation a critical time period for healing (Cheng et al., 2013). Patients should also be advised regarding appropriate lifestyle choices including smoking cessation.

Common medicolegal concerns

- Improper documentation and/or systems failure may lead to errors during the surgical intervention or postoperative management, particularly in regard to side and level of the procedure being performed.
- Expectations for symptom improvement following surgery should be discussed thoroughly with the patient to maximize trust between the health-care professional and the patient.
- Patients should be advised prior to surgery that while leg pain may often improve, many patients continue to experience chronic low back pain following a decompressive procedure.

Relevance to the advanced practice health professional

When a patient presents with low back pain, surgical intervention should not be the initial treatment method. For all patients, nonoperative management options should be exhausted prior to surgical intervention. The exception to this may be for patients who present with significant motor deficit, loss of bladder/bowel control, or foot drop secondary to a large disc herniation. These patients often undergo expeditious surgery. Education and counseling, physical therapy, anti-inflammatory and steroid treatments, and activity restriction are just a few of the effective, nonoperative strategies for symptom relief (Weinstein et al., 2006). In conjunction to any surgical intervention, the cooperation of all health-care professionals may significantly impact outcomes and the resulting quality of life for patients.

References

Besen E, Young AE, Shaw WS. Returning to work following low back pain: towards a model of individual psychosocial factors. *J Occup Rehabil.* 2015;25(1):25–37. doi: 10.1007/s10926-014-9522-9.

Bydon M, Macki M, De la Garza-Ramos R et al. Smoking as an independent predictor of reoperation after lumbar laminectomy: a study of 500 cases. *J Neurosurg Spine.* 2015;22:288–293. doi: 10.3171/2014.10.SPINE14186.

Cheng J, Wang H, Zheng W et al. Reoperation after lumbar disc surgery in two hundred and seven patients. *Int Orthop.* 2013;37(8):1511–1511. doi: 10.1007/s00264-013-1925-2.

Dasenbrock HH, Juraschek SP, Schultz LR et al. The efficacy of minimally invasive discectomy compared with open discectomy: a meta-analysis of prospective randomized controlled trials. *J Neurosurg Spine*. 2012;16(5):452–452. doi: 10.3171/2012.1.SPINE11404.

Deyo RA, Weinstein JN. Low back pain. *N Engl J Med*. 2001;344(5):363–363. doi: 10.1056/NEJM200102013440508.

Fardon DF, Williams AL, Dohring EJ, Murtagh FR, Gabriel Rothman SL, Sze GK. Lumbar disc nomenclature: version 2.0: Recommendations of the combined task forces of the North American Spine Society, the American Society of Spine Radiology and the American Society of Neuroradiology. *Spine J*. 2014;14(11):2525–2525. doi: 10.1016/j.spinee.2014.04.022.

Finch P. Technology Insight: imaging of low back pain. *Nat Clin Pract Rheumatol*. 2006;2(10):554–554. doi: 10.1038/ncprheum0293.

Greenberg, Mark S., Mark S. Greenberg. 2010. *Handbook of neurosurgery*. 7th ed. Tampa, FL: Greenberg Graphics;.

Harrington JF, French P. Open versus minimally invasive lumbar microdiscectomy: comparison of operative times, length of hospital stay, narcotic use and complications. *Minim Invasive Neurosurg*. 2008;51(1):30–30. doi: 10.1055/s-2007-1004543.

Humphreys SC, Eck JC, Hodges SD. Neuroimaging in low back pain. *Am Fam Physician*. 2002;65(11):2299–2299.

Lau D, Han SJ, Lee JG, Lu DC, Chou D. Minimally invasive compared to open microdiscectomy for lumbar disc herniation. *J Clin Neurosci*. 2011;18(1):81–81. doi: 10.1016/j.jocn.2010.04.040.

Lotke, Paul A., Joseph A. Abboud, Jack Ende. 2008. *Lippincott's primary care. Orthopaedics, Primary care series*. Philadelphia: Wolters Kluwer/Lippincott Williams & Wilkins Health.

McGregor AH, Probyn K, Cro S et al. Rehabilitation following surgery for lumbar spinal stenosis. A Cochrane review. *Spine (Phila Pa 1976)*. 2014;39(13):1044–1044. doi: 10.1097/BRS.0000000000000355.

Moore Keith L, Agur AMR. *Essential clinical anatomy*. 3rd ed. Philadelphia, PA: Lippincott Williams & Wilkins.

National Institute of Neurological Disorders and Stroke (NINDS). 2004. *Low back pain fact sheet*. Bethesda, MD: NINDS; 2014. NIH publication 15-5161.

Porchet F, Bartanusz V, Kleinstueck FS et al. Microdiscectomy compared with standard discectomy: an old problem revisited with new outcome measures within the framework of a spine surgical registry. *Eur Spine J*. 2009;18(Suppl 3):360–6. doi: 10.1007/s00586-009-0917-9.

Rasouli MR, Rahimi-Movaghar V, Shokraneh F, Moradi-Lakeh M, Chou R. Minimally invasive discectomy versus microdiscectomy/open discectomy for symptomatic lumbar disc herniation. *Cochrane Database Syst Rev*. 2014;9:Cd010328. doi: 10.1002/14651858.CD010328.pub2.

Tullberg T, Isacson J, Weidenhielm L. Does microscopic removal of lumbar disc herniation lead to better results than the standard procedure? Results of a one-year randomized study. *Spine (Phila Pa 1976)*. 1993;18(1):24–24.

van Tulder M, Koes B, Bombardier C. Low back pain. *Best Pract Res Clin Rheumatol*. 2002;16(5):761–761.

Weinstein JN, Tosteson TD, Lurie JD et al. Surgical vs nonoperative treatment for lumbar disk herniation: the Spine Patient Outcomes Research Trial (SPORT): a randomized trial. *JAMA*. 2006;296(20):2441–2441. doi: 10.1001/jama.296.20.2441.

51

ELECTIVE SPINAL SURGERY FOR LUMBAR FUSION

Nancy Thomas and Paul Park

Case vignette

A 31-year-old male presented with a 1-year history of persistent severe low back pain radiating into the left buttock, hip, and left great toe. The patient denied bowel or bladder symptoms. He underwent 6 months of conservative treatment, including therapeutic injections, without durable relief. On physical examination, motor strength was grossly normal. There was diminished left ankle reflex and decreased sensation over the left great toe. Computed tomography (CT) myelogram demonstrated evidence of bilateral L5 pars defects resulting in grade II spondylolisthesis at L5-S1 and foraminal stenosis. Standing x-rays re-demonstrated a grade II anterolisthesis of L5 on S1 (Figure 51.1). Because of his persistent symptoms, imaging findings, and failure of conservative measures, the patient was offered and elected to undergo a minimally invasive transforaminal lumbar interbody fusion (TLIF) (Figure 51.2).

Overview

Epidemiology

Low back pain is common. Five percent of the population is affected per year, with a lifetime incidence between 60% and 90% of the population. The overall prevalence of low back pain in the United States is estimated to be about 18% (Golob and Wipf, 2014).

Societal significance

Low back pain with or without radiculopathy remains one of the more difficult medical conditions to treat and has a high degree of impairment, activity limitation, and treatment cost (Eck et al., 2014). In fact, spinal disorders, including low back pain, are the most frequent cause of activity limitation in persons younger than 45 years of age. Over 14% of all new patient visits to physicians are for complaints of low back pain. From age 45 to 65, low back pain is the third most frequent cause of disability, and the economic consequences are estimated to range from $16 billion to $50 billion a year. Low back pain is responsible for 2.4 million cases of disability in the United States, with 50% becoming chronically disabled (Ma et al., 2014). The direct medical cost of low back pain was estimated to be greater than $25 billion in the United States during 1990 (Golob and Wipf, 2014). Although somewhat controversial, lumbar fusion has become an accepted treatment option for intractable back pain with or without radicular pain for patients who fail conservative care (Eck et al., 2014).

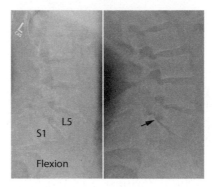

Figure 51.1 Lateral flexion (left) and extension (right) lumbosacral spine x-rays showing L5–S1 spondylolisthesis (arrowhead points to slippage of L5 over S1).

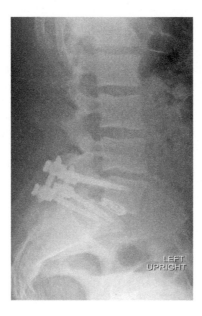

Figure 51.2 Postoperative lateral lumbosacral spine x-ray showing L5–S1 interbody cage and pedicle screw-rod instrumentation with improvement of spondylolisthesis.

Basic biologic and physiologic processes

One common purported cause of low back and leg pain is spinal degeneration. Disc degeneration, thickening and buckling of the ligamentum flavum, and facet hypertrophy contribute to spinal canal narrowing, which is generally greatest at the disc level. Disc degeneration can progress to instability of the motion segment, resulting in slippage of one vertebral body over another, which is termed *degenerative spondylolisthesis* (Katz and Harris, 2008). These degenerative processes can cause nerve root compression and produce symptoms of back pain, radiculopathy, or neurogenic claudication and are a common finding in an aging spine (Katz and Harris, 2008). Lumbar fusion with or without decompression (i.e., laminectomy) is a potential treatment option for intractable back pain with or without radicular pain for patients who fail conservative care. Beyond degeneration, other potential causes of low back pain that may be treated with lumbar fusion include congenital, traumatic, or neoplastic processes.

Anatomical review

In the lumbar spine, there are typically five vertebral bodies interconnected by intervertebral discs. The L5 vertebral body connects to the first sacral segment, which is named S1. Each disc is labeled by the adjacent vertebral bodies (e.g., the disc between the L1 and L2 vertebral bodies is termed L1-L2).

Common physical examination findings

- Abnormal posture; stooped forward
- Palpable tenderness or muscle spasms in low back region
- Difficulty walking due to lower extremity pain with possible weakness and/or sensory changes
- Sensory (including pain) and/or motor changes in a specific nerve root/dermatome distribution
- Abnormal diminished reflexes at patellae or ankles
- Watch for red flag symptoms of hyperreflexia, cauda equina syndrome, long-track signs such as Babinski, lower extremity spasticity, and clonus, which would suggest an upper motor neuron etiology and should prompt further evaluation (Suri et al., 2010)

Relevant diagnostic tests

- Standing x-rays to evaluate for alignment and structural abnormalities (e.g., fracture). Consider scoliosis x-rays for assessment of global alignment.
- Lumbar flexion and extension x-rays to evaluate for instability.
- Magnetic resonance imaging (MRI) of lumbar spine to evaluate multiplanar sagittal and axial images for structural abnormalities (e.g., disc herniation, stenosis, spondylolisthesis) affecting the neural elements (e.g., nerves). MRI is the current gold standard diagnostic study for persistent low back or leg pain.
- Lumbosacral CT to evaluate bony anatomy (e.g., pars defects, fractures) is optional.
- CT myelogram is an alternative to MRI for assessment of structural abnormalities causing nerve compression. It is typically performed when MRI is unavailable or in patients with extensive past spinal surgery with hardware that creates too much artifact on MRI, or in patients with cardiac pacemakers.
- Electromyography (EMG)/nerve conduction velocity (NCV) study to evaluate for spinal versus peripheral nerve damage.
- Bone mineral density study to evaluate bone quality (e.g., osteoporosis).

Indications for surgery

Patients with persistent mechanical back and radicular pain caused by degenerative disc disease, spondylolisthesis, lumbar spinal stenosis or spondylosis, recurrent disc herniation, lumbar deformity, or pseudoarthrosis may benefit from lumbar fusion (Mummaneni et al., 2004). Unless a significant neurologic deficit is present, surgery is offered to patients who have failed a period of nonoperative management (i.e., physical therapy and/or injections). The goal is to obtain a solid fusion of the pain-generating segment(s) using the most efficient technology with the lowest risk of complications.

Common surgical options for lumbar fusion

Fusion or arthrodesis is the process where a spinal level (e.g., L4–5) is made rigid by bone growth across the typically mobile segment. Historically, the most common method to obtain lumbar fusion has been the posterior or posterolateral fusion. In this procedure, a midline back incision is made with stripping of the paraspinal muscles to expose the posterior spine, consisting of the spinous process, lamina, facet joints, and transverse processes. Although there are many variations, in posterior fusion the lamina to be fused are decorticated so that bleeding bone is created. In posterolateral fusion, the facet joints and transverse processes are also decorticated. Bone graft is then placed on the decorticated bone to promote bone fusion. Several types of bone graft are available, including autograft and allograft. Autograft bone is bone harvested from the patient, either from the iliac crest or locally (e.g., spinous process or lamina, if a laminectomy is performed). Allograft bone is bone harvested from a cadaver that has been prepared for use as graft material. Beyond autograft and allograft bone, other options exist, including bone morphogenetic proteins.

Historically, patients were placed in a brace postoperatively to immobilize the spine so that fusion could occur, as too much motion could result in nonfusion. Failed fusion is known as a pseudarthrosis. To improve fusion rates, instrumentation can be placed to stabilize the targeted spinal segments. Presently, the most commonly used instrumentation is the pedicle screw. The pedicle screw is placed via a posterior approach and allows fixation of all three columns of the spine. After bilateral placement of a pedicle screw at each targeted vertebral body, a rod is inserted through each pedicle screw head, and a locking set-screw is applied to interconnect the screw heads in a rigid construct. The application of pedicle screw instrumentation has significantly improved fusion rates and is now the most common form of hardware used for stabilization.

In addition to posterior or posterolateral fusion, other frequently employed surgical techniques for lumbar fusion include posterior lumbar interbody fusion (PLIF), TLIF, and anterior lumbar interbody fusion (ALIF). The general rationale behind interbody fusion is to place a cage or structural allograft in the load-bearing position of the anterior and middle spinal columns, which support 80% of spinal loads and provide 90% of the osseous surface area, thereby maximally enhancing the potential for fusion (Mummaneni et al., 2004). PLIF and TLIF are typically performed via a posterior midline incision similar to the posterior and posterolateral fusion. In fact, a PLIF or TLIF will often be performed in conjunction with posterolateral fusion. Pedicle screw instrumentation is also typically employed for stabilization and to enhance fusion. In PLIF, the lamina and at least part or all of the facet joints are removed to allow access to the disc space so that a complete discectomy can be performed. Bilateral cages are typically placed in the disc space to provide anterior support in addition to bone graft to promote fusion across the disc space. TLIF involves a more lateral approach to the disc space and involves removing the lateral aspect of the lamina as well as the entire facet joint to allow access to the disc space. Similar to PLIF, a discectomy is performed, but unlike a PLIF, one cage is placed obliquely in conjunction with bone graft placement.

ALIF involves an anterior approach typically through the retroperitoneal space to allow access to the targeted disc levels. A discectomy is performed followed by insertion of either one or two cages and some form of graft material. Instrumentation can involve an anterior plate that spans the disc space fixated with vertebral body screws, or the patient can be turned prone to place pedicle screw instrumentation. Advantages of ALIF are straightforward exposure to L4 to sacrum, with best exposure of the L5-S1 intervertebral space. Approach to L4-L5 is more challenging and requires mobilization of the iliac vessels. Complications may include vascular and bowel injuries, superior hypogastric plexus injury and subsequent retrograde ejaculation, rectus muscle paresis, deep vein thrombosis, or abdominal hernia (Brau, 2002).

In recent years, minimally invasive techniques for PLIF and TLIF have become popular. With a minimally invasive PLIF or TLIF, a muscle-splitting technique is used to minimize adjacent tissue trauma while accomplishing the same radiographic and clinical outcomes as the traditional PLIF or TLIF. Another minimally invasive approach for anterior interbody fusion is lateral lumbar interbody fusion (LLIF). In LLIF, a small flank incision is typically used to enter the retroperitoneal space in conjunction with a muscle-splitting approach through the psoas muscle to access the disc space for interbody fusion. Potential complications of LLIF may include hip flexor weakness, thigh numbness, quadriceps weakness, genitofemoral neuralgia, abdominal viscera perforation, rupture of anterior longitudinal ligament, great vessel injury, kidney-ureteral injury, graft subsidence, psoas/retroperitoneal hematoma, abdominal wall paresis, or rhabdomyolysis (Dakwar et al., 2010).

Family counseling

Prognosis

In many cases, reasonable surgical outcomes may be the reduction of pain as well as improvement in mobility, function, and quality of life rather than achieving a completely asymptomatic state. Patients with neurologic deficits are more likely to develop progressive functional decline without surgery (Matsunaga et al., 2000). Overall, however, there is no guarantee that surgery will result in symptomatic improvement.

Common questions

Patients typically seek information preoperatively about the following: the surgical approach/technique, potential complications, implant type(s)/instrumentation, length of procedure, hospital stay, insurance coverage, recovery time, activity restrictions/driving, pain control, discontinuation of medications prior to surgery, expected outcomes, recurrence rate/adjacent segment disease, mobility, physical therapy, orthotic bracing, subacute rehabilitation, and return to work.

Pitfalls

- Careful patient assessment, planning, and communication often avoid or limit preventable problems and allow for optimal postoperative outcomes.
- Patient comorbidities may affect postoperative recovery or delay surgery if appropriate preoperative medical clearance or testing is not obtained (Strayer, 2009).
- Chronic pain may complicate postoperative pain control and should be addressed.
- Preoperative discussion including potential surgical risks and outcomes may limit unrealistic patient expectations, both postoperatively and long term. It is also necessary to ensure discontinuation of medications that may contribute to excessive bleeding during surgery, such as herbal or vitamin supplements, nonsteroidal medications, anticoagulants, and antiplatelet medications (Strayer, 2009).
- Adequate bone healing may be adversely affected by excessive activity during the early postoperative period, as well as use of anti-inflammatory, cytotoxic, and steroid medications. Other limitations to bone healing include use of nicotine, radiation, and systemic comorbidities such as diabetes and rheumatoid arthritis (Strayer, 2009).

Common pitfalls and medicolegal concerns

- Patient selection is key. Deciding on surgical intervention requires careful consideration of potential risks and benefits. Patients should be counseled that the benefits of surgery decline over time and that repeat operations (for same or adjacent level disease) are performed in 15%–25% of cases (Greenberg, 2010).
- Comorbidities and psychosocial factors, such as diabetes, severe cardiopulmonary disease, renal impairment, coagulopathies, obesity, poor bone quality, cancer, malnutrition, infection, chronic pain, multiple previous spine surgeries, severe depression, as well as psychosocial and secondary gain issues, may impact surgical outcome (Slover et al., 1976).
- Potential surgical complications should be discussed in detail and include infection (~10%), nerve root injury (~1%), spinal cord injury, vascular injury, damage to nearby vessels and structures that is approach-dependent, dural tear, cerebrospinal fluid leak (~10%), cage or screw misplacement or migration, pseudoarthrosis (up to 25%, depending on comorbidities), pseudomeningocele,

hematoma (~5%), blood clots, excessive blood loss, heart attack, stroke (<1%), complications of anesthesia (<1%), poor wound healing, paralysis (<1%), pain, numbness, weakness, paresthesias, neurogenic bowel/bladder, cauda equina syndrome, adjacent segment disease, coma (<1%), and death (<1%) (Nasca, 2013).

Relevance to the advanced practice health professional

Low back pain is a common medical problem. Elective lumbar fusion is an option to treat back pain with or without radicular pain for patients who fail conservative care and have concordant imaging findings. Understanding the assessment, diagnosis, and various surgical interventions to safely navigate patients through the preoperative, intraoperative, and postoperative phases is crucial to maximize outcome.

Common phone calls, pages, and requests with answers

There are several issues that the advanced practice professional may be called on to resolve during the preoperative, perioperative, or postoperative period, albeit this is not an exhaustive list:

- *How many days before surgery should I stop taking my blood thinners?*

  Approximately 5–10 days if benefit outweighs risk. Determination is usually made by the patient's cardiologist or primary care physician. Patients on aspirin therapy may continue it if considered safe for the planned surgical procedure. If it is necessary to stop antiplatelet medicines, aspirin should be withheld for 1 week before surgery and clopidogrel/prasugrel withheld for 5 days before surgery (Di Minno et al., 2009).

- *Will I become paralyzed if I do not undergo surgery?*

  Patients who present with sensory changes, muscle weakness, or cauda equina syndrome are more likely to develop functional decline without surgery (Matsunaga et al., 2000). However, paraplegia is unlikely for most other patients, since the spinal cord and conus are usually above L1.

- *How well should my postoperative pain be controlled?*

  Adequate postoperative pain management is essential, as there is growing evidence that insufficient perioperative pain management can be associated with significant adverse events including extended hospital stay, slower functional recovery, higher readmission rates, and increased health-care resource use and cost (Devin and McGirt, 2015).

- *What are my activity restrictions after surgery?*

  The typical recommendation is to gradually return to normal activities as much as possible, avoiding bending, lifting, and twisting, and no lifting greater than 5–10 pounds for 3 months. The patient should undergo radiographs at 3 months postoperatively to assess instrumentation and determine extent of fusion. A longer period may be needed, especially in noninstrumented fusions or patients with comorbidities. However, even with instrumentation, fusion may take up to a year or more to mature. With newer, less invasive techniques, postoperative immobilization usually is not needed (Strayer, 2009).

- *Do I need to wear a brace after lumbar fusion?*

  Instrumentation obviates the absolute necessity of postoperative brace wear after lumbar fusion. However, patients may be immobilized in a lumbosacral orthosis or a thoracolumbosacral orthosis, depending on factors such as bone quality.

References

Brau SA. Mini-open approach to the spine for anterior lumbar interbody fusion: Description of the procedure, results and complications. *Spine Journal.* 2002;2:216–223.

Dakwar E, Cardona RF, Smith DA, Uribe JS. Early outcomes and safety of the minimally invasive, lateral retroperitoneal transpsoas approach for adult degenerative scoliosis. *Neurosurgical Focus.* 2010;28:E8.

Devin CJ., McGirt MJ. Best evidence in multimodal pain management in spine surgery and means of assessing postoperative pain and functional outcomes. *J Clin Neurosci.* 2015;22(6):930–938.

Di Minno MN, Prisco D, Ruocco AL, Mastronardi P, Massa S, Di Minno G. Perioperative handling of patients on antiplatelet therapy with need for surgery. *Internal and Emergency Medicine.* 2009;4:279–288.

Eck C, Sharan A, Ghogawala Z, et al. Guideline update for the performance of fusion procedures for degenerative disease of the lumbar spine. Part 7: lumbar fusion for intractable low-back pain without stenosis or spondylolisthesis. *Journal of Neurosurgery:Spine* 2014;21:42–47.

Golob AL, Wipf JE. Low back pain. *Medical Clinics of North America.* 2014;98:405–428.

Greenberg MS. *Handbook of Neurosurgery, Seventh Edition.* New York, NY: Thieme; 2010.

Katz JN, Harris MB. Clinical practice. Lumbar spinal stenosis. *New England Journal of Medicine.* 2008;358:818–825.

Ma VY, Chan L, Carruthers KJ. Incidence, prevalence, costs, and impact on disability of common conditions requiring rehabilitation in the United States: stroke, spinal cord injury, traumatic brain injury, multiple sclerosis, osteoarthritis, rheumatoid arthritis, limb loss, and back pain. *Archives of Physical Medicine and Rehabilitation.* 2014;95:986–995.

Matsunaga S, Ijiri K, Hayashi K. Nonsurgically managed patients with degenerative spondylolisthesis: a 10- to 18-year follow-up study. *Journal of Neurosurgery: Spine.* 2000;93:194–198.

Mummaneni PV, Haid RW, Rodts GE. Lumbar interbody fusion: state-of-the-art technical advances. *Journal of Neurosurgery: Spine.* 2004;1:24–30.

Nasca RJ. Newer lumbar interbody fusion techniques. *Journal of Surgical Orthopaedic Advances.* 2013;22:113–117.

Slover J, Abdu WA, Hanscom B, Weinstein JN. The impact of comorbidities on the change in short-form 36 and oswestry scores following lumbar spine surgery. *Spine (Phila Pa 1976).* 1976;31:1974–1980.

Strayer A. Lumbar spine surgery: A guidee to preoperative and postoperative patient care. AANN Reference Series for Clinical Practice. Available: http://www.aann.org/pdf/cpg/aannlumbarspine.

Suri P, Rainville J, Kalichman L, Katz JN. Does this older adult with lower extremity pain have the clinical syndrome of lumbar spinal stenosis? *Journal of the American Medical Association.* 2010;304:2628–2636.

52

ELECTIVE SPINAL SURGERY FOR SCOLIOSIS AND KYPHOSIS

Khoi D. Than, Junichi Ohya, and Praveen V. Mummaneni

Case vignette

A 58-year-old woman status post a previous L3-S1 posterior spinal fusion (with interbody fusion at L4-L5 and L5-S1) presented to clinic with chronic back pain and radicular bilateral lower extremity pain. Her symptoms were mechanical in nature (i.e., worse with standing and better when sitting or supine). Her pain severely limited her activities of daily living (ADLs) to the point where she was unable to walk and was confined to a wheelchair. She treated her pain with narcotics. On neurologic examination, she was normal.

Her preoperative imaging studies included lumbar computed tomography (CT) (Figure 52.1) and scoliosis x-rays (Figure 52.2). Her CT scan demonstrated severe degenerative disc disease (DDD) at L1-L2 and L2-L3. She had a flat-back deformity, with lumbar lordosis (LL) measuring 8°. Her scoliosis films demonstrated right lateral listhesis of L2 on L3, a sagittal vertical axis (SVA) of 8.2 cm, and a pelvic incidence (PI) of 60°.

The patient was taken to the operating room for an extension of her fusion to T11 and ilium with an L3 Schwab grade 4 osteotomy and transforaminal lumbar interbody fusions (TLIFs) at L1-L2 and L3-L4. Postoperatively, she had

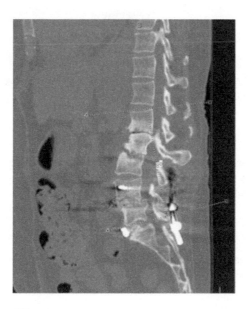

Figure 52.1   Preoperative lumbar CT scan.

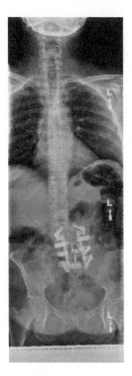 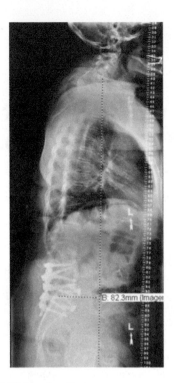

Figure 52.2   Preoperative (a) anteroposterior and (b) lateral scoliosis x-rays.

correction of her lateral listhesis, improvement of her SVA to 4.9 cm, and improvement of her LL to 51° (Figure 52.3). More importantly, she had resumed the ability to walk and stated that her surgery "made me whole again."

Overview

Epidemiology

The reported prevalence of adult scoliosis (defined as a Cobb angle greater than 10°) is as high as 68%. There are several potential causes of scoliosis and kyphosis, including degenerative, postoperative, idiopathic, and secondary to conditions such as ankylosing spondylitis.

Societal significance

Back pain affects 80% of people at some point in their lives. It is a leading cause of disability in the United States and worldwide. Although back pain is multifactorial, it is the most common symptom encountered in patients with adult scoliosis and/or kyphosis and often gets better after appropriate treatment of such conditions.

Basic biologic and physiologic processes

Previous studies have demonstrated that more than one-third of volunteers aged 50–84 years without any scoliosis developed de novo scoliosis during an average follow-up period of 12 years. Risk factors for the development of scoliosis include asymmetric intervertebral disc degeneration, rotatory subluxation, and lateral spondylolisthesis of the L3 vertebra.

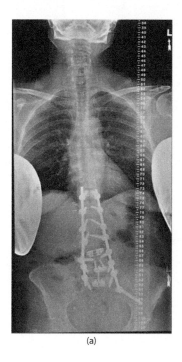
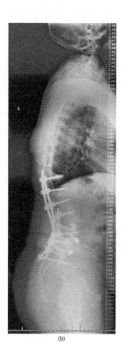

Figure 52.3 Postoperative (a) anteroposterior and (b) lateral scoliosis x-rays.

Anatomical review

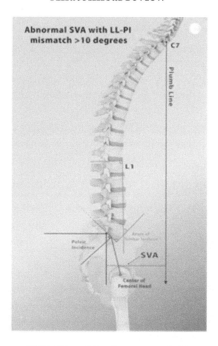

Figure 52.4 Spine with measurement of SVA, PI, and LL demonstrated. (© Ken Probst with permission.)

Common physical examination findings

- *Appearance*: Patients with kyphosis may have an obviously stooped posture. Patients with scoliosis may have an asymmetric tilt to their shoulders or hips. Patients with kyphoscoliosis may have a combination of these features.
- *Motor*: Patients with cervical involvement of their kyphosis/scoliosis may have weakness in any or all muscle groups in the upper and lower extremities. Patients whose kyphosis/scoliosis is thoracic and/or lumbar in location may have weakness in any or all muscle groups in their lower extremities only.
- *Sensory*: Patients may have loss of proprioception and/or sensation to light touch and/or pinprick in their upper extremities (cervical involvement) and/or lower extremities (thoracic and/or lumbar involvement).
- *Reflexes*: Patients may have hyperactive reflexes as a sign of cervical or thoracic myelopathy, or hypoactive reflexes as a sign of nerve root involvement.
- *Gait*: Patients may have difficulty with walking due to their pain (antalgic gait).

Relevant diagnostic tests

1. *Laboratory*: Prior to surgery, patients should have their blood drawn for
   a. Complete blood count (CBC)
   b. Basic metabolic panel (BMP)
   c. Coagulation profile

2. *Vascular/Electrophysiologic:* Rarely, patients may undergo an electromyogram (EMG) for assistance in localizing a motor deficit if it is not obvious on imaging.

3. *Radiologic:* Complete workup frequently includes
   a. Magnetic resonance imaging (MRI), which provides the best visualization of neural structures (spinal cord and nerve roots)
   b. Computed tomography (CT), which provides the best visualization of bony anatomy
   c. Scoliosis x-rays, which allow for measurement of Cobb angles, sagittal balance, and other spino-pelvic parameters
   d. Dual-energy x-ray absorptiometry (DEXA) scans should be obtained on all patients with or suspicion of osteoporosis, as the presence of this condition drastically affects surgical management.

Review of relevant interventional procedures and surgeries

Nonoperative management of sagittal and coronal imbalance can be performed in patients with good functional status and with mild pain. Physical therapy, stretching, and nonsteroidal anti-inflammatory drugs (NSAIDS) are the primary conservative treatment options. Spinal steroid injections may benefit some patients with radicular pain.

Operative treatment is recommended in patients with moderate to severe symptoms, those who fail conservative measures for pain control, and patients with neurologic deficits. Decompression without fusion can be considered in patients without evident instability, without severe sagittal imbalance, and when symptoms are secondary to nerve root compression (i.e., in patients with minimal axial low back pain). Minimally invasive decompressive techniques can be used to decrease blood loss and hospital stay. The main limitations of decompressive techniques are the inabilities to restore sagittal balance and improve axial back pain. There is also a small risk of later instability secondary to decompression.

Anterior approaches may include the ALIF (anterior lumbar interbody fusion) and LLIF (lateral lumbar interbody fusion) techniques. Potential advantages of these approaches may include indirect decompression via expanded foraminal height, as well as avoidance of posterior lumbar muscle trauma. The LLIF technique can also improve coronal spine alignment, especially from L1-L4 levels (the L5-S1 level is limited by the iliac crest), but may require a combined posterior approach. ALIF may have complications such as retrograde ejaculation or vascular injuries. LLIF has some risk of lumbar plexus injuries and rare vascular or bowel injury. In general, anterior spine techniques are useful to restore lumbar lordosis and to provide interbody fusion with indirect nerve root decompression, but most of the time will required a combined posterior approach to achieve normal or near-normal restoration of spino-pelvic measurements.

The majority of spinal deformities are treated by a posterior approach with instrumentation and fusion, with or without an anterior approach. Posterior approaches allow for direct decompression of a stenotic spinal canal or neural foramina. Advantages of the posterior approach include direct decompression, the possibility to perform lumbar interbody fusion using posterior or transforaminal techniques (PLIF or TLIF, respectively), and access to perform spinal osteotomies that can correct coronal and sagittal imbalance.

Osteotomies are used to attain coronal and sagittal deformity correction, especially in rigid deformities. The chosen osteotomy technique may vary according to the degree of correction required to restore sagittal balance. Smith-Petersen osteotomy (SPO) includes resection of the adjacent facet joints, lamina, and ligaments of the involved level and may correct up to 10° of lordosis per level. The pedicle subtraction osteotomy (PSO) consists of resection of the facet joints, lamina, pedicles, and wedge-shaped portion of the vertebral body. Closure of the PSO can result in up to 30° of lordosis correction and significant improvement of sagittal imbalance. The complication potential of PSO compared to SPO is higher, including blood loss and neurologic deficits.

In cases where there is a rigid coronal and sagittal deformity, surgeons can perform a vertebral column resection (VCR), which consists of resection of the vertebral body, adjacent discs, and all the posterior elements of the affected level, resulting in the most significant correction rate of all osteotomies but having a significant risk of new neurologic deficits and blood loss. Experienced deformity surgeons at tertiary care centers typically perform VCR for selected patients with rigid deformities.

Common grading schemes

Table 52.1 Schwab Spinal Osteotomy Classification

Grade	Anatomic resection	Description
1	Partial facet joint	Resection of the inferior facet and joint capsule at a given spinal level
2	Complete facet joint	Both superior and inferior facets at a given spinal segment are resected with complete ligamentum flavum removal; other posterior elements of the vertebra including the lamina and the spinous processes may also be resected
3	Pedicle/partial body	Partial wedge resection of a segment of the posterior vertebral body and a portion of the posterior vertebral elements with pedicles
4	Pedicle/partial body/disc	Wider wedge resection through the vertebral body; includes a substantial portion of the posterior vertebral body, posterior elements with pedicles, and resection of at least a portion of one endplate with the adjacent intervertebral disc
5	Complete vertebra and discs	Complete removal of a vertebra and both adjacent discs (rib resection in the thoracic region)
6	Multiple vertebrae and discs	Resection of more than one entire vertebra and adjacent discs

Family counseling

Prognosis

Prognosis after fusion surgery depends on many factors, but mostly on the number of levels fused. For example, after a minimally invasive one-level fusion, patients can frequently be discharged on postoperative day (POD) 2. Patients who undergo a T4-ilium fusion (14 levels), however, can spend at least one night in the intensive care unit and a week or more in the hospital. Patients who have recovered well and can manage their ADLs can be discharged to home, while patients who are older and/or have undergone bigger surgeries may require some time in acute or subacute rehabilitation. The bony fusion process, and hence patient recovery, can take at least 3 months and as long as 1 year.

Common questions

In addition to length of hospitalization, patients often ask about whether they need to wear a brace, and for how long. Although this is largely practitioner-dependent, our practice is to use a Miami J collar for cervical fusions of three levels or more, Minerva brace or cervical-thoracic orthosis (CTO) for fusions that cross the cervicothoracic junction, and thoracolumbosacral orthosis (TLSO) for fusions that cross the thoracolumbar junction. We generally keep such patients in a brace for 6 weeks.

Patients will also ask when they will be able to return to work; this, too, is dependent on the extent of surgery, the motivation of the patient, and the nature of their employment. Generally, patients are off of work for at least several weeks after surgery.

Pitfalls

One of the biggest pitfalls in the surgical management of adult scoliosis/kyphosis is unrealistic patient expectations. During their surgical consultation, patients should understand that they will still have back pain; the nature of the back pain may be different (i.e., due to the surgery rather than the disease), but it may take some time for the pain to improve as the patient heals. For neurologic symptoms such as motor weakness or sensory disturbances, it is important to not promise patients that these will improve. Generally, we inform patients that the goal of surgery is to keep symptoms from getting worse. Although often these symptoms will actually improve, it is important to not promise this to patients since such improvement is impossible to predict.

Common pitfalls and medicolegal concerns

- *Unnecessary surgery*: Develop a good understanding of surgical decision making for patients with spinal disorders.
- *Wrong-level surgery*: Check and double-check the level while in surgery.
- *Retained foreign bodies*: Check a radiograph prior to leaving the operating room and again prior to discharging the patient from the hospital.

Relevance to the advanced practice health professional

Care providers in neurosurgery must become familiar with patients with spinal disorders. Roughly three-fourths of all neurosurgical cases in the United States involve patients' spines, not their brains. As such, it is beneficial for all neurosurgical providers to thoroughly understand the management of spine patients, from preoperative workup to surgical decision making to postoperative care.

Common phone calls, pages, and requests with answers

Q: This patient had a lumbar fusion yesterday. When can we get her out of bed?

A: Early mobilization is encouraged after spine surgery. Not only does it decrease the risk of certain complications (such as deep venous thrombosis and pressure ulcers), but it also forces patients to be active and begin their route to recovery.

Q: I just had spine surgery and am in a lot of pain. What can I take?

A: Postoperatively, the mainstays of pain management are low-dose narcotics (i.e., hydrocodone, oxycodone) and muscle relaxants (i.e., baclofen, methocarbamol). One useful adjunct is transdermal patches of lidocaine or fentanyl. One medication to avoid, although useful in the preoperative management of back pain, is NSAIDs, as they have been shown to inhibit the bony fusion process.

Q: I had back surgery a few weeks ago and my incision looks a bit red. Should I be concerned?

A: Some incisional erythema is to be expected after surgery. Important information to ask of the patient includes whether the patient has been febrile, whether the redness has been worsening, whether the incision is warm to the touch, and whether the wound has had drainage. If any of these factors are present, the patient should present for attention for suspicion of underlying wound infection.

53

SPINAL TUMORS

Christine Boone, C. Rory Goodwin, Christina Hughes, and Daniel M. Sciubba

Case vignette

A 30-year-old pregnant female with a history of chronic neck and right shoulder pain for 10 years as well as difficulty with ambulation due to right-sided weakness for 4 years. She underwent a lumbar puncture to diagnose suspected influenza meningitis. After the lumbar puncture, the patient had an acute decline in strength, most notably in the right lower extremity. At arrival, she was unable to ambulate with 4/5 strength in her right upper extremity, 1–2/5 strength proximally and 2–3 strength distally in her right lower extremity, and 4+/5 strength in her left upper and lower extremities. She had positive Babinksi and positive Hoffman signs bilaterally, and she reported diffuse sensory loss in the right upper and lower extremities. Contrasted studies and computed tomography (CT) scans were contraindicated due to the pregnancy. Noncontrasted magnetic resonance imaging (MRI) revealed a right-sided intradural extramedullary-extradural lesion with severe spinal cord compression between C1 and C2 and T2 signal changes (Figure 53.1). She was taken for urgent C1 and C2 laminectomies with gross total resection of the tumor and duraplasty. Pathology revealed a cellular nerve sheath tumor with epithelioid and neuroepithelioma-like features and cystic change. She was discharged on postoperative day 5. At that time she had 5/5 strength in all muscle groups and was able to walk without assistance. She quickly weaned off all pain medications but developed postoperative positional headaches. After a discussion about the risks and alternatives to diagnostic imaging for cerebrospinal fluid (CSF) leak, she elected to attempt conservative management with bed rest, caffeine, and muscle relaxers. Postoperative imaging revealed complete resection of the tumor without evidence of recurrence.

Extradural: Metastatic spine tumors

Overview

Epidemiology: The most common tumors in the extradural space (i.e., the bony spine and related structures) are metastatic, arising primarily from breast (16.5%), lung (15.6%), and prostate (9.2%) cancers (Diagnosis and management of metastatic spine disease: A review, 2010). The spine is the most common site of metastasis to the skeleton, which is the third leading site of all metastatic disease. Men have a higher prevalence of lung and prostate cancers, which likely underlies the higher prevalence of metastatic spine tumors in men. The age of greatest incidence of metastatic extradural spine tumors, between 40 and 65 years, overlaps with that of greatest overall cancer risk (Table 53.1) (Diagnosis and management of metastatic spine disease, 2006; Diagnosis and management of metastatic spine disease: A review, 2010).

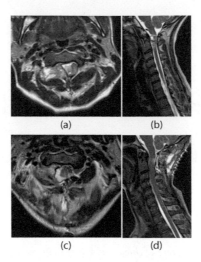

(a)   (b)

(c)   (d)

Figure 53.1 Preoperative (a) axial and (b) sagittal T2-weighted MRI demonstrating a right-sided dumbbell intra-dural extramedullary/extradural lesion with severe spinal cord compression between C1 and C2 and T2 signal changes. Postoperative (c) axial and (d) sagittal T2-weighted MRI demonstrating resection of the lesion with duraplasty.

Societal significance: Prevalence of symptomatic metastatic spine tumors will likely increase as a result of the increasing elderly population and improving cancer treatments (Diagnosis and management of metastatic spine disease. A review, 2010). Metastatic epidural spinal cord compression (MESCC) threatens patients' functional status and mobility, presenting significant societal cost. Treatment of MESCC is cost-effective, valued at nearly $31,000/year of life gained for each patient (Thomas et al., 2006).

Basic biologic and physiologic processes: The mechanism of metastatic spread, hematogenous or CSF seeding and direct extension, is associated with the biology of the primary tumor. The vertebral body is the most common site of these tumors, due to hematogenous spread through the rich blood supply of the vertebral body. Seventy percent of spine metastases emerge within the thoracic segment (Diagnosis and management of metastatic spine disease. A review, 2010).

Anatomical review: The epidural space is the compartment between the spinal canal and dural sheath. The 24 vertebrae of the spine enclose the epidural and subarachnoid spaces. The epidural space is largest in the upper thoracic spine and lumbar spinal cord. The epidural space contains fat, lymphatic structures, loose areolar connective tissue, arteries, venous plexuses, and spinal nerve roots (Fyneface-Ogan, 2012). The most common physical examination finding is pain (Diagnosis and management of metastatic spine disease, 2006; Diagnosis and management of metastatic spine disease A review, 2010) (radicular, mechanical, and local), which is the earliest complaint (83%–95% of patients). Neurologic dysfunction (motor, autonomic, or sensory) from MESCC (Diagnosis and management of metastatic spine disease, 2006; Diagnosis and management of metastatic spine disease A review, 2010) caused by encroaching tumor or bone fragments from pathological fracture, is the second most frequent symptom, and may manifest as abnormalities in gait and ambulation. Sensory dysfunction includes anesthesia, hyperesthesia, and paresthesias. Myelopathy results in sensory abnormalities in strips of areas over the thorax and abdomen. With MESCC of the thoracic spinal cord, patients may describe sensations of constriction around the chest. Autonomic dysfunction most commonly manifests as loss of normal bowel or bladder function.

Table 53.1 Summary by Tumor Type

Compartment	Tumor subtype	Age range, gender predilection	Behavior	Spine location	Presenting symptoms	Physical exam findings	Treatment	Prognosis
Extradural	Metastasis (most common type of spinal tumor)	40–65 years old, male (Diagnosis and management of metastatic spine disease, 2006; Diagnosis and management of metastatic spine disease A review, 2010)	Varies	Thoracic (Diagnosis and management of metastatic spine disease. A review, 2010)	Pain (local, radicular, mechanical), neurological dysfunction, weight loss	Gait impairment, palpable paraspinal mass (Diagnosis and management of metastatic spine disease, 2006; Diagnosis and management of metastatic spine disease A review, 2010)	Surgical resection, radio–, chemo–, pharmacotherapy	Poor, rarely curable
	Chordoma	40–60 years old, male (Ropper et al., 2012)	Malignant, low grade (Ropper et al., 2012; Sundareshan et al., 2009)	Sacrum, cervical (Ropper et al., 2012)	Neck or back pain, neurological deficit, rectal dysfunction (Sundareshan et al., 2009)	Palpable rectal mass	*En bloc* spondylectomy; refractory to radiotherapy	65% disease-free survival rate at 5 years, tendency to relapse later
	Chondrosarcoma	40 years old, male (Ropper et al., 2012)	Malignant, low grade (Ropper et al., 2012; Sundareshan et al., 2009)	Thoracic (Ropper et al., 2012)	Nocturnal pain, neurological deficit, cauda equina syndrome (CES)			Depends on severity of malignancy
	Osteosarcoma	30–60 years old, male (Ropper et al., 2012)	Malignant, high grade (Ropper et al., 2012; Sundareshan et al., 2009)	Sacrum (Ropper et al., 2012)	Indolent nocturnal back pain			Worse prognosis with metastatic disease at onset, larger tumor, sacral location (Sundareshan et al., 2009)

Compartment	Tumor subtype	Age range, gender predilection	Behavior	Spine location	Presenting symptoms	Physical exam findings	Treatment	Prognosis
	Ewing sarcoma	10–30 years old, male (Ropper et al., 2012)	Malignant, high grade (Ropper et al., 2012; Sundareshan et al., 2009)	Sacrum (Ropper et al., 2012)	Pain, local inflammation, fever, weight loss, CES, cord compression	Pelvic or sacral mass	Chemotherapy or radiotherapy	80% of patients relapse within 5 years
	Multiple myeloma/ plasmacytoma	50 years old, male (Ropper et al., 2012)	Malignant, high grade (Ropper et al., 2012; Sundareshan et al., 2009)	Thoracic (Ropper et al., 2012)	Pain, partial leg paralysis, bone fractures, neurologic deficit	Widespread osteoporosis, spinal instability	Chemotherapy and bisphosphonates, surgery for instability	Long-lasting remission, median survival: plasmacytoma—1 year; multiple myeloma—28 months
Intradural extramedullary (second most common type of spinal tumor)	Schwannoma (most common intradural spine tumor) and other neural sheath tumors	40–60 years old, none (Arnautovic and Arnautovic, 2014)	Benign (90%)	Cervical, lumbar	Back pain (nocturnal and localized or radicular) (Arnautovic and Arnautovic, 2014; Abul-Kasim et al., 2007), gradual neurological deficits, impotence (Abul-Kasim et al., 2007)	Brown–Sequard syndrome, Babinski sign, clonus, and hyperreflexia, IESCTs affect all sensory modalities	Surgical resection; postoperative adjuvant chemotherapy and radiotherapy	Good, 10% recurrence rate at 5 years post radical resection
	Meningioma	50–60 years old, women (Arnautovic and Arnautovic, 2014; Chamberlain and Tredway, 2011)	Benign	Thoracic				Good, 7% recurrence rate after total excision

Compartment	Tumor subtype	Age range, gender predilection	Behavior	Spine location	Presenting symptoms	Physical exam findings	Treatment	Prognosis
Intradural intramedullary	Ependymoma (most common)	40–50 years old, male (Koeller et al., 2000)	Benign	Cervical	Nonspecific: Pain (radicular, localized), mixed sensorimotor tract deficits	Dysesthesia, paresthesia, spasticity, torticollis, extremity weakness, Brown–Sequard syndrome, and autonomic dysfunction	Surgical resection or chemo-/radiotherapy (Chamberlain and Tredway, 2011)	Good, median overall survival: 180 months (Chamberlain and Tredway, 2011)
	Low-grade (WHO I-II) versus	Childhood, male (Koeller et al., 2000)	Malignant	Cervical			Biopsy or conservative surgical resection, adjuvant radiotherapy (Chamberlain and Tredway, 2011)	Low grade: Fair, over 70% survival at 5 years (Chamberlain and Tredway, 2011)
	High-grade (WHO III-IV) astrocytoma							High grade: 80% mortality rate within 6 months (Abul-Kasim et al., 2007)

Signs of paraneoplastic syndrome: Signs include weight loss.
Key prognostic factors
Deficits in bladder/bowel function and ambulation

  Palpable paraspinal masses (Diagnosis and management of metastatic spine disease, 2006; Diagnosis and management of metastatic spine disease A review, 2010)

  Presentation depends on systemic tumor spread, amount of bony destruction, extent of neural compression, and tumor growth rate (Diagnosis and management of metastatic spine disease, 2006; Diagnosis and management of metastatic spine disease A review, 2010)

  History remains essential to elicit risk factors (smoking, travel history, exposures, health conditions associated with heightened cancer risk) (Diagnosis and management of metastatic spine disease. A review, 2010)

Relevant diagnostic tests

Table 53.2 presents diagnostic tests and relevant findings.

Table 53.2 Diagnostic Tests and Relevant Findings

Tumor type	Laboratory	Radiologic	Vascular
Extradural metastatic	• Prostate-specific antigen assays (findings: Indicator of prostate cancer) • Blood chemistry, and blood cell counts (findings: Indicators of systemic disease, distinguish from infection)	• Gold standard: MRI with and without contrast (findings: High sensitivity to metastatic disease from high-resolution soft tissue-bone interface) • CT myelography (where MRI contraindicated), (findings: Compression of neural structures) • CT: Visualize osseous anatomy • Whole body positron emission tomography (PET) with fluorodeoxyglucose (FDG) scans: Tumor detection and staging • Radiographs: Detect extensive pathologic abnormalities (low sensitivity)	• CT angiography, MR angiography, or conventional angiography: Examine tumor-associated vasculature, preoperative embolization
Primary Extradural Tumors			
Chordoma	• Histopathology (findings: Large round cells with bubbles in cytoplasm, epithelial membrane antigen, and S-100 positive staining) (Ropper et al., 2012)	• Gold standard: MRI (findings: T1-hypo, T2-hyper, the lobulated structure forms rings and arc pattern with gadolinium enhancement, scalloping of cortical bone) (Ropper et al., 2012) • CT (findings: Sclerotic, lytic lesions)	

Tumor type	Laboratory	Radiologic	Vascular
Chondrosarcoma	• Histopathology (findings: Varies with grade, large or binucleated chondrocytes, greater atypia with higher-grade tumor) (Ropper et al., 2012; Sundareshan et al., 2009)	• Gold standard: MRI, (findings: T2-hyper, the lobulated structure forms rings and arc pattern with gadolinium enhancement (Ropper et al., 2012; Sundareshan et al., 2009) • CT (findings: Lytic lesions, scalloping and expanding bone cortex (Ropper et al., 2012) • Radiograph: (findings: Thickened cortical bone) (Ropper et al., 2012)	
Ewing sarcoma	• Histology (findings: Cells with small, uniform nuclei and indistinct boundaries between them, necrosis indicate worse prognosis) (Ropper et al., 2012; Sundareshan et al., 2009) • Blood chemistry, and blood cell counts (findings: Elevated serum lactic dehydrogenase, a reliable indicator of tumor presence and burden) (Ropper et al., 2012; Sundareshan et al., 2009)	• Radiography: Irregular pattern of bone destruction and moth-eaten, "cracked ice" appearance • CT scan: Detect osteolytic mass or metastases • MRI: T2-iso or -hyper, contrast enhancement with gadolinium (consistent with the tumor's hypercellularity) • Bone scan: Test for metastases	
Plasmacytoma/multiple myeloma	• Blood cell counts, blood chemistries, and serum/urine electrophoresis proteins (findings: Renal failure, infections, hypercalcemia, anemia, or Bence-Jones proteins) (Ropper et al., 2012; Sundareshan et al., 2009) • Bone marrow biopsies (findings: Sheets of plasma cells on histology) (Ropper et al., 2012; Sundareshan et al., 2009)	• CT or MRI. (findings: T2-hyper, T1-hypo) (Sundareshan et al., 2009) (findings: Characteristic lytic lesions with "punched out" appearance)	

Tumor type	Laboratory	Radiologic	Vascular
Intradural Extramedullary Spinal Cord Tumors			
Meningioma/schwannoma		• Gold standard: MRI with and without contrast (findings: T2-hyper, T1-iso or -hypo, enhance with contrast) (Arnautovic and Arnautovic, 2014; Abul-Kasim et al., 2007) • CT myelography (when MRI contraindicated) (Arnautovic and Arnautovic, 2014; Abul-Kasim et al., 2007) • CT scan "bone windows" (Arnautovic and Arnautovic, 2014; Abul-Kasim et al., 2007) • Meningiomas appear as solid, well-circumscribed lesions that rarely become cystic (Chamberlain and Tredway, 2011) • Schwannomas may have cystic changes and hemorrhage within the tumor and appear as focal areas of increased signal in T2-weighted images, often dumbbell shaped (Abul-Kasim et al., 2007)	

Intramedullary Spinal Cord Tumors
• Gold standard: MRI T1-weighted images reveal the solid tumor component, T2-weighted images allow visualization of cystic elements and CSF (Abul-Kasim et al., 2007; Chamberlain and Tredway, 2011)
• Radiographs: Imaging spinal deformity (Abul-Kasim et al., 2007)
• CT-myelography (where MRI contraindicated) (Abul-Kasim et al., 2007)

Tumor type	Laboratory	Radiologic	Vascular
Low-grade versus high-grade astrocytoma	Enlarged, irregularly shaped, hyperchromatic nuclei (Koeller et al., 2000)	• Off-center localization in spinal cord • Heterogeneous contrast enhancing, T1-hypo or -iso, T2-hyper	
Ependymoma	Histology: Uniform, moderately hyperchromatic nuclei and perivascular pseudorosettes (Koeller et al., 2000)	• Central localization in spinal cord • Homogeneous contrast enhancing, T1-hypo or -iso, T2-hyper • Cystic changes, syrinx, and evidence of hemorrhage (Chamberlain and Tredway, 2011)	

Abbreviations: CT, computed tomography; MRI, magnetic resonance imaging; T1-hyper, T1-weighted hyperintense; T1-hypo, T1-weighted hypointense; T1-iso, T1-weighted isointense; T2-hyper, T2-weighted hyperintense; T2-hypo, T2-weighted hypointense; T2-iso, T2-weighted isointense, CSF, cerebrospinal fluid.

Review of relevant interventional procedures and surgeries

Metastatic spine tumor surgery is most often a palliative measure. Because few cases can be cured, the goals of intervention center on neurologic function maintenance, mechanical stabilization, and pain alleviation. As many as 50% of spinal metastases necessitate treatment; however, surgery is deemed appropriate in only 5%–10% of these (Diagnosis and management of metastatic spine disease. A review, 2010).

Nonsurgical management strategies include radiation therapy, pharmacotherapy, and minimally invasive procedures. Radiation treatment can address each of the aforementioned goals of therapy. Pharmacotherapy may directly target the tumor or its secondary effects, although spinal metastases are generally refractory to tumoricidal drugs. Chemotherapy agents may be employed preoperatively to improve surgical outcomes. Spine metastases of breast or prostate origin may respond to hormone therapies, but this is not dependent on the sensitivities of the primary tumor. Analgesics, corticosteroids, and osteoclastic activity inhibitors can help relieve local pain. Minimally invasive procedures, vertebro- and kyphoplasty, also provide pain relief but are not effective to relieve compression or instability (Diagnosis and management of metastatic spine disease. A review, 2010) (Figure 53.2a–d).

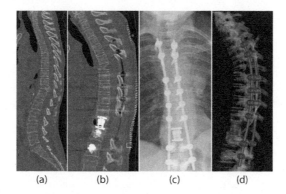

(a)   (b)   (c)   (d)

Figure 53.2 A 68-year-old female with a history of metastatic lung cancer who presents with 3-month history of back pain and inability to walk for 2 days. (a) Sagittal CT scan demonstrating pathologic compression fractures at T6 and T11. (b) The patient underwent T6 laminectomy, and T11 corpectomy with anterior cage reconstruction and T4-L1 instrumented fusion with placement of cement at T12 and L1. The patient has four lumbar vertebrae. (c) Anteroposterior x-ray and (d) 3D CT reconstruction demonstrating instrumented fusion and anterior reconstruction.

Surgery is the best option to obtain optimal resection, decompression, and stabilization. Factors considered for surgical candidacy include functional status (the best predictor of neurologic function after surgery) (Diagnosis and management of metastatic spine disease. A review, 2010), age, life expectancy (minimum of 3 months), systemic disease extent, and tumor resistance to adjuvant treatment (Donthineni, 2009).

Common grading schemes

There are several major systems of metastatic spine tumor classification; the Tomita and revised Tokuhashi schemes are considered the most functional for practical application (Choi et al., 2010). The Tomita prognostic scoring system (see Table 53.3) gives points for features corresponding to primary tumor, visceral metastasis, and bone metastasis (including to the spine) and then the points are summed. The prognostic score ranges from 2, which suggests treatment with the goal of long-term local control by surgical excision would be optimal, to 10, indicating a treatment objective of terminal care through supportive methods (Tomita et al., 2001). The Tokuhashi system uses primary tumor type, number of spine metastases, number of extraspinal bone metastases, presence of visceral metastases, overall functional status, and neurologic status of the patient to determine prognosis. Higher scores indicate better prognosis and longer life expectancy (Tokuhashi et al., 2014).

Extradural: Primary spine tumors

Table 53.3 Tomita Prognostic Scoring System

Prognostic features	0 Point	1 Point	2 Points	4 Points
Primary tumor grade	N/A	Indolent growing (breast, prostate, thyroid)	Moderate growing (kidney, uterus)	Rapidly growing (lung, liver, stomach, colon)
Visceral metastasis	None	N/A	Treatable	Untreatable
Bone metastasis	N/A	Single or isolated	Multiple	N/A

Source: Tomita K, *Spine,* 26, 298–306, 2001.

Overview

Epidemiology: Primary spinal tumors are relatively rare, comprising fewer than 10% of neoplasms arising in the bony spine. Chordoma is the most common tumor found in the sacrum. Chondrosarcoma accounts for 7%–12% of all primary spine tumors. Ewing sarcoma is the most common malignant extradural primary spine tumor in children, while plasmacytoma is the most common in adults. Family history of retinoblastoma, adolescence, and ionizing radiation exposure are among risk factors associated with primary spine tumors (Ropper et al., 2012; Sundareshan et al., 2009).

Basic biologic and physiologic processes: Chordoma arise from the remains of the notochord in vertebral bodies. Chondrosarcoma may form *de novo* or transform from existing osteosarcoma. The *de novo* lesion is indolent and low grade. Ewing sarcoma is a small round cell neoplasm thought to arise from a neural progenitor cell that frequently metastasizes. Over 90% of Ewing sarcoma tumor cells express an abnormal fusion protein leading to the production of chimeric transcription factors that promote tumor progression. Plasmacytomas/multiple myelomas are cancers of the lymphoreticular system, and within the spine they are most frequently found in the vertebral body.

Anatomical review

See previous "Anatomical Review" in the section "Extradural: Metastatic Spine Tumors."

Relevant diagnostic tests

There are a variety of primary tumor types, despite their rarity; therefore, histopathological analysis is crucial to determining tumor type, which is essential for determining optimal treatment and prognosis (Table 53.2) (Ropper et al., 2012; Sundareshan et al., 2009).

Review of relevant interventional procedures and surgeries

Treatment options include surgery, radiotherapy, and chemotherapy. Total *en bloc* resection of primary spinal column neoplasms with wide surgical margins and intact tumor capsule is ideal. The gold standard treatment for primary osseous tumors is *en bloc* spondylectomy. This management strategy requires a multidisciplinary team including thoracic surgery, orthopedic surgery, general surgery, vascular surgery, and plastic surgery, and is best undertaken by surgeons with experience in the technique (Sundareshan et al., 2009).

Adjuvant chemotherapy and radiotherapy can help prevent local recurrence. In primary tumor types that are refractory to conventional radiation treatment, osteosarcomas and chondrosarcomas, particle beam treatment may hold promise (Sundareshan et al., 2009). Surgical stabilization or decompression is indicated in situations of spinal instability or deformity. Minimally invasive techniques, kyphoplasty and vertebroplasty, are good options for pain treatment (Diagnosis and management of metastatic spine disease. A review, 2010; Ropper et al., 2012).

Common grading schemes

The most important prognostic factors for primary spine tumors include tumor histopathology, location or extent of invasion or bony destruction, size, and histologic grade (Table 53.4). The Primary Spinal Tumor Mortality Score (PSTMS) system was developed to predict poor outcomes. The total scores are categorized as follows: 0–2 points is a low mortality prognosis, 3–4 is medium, and 5–8 is high. In the PSTMS study, the estimated survival of low mortality was 96%, medium was 73%, and high was 10% at 5 years (Szövérfi et al., 2014).

Table 53.4 Primary Spinal Tumor Mortality Score (PSTMS)

Variables	0 Point	1 Point	2 Points	3 Points
Age	Under 55 y	At least 55 y		
Spinal region	Mobile spine	Sacrum		
Tumor grade	Benign	Low-grade malignancy	High-grade malignancy	Distant metastases
Spinal pain	Absent	Present		
Motor deficit	Absent	Present		
Myelopathy/CES	Absent	Present		

Source: Szövérfi Z et al., *Spine J*, 14, 2691-2700, 2014.

Intradural extramedullary spinal cord tumors (IESCTs)

Overview

Epidemiology: The second most common type of spinal tumor; the annual incidence is 0.4 per 100,000 people (Arnautovic and Arnautovic, 2014). Schwannomas represent 30% of intradural tumors and over 85% of IESCTs. Meningiomas are the second most common IESCT type. Neurofibromatosis II (NF-II) patients are predisposed to developing schwannomas and meningiomas, and multiple lesions (Abul-Kasim et al., 2007; Chamberlain and Tredway, 2011). Intradural metastases are very rare and are often due to CSF seeding (Chamberlain and Tredway, 2011; Diagnosis and management of metastatic spine disease. A review, 2010).

Basic biologic and physiologic processes: The majority of tumors are benign; nevertheless, they most commonly cause significant neurologic dysfunction due to compression of neural structures. Intradural primary tumors are derived from perineural coverings of nerve roots or from the meninges (Abul-Kasim et al., 2007). Schwannomas originate from the nerve roots in the dorsal sensory region of the cervical and lumbar spine. Meningiomas most commonly arise in the thoracic segment, possibly from dural or pial fibroblasts (Abul-Kasim et al., 2007).

Anatomical review

Intradural extramedullary space: This is located inside of the dural sheath, but outside of the actual spinal cord.

Relevant diagnostic tests

Table 53.2 presents diagnostic tests and relevant findings.

Review of relevant interventional procedures and surgeries

The goals of surgery are total tumor resection with preservation or improvement of neurological function. Attaining these goals depends on factors dictating the surgical approach, such as location within the intradural compartment and extent of neural structure involvement (Abul-Kasim et al., 2007). Partial resection may be appropriate in cases where neurologic compromise is unavoidable, often when a mass encompasses neural structures. This decision is individualized to the patient (Chamberlain and Tredway, 2011).

Nonsurgical therapies, including adjuvant chemotherapy and radiotherapy for susceptible tumors, may be appropriate postoperatively to reduce the risk of local recurrence. Radiosurgery can also be employed in cases of multiple lesions, malignant schwannoma (postoperative), and an absence of compressive myelopathy. Benign schwannoma may be managed conservatively (Chamberlain and Tredway, 2011).

In 2007, the World Health Organization (WHO) created a grading scheme for central nervous system tumors (Table 53.5) (Louis et al., 2007) that serves as a standard among clinicians across disciplines (Abul-Kasim et al., 2007).

Intramedullary spinal cord tumors (IMSCTs)

Overview

Epidemiology: Approximately 6%–8% of central nervous system tumors are IMSCTs. Ependymomas is the most common type of IMSCT. Astrocytomas make up 40% of IMSCTs, and three-quarters of these are low grade (Abul-Kasim et al., 2007; Chamberlain and Tredway, 2011).

Basic biologic and physiologic processes

Ependymomas arise from the ependymal cells lining the central canal of the spinal cord, a remnant of the embryonic ventricular structure. These tumors tend to displace nervous tissue in the cord, while astrocytic tumors are inclined to infiltrate nervous tissue, which makes these lesions poorly circumscribed (Koeller et al., 2000).

Anatomical review

Imaging is essential to identifying the tumor compartment (i.e., intramedullary versus extramedullary).

Review of relevant interventional procedures and surgeries

The approach to surgical resection varies with tumor type and characteristics. Due to their ill-defined borders, surgical treatment may be limited to the safest extent. Complete resection is seldom feasible. In some cases, the lesion is only biopsied and may be treated with radiotherapy as well (Chamberlain and Tredway, 2011). When the tumor is necrotic (high-grade astrocytoma) or an accessible tissue plane exists between the tumor and spinal cord (low-grade astrocytoma), the tumor can be separated from the healthy parenchyma with suction. Ependymomas usually have a clear tumor–spinal cord parenchymal border, which facilitates *en bloc* resection. Ependymomas can be completely excised and cured with a low risk of recurrence. The patient's neurological status may be tracked with electrophysiological monitoring during the procedure (Abul-Kasim et al., 2007).

Histologic grade and preoperative neurologic function are the most significant prognostic factors for surgical management of intramedullary spinal cord tumors. Generally, ependymomas have an excellent prognosis. High-grade astrocytomas present a poor prognosis and high mortality rate within months of diagnosis (Abul-Kasim et al., 2007; Chamberlain and Tredway, 2011).

Table 53.5 Abbreviated 2007 WHO Intradural Spinal Tumor Classification System

Tumor type	Schwannoma	Meningioma	Low-grade/High-grade astrocytoma	Ependymoma
Grade	I	I	I-II/III-IV	II

Source: Louis DN et al., *Acta Neuropathol.*, 114, 97–109, 2007.

Family counseling

In general, counseling patients with spinal tumors requires careful and open communication among physicians, patients, and caregivers. Shared decision making between these parties is key to determining the best management based on medical evidence relevant to the diagnosis and patient preferences (Diagnosis and management of metastatic spine disease. A review. 2010; Schairer et al., 2014; Csaszar et al., 2009). In IESCTs, where complete resection without neurological compromise is often impossible, partial resection is the best option. Decisions regarding the extent of resection are multifactorial and determined by patient age, neurologic status at presentation, tumor histopathology and size, and predisposition to local recurrence, such as a medical history of neurofibromatosis, in addition to the patient's concerns. Potential challenges in counseling relate to the patient's functional status, pain management, and communicating effectively with the patient.

Many patients with spinal tumors are concerned with having their normal function. They particularly want to regain or maintain ambulation (Csaszar et al., 2009; Abrahm et al., 2008). This may drive them to be overly optimistic about their condition and deny symptoms. Additionally, patients' postoperative functional status is strongly related to their preoperative function and timing of treatment after the onset of cord compression symptoms (Abrahm et al., 2008; Patchell et al., 2005). Setting expectations for patients and caregivers of postoperative function based on these preoperative factors is important.

Pain management in spine tumor patients is complex. It may arise through mechanisms related to the pathophysiology of the tumor, such as compression of foraminal stenosis in metastases or fractures from osteolytic primary tumors. The patients' emotional or psychological state can also generate or enhance pain. Effectively identifying and managing pain is difficult but vital in caring for spinal tumor patients (Csaszer et al., 2009).

Communication is vital to providing patients with the knowledge and support they need to cope and make decisions; however, it also presents opportunities for mistakes, especially with regard to language. It has been noted that a diagnosis of cancer, and particularly use of the word, "tumor," can trigger thoughts of death and even a hypnotic state in some patients. This state leads to enhanced anxiety, irritability, and reduced attention. Careful word choice is a necessary part of the communication strategy. Caregivers should also be counseled in methods of communication (Csaszer et al., 2009).

Common questions

The diagnosis of spinal cord tumor incites a multitude of questions in patients. They may ask about treatment options, timelines to undergo treatments, risks of treatment, expected functional status and pain before and after treatment, frequency of recurrence, and long-term outcome. They may also ask about how to prepare for the procedure, how to identify a spine surgeon, and costs of treatment with or without insurance.

Medicolegal concerns

- Delayed diagnosis and/or treatment of spinal cord compression is linked to decreased survival, mobility, and normal genitourinary function (Abrahm et al., 2008).
- The first sign of a spine tumor is back pain, a common and nonspecific chief complaint, to which patients and health-care providers may not attend.
- Prognosis worsens once the more specific and alarming signs of neurological dysfunction occur.

- This is a common issue in metastatic spine tumor patients. A history of cancer or conditions increasing cancer risk in a patient presenting with back pain, especially in the thoracic region, must be approached with a high suspicion of metastatic disease.
- While there is evidence that preoperative function predicts a better postoperative outcome, there is insufficient data to determine the appropriate time course of diagnosis or treatment of these spinal tumors.

Relevance to the advanced practice health professional

The patients that suffer from spinal lesions often experience significant physical impairments and immense pain. There will be challenging logistics to coordinate, need for psychosocial and physical support, and a large interdisciplinary team. Their gratitude for your compassionate care and expertise will make them some of the most rewarding patients to treat. Develop relationships with members of your institution's oncology service, therapy department, and ancillary care services (home nursing, case managers, social workers, and pastoral care). Communication within the team is crucial to providing effective, efficient care for these patients. Outcomes will vary greatly depending on the location, extent, and pathology of the lesion. It is important to promote a positive attitude while, at the same time, providing realistic expectation. Many patients feel lost amid a team of medical experts without a point of contact or continuity of care. Surgical providers are often the first contact the patient has with the medical team. The roll of the surgical midlevel will be to coordinate care and facilitate communication while the patient establishes relationships with the other members of the team.

Common phone calls, pages, and requests

1. *Does the patient need chemotherapy and/or radiation? What is the timeline for treatment?*

    The patient's need for adjunctive therapy will be based on the results of the pathology, taking into consideration the patient's goals and desires. It is important to discuss the goals of therapy and the side effects. This conversation will require the oncologist and may be best facilitated with a social worker or case manager. A general rule of thumb is that no chemotherapy or radiation should be initiated until at least 2 weeks after surgery in order to allow the surgical incision to heal and the body to recover.

    Although the oncologist will determine the treatment plan after surgery, the patient and family will often look to the surgical team for guidance. The surgical practitioners are often the first providers the patient has contact with during the battle with the disease. It is important to communicate with all members of the patient's medical team throughout the therapy in order to effectively and efficiently treat the disease.

2. *What follow-up is needed with the surgical team?*

    Care for the surgical incision is the first step during follow-up. Inspection of the wound and removal of staples or sutures may occur during the hospitalization or may require an office visit 10–14 days after surgery. Patients should have an opportunity to check in with the surgical team 2–4 weeks after discharge from the hospital to review the pathology findings and the oncologist's plan. Long-term follow-up will be determined by the institution's policies and the primary service caring for the patient. Surveillance may be performed by the surgical team or the oncologic team.

3. *Will assistive devices be required, and if so, how are they obtained?*

    The need for ambulatory assistive devices (e.g., walkers, canes, or wheelchairs), medical equipment (e.g., hospital beds or shower chairs), and bracing (e.g. cervical collars or thoracolumbosacral orthotics) will be determined on a case-by-case basis, often in conjunction with therapy services and case managers. Bracing should be obtained immediately after surgery if it is required for stabilization. Prescriptions will be required for most equipment and should be provided by the primary surgical team in order to expedite delivery. It is also important to coordinate catheter supplies, tracheostomy/ respiratory care, and nutritional needs prior to discharging the patient from the hospital. Contact your home health team, case manager, and social worker for assistance establishing services.

4. *Will rehabilitation be required?*

Most patients will benefit from a period of supervised, in-patient rehabilitation following surgical resection. Managing expectations and preparing patients for an extended period away from home will help them to establish social support and make the necessary financial arrangements prior to surgery. It is often easier for patients to transition back to home earlier rather than remain away from home longer than expected.

5. *What medications should be administered during hospitalization and dispensed prior to discharge?*

All patients should receive perioperative antibiotics; the need for long-term antibiotics will be determined by the surgeon. Perioperative steroids may help alleviate symptoms associated with edema. These should be continued postoperatively at the discretion of the surgeon in conjunction with the oncologist. Long-term anticoagulation should be considered for nonambulatory patients in order to prevent venous thrombosis and in any patient with hypercoagulopathy.

The medical team should closely monitor pain medications. It is important to counsel patients on pain medication side effects and abuse potential and to provide education on ways to differentiate the types of pain they may experience. Many oncology patients benefit from extended release formulations. Neuropathic pain responds well to the anticonvulsant class of medications, which includes drugs such as gabapentin and pregabalin. Postoperative muscular pain should be managed with muscle relaxers. Incisional pain may respond to transdermal anesthetic patches. Medications may need to be replaced intermittently to prevent tolerance. As always, pay close attention to potential interactions, as many of these patients will require a polypharmacy during their treatment.

6. *What symptoms or issues necessitate urgent evaluation?*

It is important that the patient, the patient's loved ones, and patient care staff are aware of the signs that should prompt an immediate phone call. As with any spinal condition, progressive weakness, numbness, bowel/bladder incontinence, urinary retention, and intractable pain should be evaluated immediately. After surgery, fevers/chills/sweats, erythema, edema, warmth, fluctuance and/or dehiscence at the surgical site, dizziness/loss of consciousness, shortness of breath, and swelling/pain/ redness in the lower extremities also warrant immediate evaluation. The surgical site will dictate additional concerns. If the lesion is in the cervical region, it is important to monitor for respiratory compromise and esophageal dysfunction. Thoracic lesions that require a lateral approach should be monitored for pneumothorax and hemothorax. Lumbar lesions that require an anterior approach should be monitored for intraperitoneal bleeding as well as ureteral and vascular compromise.

References

Abrahm JL, Banffy MB, Harris MB. Spinal cord compression in patients with advanced metastatic cancer: "All I care about is walking and living my life." *JAMA.* 2008;299(8):937–937. doi:10.1001/jama.299.8.937.

Abul-Kasim K, Thurnher MM, McKeever P, Sundgren PC. Intradural spinal tumors: current classification and MRI features. *Neuroradiology.* 2007;50(4):301–301. doi:10.1007/s00234-007-0345-7.

Arnautovic A, Arnautovic KI. Extramedullary intradural spinal tumors. *Contemp Neurosurg.* 2014;36(5):1–1. doi:10.1097/01.CNE.0000448459.65797.ce.

Chamberlain MC, Tredway TL. Adult primary intradural spinal cord tumors: a review. *Curr Neurol Neurosci Rep.* 2011;11(3):320–320. doi:10.1007/s11910-011-0190-2.

Choi D, Crockard A, Bunger C, et al. Review of metastatic spine tumour classification and indications for surgery: the consensus statement of the Global Spine Tumour Study Group. *Eur Spine J.* 2010;19(2):215–215. doi:10.1007/ s00586-009-1252-x.

Csaszar N, Ganju A, Mirnics ZS, Varga PP. Psychosocial issues in the cancer patient. *Spine*. 2009;34(Suppl 22):S26–S30. doi:10.1097/BRS.0b013e3181b95c55.

Diagnosis and management of metastatic spine disease. 2006;15(3):141–141. doi:10.1016/j.suronc.2006.11.002.

Diagnosis and management of metastatic spine disease. *A review.* 2010;13(1):94–94. doi:10.3171/2010.3.SPINE09202.

Donthineni R. Diagnosis and staging of spine tumors. *Orthop Clin North Am*. 2009;40(1):1–7–v. doi:10.1016/j.ocl.2008.10.001.

Fyneface-Ogan S. Anatomy and clinical importance of the epidural space. In: *Epidural Analgesia - Current Views and Approaches.* InTech; 2012. doi:10.5772/39091.

Koeller KK, Rosenblum RS, Morrison AL. Neoplasms of the spinal cord and filum terminale: radiologic-pathologic correlation. *Radiographics*. 2000;20(6):1721–1721. doi:10.1148/radiographics.20.6.g00nv151721.

Louis DN, Ohgaki H, Wiestler OD et al. The 2007 WHO classification of tumours of the central nervous system. *Acta Neuropathol*. 2007;114(2):97–97. doi:10.1007/s00401-007-0243-4.

Patchell RA, Tibbs PA, Regine WF et al. Direct decompressive surgical resection in the treatment of spinal cord compression caused by metastatic cancer: a randomised trial. *Lancet*. 2005;366(9486):643–643. doi:10.1016/S0140-6736(05)66954-1.

Ropper AE, Cahill KS, Hanna JW, McCarthy EF, Gokaslan ZL, Chi JH. Primary vertebral tumors: a review of epidemiologic, histological and imaging findings, part II: locally aggressive and malignant tumors. *Neurosurgery*. 2012;70(1):211219–discussion219. doi:10.1227/NEU.0b013e31822d5f17.

Schairer WW, Carrer A, Sing DC et al. Hospital readmission rates after surgical treatment of primary and metastatic tumors of the spine. *Spine*. 2014;39(21):1801–1801.

Sundaresan N, Rosen G, Boriani S. Primary malignant tumors of the spine. *Orthop Clin North Am*. 2009;40(1):21–21. doi:10.1016/j.ocl.2008.10.004.

Szövérfi Z, Lazary A, Bozsódi Á, Klemencsics I, Éltes PE, Varga PP. Primary spinal tumor mortality score (PSTMS): a novel scoring system for predicting poor survival. *Spine J*. 2014;14(11):2691–2691. doi:10.1016/j.spinee.2014.03.009.

Thomas KC, Nosyk B, Fisher CG et al. Cost-effectiveness of surgery plus radiotherapy versus radiotherapy alone for metastatic epidural spinal cord compression. *Int J Radiat Oncol Biol Phys*. 2006;66(4):1212–1212. doi:10.1016/j.ijrobp.2006.06.021.

Tokuhashi Y, Uei H, Oshima M, Ajiro Y. Scoring system for prediction of metastatic spine tumor prognosis. *World J Orthop*. 2014;5(3):262–262. doi:10.5312/wjo.v5.i3.262.

Tomita K, Kawahara N, Kobayashi T, Yoshida A, Murakami H, Akamaru T. Surgical strategy for spinal metastases. *Spine*. 2001;26(3):298–298.

54

POSTOPERATIVE MULTIMODAL ORAL PAIN MANAGEMENT IN THE SPINE PATIENT

Andrea L. Strayer

Postoperative pain management in the spine patient is challenging. Patient expectations, preoperative pain severity, medication use, and social support may all contribute to the postoperative pain experience by a patient. Additionally, the front-line bedside nurses' knowledge about pain and their workload may affect the patients' pain experience. Pain management requires frequent assessment and a high level of critical decision making regarding interventions to be employed. This includes making informed choices regarding pharmacologic and nonpharmacologic pain management options that are available—or should be requested and are safe for that particular patient who has undergone a certain operative procedure. This is quite challenging.

Overview of pain physiology

Pain is subjective, perceived by an individual. Different types of nociceptors—free nerve endings that detect stimuli to be interpreted as pain—are located throughout the body.

- Mechanical nociceptors are supplied by myelinated, fast-conducting A δ afferent nerve fibers.
- These fibers have a low threshold for activation (Lai et al., 2012, p. 349).
- Chemical, cold/hot, and high-intensity mechanical nociceptors are conducted on unmyelinated, slow C fibers (Lai et al., 2012, p. 349).

Tissue injury causes a cascade of events (Figure 54.1), including

- Release of inflammatory mediators
- Vasodilation
- Nociceptor activation

Nociceptor activation travels via peripheral receptors to the spinal cord dorsal horn. In the dorsal horn, neurons communicate with ultimate transmission to the central nervous system, synapsing in the thalamus, and then to the somatosensory cortex (Lai et al., 2012).

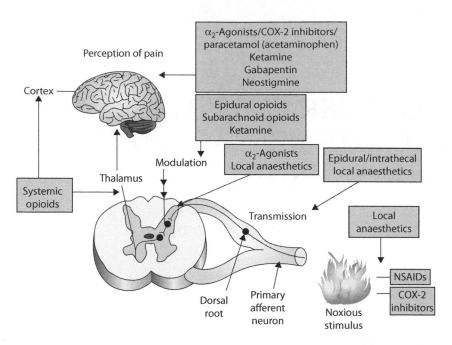

Figure 54.1 Action of analgesic at various sites of the pain pathway. (COX = cyclooxygenase.) (From Pyati S, Gan TJ. *CNS Drugs*, 21, 2007.)

Overview of peripheral and central sensitization

Activation of a cascade of events as described above leads to peripheral and central sensitization of nociceptive pathways (Figure 54.2):

Peripheral sensitization occurs from various substances from injured cells, nociceptors, enhanced capillary permeability, and generation by local enzyme activity.

Peripheral sensitization can enhance the pain responses in the central nervous system (CNS):

- Facilitates nociceptive transmission
- Leads to release of mediators within dorsal horn
- Causes neural plasticity changes with central sensitization
- Can lead to persistent postop or chronic pain

The potential of unrelieved or inadequately managed acute postsurgical pain is real. The development of persistent or chronic pain is an underrecognized problem for the postoperative spine patient who does not have adequate pain control.

The impact of pain on patients includes the following (Oderda, 2012, p. 7S; Wells et al., 2008, Chapter 17):

- Intense postsurgical pain increases the risk of developing chronic pain.
- Immunosuppression from unrelieved pain slows wound healing, delays recovery, and increases the risk of postsurgical infection.
- Sympathetic activation may predispose patients to adverse events, such as cardiac ischemia or ileus.
- Psychological impact may lead to anxiety and depression.

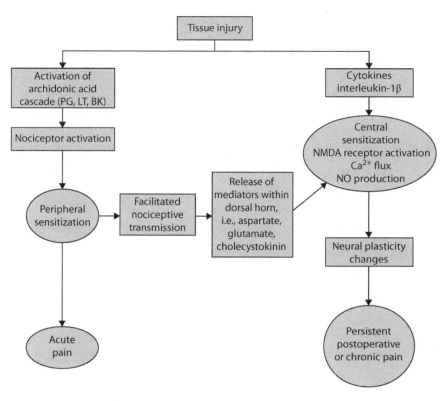

Figure 54.2 Mechanisms of peripheral and central sensitization. (BK = bradykinin; LT = leukotrienes; NO = nitric oxide; PG = prostaglandins.) (From Pyati S, Gan TJ. *CNS Drugs*, 21, 2007.)

Delayed ambulation may increase the risk of thromboembolic events and pneumonia, and delay discharge.

The patient experience may negatively affect hospital performance due to:

- Poor patient satisfaction (negative impact on reputation)
- Extended length of stay
- Increased risk of readmission
- Increased cost of care
- Increased risk of legal action

Potential financial costs are high. Thirty-day unplanned readmissions after lumbar surgery were found to be pain related in 22.4% of cases, with only wound infection more frequent at 38.6% (Pugely et al., 2014, p. 762).

Multimodal pain management

Multimodal pain management following spine surgery entails treatment directed toward a variety of sources of pain. Preemptive pain management is the pretreatment of pain, to eliminate or decrease hypersensitivity of the nociceptors. Following is a description of multimodal and preemptive pain management concepts and typical medication options.

Multimodal pain management principles

Multimodal pain management's goal is to treat postoperative pain from both peripheral and central sources, utilizing a combination of medications with the goal to decrease and minimize opioid use. By providing analgesia for postoperative pain that targets, for example, nociceptive, neuropathic, and musculoskeletal sources, the patient experiences improved pain control.

Preemptive pain management

Preemptive pain management (or preemptive analgesia) is a subconcept of multimodal pain management. Proponents of preemptive analgesia report increased postoperative pain relief and decreased opioid consumption by pretreating the patient and preventing the postoperative pain cascade of events that takes place.

Preemptive analgesia inhibits central autonomic hypersensitivity. Central hypersensitivity, as noted previously, can lead to peripheral sensitization and increased and even uncontrolled pain. Central autonomic hypersensitivity can lead to hyperalgesia from opioid use.

The type and route of preemptive analgesics utilized vary. However, the goals to fullfil the concepts of multimodal pain management are the same.

Kim and coauthors evaluated preemptive multimodal analgesia with celecoxib, pregabalin, extended-release oxycodone, and acetaminophen compared to intravenous morphine in a randomized controlled trial. The visual analogue scale was statistically significant, with scores less than control at all points after surgery. This included postanesthesia care unit; 8 hours postoperative; and then 1, 2, 3, 4, and 7 days postoperative (Kim et al., 2016).

Rajpal et al. compared perioperative oral multimodal pain management with intravenous patient-controlled anesthesia in a pre- and postintervention trial. Patients received gabapentin, acetaminophen, and long-acting oxycodone approximately 60 minutes prior to surgery and postoperatively long- and short-acting oxycodone, gabapentin, and acetaminophen. The authors found significantly less opioid consumption, lower ratings of "least pain," and patients experienced less nausea, drowsiness, interference with walking, and coughing/deep breathing (Rajpal et al., 2010).

A comprehensive assessment of the best evidence currently available for multimodal pain management after spine surgery was completed by Devin and McGirt (2015). Their evaluation is a valuable synopsis of available data.

Multimodal drugs

Acetaminophen (also known as paracetamol or APA)

The mechanism of action is not fully understood but is thought to be inhibition of cyclooxygenase (COX), predominantly COX-2. It lacks strong anti-inflammatory qualities. Also of note, a risk of hepatotoxicity exists, and any history of liver disease should be considered when prescribing.

Nonsteroidal anti-inflammatory drugs

Nonsteroidal anti-inflammatory drugs (NSAIDs) work peripherally to decrease inflammation through inhibition of the enzymes that synthesize prostaglandins. There are two types of COX inhibitors, COX-1 and COX-2. More specifically, COX acts on arachidonic acid, resulting in the synthesis of prostaglandins. COX-1 protects the gastric mucosa and plays a role in vascular hemostasis. COX-2 seems to be the major source of prostaglandins during inflammation and chronic disease (Lai et al., 2012). NSAIDs also decrease pain by central as well as peripheral mechanisms. The central mechanism may be interference with the formation of prostaglandins within the CNS; however, other theories have been postulated.

Gabapentinoids

Gabapentin and pregabalin bind to the α-2-delta subunit of N-type voltage-gated calcium channels. Here they inhibit neurotransmitter release and thus reduce excitatory neurotransmission, decreasing central hypersensitivity (Devin and McGirt, 2015, p. 934).

Yu and colleagues in a meta-analysis noted both gabapentin and pregabalin to reduce postoperative pain and opioid requirements after lumbar spine surgery (Yu et al., 2013, p. 1949–1950). Also noting positive benefit from clinical trial review, Dunn et al. (2016, p. 85) noted decreased opioid consumption and pain postoperatively, possibly improving functional status. As noted by all authors, larger trials with complex spine surgery are needed.

Opioids

The opioid mechanism of action is to bind to receptors (m and k) in the central nervous system—the brainstem, hypothalamus, limbic system, and substantia gelatinosa of the spinal cord, as well as peripherally in the gastrointestinal (GI) tract and peripheral histamine response (Lai et al., 2012, p. 352), causing reduced pain perception as well as a patient's reaction to pain. They also cause an increase in pain tolerance. The specific sites that opioids bind to can also cause adverse effects such as cognitive blunting and respiratory depression in the CNS. In the periphery, GI effects include nausea and vomiting and constipation as well as urinary retention.

Opioid-related adverse drug events

Commonly reported are urinary retention and GI and CNS disturbances. More vulnerable patient populations include anyone with comorbid conditions, age extremes, reduced hepatic or renal metabolism, and polypharmacy (Oderda, 2012).

Tramadol

Tramadol is weak mu-opioid receptor agonist, thus not exhibiting the GI or sedation side effects of traditional opioids. It releases serotonin and inhibits the reuptake of norepinephrine (Lai et al., 2012, p. 353). It may decrease the seizure threshold.

Alpha-2 receptor agonists

Clonidine and dexmedetomidine are α-2 receptor agonists, working at the spinal and supraspinal sites to provide analgesia. Dexmedetomidine provides sedation and analgesia without respiratory depression; however, this class of drugs may provide opioid-sparing effects (Dunn et al., 2016, p. 8384).

NMDA receptor antagonists

NMDA (*N*-methyl D-aspartate) receptor antagonists include ketamine, methadone, dextromethorphan, and magnesium. Their effects include prevention of central hypersensitization and reduction of opioid-induced hyperalgesia as well as opioid tolerance (Dunn, 2016, p. 82).

Common pitfalls

Every patient reacts to pain and the management of their pain differently. Thus, while protocol/guidelines are developed in any particular practice, management needs to be tailored to each individual patient. Management will require frequent evaluation and adjustment to meet that patient's needs.

Frequent education for the "front-line" nursing staff is critical to successful postoperative pain management.

Frequent communication and clear expectations with the "front-line" nursing staff are also critical to the successful postoperative pain management of patients.

Relevance to the advanced practice provider (APP)

Pain management is central to the role of the APP.

Common pages and calls

My postop lumbar fusion patient is writhing in pain, what should I do?

Assess what medications the patient was taking prior to surgery.

Assess what medications have been ordered, and what medications the patient has received after surgery.

Assess the neurologic exam, assuring there is no structural etiology for pain.

If only opioids, add multimodal pain relief including scheduled acetaminophen, gabapentin, and long- and short-acting opioids. Consider adding a muscle relaxant. Would advise not to add a benzodiazepine due to respiratory depression risk. Consider a topical such as Lidoderm. Try non-pharmacologic interventions such as heat/ice/gentle massage, mobilize.

Order continuous pulse oximetry while titrating medications. Consider vital sign and neurologic exam frequency.

My patient says his pain is a 10/10, but he cannot stay awake.

Patients can develop a hyperalgesia/paradoxical effect to opioids.

Counsel the family regarding the side effects of opioids—and the patient if he is able to participate.

Decrease opioids and evaluate for nonopioid options for pain relief, such as NSAIDs, tramadol, and nonpharmacologic interventions. Gabapentin may be used when not sedated.

Once off or significantly tapered down, patients will generally feel improved, with better pain relief.

My patient does not want oral medications after surgery. He only wants intravenous medications.

Counsel the patient regarding multimodal pain management.

Oral medications provide improved duration of pain control, with much less peaks/valleys as with intravenous medications.

Oral medications allow the patient to focus on recovery, instead of needing more medication.

Oral medication postoperative prepares the patient for going home, where the patient will complete his or her recovery.

References

Devin CJ, McGirt MJ. Best evidence in multimodal pain management in spine surgery and means of assessing postoperative pain and functional outcomes. *Journal of Clinical Neuroscience.* 2015;22:930–938.

Dunn LK, Durieux ME, Nemergut EC. Non-opioid analgesics: novel approaches to perioperative analgesia for major spine surgery. *Best Practice & Research Clinical Anaesthesiology.* 2016;30:79–89.

Kim S-I, Ha K-Y, Oh, I-S. Preemptive multimodal analgesia for postoperative pain management after lumbar fusion surgery: A randomized controlled trial. *European Spine Journal*. 2016;25:1614–1619.

Lai LT, Ortiz-Cardona JR, Bendo AA. Perioperative pain management in the neurosurgical patient. *Anesthesiology Clinics*. 2012;30:347–367.

Pugely AJ, Martin CT, Gau Y, Mendoza-Lattes S. Causes and risk factors for 30-day unplanned readmissions after lumbar spine surgery. *Spine*. 2014;39:761–768.

Pyati S, Gan TJ. Perioperative pain management. *CNS Drugs*. 2007;21:185–211.

Oderda G. Challenges in the management of acute postsurgical pain. *Pharmacotherapy*, 2012;32:6S–11S.

Rajpal S, Gordon DB, Pellino TA, et al. Comparison of perioperative oral multimodal analgesia versus IV PCA for spine surgery. *Journal of Spinal Disorders and Technology*, 2010;23:139–135.

Wells N, Pasero C, McCaffery M. Improving the quality of care through pain assessment and management. In: Hughes R.G. ed. *Patient Safety and Quality: An Evidence-Based Handbook for Nurses*. Rockville, MD: Agency for Heatlhcare Research and Quality; 2008:Chapter 17.

Yu L, Ran B, Li M. Shi Z. Gabapentin and pregabalin in the management of postoperative pain after lumbar spinal surgery. *Spine*, 2013;38:1947–1952.

55

BRACING AND ELECTRICAL STIMULATION

Kristina Shultz and Tricia Jette-Gonthier

Bracing definition, purpose, and function

Spinal orthoses are class I devices, as categorized by the U.S. Food and Drug Administration (FDA), and are classified by the region of the spine they immobilize (cervical, cervicothoracic, thoracolumbar, or lumbosacral), or their rigidity (rigid, semirigid, or flexible) (Agaabegi et al., 2010).

The purpose of an orthosis is to immobilize a motion segment and unload the forces on the segment of the spine. Instability is not a global phenomenon, rather, almost always a segmental occurrence (Benzel, 2001). Clinical instability is the inability of the spine, when under physiological loads, to preserve a relationship between vertebrae where is there no resulting damage or ensuing irritation to the spinal cord or nerve roots. Instability could potentially be associated with deformity or pain due to the structural changes (Joaquim et al., 2014).

The main functions biomechanically of an orthosis are to offer total contact, three-point pressure, endpoint control, and elevated pressure:

- *Total contact*: The more contact there is between brace and wearer, the more even the pressure distribution, and the better control there will be. As skin and soft tissues lie between the orthosis and skeletal structures, even the most rigid orthosis cannot completely immobilize the spine. There is an inverse relationship to the effectiveness of the brace between the amount of soft tissue between the spine and the surface of the brace (Benzel, 2001). Given vital structures in the neck (trachea and esophagus), greater compressive forces can be applied in the thoracolumbar spine in comparison to the cervical spine.
- *Three-point pressure*: This is needed to maintain a desired position. Effective orthoses apply sufficient pressure over bony prominences to remind the wearer to change position or maintain posture.
- *Endpoint control*: This is a firm grasp of the cephalad and caudal spinal region of interest. Motion restriction is limited in the cervical spine unless control of the head and thorax is achieved (best example of orthosis that achieves almost complete endpoint is the halo vest; greater soft tissue envelope and larger body habitus though may interfere with fit of the vest around the thorax, hence not achieving endpoint control). Control of the thorax and pelvis is necessary in restricting motion of the thoracolumbar spine.
- *Elevated pressure*: Elevated intraabdominal pressure may reduce some stress on the spine.

Another major function of all orthoses is to serve as a reminder to the patient to restrict motion.

Types of orthoses

- *Cervical*
  - Soft collar—This has little effect on restricting motion in any region of the cervical spine. *It is contraindicated for injuries with potential for instability.
  - Rigid collar—This is effective at reducing motion in the sagittal plane; less effective at reducing rotation and lateral bending (endpoint control cannot be achieved as no control of both head and thorax). It provides adequate immobilization at midcervical levels; effectiveness is lost at upper and lower segments (occiput-C2, C6-C7).
    - Points of contact: proximally with mandible and occiput; distally with clavicle and sternal notch (anteriorly), and at ~T3 spinous process (posteriorly).
  - Cervicothoracic orthoses (CTOs)—They extend further down the trunk. They provide better end-point control, but can cause greater discomfort than rigid collars.
  - Examples: Minerva, sternal-occipital-mandibular immobilizer (SOMI)
    - Halo vest—This immobilizes the spine in all three planes; it is best for immobilizing upper and lower cervical spine. But, it is associated with higher complications and mortality rates (in the elderly).

In general, the longer the construct, the greater is the restriction. When more rigid immobilization is needed, CTOs are preferred. When rigid immobilization is not needed (i.e., postop management, stable fractures), any rigid orthosis (non-CTO) may be used.

- *Thoracic*
  - Thoracolumbosacral orthosis (TLSO)—This is used to immobilize T6-L4. It can be off-the-shelf or custom molded. A custom-fit TLSO is preferred if maximum control of motion is needed. Rigidity can be increased with over-the-shoulder straps (Figure 55.1).
  - Thoracolumbar hyperextension orthoses— They are designed to unload the anterior column. There is no body shell; it provides three points of pressure—applies dorsally directed force at the sternum and pubic region, and ventrally directed force at the thoracolumbar junction (Benzel, 2001). They are most effective in limiting motion in the sagittal plane (best suited for managing traumatic or osteoporotic fxs T10-L2). They are contraindicated for unstable fractures (disruption of more than one column).

Examples include Jewett and cruciform anterior spinal hyperextension (CASH).

- *Lumbar*
  - Lumbosacral orthosis (LSO)—This is used to immobilize L3 and below. Ensure the brace is well-fitted to the pelvis to adequately support L4-L5 and L5-S1. It can be off-the-shelf or custom molded; both may be fit with thigh extension to help reduce motion (Figure 55.2).
  - Lumbar corsets—They can reduce gross trunk control (for pain control). Used when there is low tolerance to more rigid orthoses (for compression fx) and for chronic low back pain by providing abdominal support. They are never used if there is concern for instability.

Bracing indications

The use of spinal orthoses has long been a debated modality, both in the use for conservative management for traumatic and osteoporotic fractures, and for postoperative spinal fusions. Even with advancements of surgical technique and instrumentation, the use of orthoses continues to be debated.

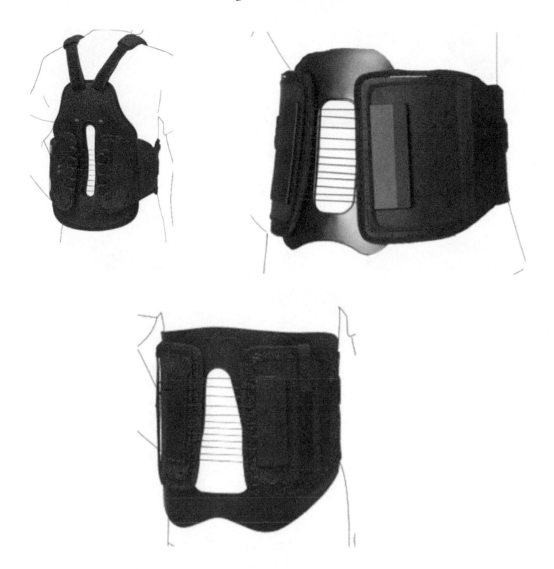

Figure 55.1   Cyberspine TLSO x4 (Premium TLSO [T2-S1] with Lateral Control), Premium Plus (Classic LSO [T9-S1]), Cybertech TriMod Standard (Classic LSO [T9-S1] with Lateral Control).

Prevention

- Neck pain—There is no evidence that the use of a cervical orthosis (soft or rigid) is beneficial in the management of axial neck pain (Agabegi et al., 2010).
- Low back pain—Orthoses are generally not indicated for primary prevention (Dailey et al., 2014).
    - They do not prevent development of low back pain in the general working population.
    - Some studies have shown that workers who used a lumbar brace for secondary prevention reported a decrease in number of days experiencing back pain as well as missed days from work.
    - For patients presenting with low back pain for 6 months or less, the use of lumbar support for 3 weeks revealed a decrease in visual analog scale (VAS) pain scores, medication usage, as well as improved functional disability (at 30–90 days).

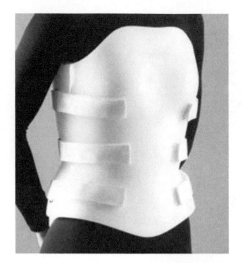
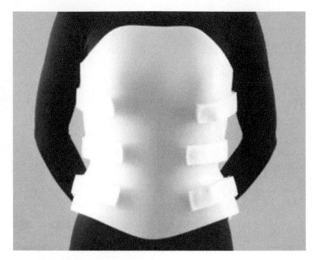
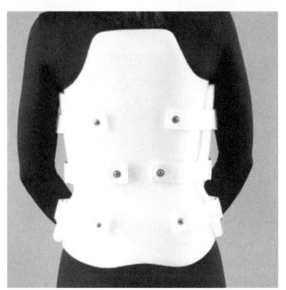

Figure 55.2 Custom TLSO Bivalve.

Fractures

- Cervical spine
  - Atlanto-occipital dislocation—highly unstable, requires surgical fixation
  - Occipital condyle fractures—can be managed with external orthoses *if* no ligamentous injury, even in the presence of cranial nerve deficits (Joaquim et al., 2014)
  - Atlas fractures (C1)—manage with external orthoses *if* no ligamentous injury (when associated with other cervical injury, the treatment is then based on this coexistent injury) (Joaquim et al., 2014)

- Axis fractures (C2)—can be further defined by anatomical location (odontoid, vertebral body, and/or posterior elements)
  - Risk factors associated with nonsurgical treatment failure: age >50, dens displacement >5 mm, comminution on the base of the odontoid process, or inability to achieve or maintain acceptable fracture alignment with external immobilization; early surgery considered if one or more risk factor
  - Fractures of the body of the axis can be treated with external immobilization (rigid collar or Minerva) as the large cancellous surface of C2 body fractures typically provide stability and fracture healing (Joaquim et al., 2014; German et al., 2005)
  - Traumatic spondylolisthesis of the axis without disruption of the ligamentous injury: use external immobilization (Joaquim et al., 2014)
- Odontoid fractures—associated with significant mortality and morbidity; most commonly occur from hyperflexion or hyperextension injury; three types (Sime et al., 2013):
  - Type 1—involves odontoid tip avulsion; considered stable
  - Type 2—occur at odontoid base (aka type 2 Dens Fracture); at higher risk of displacement; can be managed surgically or nonoperatively (debate remains in selection of operative versus nonoperative treatment)
    - Nonoperative (use external immobilization): not displaced or minimally displaced; accepted degree of displacement = fracture gap <2 mm, anteroposterior displacement <5 mm, and angulation <11°.
    - Can use rigid cervical collar or Minerva, or Halo; no statistically significant difference in bone union or risk of mortality among these various immobilization devices. Halo has shown greater rates of stable union (but higher rates of respiratory complications).
  - Type 3—extends into the axis body; considered stable
- C2-C3 ligamentous injuries; Hangman fracture
  - Most patients can be treated successfully with external immobilization.
  - Recommendations for surgery are reserved for fractures with disruption of the C2-C3 disc space and locked facets (Joaquim et al., 2014).
- Subaxial cervical spine (C3-C7)
  - Subaxial cervical spine motion segments are stabilized predominantly by facet joints and their capsules.
  - While unilateral, nondisplaced lateral mass/facet fractures historically have not been considered for surgery; nonoperative management is often unsuccessful. Surgery has been shown to be superior to orthosis in preventing rotational subluxation and loss of alignment.
    - If nonoperative management is chosen, interval imaging studies must be obtained until solid fusion is confirmed by computed tomography (CT) or flexion/extension views (Aarabi et al., 2014).
- Traumatic fractures of the thoracic and lumbar spine
  - Neurologic status is a prime consideration when considering operative versus nonoperative management.
  - Unstable fractures (i.e., fracture dislocation, flexion distraction injury, and severe burst fractures with retropulsed fragment causing a deficit) warrant surgical intervention.
    - Fixed, complete neurologic injury—surgery to provide stability
    - Incomplete spine injury—surgery to help preserve and regain neurologic function and stabilize spinal column
  - For fractures of non-load-bearing structures (spinous process, transverse process), if stable, surgery is rarely indicated (only if displaced and impinging a nerve root). Bracing is used for comfort (Chang and Holly, 2014).

- Anterior wedge compression fracture is most commonly treated with bracing for 2–3 months (prevent forward flexion, diminish load on anterior column) (Chang and Holly, 2014).
  - Monitor with standing plain films.
- Surgery if indicated for severe compression fractures with >30° local kyphosis, >50% loss of vertebral body height, *or* if three contiguous levels are involved
  - Flexion-distraction fracture (Chance fracture) may be neurologically intact, but is a highly disruptive fracture with violation of all three columns and failure of posterior ligamentous complex. Surgery is warranted (Chang and Holly, 2014).
  - Burst fractures (AO Type A3) tend to occur at the thoracolumbar junction between T11 and L2 (interface between relatively rigid segment of thoracic spine and relatively mobile segment of lumbar spine). There is no clear consensus on treatment (Chang and Holly, 2014).
    - Surgery: Significantly comminuted fractures that could result in poor loading capacity, and fractures associated with spinous process splaying—unstable
    - Bracing: Fracture with <25°–30° kyphosis, <50% loss of vertebral body height, and <50% retropulsion of bone into spinal canal
    - Can brace for 8–12 weeks with TLSO with at least three points of fixation (in relative spinal extension), with standing films every 4–6 weeks to monitor healing
    - Signs of nonoperative therapy failure: Progressive deformity, intractable back pain, any neurologic symptom (from kyphosis or loss of vertebral height)
      - While most studies support bracing in neurologically intact patients with burst fractures (Wood et al., 2015; Siebenga et al., 2006; Bailey et al., 2009), others have shown short-segment posterior fusion being superior to bracing for burst fractures (Bailey et al., 2014).

Note: While there are suggested guidelines in place, there is no clear consensus, as the data are not consistent, highlighting the importance of careful consideration with each case (Giele et al., 2009).

- Osteoporotic fractures (vertebral compression fractures [VCFs]) (Longo et al., 2012)
- Compression fractures are considered stable.
  - Bracing and cement augmentation (vertebroplasty and kyphoplasty) are two common strategies for the management of osteoporotic vertebral compression fractures in patients without neurologic impairment.
- The goal of bracing is to reduce pain by stabilizing and limiting the progression of deformity.
- Use a rigid brace (TLSO) or a Jewett or CASH brace when hyperextension is needed.
- Management is aimed at promoting healing of the fracture and preventing or minimizing hyperkyphosis (which is a common problem after osteoporotic VCFs).
- Indications for bracing or cement augmentation are not clear.
- Bracing has risks, especially in the elderly population, which need to be considered including pressure sores, diminished pulmonary capacity, and weakening of axial musculature. Brace for a finite amount of time and closely monitor for complications (Chang and Holley, 2014).

Postoperative

- A long-standing lack of consensus also exists for efficacy of postop bracing (Bible et al., 2009).
- Bracing following C1-C2 instrumented fusion can be used with consideration of bone quality (Elliott et al., 2013).
- Bracing following posterior lumbar instrumented fusion for degenerative disease has now been shown to offer no functional or radiographic benefit (Dailey et al., 2014).

Bracing considerations

The following are points to consider (Jacobson et al., 2008):

- Extrication collars (applied at the scene of an accident) are very rigid and can only be used for <24 hours (longer use increases risk for breakdown at contact areas). If immobilization is needed for more than 48 hours, change to a cervical orthosis available in your institution such as an Aspen, Miami J, or PMT.
- Diaphoretic skin or secretions can macerate skin, leading to pressure ulcers. Closed cell foam collars (Philadelphia) hold in more moisture. Consider an open cell foam collar, such as noted above, in patients with diaphoretic skin or secretions.
- Closely monitor for pressure ulcer development with cervical collar use, especially at the occiput (very little overlying subcutaneous tissue), chin, mandible, suprascapular area, ears, and over the larynx.

Bone growth stimulators

Electrical stimulation is an option for increasing the fusion rate (mechanism and efficacy still unclear) (Park et al., 2014).

There are three accepted forms (Kaiser et al., 2014):

- Direct current stimulation (DCS)—Insertion of cathodes, attached to an implanted battery, directly into the fusion substrate
- Pulsed electromagnetic field stimulation (PEMFS)—Noninvasive; delivers electromagnetic energy to the fusion by wearing an external coil (driven by electrical current); relatively benign (noninvasive), though should consider cost versus benefit
- Capacitive coupled electrical stimulation (CCES)—Noninvasive; relies on generation of an electrical field through capacitive plates (placed on patient's skin)

There is no conclusive evidence in support of bone stimulation devices; therefore, there are no clear guidelines.

The impact of stimulators is likely minimal, though there are some suggestions (Kaiser et al., 2014):

- Posterior lumbar fusions (no risk factors)—Inconclusive evidence on routine use of stimulators
- Posterior lumbar fusions *at high risk* for pseudarthrosis—May consider DCS and CCES
- Posterior lumbar *interbody* fusions *at high risk* for pseudarthrosis—May consider PEMFS
- Pseudarthrosis—PEMFS can be considered; inconclusive on its routine use for fusions

References

Agabegi SS, Asghar FA, Herkowitz HN. Spinal orthoses. *Journal of the American Academy of Orthopedic Surgery.* 2010;11:657–667.

Aarabi B, Mirvis S, Shanmuganathan K, et al. Comparative effectiveness of surgical versus nonoperative management of unilateral, nondisplaced, subaxial cervical spine facet fractures without evidence of spinal cord injury. *Journal of Neurosurgery: Spine.* 2014;20:270–277.

Bailey CS, Dvorak M F, Thomas K et al. Comparison of thoracolumbosacral orthosis and no orthosis for the treatment of thoracolumbar burst fractures: Interim analysis of a multicenter randomized clinical equivalence trial. *Journal of Neurosurgery: Spine.* 2009;11:295–303. doi:10.3171/2009.3.spine08312.

Bailey CS, Urquhart JC, Dvorak MF et al. Orthosis versus No rthosis for the treatment of thoracolumbar burst fractures without neurologic injury: A multicenter prospective randomized equivalence trial. *Spine Journal.* 2014;14:2557–2564. doi:10.1016/j.spinee.2013.10.017.

Benzel EC. Spinal bracing. In: *Biomechanics of Spine Stabilization,* first edition. Rolling Meadows, Illinois, United States: American Association of Neurological Surgeons; 2001:331–405.

Bible JE, Biswas D, Whang PG, Simpson AK, Rechtine GR, Grauer JN, Postoperative bracing after spine surgery for degenerative Cconditions: A questionnaire study. *Spine Journal.* 2009;9:309–316. doi:10.1016/j.spinee.2008.06.453.

Chang V, Holly LT, 2014. Bracing for thoracolumbar fractures. *Neurosurgery Focus.* 2014;37:E3. doi:10.3171/2014.4.FOCUS1477.

Dailey A, Ghogawala Z, Choudhri TF et al. Guideline update for the performance of fusion procedures for degenerative disease of the lumbar spine. part 14: Brace therapy as an adjunct to or substitute for lumbar fusion. *Journal of Neurosurgery: Spine.* 2014;1:91–101.

Elliott RE, Tanweer, Boah A et al. Is external cervical orthotic bracing necessary after posterior atlantoaxial fusion with modern instrumentation: Meta-analysis and review of literature. *World Neurosurgery.* 2013;7:369–374.e12. doi:10.1016/j.wneu.2012.03.022.

German JW, Hart BL, Benzel EC, Nonoperative management of vertical C2 body fractures. *Neurosurgery.* 2005; 3:516–521.

Giele BM, Wiertsema SH, Beelen A, No evidence for the effectiveness of bracing in patients with thoracolumbar fractures. *Acta Orthopaedica.* 2009;80:226–232. doi:10.3109/17453670902875245.

Jacobson TM, Tescher AN, Miers AG, Downer L. Improving practice: efforts to reduce occipital pressure ulcers. *Journal of Nursing Care Quality.* 2008;23:283–288.

Joaquim AF, Ghizoni E Tedeschi H et al. Upper cervical injuries – A rational approach to guide surgical management. *The Journal of Spinal Cord Medicine.* 2014;37:139–151. doi:10.1179/2045772313y.0000000158.

Kaiser MG, Eck JC, Groff MW et al. Guideline update for the performance of fusion procedures for degenerative disease of the lumbar spine. part 17: Bone growth stimulators as an adjunct for lumbar fusion. *Journal of Neurosurgery: Spine.* 2014;21:133–139.

Longo UG, Loppini M, Denaro L, Maffulli N, Denaro V, Conservative management of patients with an osteoporotic vertebral fracture: A review of the literature. *Journal of Bone & Joint Surgery British.* 2012;94-B:152–157. doi:10.1302/0301-620x.94b2.26894.

Park P, Lau D, Brodt ED, Dettori JR Electrical stimulation to enhance spinal fusion: A systematic review. *Evidenced Based Spine Care Journal.* 2014;5:87–94.

Siebenga J, Leferink VJM, Segers MJM et al. Treatment of traumatic thoracolumbar spine fractures: A multicenter prospective randomized study of operative versus nonsurgical treatment. *Spine.* 2006;25:2881–2890.

Sime D, Pitt V, Pattuwage L, Tee J, Liew S, Gruen R, Non-surgical interventions for the management of type 2 dens fractures: A systematic review. *ANZ Journal of SurgeryIshan.* 2013;84:320–325. doi:10.1111/ans.12401.

Wood KB, Butterman GR, Phukan R et al., Operative compared with nonoperative treatment of a thoracolumbar burst fracture without neurological deficit: A prospective randomized study with follow-up at sixteen to twenty-two years. *Journal of Bone & Joint Surgery American.* 2015;97:3–9. doi:10.2106/jbjs.n.00226.

56

POSTOPERATIVE PHYSICAL AND OCCUPATIONAL THERAPY

*Christie Stawicki, Tristan Fried, Gregory D. Schroeder, and
Alexander R. Vaccaro*

Introduction

Cervical and lumbar spine surgeries are common; however, there is no universally accepted postoperative protocol for the treatment of these patients. Furthermore, there are often multiple acceptable surgical options for the treatment of similar spine pathology, and the events in the operating room may dictate different postoperative precautions. For these reasons, it is important to discuss the postoperative precautions of each patient with the surgical team. The goal of this chapter is to describe the common hospital course and postoperative protocols for the three common spine procedures.

Lumbar microdiscectomy

A lumbar microdiscectomy is a procedure in which the herniated portion of the lumbar disc is removed, but the remaining intervertebral disc is left intact. Regardless if the surgery is done through a traditional open approach, or a "minimally invasive" approach, the incision is often less than 2 inches in length, and there is no substantial difference in the postoperative restrictions. Patients are candidates for surgery if they have a herniated disc and persistent radicular pain for greater than 6 weeks (Lurie et al., 2014). Additionally, they may be candidates for early surgical intervention if their pain is uncontrollable, or if they have profound weakness (<3/5).

Hospital course

- These are commonly outpatient surgeries that take approximately an hour; however, in older patients, patients with significant medical comorbidities, revision cases, or patients with intraoperative complications (such as a dural tear), 24 hours of observation may be necessary. Physical and occupational therapy are not commonly needed while these patients are in the hospital.
- Common complications all providers should be aware of are as follows:
  - Dural tear—If recognized in the operating room, these are often repaired and a watertight closure is performed. Symptomatic patients often complain of photophobia, nausea, positional headaches (i.e., a headache when sitting upright or standing, but no headache when lying flat), and rarely clear fluid draining from their wound (Espiritu et al., 2010). The surgical team should be notified of any patient with symptoms consistent with a symptomatic dural tear.

- The ideal postoperative protocol is still unclear. In asymptomatic patients, some surgeons will not alter the postoperative management, while other surgeons will choose to treat all patients with a dural tear with flat bed rest for at least 24 hours. All patients with a symptomatic dural tear should be treated with flat bed rest for approximately 24 hours. Bed rest for longer than 24 hours has been associated with an increased risk of medical complications (Radcliff et al., 2016).
- New neurologic deficit—The surgical team should be notified immediately if a patient has a new or worsened neurologic deficit, as advanced imaging or surgical intervention may be warranted.
- As with any surgery, other surgical or anesthesia-related complications such as infection, deep vein thrombosis, pulmonary embolism, or cardiac/pulmonary complications may occur; however, these are rare.

Common postoperative protocols

- The role for postoperative restrictions after a lumbar microdiscectomy is unclear. Traditionally, patients have been counseled against heavy lifting, significant lumbar rotation, and strenuous activity for 4–6 weeks. However, in a study designed to assess the feasibility of removing activity restrictions postoperatively, patients were advised to return to regular activity when they felt able. This approach allowed 98% of patients to return to work 1–2 weeks after their procedure and did not cause additional complications (Carragee et al., 1996).
- The need for postoperative therapy is also unclear; however, participation in standardized training and exercise that begins 4 weeks following surgery has been shown to decrease postoperative disability (Danielsen et al., 2000). Furthermore, incorporating specific exercises to improve strength, endurance, and mobility of the trunk muscles can significantly improve short-term pain, disability, and spinal function (Dolan et al., 2000).

Posterior lumbar decompression and fusions

A lumbar fusion for degenerative pathology (i.e., not trauma/tumor/infection) is performed when the patient has significant compression of the neurologic elements with associated instability (spondylolisthesis, scoliosis, or iatrogenic). This can present as neurogenic claudication or radicular symptoms, which may or may not be associated with low back pain. Surgical intervention is designed to address the neurologic symptoms, not axial back pain. Various surgical techniques have been implemented; however, almost all lumbar fusions performed in the United States today are done with the addition of posterior instrumentation (Kepler et al., 2014). In addition to the posterior fusion, often the intervertebral disc is removed and an interbody fusion is performed. This can be done anteriorly (anterior lumbar interbody fusion [ALIF]), laterally (lateral lumbar interbody fusion [LLIF]), or through one of two posterior approaches (posterior lumbar interbody fusion [PLIF] or transforaminal lumbar interbody fusion [TLIF]). This chapter focuses on posterior fusions, and the hospital course and postoperative restrictions are not affected by the addition of an interbody fusion.

Hospital course

- Almost all patients who undergo a lumbar decompression and fusion will require an admission for 2–3 days. Prior to being discharged, patients must have their pain controlled, be tolerating a diet, be passing flatus, and demonstrate the ability to perform activities of daily living (ADLs).

Treatment from occupational and physical therapists is often needed to help patients be able to perform their ADLs.

- Changes in paraspinal muscle structure and function can occur as a result of the surgery. Consequently, reduced trunk strength and lack of mobility are common postoperatively. The implementation of therapy is vital to regain muscle strength and function, and to maintain mobility (Tarnanen et al., 2014).
- The use of a brace postoperatively is controversial; however, in an instrumented lumbar fusion, the construct should be stable with or without a brace. Because of this, the most recent guidelines from the American Association of Neurological Surgeons recommended against the routine use of a brace postoperatively in patients who underwent an instrumented lumbar fusion. In spite of this, some surgeons still routinely use a brace, predominately as a comfort measure for patients (Dailey et al., 2014).

- Common complications all providers should be aware of include the following:
  - Similar to patients who undergo a microdiscectomy, dural tears, neurologic deficits, and other medical complications can occur in patients undergoing a lumbar fusion. These complications should be handled similarly in all patients.
  - Early hardware failure
    - Early hardware failure is rare in lumbar fusions, and the instrumentation should be strong enough to allow for the patient to work with the therapist. However, all health-care professions should be aware when instrumentation has been used, and they should notify the surgical team if the patient feels the hardware is moving.

Common postoperative protocols

- As discussed above, the routine use of a brace postoperatively is controversial but likely is unnecessary (Dailey et al., 2014).
- Patients should avoid activities such as heavy lifting, contact sports, and running for at least the first 6 months after surgery (Abbott et al., 2010). It is controversial if patients with a lumbar fusion should ever return to heavy lifting or contact athletics.
- Physical therapy is needed for most patients after a lumbar fusion.
  - In an attempt to maintain stability of the lumbar spine in a neutral position, strengthening exercises can be performed to reduce strain on the fused area.
  - Walking and dynamic exercises, as well as strengthening of the paraspinal, abdominal, and leg muscles are common focal points during rehabilitation. Functional movements that mimic the trunk muscles such as pushing and pulling can also be beneficial.
  - Stability of the lumbar spine and lumbo-pelvic complex is critical; therefore, strengthening of trunk muscles is essential. Additionally, focus on stretching of the lower back and cardiovascular aerobic exercise can facilitate recovery.

Anterior cervical discectomy and fusion (ACDF)

An ACDF is one of the most common and successful spine surgeries. It is commonly done for one- and two-level pathology, but it can be done at three or more levels as well. Furthermore, rather than just removing the intervertebral disc, the entire vertebral body can also be removed from the anterior approach. While the incisions often look the same, the postoperative course, restrictions, and possible complications significantly change as the complexity of the surgery increases. Therefore, it is critical that all health-care professionals understand the extent of the surgery that was performed. The management of patients with complex cervical spine pathology is beyond the scope of this chapter; instead, it focuses on the postoperative protocol for patients who undergo either a one- or two-level ACDF. The two major indications for this procedure are persistent cervical radiculopathy (compression of the nerve root) or cervical myelopathy (compression of the spinal cord).

Hospital course

- Most patients who undergo an ACDF will go home the next day. More recently, some surgeons have been sending these patients home the same day. The need for patients to stay overnight after a routine ACDF is unclear (Garringer and Sasso, 2010).
- Regardless if patients stay overnight, the role for physical or occupational therapy in the hospital is limited.
- The need for a cervical collar in these patients is controversial. In one small, randomized trial, there was no benefit to a collar in patients undergoing a single-level ACDF. However, the efficacy has not been evaluated in two-level fusions. Furthermore, many surgeons use a brace for comfort as well as to help remind the patient and the caretakers that the patient has recently had cervical spine surgery (Campbell, 2009).
- Common complications all providers should be aware of include the following:
    - Like all previously mentioned spine cases, dural tears (while much more rare after an ACDF), neurologic injuries, and medical complications can occur. Importantly, neurologic injuries in the cervical spine may be devastating, as the spinal cord may be injured.
    - Dysphagia—This complication is almost ubiquitous in patients who have an ACDF (Joaquim et al., 2014). Immediately after surgery, patients will often have a hoarse throat and a difficult time swallowing. Patients should be encouraged to eat slow and thoroughly chew their food.
    - Retropharyngeal hematoma—This rare complication can be fatal if not diagnosed quickly (O'Neill et al., 2014). It is critical to understand that while minor hoarseness and dysphagia are common, difficulty breathing is not. A surgeon should be notified immediately if any patient has a difficult time breathing, as this may be a surgical emergency.
    - Horner syndrome—This rare complication can occur if the stellate ganglion is damaged. Patients present with ipsilateral decreased pupil size, a drooping eyelid, and decreased forehead sweating (Cody et al., 2014). The surgeon should be notified immediately if a patient is found to have Horner syndrome.

Common postoperative protocols

- As discussed above, the utility of a cervical collar is controversial.
- Therapy after surgery is often patient directed. Patients should begin with short walks and slowly expand to walking greater distances each day as tolerated. In some cases, formal rehabilitation may be necessary if the patient is significantly deconditioned.
- Patients should avoid heavy lifting and strenuous activity until the fusion is completely healed (often 6–12 months), and they have regained full cervical strength and range of motion.

Common pitfalls and medicolegal concerns

- A new or worsened postoperative neurologic deficit should never be ignored. These should all be reported to the attending surgeon, as advanced imaging or surgical management may be necessary.

- All patients who have spine surgery may have medical complications, and it is important to thoroughly investigate any possible complication.
- After an ACDF, difficulty breathing may be a sign of a retropharyngeal hematoma. This is a surgical emergency.

Relevance to the advanced practice health professional

- This chapter highlights the expected postoperative course, possible complications, and postoperative therapy needs of patients undergoing three common spine surgeries. Any advanced practice health professional taking care of these patients should have a solid understanding of this chapter; however, as the exact postoperative protocols of surgeons can vary widely, it is also critical that the advanced practice health professional has excellent communication with the treating surgeon.

Common phone calls, pages, and requests with answers

- Call—The patient who just underwent a microdiscectomy developed a terrible headache when he was getting dressed to go home. Is it still OK for the patient to go home?
  - Answer—This patient has one of the classic signs of a dural tear. While it is possible that the patient has a headache from the narcotics, this should be investigated further before the patient is discharged.
- Call—The patient who just had an ACDF is complaining of difficulty moving his left arm. What should we do?
  - Answer—Contact the surgeon immediately, and obtain magnetic resonance imaging (MRI). The patient may have a C5 nerve root palsy that occurs sometimes after cervical spine surgery, but a hematoma cannot be excluded and if left untreated could lead to spinal cord compression and paralysis.
- Call—The patient who had an ACDF has a hoarse voice and some difficulty swallowing. What should I do?
  - Answer—Reassure the patient that this is common and resolves spontaneously in most patients. It is important that patients take small bites and thoroughly chew their food.
- Call—The patient who had an ACDF is having a difficult time breathing. What should I do?
  - Answer—Call the surgeon immediately. The patient may have a retropharyngeal hematoma. This is a surgical emergency.
- Call—The patient who underwent a one-level instrumented lumbar fusion for a degenerative spondylolisthesis is afraid to move without his brace on. Does he need to wear a brace at all times?

  - This is somewhat controversial, so you should talk to the attending surgeon; however, with instrumentation, the construct is usually stable. While the brace may give the patient comfort, he often does not need to wear it at all times.

References

Abbott AD, Tyni-Lenne R, Hedlund R. Early rehabilitation targeting cognition, behavior, and motor function after lumbar fusion: A randomized controlled trial. *Spine (Phila Pa 1976)*. 2010;35:848–857.

Campbell MJ, Carreon LY, Traynelis V, Anderson PA. Use of cervical collar after single-level anterior cervical fusion with plate: is it necessary? *Spine (Phila Pa 1976)*. 2009;34:43–48.

Carragee EJ, Helms E, O'Sullivan GS. Are postoperative activity restrictions necessary after posterior lumbar discectomy? A prospective study of outcomes in 50 consecutive cases. *Spine (Phila Pa 1976)*. 1996;21:1893–1897.

Cody JP, Kang DG, Tracey RW, Wagner SC, Rosner MK, Lehman RA, Jr. Outcomes following cervical disc arthroplasty: A retrospective review. *J Clin Neurosci*. 2014;21:1901–1904.

Dailey AT, Ghogawala Z, Choudhri TF, et al. Guideline update for the performance of fusion procedures for degenerative disease of the lumbar spine. Part 14: brace therapy as an adjunct to or substitute for lumbar fusion. *J Neurosurg Spine*. 2014;21:91–101.

Danielsen JM, Johnsen R, Kibsgaard SK, Hellevik E. Early aggressive exercise for postoperative rehabilitation after discectomy. *Spine (Phila Pa 1976)*. 2000;25:1015–1020.

Dolan P, Greenfield K, Nelson RJ, Nelson IW. Can exercise therapy improve the outcome of microdiscectomy? *Spine (Phila Pa 1976)*. 2000;25:1523–1532.

Espiritu MT, Rhyne A, Darden BV, 2nd. Dural tears in spine surgery. *J Am Acad Orthop Surg*. 2010;18:537–545.

Garringer SM, Sasso RC. Safety of anterior cervical discectomy and fusion performed as outpatient surgery. *J Spinal Disord Tech*. 2010;23:439–443.

Joaquim AF, Murar J, Savage JW, Patel AA. Dysphagia after anterior cervical spine surgery: a systematic review of potential preventative measures. *Spine J*. 2014;14:2246–2260.

Kepler CK, Vaccaro AR, Hilibrand AS, et al. National trends in the use of fusion techniques to treat degenerative spondylolisthesis. *Spine (Phila Pa 1976)*. 2014;39:1584–1589.

Lurie JD, Tosteson TD, Tosteson AN, et al. Surgical versus nonoperative treatment for lumbar disc herniation: Eight-year results for the spine patient outcomes research trial. *Spine (Phila Pa 1976)*. 2014;39:3–16.

O'Neill KR, Neuman B, Peters C, Riew KD. Risk factors for postoperative retropharyngeal hematoma after anterior cervical spine surgery. *Spine (Phila Pa 1976)*. 2014;39:E246–252.

Radcliff KE, Sidhu GD, Kepler CK, et al. Complications of flat bed rest after incidental repair. *J Spinal Disord Tech*. 2016;29(7):281–284.

Tarnanen SP, Neva MH, Hakkinen K, et al. Neutral spine control exercises in rehabilitation after lumbar spine fusion. *J Strength Cond Res*. 2014;28:2018–2025.

57

COMMUNITY-ACQUIRED SPINAL INFECTIONS

Tammy L. Tyree and Luis M. Tumialán

Case vignette

A 55-year-old man with a history of obesity, hypertension, and tobacco abuse presented to the emergency department with a 5-day history of intermittent chills, rigors, night sweats, and severe thoracic back pain radiating to his left arm. He reported injuring his hand on coral while scuba diving, and then he developed a palmar abscess after repeated use of a hot tub. In the emergency department, his temperature was 100°F, white blood cell count was 1.5×10^9/L, erythrocyte sedimentation rate (ESR) was 95 mm/hr, and C-reactive protein (CRP) was 15.4 mg/L. Magnetic resonance imaging (MRI) with and without contrast revealed a left paracentral enhancing epidural abscess spanning from C5 down to T1 with associated phlegmon (Figures 57.1a-b and 57.2). The patient underwent drainage with hemilaminectomy and decompression of the epidural abscess. Blood cultures were negative. Intraoperative cultures grew Salmonella sp. He was treated with intravenous (IV) ceftriaxone for 6 weeks. By the third postoperative month, he had returned to his previous level of functioning.

Overview of spinal infections

Epidemiology

Spinal infections—other than meningitis—are uncommon. The incidence of discitis has been approximately 2 cases per 100,000 patients per year (Hopkinson et al., 2001), although a recent study suggests that the current rate of pyogenic spondylodiscitis is about 4 cases per 100,000 persons (Kehrer et al., 2014). The rate of spontaneous spinal infections in patients aged 65 years and older can be as high as 9.8 in 100,000 persons (Hutchinson et al., 2009). Spinal epidural abscesses occur in 1.5 to 2.8 cases per 10,000 hospital admissions (Danner et al., 1987; Hawkins et al., 2013). The increased rates of these infections may be due to an aging population, increased use of spinal instrumentation, increased IV drug abuse, and improvements in diagnostic techniques that are identifying infections more accurately and earlier in their course (Hopkinson et al., 2001; Danner et al., 1987; Kehrer et al., 2014). Risk factors for spinal infection include invasive procedures (reportedly responsible for up to 41% of cases), preexisting infection (e.g., endocarditis and tuberculosis), IV drug abuse, immunosuppression (e.g., HIV or chronic prescription corticosteroid use), malnutrition, male sex, travel to endemic geographic areas (*Brucella* sp.), trauma, and other comorbidities (i.e., diabetes mellitus, hypertension, chronic renal failure, cancer, alcoholism, cirrhosis, sickle cell anemia, and organ transplantation) (Hopkinson et al., 2001; Danner et al., 1987; Duarte et al., 2013; Kim et al., 2010; Karadimas et al., 2008; Cottle et al., 2008).

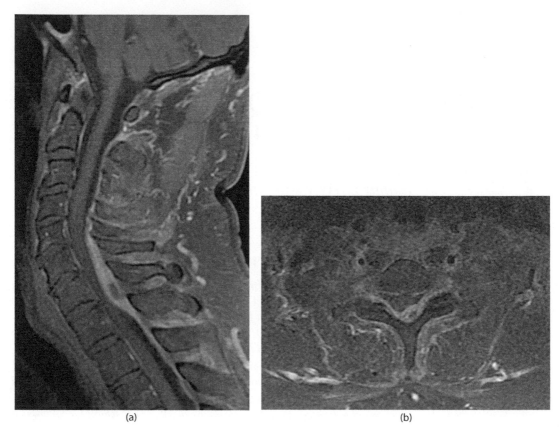

(a)

(b)

Figure 57.1 (a) MRI with gadolinium contrast. Sagittal view of the cervical spine demonstrating an enhancing fluid collection consistent with an abscess. (b) Axial MRI with gadolinium contrast demonstrating enhancing fluid collection causing compression of the spinal cord. (Used with permission from Barrow Neurological Institute, Phoenix, Arizona.)

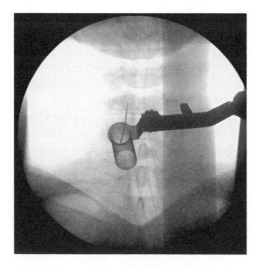

Figure 57.2 Anteroposterior fluoroscopic image demonstrating minimal access port in position for decompression. (Used with permission from Barrow Neurological Institute, Phoenix, Arizona.)

The three most common community-acquired spinal infections are discitis (or spondylodiscitis), osteomyelitis, and epidural abscess. Other spinal-related infections that are less common include paravertebral abscess, psoas abscess, and acute necrotizing myelitis. Meningitis is covered elsewhere in this book. This chapter focuses on community-acquired spontaneous spinal infections.

Discitis is an infection of the intervertebral disc space that, in adults, is most often caused by an invasive procedure; spontaneous discitis is uncommon in adults (Honan et al., 1996). Osteomyelitis typically occurs from the progression of discitis to adjacent vertebral endplates; however, the medical literature frequently groups discitis and osteomyelitis as a single entity. Discitis and osteomyelitis can further be delineated into pyogenic (pus-forming) or nonpyogenic types. Nonpyogenic etiologies include—but are not limited to—*Mycobacterium, Brucella* sp., *Candida tropicalis,* and fungal organisms such as *Aspergillus* sp., *Blastomyces* sp., and *Coccidioides* sp. (Greenberg, 2010). These nonpyogenic infections can occur spontaneously or postoperatively. An epidural abscess is a collection of purulent material between the dura mater of the spinal cord and the vertebral canal.

Societal significance

Data suggest a mortality rate of up to 15% for patients with spinal epidural abscesses and mortality rates between 2% and 20% for those with discitis and osteomyelitis (Parkins et al., 2008; Cottle et al., 2008; Kourbeti et al., 2008; Butler et al., 2006). Prognosis for recovery correlates with level of function at the time of diagnosis (Danner et al., 1987). Patients with epidural abscesses who present with weakness or paralysis have worse prognoses than patients who present with no deficit or radicular pain only (Danner et al., 1987). Other predictors of a poor prognosis include debilitating comorbidities (Solis Garcia del Pozo et al., 2007; Duarte et al., 2013), advanced age, cervical or thoracic involvement, infection with methicillin-resistant *Staphylococcus aureus*, alcohol or IV drug abuse, HIV infection, and the interval between onset of symptoms and treatment (Turunc et al., 2007; Solis Garcia del Pozo et al., 2007; Duarte et al., 2013; Kehrer et al., 2014). Prompt initiation of targeted antimicrobial therapy can improve outcomes (Cottle et al., 2008; Karadimas et al., 2008).

Basic biologic and physiologic processes

There are two routes of pathogen spread for community-acquired spinal infections: (1) hematogenous spread, and (2) dissemination by infection from adjacent tissue (Duarte et al., 2013). The pathophysiology of discitis and osteomyelitis differs with age because children have vascular channels in disc spaces that typically disappear by adulthood (Honan et al., 1996; Cottle et al., 2008). Infections can be spread directly through these vascular channels, depositing microbial emboli into the disc space. Adult disc spaces are avascular and require permeation of infectious organisms through vertebral metaphysis into the disc space (Fernandez et al., 2000; Kourbeti et al., 2008; Reiss-Zimmermann et al., 2010; Lehovsky, 1999).

The spine segments most susceptible to spondylodiscitis and osteomyelitis are the lumbar vertebrae, followed by the thoracic and then the cervical vertebrae, although tuberculosis more commonly affects the thoracic spine (Fernandez et al., 2000; Hopkinson et al., 2001; Karadimas et al., 2008; Kehrer et al., 2014; Kim et al., 2010; Kourbeti et al., 2008). The thoracic spine is the most common site for spinal epidural abscesses, followed by the lumbar and then the cervical spine (Danner et al., 1987).

Epidural abscesses are frequently caused by untreated osteomyelitis or discitis, and they involve collections of microorganisms (alive or dead), destroyed tissue, and white blood cells (Lehovsky, 1999). This pus can be enveloped by a membrane, forming loculations. This fluid collection can exert pressure on the spine.

Multiple organisms are responsible for spinal infections, but up to 50% of these cases have no organism identified (Greenberg, 2010). Initial treatment should be directed toward any presumed organisms, so a detailed patient history and thorough physical examination are imperative. The following events or comorbidities may help identify the causative agent:

- Recent invasive procedure (*S. aureus, Staphylococcus epidermidis,* or *Propionibacterium acnes*)
- Recent infection, such as urinary tract infection (*Escherichia coli, Proteus* sp.), or respiratory tract infection (*Streptococcus pneumoniae*)
- Any unusual oral mucosa or skin lesions
- Dental caries or dental procedures (*Streptococcus* sp.)
- Parenteral injections, such as IV drug use (*Pseudomonas aeruginosa, S. aureus*)
- Endocarditis (acute [*S. aureus*]; subacute [*Streptococcus* sp.])
- Penetrating or blunt trauma
- Chronic medical comorbidities
- Immigration from endemic areas (*Brucella* sp., *Salmonella* sp., fungi, or parasites)
- Alcohol abuse (*Klebsiella pneumoniae*)

The most common causative organisms of spinal epidural abscesses include the following:

- *S. aureus* (both methicillin sensitive and methicillin resistant) is the most common organism cultured in more than 50% of cases (Greenberg, 2010; Karadimas et al., 2008)
- *Streptococcus* sp. (both aerobic and anaerobic) is the second most common organism
- *E. coli*
- *P. aeruginosa*
- *Diplococcus pneumoniae*
- *Serratia marcescens*
- *Enterobacter* sp.
- *Corynebacterium* sp.
- *Enterococcus* sp.
- *C. albicans*
- *S. epidermidis*

Less common organisms include *Propionibacterium acnes, Finegoldia magna* (formerly *Peptostreptococcus magnus*), *Actinomyces* sp., *Proteus mirabilis, Salmonella enterica* subsp. *enterica* serovar Enteritidis (formerly *S. enteritidis*), *Lactobacillus* sp., and group G *Streptococcus* (Karadimas et al., 2008; Greenberg, 2010; Parkins et al., 2008).

The most common causative organisms for vertebral osteomyelitis and discitis include the following:

- *S. aureus* (the most common, found in 40%–50% of positive culture results) (Greenberg, 2010; Hopkinson et al., 2001)
- Other *Staphylococcus* sp.
- *E. coli*
- Viridans streptococci
- Anaerobic *Streptococcus* sp.
- *P. aeruginosa*
- *Mycobacterium tuberculosis*
- *Brucella melitensis* (Karadimas et al., 2008)
- *Proteus* sp.
- *Candida albicans*

Anatomical review

When an abscess occupies the cervical epidural space, it can cause thrombosis of the veins (Figure 57.3). This, in turn, may cause irreversible neurologic deficits. Abscesses in the lumbar epidural space most likely are a result of regional spread from discitis (Figure 57.4).

Common physical examination findings

The most common presenting symptom is pain in the area of spinal involvement. Pain associated with spinal infection is frequently exacerbated by movement and radiates to the extremities; it may worsen at night (Greenberg, 2010). Fever, chills, night sweats, numbness, anorexia, and weight loss may also be present (Cottle et al., 2008; Fernandez et al., 2000; Hopkinson et al., 2001; Karadimas et al., 2008; Kehrer et al., 2014). Physical examination findings include hyperthermia, localized point tenderness, paravertebral muscle spasm with associated impaired mobility, weakness, incontinence, urinary retention, and decreased deep tendon reflexes (Cottle et al., 2008; Duarte et al., 2013; Hopkinson et al., 2001; Kehrer et al., 2014; Lehovsky, 1999). In addition, patients may present with kyphotic deformities or swelling around the affected area (Duarte et al., 2013).

Relevant diagnostic tests

Laboratory tests

- Complete blood cell count with white blood cell count differential
- ESR (to diagnose and monitor treatment progress)
- CRP (Simon et al., 2004)

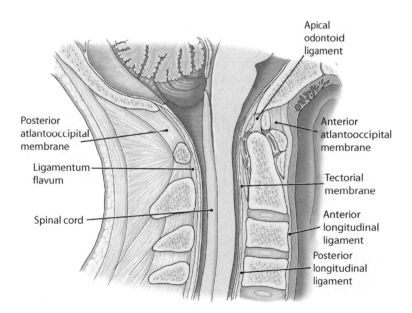

Figure 57.3   The cervical epidural space. When the epidural space is occupied by an abscess, it may lead to thrombosis of the veins, which can cause irreversible neurologic deficits. (Used with permission from Barrow Neurological Institute, Phoenix, Arizona.)

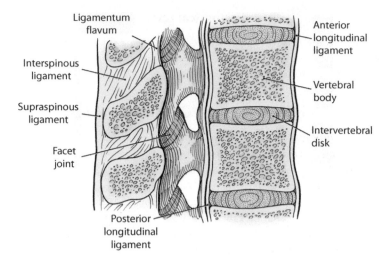

Figure 57.4 The lumbar epidural space. Most lumbar epidural abscesses result from regional spread from discitis. (Used with permission from Barrow Neurological Institute, Phoenix, Arizona.)

- Procalcitonin (Simon et al., 2004; Schwarz et al., 2000)
- Culture and sensitivity of abscess material, bone, and disc (if needle biopsy or surgery is performed)
- Blood cultures (may be positive in a large percentage of patients) (Danner et al., 1987)

Radiologic tests

Radiographs

Plain radiographs of any affected spine segments should be obtained to identify disc space narrowing, end-plate changes, and vertebral body destruction (Osenbach et al., 1990). Changes on plain radiographs may be delayed up to 8 weeks after onset of infection (Lehovsky, 1999).

Computed tomography

Computed tomography (CT) is the best imaging modality for revealing bony destruction. Abscesses are much easier to identify on a CT scan with IV contrast. CT scans are also used for percutaneous needle biopsy of the area in question (Duarte et al., 2013; Osenbach et al., 1990; Varma et al., 2001).

Magnetic resonance imaging

MRI with and without contrast should be conducted to examine the segment of the spine that is affected. Signal change representing edema is the best method of identifying abscess formation (Osenbach et al., 1990). MRI is about 95% accurate in the diagnosis of spinal infections and epidural abscesses (Lury et al., 2006). Positive findings may include hyperintensity of T2-weighted images due to edema. There may be hypointensity of T1-weighted images due to replacement of marrow fat by edema. Contrast enhancement will help delineate infection (Lury et al., 2006). Abscess formation may show up as an enhancing fluid collection that encroaches on the thecal sac or on spinal nerves. A rim of enhancement may also be visible (Lury et al., 2006).

Nuclear medicine bone scan

A nuclear medicine bone scan may be conducted to evaluate the patient for increased uptake of isotope at the site of the infection (Varma et al., 2001; Greenberg, 2010). A bone scan can detect infection as early as 2 days after symptom onset (Lehovsky, 1999).

In general, however, imaging lags behind both onset and resolution of infection and symptoms (Lehovsky, 1999; Lury et al., 2006). An emergency department protocol for MRI as the primary method to evaluate patients for spinal abscesses may be discussed with hospital representatives.

Review of relevant interventional procedures and surgeries

Typically, a CT-guided biopsy and blood cultures are performed. If a pathogen is identified, targeted antimicrobial therapy is initiated. If no pathogen is identified, surgical biopsy may be considered. If a pathogen is still not identified after surgical biopsy, empiric antimicrobial treatments are initiated, taking into consideration any elements of the detailed patient history and physical examination as outlined above. Antimicrobial treatment typically involves a period of IV medication, followed by oral antibiotics (Cottle et al., 2008; Lehovsky, 1999; Osenbach et al., 1990). The duration of antimicrobial treatment varies, depending on the causative organism and the response of the patient. Infectious diseases and pain management specialists should be consulted, and spinal immobilization should be considered.

Surgery

The goal of surgery for patients with spinal infections is to decompress the spine and nerves to prevent long-term sequelae, to stabilize the spine when severe bony destruction and/or kyphosis have occurred, to manage severe pain, to drain abscesses, and to obtain open biopsies to identify the pathogen (Cottle et al., 2008; Lehovsky, 1999; Osenbach et al., 1990). Some authors suggest that débridement and fusion are more effective in preventing postinfection sequelae such as delayed kyphosis and chronic back pain (Hadjipavlou et al., 2000). Indications for surgical treatment include extensive vertebral destruction with kyphosis or instability, presence of epidural abscess, progression of neurologic deficits, intractable pain, and lack of response to conservative medical management (e.g., persistent fever, pain, and laboratory markers of infection) (Karadimas et al., 2008; Lehovsky, 1999).

Family counseling

Prognosis

Patients may present with vague complaints and are often difficult to diagnose. As few as 18% of patients with epidural abscess may be diagnosed correctly (Danner et al., 1987). Outcomes are based on prompt initiation of targeted antimicrobial therapy, neurologic function at the time of presentation, and preexisting comorbidities (Solis Garcia del Pozo et al., 2007; Cottle et al., 2008; Danner et al., 1987; Karadimas et al., 2008). Outcomes improve with early diagnosis (Karadimas et al., 2008). Spine infection should be considered in any patient presenting with new-onset back pain, even without infectious indicators such as fever or abnormal laboratory values.

Common questions

Q: How did I get this infection?
A: Certain coexisting conditions can contribute to spontaneous spine infections, such as chronic comorbid illnesses (e.g., diabetes mellitus, renal failure, tuberculosis, endocarditis, sickle cell anemia, immune

disease, or an infection elsewhere in your body). Any of these conditions may contribute to such an infection. However, in up to 50% of spinal infection cases, we never identify the actual cause.

Q: Will I have this much back pain forever?

A: The hope and goal of treatment is that your back pain will improve over time as treatment goes on.

Q: What if the medications don't work?

A: If there is progression of your symptoms or bony destruction despite antimicrobial therapy, you may require some type of surgery to drain the infection and to stabilize your spine. Our hope is that the medication will be effective and that surgery will not be required.

Common pitfalls and medicolegal concerns

- Failure to obtain an accurate and detailed medical history from the patient and/or to conduct a comprehensive physical examination should empiric antibiotic therapy be indicated
- Initiation of antibiotic therapy prior to obtaining blood and tissue samples for culture and sensitivity testing
- Failure to recognize the patient's worsening neurologic condition or the worsening of infectious markers that may warrant surgical intervention

Relevance to the advanced practice health professional

A detailed medical history and a comprehensive physical examination of the patient are keys to early diagnosis of discitis, osteomyelitis, and epidural abscesses. Prompt diagnosis and targeted antimicrobial treatment are known to decrease long-term sequelae such as chronic pain, deformity, and neurologic debilitation. Delayed diagnosis and treatment may necessitate surgery that could have been prevented with immediate treatment.

Common telephone calls, pages, and requests with answers

Question from nurse caring for patient with discitis: "The patient's ESR has not come down despite two weeks of IV antibiotic treatment. She reports that her back pain continues to improve. What should be done?"

Answer: The laboratory markers of infections, and sometimes the repeated imaging, lag behind clinical improvement. We know that CRP frequently normalizes more quickly. An indication of good response to treatment is a 50% drop in the CRP level each week (Grados et al., 2007).

Question from an intensive care unit nurse caring for a patient with a possible epidural abscess: "Radiology will not be able to do the patient's CT-guided biopsy until tomorrow morning. Should I start her on antibiotics now since there is going to be a delay?"

Answer: No, do not start antibiotics until the biopsy is performed to try to isolate the organism. Although we understand the importance of prompt treatment with antibiotics, we also know that the most success with treatment is when a causative organism is identified prior to initiation of antibiotics. In the absence of impending sepsis, we should wait to prescribe antibiotics until a culture is taken (Osenbach et al. 1990).

References

Butler JS, Shelly MJ, Timlin M, Powderly WG, O–Byrne JM. Nontuberculous pyogenic spinal infection in adults: A 12-year experience from a tertiary referral center. *Spine*. Nov 1 2006;31(23):2695–700.

Cottle L, Riordan T. Infectious spondylodiscitis. *Journal of Infection*. Jun 2008;56(6):401–12.

Danner RL, Hartman BJ. Update on spinal epidural abscess: 35 cases and review of the literature. *Reviews of Infectious Diseases.* Mar–Apr 1987;9(2):265–274.

Duarte RM, Vaccaro AR. Spinal infection: State of the art and management algorithm. *European Spine Journal.* Dec 2013;22(12):2787–2799.

Fernandez M, Carrol CL, Baker CJ. Discitis and vertebral osteomyelitis in vchildren: An 18-year review. *Pediatrics.* Jun 2000;105(6):1299–1304.

Grados F, Lescure FX, Senneville E, Flipo RM, Schmit JL, Fardellone P. Suggestions for managing pyogenic (non-tuberculous) discitis in adults. *Joint, Bone, Spine Revue du Rhumatisme.* Mar 2007;74(2):133–139.

Greenberg MS. *Handbook of Neurosurgery,* 7th ed. Thieme Medical Publishers; 2010.

Hadjipavlou AG, Mader JT, Necessary JT, Muffoletto AJ. Hematogenous pyogenic spinal infections and their surgical management. *Spine.* Jul 1 2000;25(130:1668–1679.

Hawkins M, Bolton M. Pediatric spinal epidural abscess: A 9-year institutional review and review of the literature. *Pediatrics.* Dec 2013;132(6):e1680–1685.

Honan M, White GW, Eisenberg GM. Spontaneous infectious discitis in adults. *American Journal of Medicine.* Jan 1996;100(1):85–89.

Hopkinson N, Stevenson J, Benjamin S. A case ascertainment study of septic discitis: Clinical, microbiological and radiological features. *QJM.* Sep 2001;94(9):465–740.

Hutchinson C, Hanger C, Wilkinson T, Sainsbury R, Pithie A. Spontaneous spinal infections in older people. *Internal Medicine Journal.* Dec 2009;39(12):845–848.

Karadimas E, Bunger JC, Lindblad BE, et al. Spondylodiscitis. a retrospective study of 163 patients. *Acta Orthopaedica.* Oct 2008;79(5):650–659.

Kehrer M, Pedersen C, Jensen TG, Lassen AT. Increasing incidence of pyogenic spondylodiscitis: A 14-year population-based study. *Journal of Infection.* Apr 2014;68(4):313–320.

Kim CJ, Song KH, Jeon JH et al. A comparative study of pyogenic and tuberculous spondylodiscitis. *Spine.* Oct 1 2010;35(21):E1096–100.

Kourbeti IS, Tsiodras S, Boumpas DT. Spinal infections: Evolving concepts. *Current Opinion in Rheumatology.* Jul 2008;20(4):471–479.

Lehovsky J. Pyogenic vertebral osteomyelitis/disc infection. *Bailliere's Best Practice & Research. Clinical Rheumatology.* Mar 1999;13(1):59–75.

Lury K, Smith JK, Castillo M. Imaging of spinal infections. *Seminars in Roentgenology.* Oct 2006;41(4):363–379.

Osenbach RK, Hitchon PW, Menezes AH. Diagnosis and management of pyogenic vertebral osteomyelitis in adults. *Surgical Neurology.* Apr 1990;33(4):266–275.

Parkins MD, Gregson DB. Community-acquired serratia marcescens spinal epidural abscess in a patient without risk factors: Case report and review. *Canadian Journal of Infectious Diseases & Medical Microbiology / AMMI Canada.* May 2008;19(3):250–252.

Reiss-Zimmermann M, Hirsch W, Schuster V, Wojan M, Sorge I. Pyogenic osteomyelitis of the vertebral arch in children. *Journal of Pediatric Surgery.* Aug 2010;45(8):1737–1740.

Schwarz S, Bertram M, Schwab S, Andrassy K, Hacke W. Serum procalcitonin levels in bacterial and abacterial meningitis. *Critical Care Medicine.* Jun 2000;28(6):1828–1832.

Simon L, Gauvin F, Amre DK, Saint-Louis P, Lacroix J. Serum Procalcitonin and C-reactive protein levels as markers of bacterial infection: A systematic review and meta-analysis. *Clinical Infectious Diseases.* Jul 15 2004;39(2):206–217.

Solis Garcia del Pozo J, Vives Soto M, Solera J. Vertebral osteomyelitis: Long-term disability assessment and prognostic factors. *Journal of Infection.* Feb 2007;54(2):129–134.

Turunc T, Demiroglu YZ, Uncu H, Colakoglu S, Arslan H. A comparative analysis of tuberculous, brucellar and pyogenic spontaneous spondylodiscitis patients. *Journal of Infection.* Aug 2007;55(2):158–163.

Varma R, Lander P, Assaf A. Imaging of pyogenic infectious spondylodiskitis. *Radiologic Clinics of North America.* Mar 2001;39(2):203–213.

58

IATROGENIC SPINAL INFECTIONS

Khalid Al-Rayess, Michael Virk, and Praveen V. Mummaneni

Epidemiology

Surgical site infections (SSIs) are one of the most common hospital-acquired infections in the postoperative period (Weinstein et al., 2000). The reported incidence of SSIs in adults undergoing spinal operations ranges from 0.7% to 16% (Weinstein et al., 2000). There are three different types of SSIs defined by the Centers for Disease Control and Prevention (CDC), and these are classified as either incisional or organ/space (Horan et al., 1992). Incisional infections are subclassified as superficial or deep. Superficial infections are limited to dermal and subcutaneous tissue, while deep infections involve subfacial tissues (Horan et al., 1992). Organ/space SSIs involve bone, disc, and/or the epidural space (Horan et al., 1992). The largest study that looked at incidence of SSIs following spine surgery was conducted by Smith and colleagues and included a total of 108,419 patients from 2004 to 2007. They found that infections were superficial in 0.8% of cases and 1.3% deep (Smith et al., 2011). Furthermore, they found that the infection rate among adults varied depending on the location of spine surgery (Smith et al., 2011). The highest rates were for thoracic procedures at 2.1%, then lumbar at 1.6%, and finally cervical at 0.8% (Smith et al., 2011).

Spinal infections are often caused by either bacteria or fungi. The majority of spinal infections are bacterial organisms. The most frequent bacterial pathogen is *Staphylococcus aureus*, which has an incidence range between 30% and 80% (Sobottke et al., 2008). In addition, Gram-negative organisms such *Escherichia coli* are responsible for up to 25% of spinal infections (Sobottke et al., 2008). Overall, the most frequent pathogens found in SSIs are *Staphylococcus aureus*, *Escherichia coli*, *Streptococcus sanguis*, *Pseudomonas aeruginosa*, *Staphylococcus agalactiae*, and *Staphylococcus epidermis* (Sobottke et al., 2008).

There are many risk factors that contribute to the development of these organisms. Some of these are modifiable, while others are not. The greatest risk factors are immunocompromise, diabetes, poor nutritional status, obesity, intravenous drug use history, age greater than 70, and a history of prior SSIs (Koutsoumbelis et al., 2011). Procedure-specific risk factors encompass duration of surgery, intraoperative blood loss, use of instrumentation, multiple stage interventions, number of levels fused, and prolonged preoperative hospital stay (Koutsoumbelis et al., 2011). The Surgical Invasiveness Index (SII) is a validated instrument that accounts for the number of levels arthrodesed, decompressed, or instrumented, as well as the approach (Mirza et al., 2008). Higher SII scores (range: 0–48) indicate more invasive surgery and are associated with a great risk of infection (Mirza et al., 2008). Mirza and colleagues demonstrated that patients with an index of 1 through 5 developed SSIs in 2% of cases, but a group of patients with an index greater than 25 had a rate of 11% (Mirza et al., 2008). Thus, whenever possible, patients should be optimized preoperatively to reduce modifiable risk factors as much as possible. Additionally, for patients with several nonmodifiable risk factors, surgical procedures should be selected that minimize invasiveness and subsequent risk.

Presentation

Diagnosis of spinal infections requires support by clinical, laboratory, and imaging findings. Early diagnosis of SSI following spine surgery is crucial to initiate treatment and prevent further progression. The typical symptoms of SSI include fever and signs of inflammation such as tenderness, erythema, swelling, and warmth (Jensen et al., 1997). However, the most common symptom is wound drainage with an incidence of 68.2% (Pull ter Gunne et al., 2010).

Patients show symptoms on average 28.7 days after spinal surgery (Pull ter Gunne et al., 2010). Superficial infections present earlier than deep infections and are characterized by pain, swelling, redness, and drainage (Jensen et al., 1997; Pull ter Gunne et al., 2010). Deep infections present with more constitutional symptoms including fever, myalgia/arthralgia, pain, and malaise/fatigue. In addition, deep infections have a longer latency than superficial infections and can progress to discitis, osteomyelitis, or epidural (Jensen et al., 1997).

There are several modalities used to diagnose SSIs. Acute phase reactants may be helpful screening tools; however, it is important to note that they need to be evaluated with respect to the time of surgery and are nonspecific. For example, erythrocyte sedimentation rate (ESR) remains elevated for up to 6 weeks after surgery, while C-reactive protein (CRP) normalizes within 2 weeks (Heller, 1992). Elevated ESR and CRP levels are sensitive indicators of any infection and serve as good markers with which to trend the status of infections over time (Heller, 1992). ESR levels can be altered by patient's age and nutrition and may change during the day (Assicot et al., 1993). Thus, CRP is more predictable and responsive in the early postoperative period than ESR (Assicot et al., 1993). In addition, procalcitonin is a precursor of calcitonin, and elevated levels are found in patients with severe bacterial infections (Assicot et al., 1993). In some cases, it has been shown to be more reliable than CRP in the postoperative period with sensitivity of 92% for infection (Nie et al., 2011).

Out of all the imaging modalities, MRI is the most useful to study and diagnose spinal infections. It is the most sensitive (93%) and specific (96%) and has the ability to identify the involvement of surrounding soft tissues (Massie et al., 1992). When using MRI, gadolinium must be used because it improves the accuracy of MRI (Massie et al., 1992). When performing an MRI, any of these findings in a patient may suggest infection: diminished disk height, vertebral body, and disk space; decreased intensity on T1-weighted images, and increased signal intensity on T2-weighted imaging secondary to edema; and endplate definition loss (Figures 58.1 and 58.2) (Massie et al., 1992). Contrast-enhancing pockets or rim-enhancing lesions are also suspicious for infection. Diffusion-weighted imaging demonstrating restriction is also highly suggestive of infection.

The gold standard to diagnose infection is by culture obtained intraoperatively under sterile conditions (Bassewitz et al., 2000). Such cultures are not only helpful to diagnose infection, but also identify a specific pathogen and its drug sensitivities (Bassewitz et al., 2000). Treatment options can be selected based on these sensitivities. Cultures obtained at the bedside by probing an open wound are generally contaminated by skin flora and are of little utility.

Prevention

Preoperative patient optimization can dramatically decrease the rate of SSIs; such prehabilitation consists of lowering pre-op HbA1c, decreasing BMI <30, achieving smoking cessation, weaning off or decreasing steroid use, increasing albumin and vitamin D levels via nutrition/supplementation, optimizing skeletal health and bone density, as well as prescreening for the presence of common pathogens like methicillin-resistant *Staphylococcus aureus* (MRSA) and vancomycin-resistant enterococcus (VRE).

Presurgical precautions are also important. Patient skin antisepsis is recommended at multiple time points with presurgery washes and intraoperative skin preparations (Malangoni, 1997). Common antiseptics generally consist of iodine- and chlorhexidine-based products (Malangoni, 1997). Iodine-based surgical antiseptics are effective against a wide range of Gram-positive and Gram-negative organisms, as well as fungi and viruses (McLure, 1992). Chlorhexidine gluconate has a broad activity against Gram-positive

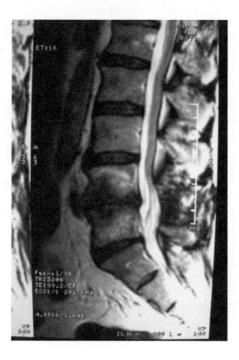

Figure 58.1   Disc space infection at L4/5.

and Gram-negative bacteria, yeasts, and some lipid-enveloped viruses, but fungal coverage is reduced compared to iodine-based antiseptics (Milstone , 2008). Proper surgical handwashing technique with chlorhexidine or iodine scrubs is essential (Tanner et al., 2008). Avoidance of intraoperative containment sources include C-arm, scrubs, gowns, microscopes, graft materials, and implants (Kim et al., 2010). Thus, in the operating room, strict adherence to sterile technique is mandatory.

Also, to prevent SSIs various antibiotic drugs have been assessed as prophylaxis. Potent antibiotics against Gram-positive bacteria like intravenous cephalosporins are used (Doyon et al., 1987). However, intravenous cephalosporins cover less than half of today's staphylococci. Vancomycin is used as prophylaxis for MRSA (Klevens et al., 2002). Since vancomycin needs a higher concentration *in vitro* to be effective, vancomycin powder has been recently introduced into spinal surgery. Khan et al. performed a comprehensive search of clinical studies that identified that vancomycin powder significantly reduced the incidence of SSI after spinal surgery by 2.8% (Khan et al., 2014). The use of prophylactic drains is also common. The advantages of postoperative drain include evacuation of the postoperative hematoma and seroma, thus decreasing the risk of infection and wound breakdown (Weinstein et al., 2000). In addition to drains and vancomycin powder, postoperative wound complications have been lowered by 6.8% after closure of spinal wounds with local muscle flaps (Cohen et al., 2016). Specifically, these spinal reconstructions were performed by use of local muscles and include the paraspinous, trapezius, latissimus, thoracolumbar, and superior gluteal flaps to close the wound (Cohen et al., 2016).

Treatment

Spinal infections are difficult to manage and require careful diagnosis of infection. If the spinal infection is diagnosed as a superficial infection, the infection is usually treated with oral antibiotics for 2 weeks (Weinstein et al., 2000). For deeper infections, surgical incision and drainage with cultures may be necessary (Weinstein et al., 2000). If the diagnosis is a deep wound infection, the patient is brought to the operating

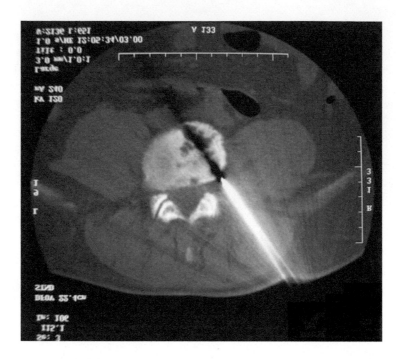

Figure 58.2 Percutaneous biopsy of the disc.

room where the wound is débrided and irrigated under sterile conditions with anesthesia (Malangoni, 1997). These patients are then treated with IV antibiotics for 6–8 weeks (Weinstein et al., 2000). In rare, severe cases, the wound may be packed open and redébrided in 2–4 days (Malangoni, 1997). To improve wound healing, the use of suction irrigation or vacuum-assisted closures (VACs) are being used. Mehbod and colleagues showed that after use of the VAC for 7 days, the wound can be closed without adverse effects or need for removal of hardware (Labler et al., 2006). Suppressive antibiotic therapy is administrated for anaerobes, which consists of oral administration of sulfamethoxazole, trimethoprim or doxycycline (Weinstein et al., 2000). However, for patients who have hardware that cannot be removed with deep infections, long-term suppressive antibiotics are given by mouth after 6–8 weeks of IV antibiotics (Picada et al., 2000).

Conclusion

SSIs following spinal surgery have been reported to occur in up to 16% of cases. Patient prehabilitation prior to surgery, intraoperative skin antisepsis and wound antibiosis, drains, and closure techniques have all been shown to decrease this rate. When infections do occur, recognizing the symptoms, laboratory results, and imaging data facilitate early detection. Oral antibiotics are often sufficient treatment for superficial infections. For deep infections, however, surgical débridement and washout with postoperative IV antibiotics followed by long-term suppressive treatment may be required.

References

Assicot M, Gendrel D, Carsin H, et al. High serum procalcitonin concentration in patients with sepsis and infection. *Lancet.* 1993;341:515–518.

Bassewitz HL, Fishgrund JS, Herkowitz HN. Postoperative spine infections. *Semin Spine Surg.* 2000;12:203–211.

Cohen LE, Fullerton N, Mundy LR. Optimizing Successful Outcomes in Complex Spine Reconstruction Using Local Muscle Flaps. *Plastic and Reconstructive Surgery.* 2016;137(1):295–301.

Doyon F, Evrard J, Mazas F, Hill C. Long-term results of prophylactic cefazolin versus placebo in total hip replacement. *Lancet.* 1987;1:860.

Heller JG. Postoperative infections of the spine. In: Rothman RH, Simeone FA, eds. *The spine.* Philadelphia: WB Saunders; 1992:1817–1837.

Horan TC, Gaynes RP, Martone WJ, Jarvis WR, Emori TG. CDC definitions of nosocomial surgical site infections, 1992: A modification of CDC definitions of surgical wound infections. *Infect Control Hosp Epidemiol.* 1992;13(10):606–608

Jensen AG, et al. Increasing frequency of vertebral osteomyelitis following *Staphylococcus aureus* bacteraemia in Denmark 1980–1990. *J Infect.* 1997;34(2):113–118.

Khan NR, Thompson CJ, DeCuypere M, et al. A meta-analysis of spinal surgical site infection and vancomycin powder. *J Neurosurg Spine.* 2014;21(6):974–83.

Kim DH, Spencer M, Davidson SM, et al. Institutional prescreening for detection and eradication of methicillin-resistant *Staphylococcus aureus* in patients undergoing elective orthopedic surgery. *J Bone Joint Surg Am.* 2010;92:1820–1826

Klevens RM, Edwards JR, Richards CL, Jr., et al. Estimating health care- associated infections and deaths in U.S. hospitals, 2002. *Public Health Rep.* 2007;122:160–166.

Koutsoumbelis S, Hughes AP, Girardi FP, et al. Risk factors for postoperative infection following posterior lumbar instrumented arthrodesis. *J Bone Joint Surg Am.* 2011;93:1627–1633.

Labler L, Keel M, Trentz O, et al. Wound conditioning by vacuum assisted closure (V.A.C.) in postoperative infections after dorsal spine surgery. *Eur. Spine J.* 2006:15:1388–1396.

Massie JB, Heller JG, Abitbol JJ, McPherson D, Garfin SR. Postoperative posterior spinal wound infections. *Clin Orthop Relat Res.* 1992;(284):99–108.

Malangoni MA, editor. *Critical Issues in Operating Room Management.* Philadelphia: Lippincott-Raven; 1997.

McLure AR, Gordon J. In-vitro evaluation of povidone-iodine and chlorhexidine against methicillin-resistant *Staphylococcus aureus. J Hosp Infect.* 1992;21:291–299.

Milstone AM, Passaretti CL, Perl TM. Chlorhexidine: Expanding the armamentarium for infection control and prevention. *Clin Infect Dis.* 2008;46:274–281.

Mirza SK, Deyo RA, Heagerty PJ, et al. Development of an index to characterize the "invasiveness" of spine surgery: Validation by comparison to blood loss and operative time. *Spine.* 2008;33(62):3651–3661.

Nie H, Jiang D, Ou Y, et al. Procalcitonin as an early predictor of postoperative infectious complications in patients with acute traumatic spinal cord injury. *Spinal Cord.* 2011;49:715–720.

Picada R, Winter RB, Lonstein JE, et al. Postoperative deep wound infection in adults after posterior lumbosacral spine fusion with instrumentation: incidence and management. *J Spinal Disord.* 2000;13:42–45.

Pull ter Gunne AF, Mohamed AS, Skolasky RL, et al. The presentation, incidence, etiology, and treatment of surgical site infections after spinal surgery. *Spine.* 2010;35:1323–1328.

Smith JS, Shaffrey CI, Sansur CA, Berven SH, Fu KG, Broadstone PA. "Rates of infection after spine surgery based on 108,419 procedures." *Spine.* 2011;36:556–6310.

Sobottke R, et al. Current diagnosis and treatment of spondylodiscitis. *Dtsch Arztebl Int.* 2008;105(10):181–187.

Swenson BR, Hedrick TL, Metzger R, et al. Effects of preoperative skin preparation on postoperative wound infection rates: A prospective study of 3 skin preparation protocols. *Infect Control Hosp Epidemiol.* 2009;30:964–971.

Tanner J, Swarbrook S, Stuart J. Surgical hand antisepsis to reduce surgical site infection. *Cochrane Database Syst Rev.* 2008

Weinstein MA, McCabe JP, Cammisa FP., Jr.. Postoperative spinal wound infection: A review of 2,391 consecutive index procedures. *J Spinal Disord.* 2000;13:422–426

59

SPINAL FLUID LEAKAGE

Vincent J. Alentado and Michael P. Steinmetz

Case vignette

A nurse from the spine surgery postoperative floor calls to tell you that she is concerned about a new increase in the amount of fluid soaking the bandage of your postoperative patient. The patient is postoperative day 2 from a large lumbar fusion revision surgery. The patient informs you that, in addition to his low back pain from the surgery, he has noticed a new headache that is worse when he sits up in his bed. You examine the bandage covering the wound and notice a red-tinged circle with a surrounding halo of clear fluid. You recognize the patient's positional headache and the classic "target sign" on the patient's bandage as likely representative of a cerebrospinal fluid (CSF) leak. You order magnetic resonance imaging (MRI), which confirms your suspicions (Figure 59.1). With the diagnosis confirmed, you place a lumbar drain and start the patient on prophylactic antibiotics.

Overview

Epidemiology

A CSF leak is a relatively rare postoperative complication following spinal surgery (Mayfield, 1976, p. 435). A CSF leak can result in significant morbidity and possible mortality if untreated. A CSF leak is most commonly encountered following incidental durotomy during either anterior or posterior spinal surgery. Incidental durotomy is an often underreported complication of spinal surgery with an incidence between 3% and 14%. The vast majority of incidental durotomies are identified and contained intraoperatively without significant morbidity. However, an incidental durotomy may turn into a CSF cutaneous fistula if watertight closure of the dura is not achieved intraoperatively or if the durotomy goes unnoticed during the procedure. Overall, the incidence of CSF cutaneous fistula requiring reoperation after spinal surgery is 0.3% (Mayfield, 1976, p. 435). However, the incidence of CSF leak increases to 43% following surgery after spinal radiation surgery, and 13% after surgery for tethered spinal cord (Zide et al., 1987, p. 62). CSF leaks following spinal surgery are most commonly encountered in the lumbosacral region due to the anatomy and higher incidence of surgeries in this region of the spine.

Societal significance

Although most incidental durotomies are repaired intraoperatively without significant postoperative morbidity, persistence of spinal fluid leaks may lead to pseudomeningocele formation, arachnoiditis, intracranial hypotension, neural element herniation, wound dehiscence, fistula formation, and infection. The presence of CSF leak therefore requires immediate intervention be taken to stop the leak. Even when adequately

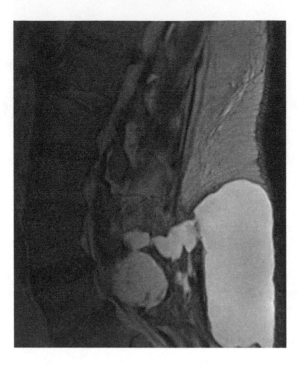

Figure 59.1   Large CSF cutaneous fistula in a patient who presented with postoperative wound drainage.

treated, spinal fluid leaks contribute to increased postoperative morbidity, prolonged hospitalization, and increased cost of care. These factors are further worsened in cases where conservative management fails and additional surgery is needed to repair the leakage.

Basic biologic and physiologic processes

A dural tear is the initial event that leads to postoperative CSF leak. If a watertight dural closure is not achieved during surgery, CSF may drain through the surgical tract to create a CSF cutaneous fistula. Cutaneous CSF fistulas most commonly occur in the immediate postoperative period 1–7 days after surgery. Not all incidental durotomies proceed to becoming CSF leaks. Rather, any process that disrupts dural or wound healing may predispose to CSF leakage. This includes scar tissue, irradiation, localized infection, or foreign bodies. Patient risk factors include nutritional deficits, endocrine disorders, chronic diseases, and steroids. An upright posture, coughing, sneezing, or Valsalva maneuver may increase leakage from fistulas due to the transient increase in CSF pressure.

Anatomical review

Three separate membranes, known as the meninges, cover the central nervous system. The dura mater is the thickest, outermost layer. It is a dense, fibrous sheath that forms around the brain and spinal cord. The arachnoid mater is the middle layer of meninges that loosely adjoins the dura mater. The potential space between the dura and arachnoid layers is known as the subdural space. The arachnoid layer is connected to the innermost pia mater by fine trabeculae. The space between the arachnoid mater and pia mater creates a true space known as the subarachnoid space. The subarachnoid space is filled with CSF, which provides nourishment and protection to the central nervous system (CNS).

Common physical examination findings

- Postural or persistent headache
- Dizziness
- Unrelenting back pain
- Cranial nerve root entrapment
- Fluctuations in conscious state
- Watery discharge that is augmented by upright posture or Valsalva
- Clear halo that surrounds central pink stain on an absorbent surface
- Wound swelling

Relevant diagnostic tests

Laboratory

- Glucose content of CSF will be greater than or equal to half serum glucose levels
- Immunofixation of ß2-transferrin is specific for CSF

Vascular/Electrophysiologic/Radiologic

- MRI and computed tomography (CT) will help localize the CSF leak.
  - MRI is superior because of soft tissue enhancement.
- For operative planning, intrathecal dye may be injected into the subarachnoid space, and then a CT scan is performed to visualize a CSF leak.
- For slow or intermittent leaks, radionuclide myelography may better visualize leakage.

Review of relevant interventional procedures and surgeries

Most cases of postoperative CSF leak can be managed via nonoperative methods. Initial management of CSF leak includes laying the patient flat to more evenly distribute CSF pressure. If positioning alone does not relieve or improve the leak within 24 hours, other nonoperative interventions are warranted. The type of nonoperative treatment implemented depends on the size and location of the leak. A small, localized leak may be resolved by placing a single subcutaneous stitch to close the fistula tract to the skin.

Persistent leaks require CSF diversion through external drainage. This is most commonly done via a lumbar drain. In order to place a lumbar drain, a 19-gauge catheter is threaded percutaneously through a 17-gauge Tuohy needle that has been inserted into the lumbar subarachnoid space. Initial insertion of the Tuohy needle is performed in analogous fashion to a lumbar puncture. After 10–20 cm of the catheter has been threaded through the needle, the needle is removed over the catheter. The proximal end of the catheter is then connected to a sterile drainage system. The site of catheter insertion into the skin should be covered with a waterproof dressing, and the catheter should be taped to prevent disconnection or pulling. Some providers suggest that antibiotics should be administered while the catheter is within the subarachnoid space; however, evidence of the utility of this measure is lacking. Drainage should be continued for 3–5 days after the leak has stopped in order to maximize healing potential. Daily samples of CSF should be obtained for culture, Gram stain, cell count with differential, glucose, and protein. If antibiotics were used, they should be continued 8–24 hours after removal of the catheter. If the patient gets out of bed, the drain should be temporarily clamped to prevent sudden overdrainage.

If the leak is a low- or normal-pressure leak, a percutaneous epidural blood patch may also be used to seal the leak. A percutaneous blood patch has a theoretically smaller risk of infection and earlier mobilization compared with CSF diversion. A blood patch is performed by injecting 10–25 mL of fresh autologous blood into the epidural space near the drainage site. This blood forms an occlusive clot over the dural breach and increases extradural tissue pressure, allowing for adequate healing in some cases.

When nonoperative interventions fail, or if a patient has significant symptoms, a revision surgery may be indicated.

Common grading schemes

There is no grading system for CSF leaks. Rather, CSF leaks are categorized based on their timing of presentation. CSF leaks may be categorized as traumatic or nontraumatic. Acute leaks happen within a week of trauma, whereas delayed leaks occur weeks to months postoperatively.

Family counseling

Prognosis

The prognosis following CSF leaks is favorable. CSF diversion is successful at alleviating a cutaneous fistula in 90%–100% of cases. However, CSF leaks are associated with a 10% chance of infection, which may lead to further complications such as meningitis. Furthermore, 60% of patients with lumbar drainage complain of significant postural headaches during their treatment course.

Common questions

- *How does the body compensate for the leaking CSF?*
  - The intracranial hypotension that causes postural headache in cases of CSF leak is compensated for by increased CSF production within the brain.
- *What is the rate of reoccurrence of CSF leak?*
  - 10% of CSF leaks will recur over 10 years. Typically, the cutaneous fistula is at a different location than the original leak.

Pitfalls

Since CSF leaks are relatively uncommon, and drainage from a postoperative spinal wound is expected, CSF leaks may often be missed until they have progressed significantly. Therefore, a high index of suspicion is required for prompt diagnosis of CSF leak. Failure to recognize CSF leak could cause postoperative wound infection, meningitis, and delayed wound healing. Furthermore, excessive CSF drainage may cause intracranial complications such as subdural hematoma or cranial nerve compression.

Common pitfalls and medicolegal concerns

- A study reviewing malpractice lawsuits related to spinal operations observed that incidental durotomy was the second most common (16%) complaint identified (Goodkin and Laska, 1995, p. 4).

Relevance to the advanced practice health professional

CSF leaks are a relatively rare postoperative complication following spinal surgery. Often, these leaks initially go undiagnosed because of the normal surgical site pain and drainage that accompany all spinal procedures. However, early diagnosis of CSF leakage is extremely important in preventing adverse outcomes related to the leak. Advanced practice health professionals should therefore be able to recognize the signs and symptoms of CSF leak, which is vital in early detection and treatment of this complication.

Common phone calls, pages, and requests with answers

- *Are antibiotics for patients with cutaneous fistula necessary?*
  - Most of this evidence related to antibiotics for CSF leak is extrapolated from rhinorrhea or otorrhea where evidence does not support their administration. If antibiotics are administered, a broad-spectrum antibiotic is recommended.

- *A patient's postural headache is not improving after insertion of the lumbar drain.*
  - The lumbar drain facilitates healing by redistributing pressure away from the injured dura at the site of the initial CSF leak. However, the lumbar drain creates a similar decrease in CSF levels that is responsible for the postural headache seen during CSF leak. These headaches can be treated with caffeine and pain medications, as appropriate.

References

Goodkin R, Laska LL. Unintended 'incidental' durotomy during surgery of the lumbar spine: Medicolegal implications. *Surgical Neurology.* 1995;43(1):4–12; discussion 12–14.

Mayfield FH. Complications of laminectomy. *Clinical Neurosurgery.* 1976;23:435–39.

Zide BM, Wisoff JH, Epstein FJ. 1987. Closure of extensive and complicated laminectomy wounds operative technique. *Journal of Neurosurgery.* 1987;67(1):59–64. doi:10.3171/jns.1987.67.1.0059.

60

PERCUTANEOUS SPINAL INTERVENTIONS AND PAIN MANAGEMENT

Eric Mayer and Karen Bond

Introduction

Spinal disorders that include back pain and neck pain are common and costly. Chief presenting complaints of back and neck pain are among the top three types of visits to primary care and emergency physicians and among the top five reasons to seek specialty care (Martin et al., 2008). Radiating pain to arm or leg (known as radicular pain) is a less common presenting symptom but accounts for a significant amount of lost work time and lost productivity. The point prevalence for neck and back pain is between 30% and 50% with lifetime prevalence exceeding 85%. Familiarity with the continuum of treatment options for axial back/neck pain, radiating arm/leg pain, and common misdiagnoses will aid all advanced practice providers in providing more valuable care. Although the majority of back pain is self-limiting, with symptom improvement or resolution within 30 days with conservative therapy, about 10% of patients do not realize improvement in their symptoms and would benefit from further intervention. There are three basic principles of acute low back or neck pain demonstrated in the literature:

1. In the majority of cases of acute low back and neck pain, a precise anatomic diagnosis is never identified (Carragee et al., 2006).
2. The natural history of acute low back and neck pain is extremely favorable with spontaneous resolution within 30 days in most patients.
3. Serious causes of low back pain such as fracture, infection, malignancy, cauda equina, or spinal cord injury are extremely rare but should be suspected in the presence of "red flag" screening.

Conversely, there are several principles that encourage early diligence to maximize benefit to the patient:

1. Bed rest exceeding 48 hours has been implicated in being a leading contributor to chronic, disabling spinal pain (Deyo et al., 1986).
2. Early prescriptions for opioid narcotic medication, particularly for work-related pain, increase the risk for poor outcome, the duration of absence from normal function (Volinn et al., 2009), and the likelihood of prolonged disability (Franklin et al., 2008).
3. Reasons for prolonged disability include the following: Most commonly, unrecognized, complicating psychosocial issues; previously unrecognized pathology; and excessive passive treatment modalities (e.g., prolonged bed rest and passive forms of therapy) (Klenerman et al., 1995). Intuitive

identification of these salient features before the advantage of the subacute timeframe (6–12 weeks) will reduce the burden of care.

The most important message is that persistent functional disability related to back and neck pain that exceeds 3 months increases the likelihood of disability (Chou et al., 2007). There are very few instances in which a patient with back pain or radiculopathy would require a referral directly to a spine surgeon (Daffner et al., 2010). Importantly, early referral for spinal surgery has not been shown to significantly improve outcomes at 1 year or beyond (Weinstein et al., 2006). Patients with the best postsurgical outcomes are typically those who have tried and failed one (or more) type of conservative or minimally invasive form of treatment (Chou et al., 2009). Immediate referral to a spine surgeon is indicated in the face of red flags (bowel or bladder incontinence, high clinical suspicion for spinal fracture, high clinical suspicion for infection, progressive weakness, paralysis, and high clinical suspicion for malignancy). This chapter outlines the most common therapeutic options that are available for axial and radicular spinal pathology.

After a thorough interview and examination of the patient, the clinician must differentiate between axial spinal pain and radicular pain, for this will guide most future treatment options. Going forward, we divide the sections into axial versus radicular pain with a discussion of possible confounding features that we term *masqueraders*.

Axial back pain

Axial back pain can be defined as back pain that is at the midline or just lateral to the midline. Axial back pain can be mechanical, myofascial, inflammatory, or a combination. The history of patients with mechanical back pain will often include some type of abnormal stress on the muscles that support and move the vertebral column, usually due to deconditioning, posture, excessive weight, improper body mechanics, overuse, or trauma. As stated above, in most cases, the pain is idiopathic, and an anatomic cause will not be adequately determined. Importantly, in cases of axial back pain, there is a *normal* neurologic exam.

The role of imaging in axial back pain

- If there has been significant trauma to the spine, or if there is tenderness on palpation to the vertebrae on physical examination, x-ray may be considered to identify a fracture.
- In the absence of trauma, x-ray may not be helpful; though incidental findings of spinal curves, occult fractures, congenital variations, or degenerative changes may be discovered.
- If the patient fails to make meaningful improvement in functional/work status, objective testing in physical therapy, or pain scores in 4–8 weeks, advanced imaging to determine a pain-generator is advocated.

Etiology of axial back pain

Axial back pain has four main etiologies:

1. *Facet joint–mediated pain*
   - Lumbar facet arthropathy can present as pain in the lower back and may refer to the posterior thigh.
   - Cervical facet arthropathy may present as pain in the neck, trapezius, or shoulder blades, and may include headache.
   - Facet-mediated pain in cervical and lumbar spine may also be related to incidental discoveries like spondylolysis, spondylolisthesis, congenital hemifusion, limbus vertebrae, or limbus discs.

2. *Sacroiliac (SI) joint-mediated pain:* This is characterized by pain directly over the affected sacroiliac (SI) joint and may refer to the ipsilateral buttock, lateral hip, lateral thigh, or groin.
3. *Myofascial neck or back pain:* This is either idiopathic or due to mechanical sprain/strain and follows the distribution of one or more muscles involved in a particular action.
4. *Discogenic pain:* Pain is typically worse with flexion, improved with extension, and tends to be deep and agonizing in quality; it may resolve only with prolonged recumbent positioning.

Due to the multiplicity of etiologies involved in low back and neck pain, the definitive diagnosis of true discogenic pain can be difficult. Both discography and magnetic resonance imaging (MRI) are used for this purpose, but proper diagnostic testing remains controversial with literature showing both poor positive and negative predictive values (PPV/NPV) from MRI and discography. Among the most contentious aspects of discography's ability to diagnose discogenic pain is the fact that severely damaged discs do not always cause pain, and minimally damaged discs may cause severe pain. Moreover, the test has been implicated in potentially accelerating disc degeneration (Figure 60.1).

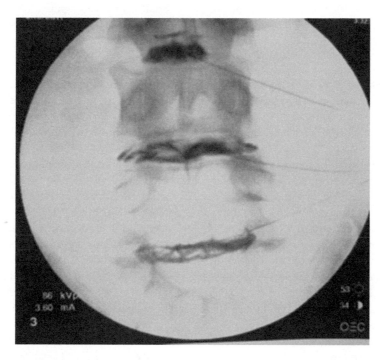

Figure 60.1 Discography is a diagnostic procedure whereby contrast dye is injected into the disc using fluoroscopic guidance with the objective of increasing intradiscal pressure in order to replicate symptoms and thus identify a specific disc as a source of pain.

Treatments for axial back pain

-   *Initial, noninvasive treatment:* The initial treatment for all types of mechanical axial back pain is straightforward and may include one or all of the following, depending on the severity of the symptoms:
    -   Appropriate education about the favorable prognosis of acute axial pain, encourage return activity including work (even in a modified capacity), and discourage prolonged rest.

- Physical therapy may be beneficial in only select patients in the first 2–4 weeks (Gellhorn et al., 2012); it has been shown to reduce functional inhibition (Fritz et al., 2003), disability, and work absence after 4 weeks (Long et al., 2004).
- Nonsteroidal anti-inflammatory drugs (NSAIDS) have been shown in the literature to be more effective than placebo in allowing a patient to return to normal function and to relieve pain (Chou et al., 2007).
- Skeletal muscle relaxants (SMRs) are more effective in combination with NSAIDs than NSAIDs alone. Meaningful efficacy of SMRs regresses after approximately 2 weeks. Carisoprodol (Soma) poses a high risk for physical and psychological dependence, abuse, and harm and should therefore be avoided. Cyclobenzaprine should be avoided in patients who are taking tramadol or selective serotonin reuptake inhibitors (SSRIs) due to the rare but potentially devastating risks associated with "serotonin syndrome."
- Membrane stabilizers (i.e., gabapentin, pregabalin) show limited evidence for use in axial neck or back pain.
- Psychiatric assistance with education about "hurt versus harm" should be consistently delivered by any health-care provider with possible referral for formal cognitive behavioral therapy or other psychological intervention to reduce pain inhibition behaviors.
- Watchful waiting

- *Joint injections*: Cervical or lumbar facet joint pain has been shown to be the source of pain in 15%–40% of patients. Controversy regarding the efficacy of certain forms of physical therapy alone, in combination with intraarticular injections, medial branch blocks, or radiofrequency rhizotomy of medial branch/dorsal rami nerves has not been resolved in the literature. Clinical consultation with an interventional spine specialist (physiatry, anesthesia, or radiology) is an option. Additional injections after the first injection should be contingent upon >50% improvement sustained more than 4 weeks, with concomitant improvement in functional/work status, or complete elimination of pain symptoms for a minimum of 1 week following single joint injection.
- *SI joint injections*: These may be used for clinical evidence of reproduction of pain with 2–3/6 provocative maneuvers concordant with pain centered over posterior superior iliac spine (PSIS), or SI joint. When not combined with steroids, SI joint injections can be diagnostic, to differentiate SI joint (from lower lumbar facet joints or intrinsic hip pathology) as the cause of referred low back pain. SI joint injections may be therapeutic when steroid is added, to treat SI joint pain. Available literature indicates that therapeutic SI injections have variable longevity when not combined with specific physical therapy.
- Articular joint (facet) injections:
  - Aggressive investigation for unrecognized structural causes of pain should be performed to eliminate "masquerader" like "hip-spine" syndrome or "shoulder-neck" syndrome, well described by Ian McNab in the 1970s.

    - Radiologically guided, diagnostic and possibly therapeutic intraarticular joint injection with ultrasound, fluoroscopy, computed tomography (CT), or MRI is particularly useful in identifying and possibly eliminating persistent nonspinal causes of pain.
    - Intraarticular injections should be combined with physical therapy to improve durability of functional improvement and pain relief.

- Minimally invasive intradiscal therapies

- Thermal therapies, annular repair, intradiscal platelet-rich plasma (PRP), and intradiscal stem cells are unproven in efficacy, with only one level II study on intradiscal electrothermal annuloplasty (IDEA; or intradiscal electrothermal therapy, IDET) performed. While this remains a robust area of study at the publication of this chapter, there remains much greater hope and hype rather than evidence or efficacy.

Radicular pain

Radicular pain is pain referred from a spinal nerve root along one or more dermatomes or myotomes of an extremity. In the case of spinal disc hernation/extrusion upper/lower limb pain is usually greater and more intense than axial spine pain. Weakness may or may not be present with a radiculitis, but it should provide heightened concern for advanced imaging and referral to a spine specialist if weakness is progressive or accompanied by bowel or bladder incontinence. Proper diagnostic testing is important to determine if the extremity pain is the result of nerve root inflammation, compression, or some other confounding peripheral cause (e.g.. peripheral neuropathy, carpal tunnel, ulnar neuropathy, brachial/lumbar plexopathy, amyotrophy, etc.). Common mimics of lumbar radiculopathy include inflammatory bursitis, iliotibial band syndrome, rotator cuff syndrome, femoral acetabular impingement, osteoarthritis of the hip/shoulder, elbow/knee/wrist pathology, trochanteric bursitis, or hip fracture.

The role of imaging in radicular pain

In the absence of extreme pain, weakness, or persistent objective sensory deficit with reflex abnormality, imaging is not recommended (Chou et al., 2011). If the patient has failed at least 4 weeks of conservative therapy, or if there are neurologic or sensory abnormalities present along with complaints of pain, MRI or CT scan are indicated. MRI is the study of choice for radicular pain, but for patients for whom MRI is contraindicated, standard CT or a CT myelogram is usually a suitable alternative.

Treatments for radicular pain

- *Initial, noninvasive treatment*: Like axial back pain, radicular pain may be self-limited. Initial therapy for radicular pain is similar to that for axial back pain and may include the following:
  - *Physical therapy*: Literature shows particular efficacy with directional therapy (often known as "McKenzie-based programs") (Donelson, 2011), core strengthening, and aerobic exercise (Gellhorn, 2012). Avoidance of "passive therapy" is encouraged with poor efficacy noted with E-Stim, traction, "cold-laser," dry needling, and trigger points.
  - *Manipulation*: A cohort of uncontrolled studies and "case series" has suggested a benefit from chiropractic or osteopathic manipulation to improve cervical or lumbar radiculopathy. No high-quality prospective randomized study exists showing objective clinical efficacy from manipulation improving functional or utility outcomes in radiculopathy. Moreover, several case reports associate cervical manipulation with serious vascular and mechanical complications including radiculopathy, and myelopathy, vertebral artery injury. Increased risk of serious harm from spinal manipulation with hands or devices (e.g., DRX or VAX) makes these methods controversial. In the absence of clear efficacy and possible risk, manipulation to reduce symptoms associated with radiculopathy is not recommended.
  - *Membrane stabilizers* (i.e., gabapentin, pregabalin, Topiramate, etc.): Use of this heterogeneous group of medications that include antiepileptics and antidepressant medications may have indications for neuropathic pain (Yaksi et al., 2007). Specific use for radiculopathy is considered by many to be

U.S. Food and Drug Administration (FDA) "off-label." These medications are generally considered to be superior to opioids and NSAIDs for neuropathic pain (Chou et al., 2007).

- *NSAIDs and SMRs*: Barring any contraindications, it is recommended to use NSAIDS, SMRs, or acetaminophen. Consider limiting the use of such medications to a 2-week trial and only continuing if clear efficacy is endorsed by the patient.
- *Oral corticosteroid taper*: Despite the presence of only three moderate-evidence studies supporting the use of oral steroids, a clinician may consider a tapering course of oral steroid medications in a carefully selected group of patients who do not improve promptly with modalities listed above in the first 4 weeks and have consistent functional inhibition. Patients with diabetes, hypertension, or coronary artery disease must be cautioned about side effects, and there are rare, idiopathic examples of avascular necrosis in peripheral joints.

  - *Opiate analgesics*: Opioids may be considered as a last-line option for severe/disabling acute or chronic acute back pain that has been refractory to other pharmaceutical treatment. If prescribed, the course of treatment should not exceed 2 weeks. In the setting of chronic, unremitting pain, consultation with a pain management provider or an interdisciplinary pain program is advisable. Recent evidence of increased lifetime risk of abuse, misuse, diversion, and associated disability are reported in the medical literature along with other risks including gonadal suppression, increased fracture risk, and central sensitization. The use of prescription monitoring programs, compliance monitoring, and regular assessment of the "four A's" of opioid analgesia—activities of daily living, analgesia, adverse effects, and aberrant drug use—is necessary. Tramadol is a weak opioid that may be considered as an opioid alternative, although no high-quality studies show risk reduction with use of this medication.

Epidural steroid injections (ESIs)

For patients who have failed 4 weeks of initial conservative treatment, epidural steroid injection may be considered. In epidural steroid injections, a combination of short-acting anesthetic and long-acting steroid are injected directly into the epidural space at the level of known or suspected spinal pathology. Advanced imaging (MRI or CT) is strongly recommended prior to an attempt at ESI, as aberrant vascular and congenital findings can lead to harm. It is important to note that the ESI does not alter the lesion but has shown efficacy in improving function, improving work attendance, and reducing symptoms (Armon et al., 2007). Selection of the type of ESI performed is made based on the patient's individual pathology and anatomy. ESIs must be done by a highly trained practitioner, and it is strongly advised if not required by many insurance plans that injections be done with radiologic guidance (fluoroscopy) to avoid complications of epidural hematoma, neural injury, dural puncture, or nerve damage (Kolstad et al., 2005). The expectations are that there should be at least a 50% postinjection reduction in reported pain symptoms, and that symptom relief should last up to 3 months. Failure to achieve at least a 50% reduction in pain symptoms for 30 days should preclude a second injection. More than three steroid injections in a 6- to 12-month period should be avoided due to potential side effects of corticosteroids. There are three main types of ESIs:

- *Transforaminal injection*: A combination of anesthetic and steroid is injected directly into the neuroforamen in proximity to the affected nerve root.
- *Intralaminar injection* (aka "midline" epidural injection): A combination of anesthetic and steroid is injected directly into the epidural space between the lamina, at the midline.
- *Caudal injection*: A combination of anesthetic and steroid is injected via a needle inserted into the sacral hiatus, which leads to the epidural space.

- *Complications of epidural steroid injections*: The potential complications of ESIs include
  - Infection
  - Dural puncture
  - Bleeding
  - Nerve damage
  - Allergic reaction to medication or contrast dye
  - Inadvertent vascular uptake of anesthetic

    - *Side effects of corticosteroids*: Although usually less pronounced than with steroids that are given orally, the common side effects of steroids may be produced in patients who receive ESIs (i.e., increased serum glucose levels in diabetics).

- *Surgery*: Although the majority of patients do well with conservative treatment, referral to a spine surgeon (either neurosurgeon or orthopedic surgeon specializing in the spine) is indicated under the following circumstances:

  - Radicular pain, with correlating lesion on imaging, with progressive neurologic deficit that has been refractory to any of the above treatment modalities.
  - Neurogenic claudication, with correlating lesion on imaging, that has been refractory to conservative treatment.
  - Cases of myelopathy or rapid neurologic decline. If a patient exhibits these "red flags," do not start conservative therapy but refer directly to a surgeon.

    - Gait disturbance
    - Hand clumsiness
    - Bowel or bladder dysfunction

Conclusion

Because of the multitude of etiologies for pain originating from the spine, as well as the presence of "masqueraders" of spinal pain, the practitioner must take great care in differentiating spinal pain from pain of other sources through careful history and physical examination. Although treatment options for various spinal pathologies are varied, there are several common dos and don'ts when treating these patients.

Do:

- Monitor the patient for the presence of red flags (bowel or bladder incontinence, progressive weakness, paralysis, or high clinical suspicion for fracture, infection, or malignancy).
- Refer directly to a spine surgeon in the presence of red flags.
- Follow a continuum of care, progressing from most conservative to most invasive.
- Encourage early activity.
- Monitor the patient frequently to encourage active participation of the patient in his or her own care and to monitor either positive or negative progression of condition.
- Strongly consider use of available outcomes assessment tools (EQ-5D, PDQ, ODI, STaRT) to aid clinical decision making.
- Consider advanced imaging and/or referral to a qualified spine interventionist if there is not at least 50% improvement in symptoms after 4–6 weeks of conservative management.

Don't:

- Prescribe an opioid early in the course of treatment.
- Recommend prolonged rest or prolonged work absences.
- Prescribe opioids for chronic pain; refer to a qualified pain management provider.
- Recommend a "series" of injections without clinical reassessment.

References

Armon C, Argoff CE, Samuels J, Backonja MM. Therapeutics and Technology Assessment Subcommittee of the American Academy of Neurology. Assessment: Use of epidural steroid injections to treat radicular lumbosacral pain: Report of the Therapeutics and Technology Assessment Subcommittee of the American Academy of Neurology. *Neurology.* 2007;68(10):723–729.

Carragee E, Alamin T, Cheng I, Franklin T, van den Haak E, Hurwitz E. (2006b). Are first-time episodes of serious LBP associated with new MRI findings? *The Spine Journal (TSJ).* 2006;6:624–635.

Chou R, Baisden J, Carragee EJ, Resnick DK, Shaffer WO, Loeser JD. Surgery for low back pain: A review of the evidence for an American Pain Society Clinical Practice Guideline. *Spine.* 2009;34(10):1094–1109.

Chou R, Huffman LH; American Pain Society; American College of Physicians. Medications for acute and chronic low back pain: A review of the evidence for an American Pain Society/American College of Physicians clinical practice guideline. *Ann Intern Med.* 2007;147(7):505–514.

Chou R, Qaseem A, Owens DK, Shekelle P; Clinical Guidelines Committee of the American College of Physicians. Diagnostic imaging for low back pain: Advice for high-value health care from the American College of Physicians. *Ann Intern Med.* 2011;154(3):181–189.

Chou R, Qaseem A, Snow V, et al. Clinical Efficacy Assessment Subcommittee of the American College of Physicians; American College of Physicians; American Pain Society Low Back Pain Guidelines Panel. Diagnosis and treatment of low back pain: A joint clinical practice guideline from the American College of Physicians and the American Pain Society. *Ann Intern Med.* 2007;147(7):478–491.

Daffner SD, Hymanson HJ, Wang JC. Cost and use of conservative management of lumbar disc herniation before discectomy. *Spine J.* 2010;10:463–468.

Deyo R, Diehl A, Rosenthal M. How many days of bed rest for acute low back pain? *New England J Med,* 1986;315:1064–1070.

Donelson R. Mechanical diagnosis and therapy for radiculopathy. *Phys Med Rehabil Clin N Am.* 2011;22(1):75–89.

Franklin GM, Stover BD, Turner JA, Fulton-Kehoe D, Wickizer TM. Disability Risk Identification Study Cohort. Early opioid prescription disability among workers with back injuries: The Disability Risk Identification Study Cohort. *Spine.* 2008;33(2):199–204.

Fritz JM, Delitto A, Erhard RE. Comparison of classification-based physical therapy with therapy based on clinical practice guidelines for patients with acute low back pain: A randomized clinical trial. *Spine.* 2003;28(13):1363–1371; discussion 1372.

Gellhorn AC, Chan L, Martin B, Friedly J. Management patterns in acute low back pain: The role of physical therapy. *Spine.* 2012;37(9):775–782.

Klenerman L, Slade P, Stanley I, et al. The prediction of chronicity in patients with acute attack of low back pain in a general practice setting. *Spine* 1995;20:478–484.

Kolstad F, Leivseth G, Nygaard OP. Transforaminal steroid injections in the treatment of cervical radiculopathy. *A prospective outcome study. Acta Neurochir (Wien).* 2005;147(10):1065–1070.

Long A, Donelson R, Fung T. Does it matter which exercise? A randomized control trial of exercise for low back pain. *Spine.* 2004;29(23):2593–2602.

Martin BI, Deyo RA, Mirza SK, et al. Expenditures and health status among adults with back and neck problems. *JAMA.* 2008;299(6):656–664.

Volinn E, Fargo JD, Fine PG. Opioid therapy for nonspecific low back pain and the outcome of chronic work loss. *Pain.* 2009;142(3):194–201.

Weinstein JN, Tosteson TD, Lurie JD, et al. Surgical vs nonoperative treatment for lumbar disk herniation: The Spine Patient Outcomes Research Trial (SPORT): A randomized trial. *JAMA.* 2006;296(20):2441–2450.

Yaksi A, Ozgönenel L, Ozgönenel B. The efficacy of gabapentin therapy in patients with lumbar spinal stenosis. *Spine.* 2007;32(9):939–942.

PART VII

Clinical Pathologies and Scenarios: Neurology

61

ACUTE ISCHEMIC STROKE

Nicole Bennett

Case vignette

A 67-year-old female was with friends and suddenly slumped over, unable to speak. 911 was called, and emergency medical services (EMS) arrived within 10 minutes of symptom onset. Paramedics confirmed a positive Cincinnati Stroke Scale with right facial droop, right upper extremity pronator drift, and difficulty speaking. Her blood glucose was 110. While en route to the local emergency department (ED), EMS notified the ED of a possible stroke patient.

Upon receiving the EMS call, the ED activated their internal Stroke Code, alerting radiology, laboratory, nursing, pharmacy, and providers of a possible stroke patient. The team was waiting in the computed tomography (CT) suite when she arrived. The ED provider began an initial exam, a nurse placed an IV, and labs were sent. Her neurologic exam was significant for a left gaze preference, right facial droop, right arm and right leg without movement, and 0/5 strength. She was alert, though unable to verbalize or follow commands. Blood pressure 181/78, heart rate 60, respiratory rate 16; electrocardiogram demonstrated a normal sinus rhythm. The noncontrast head CT revealed no intracranial hemorrhage; however, a dense artery sign was noted in the left middle cerebral artery (Figure 61.1).

A telestroke consult was completed with a vascular neurologist, and intravenous-alteplase was recommended. The bolus and drip were started within 45 minutes of the patient's ED arrival. While the IV-alteplase was infusing, she was air transported to the nearest Comprehensive Stroke Center for consideration of neuroendovascular treatment of suspected embolus. Upon arrival, the patient was able to move her right upper extremity but was without return of right lower extremity strength or speech. CT angiography and CT perfusion were emergently completed on arrival, demonstrating a large vessel occlusion of the left middle cerebral artery and critical stenosis of the left internal carotid artery.

Neuroendovascular intervention with balloon angiography to open the stenosed left internal carotid artery was emergently completed. A Stentriever could then be used to remove the clot. Postprocedure, imaging showed complete resolution of blood flow to the left middle cerebral artery. She was taken to the neuroscience intensive care unit (Neuro-ICU) for recovery.

Examination the following morning revealed only mild arm and leg weakness (4/5) and a left pronator drift as well as moderate expressive aphasia, though improved from preoperatively. A repeat head CT was completed showing no hemorrhagic transformation and only a small area of infarct in the deep basal ganglia. She was started on aspirin 81 mg and atorvastatin 80 mg for secondary stroke prevention. Etiology of her stroke was attributed to atherosclerosis of her left internal carotid artery, which caused an artery-to-artery embolism. She discharged to acute rehabilitation, and a carotid endarterectomy was planned in the next several weeks.

Introduction

Stroke is the fifth leading cause of death in the United States (National Center for Health Statistics, 2016). It is estimated that someone in the United States has a stroke every 40 seconds, and the economic burden exceeds $34 billion annually. Over the past 10 years, there has been a sharp decrease in the death rate from stroke, thought to be related to prevention education, improved access to early treatment, increased use of thrombolytics, etc. Despite this, stroke remains the leading cause of disability (Jauch et al., 2013; Mozaffarian et al., 2016).

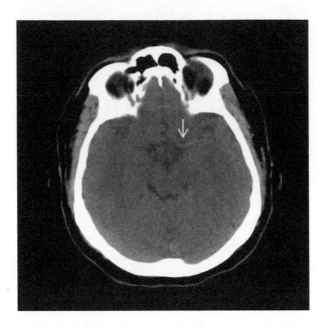

Figure 61.1 Left middle cerebral artery, dense artery sign.

Ischemic stroke occurs when there is a blockage of blood flow to the brain and accounts for greater than 80% of all strokes. Tissue plasminogen activator (IV-alteplase), approved by the U.S. Food and Drug Administration in 1996, remains the only pharmacologic agent available for emergent use, and must be given within 3–4.5 hours of symptom onset. Since IV-alteplase approval, research has continued to advance the science of initial stroke treatment, with technological improvements in imaging modalities and innovative device design. Notably, in 2015, the first positive trials substantiating the benefit of early endovascular intervention were published. Time to treatment, however, continues to be a constraining factor.

Time is brain!

Early identification of symptoms is paramount to receiving treatment necessary to improve functional outcomes in stroke. The current American Heart Association's (AHA) public education campaign is "*Spot a Stroke FAST*" with symptoms including

- **F**acial drooping
- **A**rm weakness or numbness
- **S**peech difficulty
- **T**ime to call 911

Continual public education campaigns are necessary to ensure knowledge of stroke signs and symptoms, as message retention can wane over time (Wall et al., 2008). It is estimated that IV-alteplase is given in only 6%–8% of eligible patients, with the reasons being complex, though commonly associated with delay in presenting to the ED within the time window (Demaerschalk et al., 2016). Community education should also stress calling 911, as Fussman and colleagues (2010) found that even in persons with adequate knowledge of stroke signs and symptoms, there was a disconnect with them activating EMS.

Prehospital care

Timely treatment relies not only on community awareness of stroke, but also on early identification by prehospital providers and hospital prenotification of a potential stroke patient. Research demonstrates that with hospital prenotification, more patients undergo timely evaluation, have shorter time to drug administration, and more eligible patients are treated with IV-alteplase (Lin et al., 2012). Evidence-based stroke scales to aid in stroke symptom recognition commonly include the Cincinnati Prehospital Stroke Scale (CPSS) or Los Angeles Prehospital Stroke Screen (LAPSS), though others exist (Brandler et al., 2014).

After initial patient assessment and stabilization, the next priority is for EMS to determine the time the patient was last known well without neurologic symptoms. This is considered to be one of the most critical pieces of information as it will determine treatment options available (Jauch et al., 2013). It is important to interview family members, caregivers, and witnesses to get an accurate understanding of when the patient was last seen at baseline (Crocco et al., 2007). For example, if the patient woke up with weakness, the last known well would be before bed the previous night. However, if the patient woke up to use the bathroom at 5 a.m. and was without symptoms, the last known well would be many hours less and potentially place the patient in the window for IV-alteplase or endovascular intervention. EMS providers should also obtain any pertinent medical history and phone numbers of family members in case of questions in the ED.

Determining the appropriate hospital for transport can be exceedingly complex, with patient preference, insurance issues, and hospital capability playing a factor. According to the most recent Stroke Systems of Care Guidelines, EMS should have knowledge of their local hospitals' capabilities of providing stroke

Table 61.1 Symptoms Associated with Vascular Territory

Anterior circulation	*Posterior circulation*
Middle cerebral artery (MCA)	Vertebral artery, posterior inferior cerebellar artery
• Aphasia (dominant hemisphere)	(PICA), anterior inferior cerebellar artery (AICA)
• Contralateral hemispatial neglect (nondominant hemisphere)	• Ataxia or incoordination
	• Vertigo
• Contralateral motor/sensory loss in face, arm, leg	• Nausea/vomiting
• Contralateral hemispatial neglect or anosognosia (lack of awareness of deficits)	• Nystagmus, diplopia, dysconjugate gaze
	• Dysphagia, dysarthria, dysphonia
• Homonymous hemianopia	• Lateral medullary syndrome/ Wallenberg syndrome:
• Eye deviation toward the side of the stroke	crossed findings of loss of pain and temperature to
Anterior cerebral artery (ACA)	ipsilateral face and contralateral trunk
• Contralateral motor/sensory loss with leg greater than arm or face	Basilar artery
	• Sudden loss of consciousness
• Abulia or personality changes	• Locked-in syndrome
Carotid artery	• Gaze paresis or intranuclear ophthalmoplegia (INO)
• Similar to MCA symptoms	• Abnormal respirations
• Horner syndrome: ptosis, pupillary constriction and anhidrosis	Posterior cerebral artery
	• Homonymous hemianopia
• Monocular vision loss related to amaurosis fugax or central retinal artery occlusion	• Visual agnosia
	• Chorea
	• Weber syndrome: ipsilateral third nerve palsy with contralateral hemiplegia

Source: Adapted from Pare JR, Kahn JH. *Emerg Med Clin North Am.* 2012;30:601-615; Baumann J. *AANN Comprehensive Review for Stroke Nursing.* Chicago: American Association of Neuroscience Nursing; 2014; Merwick A, Werring D. *BMJ.* 2014;348:g3175.

Note: Right-handed and most left-handed people (70%–80%) are left hemisphere dominant, meaning symptoms of aphasia arise from the left hemisphere, whereas neglect is a result of injury to the right hemisphere.

care. They should seek care at a facility with the highest level of stroke care, but should not bypass the closest facility to go to a higher-level facility if such a diversion would add more than 15–20 minutes to the transportation time. This remains a hotly debated topic, and decisions may be controlled by local rules and regulations (Higashida et al., 2013).

Emergency department evaluation and triage

EDs should have an established stroke response (Stroke Code) based on EMS prenotification. Also critical is efficient ED triage to recognize stroke symptoms in patients who present by private car. Having a predefined process ensures standards of care within an organized protocol are carried out with a goal of door-to-needle (IV-alteplase) time of 60 minutes from hospital arrival.

Stroke codes activation protocols should have sensitivity for detecting subtle signs of stroke. This may include symptoms such as dizziness, ataxia, nausea and vomiting, diplopia, visual field deficits, dysarthria, or dysphagia. These can be difficult to distinguish from a peripheral process and can be associated with stroke occurring in the posterior vascular territories supplying the brainstem, cerebellum, and occipital cortex (Merwick and Werring, 2014; Baumann, 2014).

Diagnostic uncertainty with stroke is common due to anatomical variations of the brain, causing stroke in the same vascular territory to present differently among patients. Moreover, nontraditional symptoms such as confusion and emotional lability, or subtle, mild symptoms can also be present, confounding a stroke assessment. In general, stroke symptoms tend to be negative, meaning loss of symptoms (limb weakness or vision loss) rather than positive (limb shaking or flashing lights) (Edlow and Selim, 2011). Stroke strikes suddenly and symptoms are usually maximal at onset, though fluctuation can occur (Nouh et al., 2014). Refer to Table 61.1 for symptoms associated with vascular territories.

Initial evaluation in the ED should occur expeditiously, with stroke patients given the same priority as trauma or myocardial infarction patients. Many hospitals have found that taking arriving patients to the CT suite, rather than an ED room, improves door to IV-alteplase time. Initial neurologic exams, lab draws, and IV access can be performed as the scanner is readied. Airway, breathing, and circulation (ABCs) and vital signs should also be part of the initial assessment as rapid deterioration can occur. Critical assessments and testing that occur in the first hour are discussed in the following sections (Jauch et al., 2013; Summers et al., 2009).

Neuro assessment

An initial neurologic assessment should be brief but thorough. The National Institute of Health Stroke Scale (NIHSS) is the most widely used tool for assessing stroke and is recognized as valid and reliable in initial stroke assessment as well as in evaluating outcomes after treatment.

Pertinent medical history

In addition to last known well and circumstances surrounding onset of symptoms, other medical history that should be obtained includes the patient's risk factors for stroke, such as hypertension, diabetes, atrial fibrillation, dyslipidemia, history of stroke or seizure, as well any history of recent trauma, myocardial infarction, surgeries, or other recent medical treatment received.

Brain imaging

A noncontrast head CT is required prior to fibrinolytics to assess for intracranial bleeding. The recommended door-to-imaging time is 25 minutes, with interpretation by 45 minutes.

With advances in endovascular treatment options, vascular and perfusion studies are also beneficial to aid in determining possible interventions but should not delay IV-alteplase administration.

Oxygenation

Supplemental oxygen does not need to be applied unless oxygen saturations are less than 92%. Most stroke patients maintain alertness; however, a loss of consciousness or rapid deterioration should raise suspicion for intracranial hemorrhage or basilar artery involvement. This may necessitate the need for airway support and ventilatory assistance.

Blood pressure

Permissive hypertension is generally allowed to facilitate cerebral perfusion, and care should be taken to avoid hypotension as this may worsen cerebral ischemia. Current guidelines recommend blood pressures not be treated until 220/120 for those patients not receiving IV thrombolytics, unless there is evidence of end organ damage such as cardiac ischemia. For patients eligible for thrombolytics, blood pressure needs to be <185/110. Labetalol or nicardipine are reasonable options for treatment.

Glucose

Most EMS personnel will have established an initial blood glucose level via fingerstick. Hypoglycemia can mimic stroke, and treatment should be initiated. Treatment of hyperglycemia is also recommended due to unfavorable outcomes.

Labs and IV access

The only lab result required before fibrinolytic administration is glucose. International normalized ratio (INR), partial thromboplastin (PTT), and platelet count results are not required unless the patient has been on anticoagulants such as warfarin, or a bleeding disorder is suspected. Note with the novel oral anticoagulants (NOACs), PTT and INR are not helpful in determining therapeutic levels. Other lab tests to consider in the acute phase to aid in diagnosis include complete blood counts, electrolytes (imbalance can mimic stroke symptoms), renal function studies, and cardiac enzymes. IV access should be obtained, if not done by EMS, and two to three are preferred. If the patient is noted to be hypotensive, non-dextrose-containing IV fluids can be started.

Cardiac monitoring and electrocardiogram

EMS should initiate cardiac monitoring, continuing during emergency evaluation. It is not uncommon to have both acute stroke and myocardial infarction simultaneously, with one precipitating the other. Monitoring should continue during hospitalization to assess for atrial fibrillation or other arrhythmias. An electrocardiogram (ECG) can also be obtained upon admission but should not delay fibrinolytic therapy.

Telemedicine considerations

Establishing telestroke consultation protocols has been shown to improve rates of IV-alteplase administration for eligible patients. This technology provides stroke expertise in smaller community hospitals and in geographically remote areas, where neurologic expertise is typically unavailable on an emergent basis (Amorim et al., 2013).

IV Thrombolytic administration

IV-alteplase is currently the only acute medical therapy available for patients presenting 3–4.5 hours from stroke onset, and its use is widely accepted. In addition to moderate to severe stroke, use should be strongly considered in those with fluctuating symptoms who do not improve to a nondisabling state, unless other contraindications are present. This includes symptoms such as isolated aphasia, significant weakness of extremities, visual disturbance, or a deficit considered potentially disabling in the view of the patient. Time should not be wasted waiting for further improvement to take place (Levine et al., 2013). Once inclusion/exclusion criteria for IV-alteplase have been reviewed and the patient determined to be eligible, consent is obtained from the patient or appropriate proxy. It is permissible to administer if no proxy is present (Jauch et al., 2013).

IV-alteplase is weight based: 0.9 mg/kg; maximum dose of 90 mg. Administration includes an initial bolus of 10% followed by an infusion of the remaining 90% over 1 hour. Post IV-alteplase monitoring includes vital signs and neurologic assessments with recommended frequency of every 15 minutes for the first 2 hours, every 30 minutes for 6 hours, and then hourly until 24 hours from IV-alteplase administration. Blood pressure should be maintained at <180/105. This may require single doses of labetalol or a continuous infusion of medications such as nicardipine (Jauch et al., 2013).

The major risk associated with IV-alteplase is bleeding, particularly symptomatic intracranial hemorrhage (sICH). Rates of bleeding complications are low, even in patients whose symptoms were later attributed to stroke mimics such as complicated migraine, seizure, or conversion disorder (Lewandowski et al., 2015). Signs of sICH include the following:

- Decrease in level of consciousness
- Deterioration in neurologic exam
- New onset of headache
- New-onset nausea and vomiting
- Elevation in blood pressure

For onset of any of these symptoms, discontinue the infusion and obtain STAT head CT. It is beneficial to have a hemorrhagic transformation algorithm for post-IV-alteplase patients to facilitate diagnostics and treatment (Summers et al., 2009).

Another complication of IV-alteplase, though rare, is the risk for orolingual angioedema. This is swelling to the lips and tongue, with potential for airway compromise, and is often associated with patients also taking angiotensin-converting enzyme (ACE) inhibitors (Yayan, 2013). Treatment should include stopping the infusion and administering corticosteroids, antihistamines, and possibly epinephrine, depending on severity (Correia et al., 2015). Though infrequent, it is beneficial to have these medications ordered, as needed and in the same order set as IV-alteplase, to facilitate prompt treatment in the event of an allergic reaction.

Endovascular trials

Prior to 2015, IV-alteplase remained the sole medical therapy for treatment of acute ischemic stroke. Several trials regarding mechanical recanalization treatment of blocked cerebral blood vessels had been completed (SYNTHESIS, IMS-III, MR RESCUE); however, their outcomes at 3 months failed to show superior efficacy when compared with IV-alteplase. Then in 2015 came a trial from the Netherlands, the Multicenter Randomized Clinical Trial of Endovascular Treatment for Acute Ischemic Stroke, otherwise known as MR. CLEAN. This was the first trial to show superior outcomes with endovascular therapy when compared to standard medical therapy. Result of other trials, including EXTEND-IA, ESCAPE, and SWIFT PRIME, soon followed, showing similar results (Beadell et al., 2015). It is important to note that patients should still receive IV-alteplase as soon as possible from symptom onset, regardless of the possibility for endovascular intervention. In each of the positive endovascular trials, patients with the best outcome at 3 months received both IV-alteplase as well as endovascular care (Powers et al., 2015).

While these trials focused on anterior circulation stroke, endovascular therapy for basilar artery thrombosis should be considered. There are currently no randomized control trials for this population; however, several retrospective case studies have shown benefit from use of mechanical thrombectomy as well as an extended time window beyond the established 6 hours, given their poor prognosis (van Houwelingen et al., 2016).

Patient selection criteria for endovascular care are outlined in the 2015 Focused Update of the 2013 Guideline for the Early Management of Patients with Acute Ischemic Stroke Regarding Endovascular Treatment and include the following (Powers et al., 2015):

- Acute ischemic stroke receiving IV-alteplase within 4.5 hours of onset
- Age ≥18 years
- Prestroke modified Rankin score of 0–1
- Causative occlusion of the internal carotid artery or proximal middle cerebral artery (MCA)
- NIHSS score of ≥6
- ASPECTS score of ≥6
- Treatment can be initiated (arterial puncture) within 6 hours of symptom onset

For patients who meet these criteria, prompt transfer to a Comprehensive Stroke Center should be arranged. Current guidelines recommend patients receive IV-alteplase prior to transfer, as outcomes have been shown to be similar for patients needing a "drip and ship." Predetermined transfer criteria and policies should be established to assure a smooth transition when transfer is needed (Higashida et al., 2013).

Hospital care

Ischemic stroke patients have been shown to have better functional outcomes when admitted to a specialized stroke unit after initial triage. Nursing interventions include patient and family education, complication surveillance, and prevention and coordination of the multidisciplinary team to ensure a smooth discharge. Evaluations by physical, occupational, speech/cognition, and swallow therapists are important to maximize the patient's functional recovery and determine discharge destination to acute rehabilitation, skilled nursing facility, or home with outpatient therapy or home health care.

Level of care should be determined by the clinical severity of the stroke and risk for decompensation. An ICU is appropriate for the first 24 hours after IV-alteplase administration, as well as those at high risk for cerebral edema, such as younger stroke patients with large MCA territory infarcts or stroke occurring in the cerebellum. In these cases, it is beneficial to be in an organization with neurosurgical procedure capability such as hemicraniectomy. For patients not receiving fibrinolytics and for which the risk of cerebral edema is low, a neuroscience general care unit, with nurses trained in caring for stroke patients, is appropriate.

Diagnostic tests during hospitalization provide valuable information to aid in determining etiology of stroke and drive subsequent treatment decisions. Testing typically includes the following (Summers et al., 2009):

- Neck vessel imaging: Computed tomography angiography (CTA), magnetic resonance imaging (MRI), or carotid ultrasound to evaluate for stenosis
- ECG and cardiac monitoring: To evaluate for atrial fibrillation or other arrhythmias
- Echocardiogram: To evaluate the structures of the heart and the presence of thrombus or other structural abnormality
- Laboratory testing including HgbA1c, lipid and thyroid levels

Complications are common after stroke, hindering recovery and impacting functional outcomes. Nurses with expertise in stroke care have the knowledge and experience in prevention strategies and implementing interventions for complications as they arise.

Aspiration

It is estimated that 42%–67% of patients with stroke exhibit dysphagia. Dysphagia screening in stroke patients is critical to prevent adverse outcomes including aspiration, pneumonia, inadequate hydration/nutrition, and mortality. Patients should be kept NPO (nothing by mouth), until a swallow assessment can be completed. Many nursing-administered bedside swallow screens exist and have been successfully implemented in emergency departments and neuro stroke units. Prompt screening and referral to swallow therapist ensure optimal patient outcomes and improved patient satisfaction (Donovan et al., 2013). A nasogastric tube may need to be placed for patients with significant dysphagia to maintain hydration and nutrition, and a conversation with patient and family regarding the desire for long-term feeding tube placement should take place (Jauch et al., 2013). The patient's head of bed should be kept at least 30° to help handle oral secretions and prevent aspiration (Summers et al., 2009).

Urinary tract infection

Urinary retention is common after stroke and can increase the prevalence of urinary tract infection (UTI), which negatively impacts outcomes. Nursing interventions to avoid UTIs include avoidance of urinary catheters, bladder scanning to assess for retention, and implementation of bladder retraining. Prophylactic antibiotics are not recommended. Signs of a UTI may include urinary frequency, pain with urination, suprapubic pain, fever, or changes in neurologic status, such as delirium (Summers et al., 2009; Jauch et al., 2013).

Hyperglycemia

Elevated blood glucose levels are common after stroke, and hyperglycemia has been known to worsen outcomes. Current recommendations are to aim for blood glucose levels in a range of 140–180 mg/dL and to closely monitor and prevent hypoglycemia. Due to the frequency of contrast administration for diagnostic imaging, it is reasonable to hold metformin during hospitalization to avoid kidney injury (Jauch et al., 2013).

Venous thromboembolism

The incidence of venous thromboembolism (VTE) among patients with ischemic stroke is high, and pulmonary embolism (PE) remains the third-highest cause of fatality in stroke. Interventions include early mobilization and hydration as well as prophylaxis with either unfractionated heparin or low molecular weight heparin. External compression devices are also an option for those in whom antithrombotic agents are contraindicated, such as the first 24 hours after IV-alteplase. Graduated compression stockings are associated with skin breakdown and have not been shown to be effective in preventing VTE (Field and Hill, 2012).

Stroke etiology and treatment

The etiology of stroke is important to understand as it can drive subsequent treatment strategies. The most common stroke mechanisms include large vessel disease, small vessel disease, and cardioembolic, though other categories exist. Each group has associated risk factors and specific medical and/or surgical options.

Large vessel disease and atherosclerosis

Atherosclerosis, or plaque buildup, can develop in the large carotid and vertebral arteries leading to the brain. This plaque can either narrow the lumen to restrict blood flow or can also develop thrombus that can break off and cause artery-to-artery embolism and infarction (Livesay and Hickey, 2014). Patients with symptomatic carotid stenosis greater than 70% may benefit from surgical intervention to reopen narrowed vessels. This can be achieved by carotid endarterectomy or carotid stenting. The type of surgery depends on many factors, including location of the stenosis and comorbidities of the patient. Timing of the surgery does not need to be emergent, but within 2 weeks is recommended (Kernan et al., 2014).

Atherosclerosis of the vertebral arteries should be treated medically with antiplatelet and statin medications. Surgical interventions have not been shown to be superior to medical therapy in vertebral artery stenosis but may be explored for patients who fail medical therapy (Kernan et al., 2014).

Similarly, intracranial atherosclerosis should also be managed medically with antiplatelet and statin medications. There are current studies underway to determine if these patients may benefit from dual anti-platelet therapy. No surgical intervention has been shown to be effective (Kernan et al., 2014).

Small vessel disease

Small vessel disease, or lacunar stroke, is occlusion of smaller penetrating arteries caused by lipohyalin-osis and microatheroma formation. This is most commonly found in the deeper structures of the brain including basal ganglia, thalamus, and internal capsule. Diabetes, hypertension, and smoking are strongly associated with the development of small vessel disease. Treatment consists of antiplatelet agents, statin medications, and management of modifiable risk factors (Livesay and Hickey, 2014).

Cardioembolic

Embolism arising from the heart causes up to 30% of ischemic stroke, and atrial fibrillation is the most common reason for embolism formation. Other cardiac sources include aortic arch atherosclerosis, valvular disease, atrial or ventricular thrombus, etc. For atrial fibrillation, current guidelines recommend anticoag-ulation with warfarin or a newer anticoagulant (Arboix and Ali, 2011).

Cryptogenic

About 25% of strokes are considered cryptogenic and lack an obvious etiology. Further workup may include hypercoagulable studies, long-term cardiac monitoring to evaluate for paroxysmal atrial fibril-lation, and additional paradoxical embolism evaluation, such as lower extremity ultrasound. This may be beneficial for patients with known patent foramen ovale (PFO) or atrial septal defect, as theoretically, a VTE can be transmitted through the PFO and into arterial circulation (Dalen and Alpert, 2016).

Less common causes

About 5% of strokes are caused for other reasons including carotid dissection, nonatherosclerotic vascu-lopathies, hypercoagulable states, hematologic disorders, arteritis, or vasospasm (Livesay and Hickey, 2014). Imaging and laboratory testing are typically needed to confirm these less common diagnoses.

Secondary stroke prevention interventions

Once etiology has been established, prevention of future strokes becomes the center of focus. Interventions include initiation of new medications, education about personal modifiable risk factors, and discussion of any potential surgical procedures based on results of diagnostic studies. Nursing as well as the multidisciplinary team need to be aware of each patient's risk factors for stroke so education can be tailored.

Antiplatelet/Anticoagulant

Oral administration of aspirin should begin within 24–48 hours after stroke unless a reason for anticoagulation, such as atrial fibrillation, has been found. Aspirin has been shown to decrease mortality and should continue indefinitely. For patients initiated on anticoagulants, the side effects of bleeding should be discussed as well as any lab testing that might be needed (Summers et al., 2009).

Antihypertensives

Treating high blood pressure is one of the most important risk reduction strategies for secondary stroke prevention. Antihypertensives should be considered for blood pressure higher than 140/90. This should be in combination with other lifestyle modifications including weight reduction and dietary changes such as reduction in salt intake with the Dietary Approaches to Stop Hypertension (DASH) diet (Kernan et al., 2014). For patients with known hypertension, antihypertensives can be restarted within 24 hours of stroke if the neuro exam is stable (Jauch et al., 2013).

Statin therapy

Dyslipidemia is commonly associated with ischemic stroke. Statins reduce blood cholesterol levels as well as reduce inflammation that is thought to contribute to atherosclerosis formation (Ridker et al., 2009). Current American College of Cardiology (ACC)/American Heart Association (AHA) guidelines state that for patients younger than 75 years, high-intensity statin should be prescribed regardless of lipid levels. Though there is no longer a goal low-density lipoprotein (LDL) level, subsequent lipid level measurements can monitor adherence to drug regimen. Baseline liver enzyme should be evaluated upon initiation and does not need to be trended unless the patient is symptomatic (Stone et al., 2013).

Diabetes management

Diabetes is a known risk factor for ischemic stroke and has been implicated in development of atherosclerosis and lipohyalinosis. Glucose control is recommended to be near-normoglycemic levels to reduce microvascular complications, and more rigorous control of blood pressure and lipids should also be considered for the patient with diabetes. Patients should be screened via HgbA1c level with a goal of <7%. Consult to diabetes management services may be warranted to improve patient glycemic control (Summers et al., 2009).

Healthy lifestyle modifications

Encourage patients who are able to engage in 30–40 minutes of moderate-intensity exercise most days of the week. Screen patients for obesity, and discuss healthy body mass index (BMI) levels. Even small decreases in weight have been shown to reduce cardiovascular risk. Encourage a diet rich in fruits and vegetables, whole grains, lean meats, and low-fat dairy (Kernan et al., 2014).

Smoking cessation

Cigarette smoking has been shown to be an independent risk factor for stroke. Counseling and nicotine and oral smoking cessation medications have been shown to be beneficial in assisting with quitting (Kernan et al., 2014).

Conclusion

Caring for patients after an ischemic stroke is both challenging and rewarding. Practices are driven by evidence-based guidelines, and the science is continually evolving. An interdisciplinary, team-based approach to care is essential to achieving the best outcomes for patients, and nursing plays a pivotal role in navigating patients and families through this life-altering event.

References

American Heart Association/American Stroke Association. Four letters: F-A-S-T. Three numbers: 9-1-1. http://www.strokeassociation.org/STROKEORG/WarningSigns/Stroke-Warning-Signs-and-Symptoms_UCM_308528_SubHomePage.jsp, accessed November 20, 2016.

Amorim E, Shih MM, Koehler SA et al. Impact of telemedicine implementation in thrombolytic use for acute ischemic stroke: the University of Pittsburgh Medical Center telestroke network experience. *J Stroke Cerebrovasc Dis.* 2013;22(4):527–531. doi:10.1016/j.jstrokecerebrovasdis.2013.02.004.

Arboix A, Alio J. Cardioembolic stroke: clinical features, specific cardiac disorders and prognosis. *Curr Cardiol Rev.* 2010;6(3):150–161. doi:10.2174/157340310791658730.

Baumann J. Hyperacute care. In: Livesay S ed. *AANN Comprehensive Review for Stroke Nursing.* 1st ed. Chicago, IL: American Association of Neuroscience Nursing; 2014: pp. 61–82.

Beadell NC, Bazan T, Lutsep H. The year embolectomy won: a review of five trials assessing the efficacy of mechanical intervention in acute stroke. *Curr Cardiol Rep.* 2015;17(11):102. doi:10.1007/s11886-015-0657-x.

Brandler ES, Sharma M, Sinert RH, Levine SR. Prehospital stroke scales in urban environments: a systematic review. *Neurology.* 2014;82(24):2241–2249.

Correia AS, Matias G, Calado S, Lourenco A, Viana-Baptista M. Orolingual angiodema associated with alteplase treatment of acute stroke: a reappraisal. *J Stroke Cerebrovasc Dis.* 2015;24(1):31–40. doi:10.1016/j.jstrokecerebrovasdis.2014.07.045

Crocco TJ, Grotta JC, Jauch EC, et al. EMS management of acute stroke--prehospital triage (resource document to NAEMSP position statement). *Prehosp Emerg Care* 2007;11(3):313–317. doi:10.1080/10903120701347844

Dalen JE, Alpert JS. Cryptogenic strokes and patent foramen ovales: what's the right treatment? *Am J Med.* 2016;129(11):1159–1162. doi:10.1016/j.amjmed.2016.08.006

Demaerschalk BM, Kleindorfer DO, Adeoye OM, et al. Scientific rationale for the inclusion and exclusion criteria for intravenous alteplase in acute ischemic stroke: a statement for healthcare professionals from the American Heart Association/American Stroke Association. *Stroke.* 2016;47(2):581–641. doi:10.1161/str.0000000000000086

Donovan NJ, Daniels SK, Edmiaston J, Weinhardt J, Summers D, Mitchell PH; American Heart Association Council on Cardiovascular Nursing and Stroke, Council Dysphagia screening: state of the art: invitational conference proceeding from the State-of-the-Art Nursing Symposium, International Stroke Conference 2012. *Stroke.* 2013;44:e24–e31.

Edlow JA, Selim MH. Atypical presentations of acute cerebrovascular syndromes. *Lancet Neurol.* 2011;10(6):550–560. doi:10.1016/s1474-4422(11)70069-2

Field TS, Hill MD. Prevention of deep vein thrombosis and pulmonary embolism in patients with stroke. *Clin Appl Thromb Hemost.* 2012;18(1):5–19. doi:10.1177/1076029611412362

Fussman C, Rafferty AP, Lyon-Callo S, Morgenstern LB, Reeves MJ. Lack of association between stroke symptom knowledge and intent to call 911: a population-based survey. *Stroke.* 2010;41(7):1501–1507. doi:10.1161/strokeaha.110.578195

Higashida R, Alberts MJ, Alexander DN et al. Interactions within stroke systems of care: a policy statement from the American Heart Association/American Stroke Association. *Stroke.* 44(10):2961–2984. doi:10.1161/STR.0b013e3182a6d2b2

Jauch EC, Saver JL, Adams HP et al. Guidelines for the early management of patients with acute ischemic stroke: a guideline for healthcare professionals from the American Heart Association/American Stroke Association. *Stroke.* 2013;44(3):870–947. doi:10.1161/STR.0b013e318284056a

Kernan WN, Ovbiagele B, Black HR et al. Guidelines for the prevention of stroke in patients with stroke and transient ischemic attack: a guideline for healthcare professionals from the American Heart Association/American Stroke Association. *Stroke.* 2014;45(7):2160–2236. doi:10.1161/str.0000000000000024

Levine SR, Khatri P, Broderick JP. Review, historical context, and clarifications of the NINDS rt-PA stroke trials exclusion criteria: part 1: rapidly improving stroke symptoms. *Stroke.* 2013;44(9):2500–2505. doi:10.1161/strokeaha.113.000878

Lewandowski C, Mays-Wilson K, Miller J et al. Safety and outcomes in stroke mimics after intravenous tissue plasmino-gen activator administration: a single-center experience. *J Stroke Cerebrovasc Dis.* 2015;24(1):48–52. doi:10.1016/j.jstrokecerebrovasdis.2014.07.048

Lin CB, Peterson ED, Smith EE et al. Emergency medical service hospital prenotification is associated with improved evaluation and treatment of acute ischemic stroke. *Circ Cardiovasc Qual Outcomes.* 2012;5(4):514–522. doi:10.1161/circoutcomes.112.965210

Livesay S, Hickey J. Transient ischemic attacks and acute ischemic stroke. In: Hickey JV, ed. *The Clinical Practice of Neuro-logical and Neurosurgical Nursing.* 7th ed. Philadelphia, PA: Lippincott Williams & Wilkins; 2014:511–541

Merwick A, Werring D. Posterior circulation ischaemic stroke. *BMJ.* 2014;348:g3175. doi:10.1136/bmj.g3175

Mozaffarian D, Benjamin EJ, Go AS et al. Heart disease and stroke statistics-2016 update: a report from the American Heart Association. *Circulation.* 2016;133(4):e38–e360.

National Center for Health Statistics. *Health, United States, 2015: with Special Feature on Racial and Ethnic Health Dispar-ities.* Hyattsville, MD: National Center for Health Statistics (US); 2016.

Nouh A, Remke J, Ruland S. Ischemic posterior circulation stroke: a review of anatomy, clinical presentations, diagno-sis, and current management. *Front Neurol.* 2014;5:30. doi:10.3389/fneur.2014.00030

Pare JR, Kahn JH. Basic neuroanatomy and stroke syndromes. *Emerg Med Clin North Am.* 2012;30(3):601–615. doi:10.1016/j.emc.2012.05.004

Powers WJ, Derdeyn CP, Biller J et al. American Heart Association/American Stroke Association focused update of the 2013 guidelines for the early management of patients with acute ischemic stroke regarding endovascular treatment: a guideline for healthcare professionals from the American Heart Association/American Stroke Association. *Stroke.* 2015;46(10):3020–3035.

Ridker PM, Danielson E, Fonseca FA et al. Reduction in C-reactive protein and LDL cholesterol and cardiovascular event rates after initiation of rosuvastatin: a prospective study of the JUPITER trial. *Lancet.* 2009;373(9670):1175–1182. doi:10.1016/s0140-6736(09)60447-5

Smith EE, von Kummer R. Door-to-needle times in acute ischemic stroke: how low can we go? *Neurology.* 2012;79:296–297.

Stone NJ, Robinson JG, Lichtenstein AH et al. 2013 ACC/AHA guideline on the treatment of blood cholesterol to reduce atherosclerotic cardiovascular risk in adults: a report of the American College of Cardiology/American Heart Association Task Force on Practice Guidelines. *J Am Coll Cardiol.* 2013;63(25 Pt B):2889–2934. doi:10.1016/j.jacc.2013.11.002

Summers D, Leonard A, Wentworth D et al. Comprehensive overview of nursing and interdisciplinary care of the acute ischemic stroke patient: a scientific statement from the American Heart Association. *Stroke.* 2009;40(8):2911–2944. doi:10.1161/strokeaha.109.192362

van Houwelingen RC, Luijckx GJ, Uyttenboogaart M. Intra-arterial treatment for basilar artery occlusion-reply. *JAMA Neurol.* 2017;74(1):130–131. doi:10.1001/jamaneurol.2016.4870

Wall HK, Beagan BM, O'Neill J, Foell KM, Boddie-Willis CL. Addressing stroke signs and symptoms through public education: the Stroke Heroes Act FAST campaign. *Prev Chronic Dis.* 2008;5(2):A49.

Yayan J. Onset of orolingual angioedema after treatment of acute brain ischemia with alteplase depends on the site of brain ischemia: a meta-analysis. *N Am J Med Sci.* 2013;5(10):589–593. doi:10.4103/1947-2714.120794

62

DELIRIUM

Colleen M. Foley

Case vignette

Edith is an 85-year-old female who presents to the emergency department after an unwitnessed fall from standing while at her assisted living facility (ALF). Her past medical history includes hypertension, diabetes type 2, hyperlipidemia, and dementia. Edith needs assistance with all instrumental activities of daily living (IADLs) and some assistance with bathing. She is typically pleasant without any behavioral disturbances. Edith was a professor of botany, widowed, and has a son. She arrived with her hearing aids and glasses; she endorses a headache and dizziness. On exam she appears confused and anxious, her neurologic exam is otherwise nonfocal. Edith's labs and chest x-ray were unremarkable except for a sodium of 152. Her head computed tomography (CT) scan demonstrated a subdural hematoma not causing mid-line shift. She was admitted to the general care unit for intravenous (IV) fluid to correct her sodium and serial neurologic assessments. Overnight, Edith became aggressive with staff, trying to get out of bed multiple times while staff were encouraging her to go back to bed. At 2 a.m. she hit the nurse collecting laboratory studies. Overnight Edith received 5 mg intramuscular (IM) haloperidol and 2 mg IM lorazepam. As the provider, you are wondering what triggered her mental status changes: delirium dementia with behaviors or worsening subdural hematoma.

Delirium

Definition

Delirium is an abrupt change in cognitive function from a patient's baseline. Clinical features include a waxing and waning pattern, inattention, and disorganized thinking. A patient's level of consciousness may or may not be affected.

Types

There are three different types of delirium: hyperactive, hypoactive, and mixed. The hyperactive form is what most providers attribute to delirium. Patients are described as "agitated," exhibiting behaviors such as hitting, kicking, or grabbing—causing significant stress to staff. Alternatively, hypoactive delirium patients are described as "sleepy"—although concerning for the patient, this tends not to be problematic for staff as patients are not disrupting care. Often misdiagnosed as dementia or depression, hypoactive delirium has an increased mortality rate compared to hyperactive delirium (Yang et al., 2009, p. 252). Mixed delirium is a pattern of fluctuating hyperactive/hypoactive. A patient may present with hyperactive delirium, changing to hypoactive. Staff may interpret this as "improved;" however, the patient is continuing to fluctuate between two forms of delirium.

Epidemiology

Delirium is common in health care, especially in older adult populations:

- 10%–31% of older adults admitted are delirious, while 11%–42% develop delirium while hospitalized (Siddiqi et al, 2006, p. 355)
- 80% of ventilated patients in the intensive care unit (ICU) setting are delirious (Vanderbilt Medical University, 2013)
- 27% of patients on stroke units are delirious (Hospital Elder Life Program, 2015)

Pathophysiology

The pathophysiology of delirium is not well understood. Multiple mechanisms may contribute to its pathogenesis (Fong et al, 2009, p. 211-212).

Neurotransmission: The cholinergic system impacts attention and cognition. In particular, decreases in acetylcholine may lead to the development of delirium. Medications with anticholinergic side effects lead to an increased risk of development or worsening of delirium.

Inflammation: Proinflammatory cytokines may induce delirium. Patients who experience insults (i.e., infection, trauma, or surgery) release proinflammatory cytokines. Proinflammatory cytokine levels have been shown to be higher in patients who experience delirium.

Acute stress response: Delirium may be triggered by high levels of cortisol. Elevated levels of cortisol have been found in patients with postoperative delirium. Cortisol may already be higher in older adults, so be aware that providing additional steroids may further increase risk of delirium.

Neuronal injury: Patients may experience multiple neuronal injuries in the hospital setting. For example, metabolic disturbances and hypoxia can lead to oxygen deprivation to the brain cells. The release of neurotransmitters can become impaired, which may play a role in the development of delirium.

Impact on patients

Delirium leads to poor outcomes: increased cost, worsened cognition, increased risk of falls, institutionalization, and increased mortality.

Cost: Delirium increases cost of patient care. Hospitalization costs rise due to increased length of stay and increased nursing care needs. Delirium can cost $2500 per patient per hospitalization totaling approximately $6.9 billion annually in Medicare costs. Posthospitalization care costs increase as a result of institutionalization and rehabilitation. Posthospitalization care, which can range from $60,000 to $64,000 per patient, totals $38 billion to $152 billion nationally (Fong et al, 2009, p. 217).

Cognition: Often delirium is thought to be reversible; however, delirium may cause cognitive decline in some patients. A study by Pandharipande and colleagues (Pandharipande et al., BRAIN-ICU Study Investigators 2013, p. 1309 and 1311) found that patients who experienced delirium in the ICU are at high risk of cognitive impairments at 12 months. The deficits occurred in both younger and older adults. Prolonged delirium was associated with worsened long-term cognition.

Falls: Delirium increases the risk of patient falls. In a study by Mangusan and colleagues (Mangusan et al., 2015, p. 160), patients with postoperative delirium were four times more likely to fall. Alternatively, a meta-analysis by Hshieh and colleagues (Hshieh et al., 2015, p. E5) found the odds of falling decreased by 62% when utilizing nonpharmacologic strategies to prevent delirium. Side effects of medications used in the management of delirium increase fall risk. Additionally, delirious patients are challenging to mobilize, contributing to deconditioning and increasing fall risk.

Institutionalization: Patients who experience functional decline are more likely to discharge to a skilled facility instead of home (Witlox et al., 2010, p. 447).

Death: Patients who develop delirium have an increased risk of death, three times more likely within 1 year, as compared to those whose delirium resolved (Kiely et al., 2009, p. 59).

Identification of delirium

Despite delirium's serious consequences for patients and costs to health care, it is underrecognized. Approximately two-thirds of physicians and two-thirds of nurses do not recognize delirium (Hospital Elder Life Program, 2015). While asking a patient orientation questions (i.e., what is your name? what is the date? etc.) may be part of a mental status assessment, it is not a reliable method to identify delirium; therefore, providers should utilize standardized tools. The most widely used tool to identify delirium is the Confusion Assessment Method (CAM), which has a high sensitivity and specificity (Wei et al., 2008, p. 829). The CAM may be used in multiple settings, including a CAM specific to the ICU. In general, if the confusion has an acute onset and fluctuates, it is likely delirium.

For more information on the Short-Form CAM, please go to http://www.hospitalelderlifeprogram. org. For more information on the CAM-ICU, please go to http://www.icudelirium.org.

Delirium development

A single factor can lead to delirium development; however, more often, the cause for delirium is multifactorial. Underlying causes such as an infection, electrolyte imbalance, and deliriogenic medications combined with underlying risk factors contribute to delirium. See Table 62.1 for a pneumonic tool to help providers consider different causes of delirium.

Patients' underlying risk factors play a significant role in delirium development. A greater number of modifiable and nonmodifiable risk factors increases the likelihood of developing delirium. Please refer to Table 62.2 for a list of risk factors. Anyone is at risk for delirium; however, delirium typically affects the older adult population more, especially those with dementia.

Edith's risk factors—advanced age, comorbidities, subdural hematoma (SDH), electrolyte imbalance, poor vision/hearing, impaired cognition, and the use of tethers—increased her likelihood of developing delirium.

If delirium is suspected

- Complete a delirium screening tool, such as the CAM
- Perform vital signs
- Complete a physical exam with a focus on a patient's mental status and neurologic exam

Table 62.1 Pneumonic Device for Underlying Causes of Delirium

D	rugs, dehydration
E	lectrolyte imbalances
L	ack of sleep
I	nfection
R	estraints, reduced hearing or vision, reduced mobility
I	ntracranial problems
U	rinary/fecal issues
M	alnutrition

Table 62.2 Nonmodifiable and Modifiable Risk Factors for Delirium

Nonmodifiable risk factors
- Dementia or cognitive impairment
- Over 65 years of age
- History of neurologic disease
- History of delirium
- Multiple comorbidities
- Chronic renal or hepatic impairments

Modifiable risk factors
- Sensory impairment (visual or hearing)
- Immobilization
- Tethers/restraints
- Acute neurologic disease
- Current illness
- Electrolyte abnormalities
- Surgery
- Environment
- Pain
- Emotional distress
- Sleep deprivation
- Certain medications

- Collect labs and diagnostics, based on physical findings:
  - Complete blood count
  - Metabolic panel
  - Liver panel
  - Thyroid function
  - Serum drug levels
  - Arterial blood gas
  - Blood cultures
  - Chest x-ray
  - Electrocardiogram

- These tests are not typically ordered unless there is strong evidence:
  - Brain imaging is not useful unless focal neurologic findings or head trauma
- Spinal fluid analysis is not useful unless evidence of meningitis
  - EEG is not useful unless evidence of seizures

Delirium management

1. *Prevention*: Delirium prevention is the goal. An estimated 30%–40% of delirium is preventable (Hospital Elder Life Program, 2015). Nonpharmacologic and targeting interventions to the patients' modifiable risk factors may help prevent delirium (Hshieh et al., 2015, p. E8; Inouye et al., 1999 p. 673). See Table 62.3 for interventions to consider. Currently no evidence supports the use of medications to prevent the onset of delirium (Fong et al, 2009, p. 214). Avoiding medications that can induce or perpetuate delirium may also prevent the onset or worsening of delirium (American Geriatrics Society Expert Panel on Postoperative Delirium in Older Adults, 2015, p. 146). If a patient does require a deliriogenic medication for dangerous behaviors, providers should consider starting with the lowest effective dose. Common medications that induce or perpetuate delirium include

a. Medications with strong anticholinergic properties, such as oxybutynin, diphenhydramine, prochlorperazine, and promethazine

b. Opioids

c. Steroids

d. Benzodiazepines

e. Sedative hypnotics

2. *Treat underlying cause(s)*: Once a patient has developed delirium, typically an underlying cause(s) can be identified and treated. See Table 62.1 for primary causes of delirium.

Table 62.3 Nonpharmacologic Recommendations for Delirium Prevention and Treatment

Modifiable risk factor	Intervention
Sensory impairment	• Use eyeglasses, hearing aids, or voice amplifiers. • Patients without glasses and poor vision, ensure slow approach, explain actions, and attempt to get in line of patient's sight carefully. • Patients without hearing aids or voice amplifiers, ensure words are spoken in deep voice with good enunciation. Use teach-back to ensure understanding/patient was able to hear what was told. • If the patient hears better out of one ear versus the other, speak into the better ear.
Functional decline	• Optimize mobility and self-care ability. • Ensure patient is ambulating, unless there is a specific medical indication he or she is unable (i.e., lower extremity fracture, unable to ambulate at baseline). • Do not allow older adults to stay in bed or only get up to the chair during their hospital stay (American Academy of Nursing's "Choosing Wisely" guidelines) • Avoid bed rest unless medically necessary.
Tethers: Restraints, catheter, intravenous lines, drains, chest tubes, etc.,	• Avoid use of tethers, if possible; if unable, discontinue as soon as possible. • Avoid physical restraints to manage behavioral symptoms of hospitalized older adults with delirium (AGS Choosing Wisely Workgroup, 2014, p. 957).★ • Do not place or maintain urinary catheters unless there is a specific medical reason to do so (American Academy of Nursing's "Choosing Wisely" guidelines)

Dehydration or poor nutrition	• Assure adequate hydration:
	  • Encourage adequate fluid intake.
	  • Ensure there is a cup of water at bedside and patient is encouraged to take a sip every time staff enters the room.
	  • Monitor sodium levels.
	  • Be aware of prolonged NPO status.
	• Assure adequate nutrition:
	  • Consider liberalizing diet if variety (i.e., diabetic) or consistency (thickened liquids) contributing to poor intake. Please note this may prompt a risk versus benefit discussion.
	  • Be aware of prolonged NPO status.
	  • Alternative routes of nutrition should be carefully considered. Although nutrition is a critical part of healing, tubes increase delirium risk or worsen delirium.
	• Encourage good meal hygiene:
	  • Up to chair for all meals.
	  • Deinstitutionalize food before bringing meal into room (i.e., remove covers, set up silverware).
	  • Request food the patient may enjoy.
	  • Organize food tray/table to help create an appropriate mealtime setting (i.e., remove urinal, gauze, etc.).
	  • If possible, create a more social mealtime environment (i.e., volunteers, family).

(Continued)

Table 62.3 (Continued) Nonpharmacologic Recommendations for Delirium Prevention and Treatment

Modifiable risk factor	Intervention
Disorientation	• Reorient patient and communicate clearly.
	• Ensure clock and patient communication board are accurate with correct date, location, and reason for admission. Refer to this often with patient.
	• If patient disagrees with reorientation and triggers a disagreement, do not argue, try redirection.
	• Encourage patient to participate in meaningful conversations and activities.
	• Discuss topics the patient enjoys, discuss current events, play word games, and read magazines or newspapers as the patient is able.
Hospital environment	• Encourage the presence of family members for reassurance.
	• Encourage the family to bring in familiar objects, pictures, quilts, etc.
	• Declutter room.
	• Decrease noise.
Sleep deprivation	• Normalize sleep–wake cycle.
	• For nighttime:
	• Aim for uninterrupted periods of sleep at night.
	• Avoid noise in hallways.
	• Keep the room dim.
	• Do not wake the patient for routine care unless the patient's care or condition specifically requires it (American Academy of Nursing's "Choosing Wisely" guidelines).
	• Consider warm milk, noncaffeinated tea, back massage for sleep rather than a sedative hypnotic (McDowell et al., 1998, p. 703).
	• For daytime:
	• Discourage too much daytime napping.
	• Expose the patient to ambient light.
	• Take the patient outside during the daytime if possible.
	• During the day, keep the room well lighted with lights on and shades open.
	• Ask family to come during the day or consider utilizing a volunteer to help keep the patient engaged.
Pain	• Treat pain with nonpharmacologic modalities:
	• Heat or cold
	• Distraction
	• Music
	• Consider scheduling acetaminophen to help decrease the need of opioid.
	• If opioids are needed, start with the lowest effective dose ("start low and go slow"), continue to use nonpharmacologic modalities.
	• Ensure adequate kidney function to avoid excessive opioid buildup.
Behaviors	• Avoid triggers that lead to agitation.
	• Avoid overstimulating environment.
	• Try music, massage, appropriate TV stations, and relaxation techniques.
	• If an intervention, such as checking vital signs, increases a patient's agitation, wait and reapproach later.
	• Attempt redirection.
	• Discuss patient's hobbies or enjoyments.
	• If patient becomes agitated, try changing the topic to a subject the patient enjoys discussing.
	• Stay calm with a relaxing voice.
	• Do not argue with the patient.

3. *Nonpharmacologic interventions*: Nonpharmacologic interventions are the cornerstone treatment of delirium. See Table 62.3 for methods to consider.

4. *Medications for delirium*: Consider a medication for delirium *only* if a patient is a danger to themselves or others. If medications are initiated, nonpharmacologic interventions continue. Medications for delirium typically include antipsychotics (typical, i.e., haloperidol; atypical, i.e., quetiapine, olanzapine) or benzodiazepines. However, there is no consistent evidence regarding the effectiveness of medications in the treatment of delirium (Inouye, Westendorp, and Saczynski, 2014, p.917).

   a. There is no U.S. Food and Drug Administration (FDA)-approved medication for treatment of delirium. Antipsychotics used for delirium are off-label use and have a block box warning associated with them when used in the older adult population due to the increased risk of mortality.

   b. Medications should not be used to treat hypoactive delirium (American Geriatrics Society Expert Panel on Postoperative Delirium in Older Adults, 2015, p. 147).

   c. Benzodiazepines should not be used as first-line treatment for delirium unless they are specifically indicated, such as for alcohol or benzodiazepine withdrawal (American Geriatrics Society Expert Panel on Postoperative Delirium in Older Adults, 2015, p. 147).

   d. Typical and atypical antipsychotics increase risk of prolonged QTC interval, and thus increase risk of arrhythmia development.

   e. In general, antipsychotics should be avoided in patients with Lewy body dementia (LBD). Typical antipsychotics in patients with LBD may increase risk of mortality (McKeith et al., 1992, p. 917), and they may be particularly sensitive to all antipsychotics (Weintraub and Hurtig, 2007, p. 1495 and 1496).

   f. In general, antipsychotics should be avoided for Parkinson disease as they can worsen the motor aspects of parkinsonism; however, if a medication is needed, quetiapine could be considered (Weintraub and Hurtig, 2007, p. 1496).

Table 62.4 Medications for Hyperactive Delirium

Pharmacologic therapy of agitated delirium

Agent	Mechanism of action	Dosage	Benefits	Adverse events	Comments
Haloperidol[OL]	Antipsychotic	0.25–1 mg po, IM, or IV q4h prn for agitation	Relatively nonsedating; few hemodynamic effects	EPS, especially if >3 mg/d	Usually agent of choice[a]
Risperidone[OL]	Second-generation antipsychotic	0.25–1 mg po q4h prn for agitation	Similar to haloperidol	Might have slightly fewer EPS than haloperidol	Small trials[b]
Olanzapine[OL]	Second-generation antipsychotic	2.5–5 mg po, SL, or IM q12h, max dosage 20 mg q24h (cannot be given by IV infusion)	Fewer EPS than haloperidol	More sedating than haloperidol	Small trials[b]; oral formulations less effective for acute management
Quetiapine[OL]	Second-generation antipsychotic	25–50 mg po q12h	Fewer EPS than haloperidol; can be used in patients with parkinsonism	More sedating than haloperidol; hypotension	Small trials[b]

(*Continued*)

Table 62.4 (Continued) Medications for Hyperactive Delirium

Pharmacologic therapy of agitated delirium

Agent	Mechanism of action	Dosage	Benefits	Adverse events	Comments
Lorazepam[OL]	Benzodiazepine	0.25–1 mg po or IV q8h prn for agitation	Use in sedative and alcohol withdrawal; history of neuroleptic malignant syndrome	More paradoxical excitation, respiratory depression than haloperidol	Generally should not be used; see "page 10" for specific indication

Source: Marcantonio ER. Geriatrics Review Syllabus: A Core Curriculum in Geriatric Medicine, American Geriatrics Society, New York, 2016. With permission.

Note: EPS = extrapyramidal symptoms.

Use of all of these drugs for delirium is an off-label indication. Because of the small number and size of trials investigating the use of these agents in the treatment of agitation in delirium, the SOE = B.

[a] In a randomized trial comparing haloperidol, chlorpromazine, and lorazepam in the treatment of agitated delirium in young patients with AIDS, all were found to be equally effective in treating symptoms of psychosis, but haloperidol had the fewest adverse events.

[b] Second-generation antipsychotics have been tested primarily in small equivalency trials with haloperidol and recently in small placebo-controlled trials in the ICU. The FDA requires a black box warning for all second-generation antipsychotics because of the increased risk of cerebrovascular events, stroke, and mortality in patients with dementia. First-generation antipsychotic agents also have an FDA black box warning regarding an increase in all-cause mortality among patients with dementia.

  g. See Table 62.4 for medications to consider in delirium management from the American Geriatrics Society.

  h. In light of considerable side effect profile, antipsychotics for delirium should be reviewed daily and a plan for discontinuing established prior to discharge.

 5. *Involve patient's support system*: Despite deliriums commonplace in health care, family commonly express, "I had no idea this would happen." Good communication and education with family is critical, especially as their involvement is a key strategy in delirium prevention and treatment. Support and educate families about delirium so families are better able to support the patient.

Trajectory

Delirium is thought to be reversible, although severe, prolonged delirium may have permanent cognitive effects. Following full treatment with clinical improvement, delirium may linger for weeks to months—its trajectory can be challenging to predict. Brain imaging in the neuroscience patient may demonstrate improvement overall; however, delirium may continue to wax and wane.

Conclusion

The cause of Edith's confusion was likely delirium compared to worsening of her dementia as she had an acute change in cognition. The main contributor for developing delirium was the SDH and hypernatremia. Along with her SDH, other nonmodifiable risk factors were her age, previous comorbidities, and impaired cognition. Modifiable risk factors included a new environment, tethers, comorbidities, poor hearing, and poor vision.

 Risk factors the team providing care for Edith could have addressed are as follows:

- Ensured her glasses and hearing aids were being used at all times.
- Provided continued reorientation.

- Ambulated Edith instead of encouraging her to go back to bed.
- Discussed botany or her son may have served as a distraction when Edith became agitated.
- Avoided triggers, which in her case was collecting laboratory studies. By avoiding the trigger, Edith may not have hit the nurse, which may have prevented the administration of the antipsychotic and benzodiazepine.
- The medication choices for Edith were inappropriate. She received 5 mg haloperidol and 2 mg lorazepam. Ideally the medication could have been avoided; however, if a medication was necessary, 0.25–1 mg haloperidol would have been a more appropriate choice, and the benzodiazepine should not have been administered as it may perpetuate the delirium.

Edith's story is unfortunately a common scenario in health care. Delirium negatively impacts patients, families, and health-care systems, and is underrecognized. Delirium is preventable; however, once delirium strikes, it is challenging to manage.

In the neuroscience population, delirium is more challenging. The additional neuronal injury creates a diagnostic and treatment complexity. Patients with a chronic or acute neurologic process are at increased risk for developing delirium. The trajectory of delirium's course is more difficult to predict. Unfortunately, data are lacking about delirium in neurologic and neurosurgical patients; however, treatment parallels other patients with delirium.

Resources providers and other staff may find helpful include

- American Geriatric Society—http://www.americangeriatrics.org/
- ICU Delirium and Cognitive Impairment Study Group—http://www.icudelirium.org/
- Hartford Institute for Geriatric Nursing—http://hartfordign.org/
- Hospital Elder Life Program—http://www.hospitalelderlifeprogram.org/
- ConsultGeri.org—http://consultgerirn.org/

References

American Geriatrics Society Expert Panel on Postoperative Delirium in Older Adults. American Geriatrics Society abstracted clinical practice guideline for postoperative delirium in older adults. *J Am Geriatr Soc.* 2015;63(1):142–150. doi:10.1111/jgs.13281.

Confusion Assessment Method. Copyright 1988, 2003, Hospital Elder Life Program. Not to be reproduced without permission. Adapted from: Inouye SK, et al. Ann Intern Med. 1990;113:941–948.

Ely Wesley E. CAM-ICU. Vanderbilt University Medical Center. *Revised* March 2014.

Fong TG, Tulebaev SR, Inouye SK. Delirium in elderly adults: diagnosis, prevention and treatment. *Nat Rev Neurol.* 2009;5(4):210–220. doi:10.1038/nrneurol.2009.24.

Hospital Elder Life Program. *Why delirium is important.* http://www.hospitalelderlifeprogram.org/for-clinicians/why-delirium-is-important/ Accessed August 17, 2015.

Hshieh TT, Yue J, Oh E et al. Effectiveness of multicomponent nonpharmacological delirium interventions: a meta-analysis. *JAMA Intern Med.* 2015;175(4):512–520. doi:10.1001/jamainternmed.2014.7779.

ICU Delirium and Cognitive Study Group. 2013. Delirium: assess, prevent and manage. http://www.icudelirium.org/delirium.html.

Inouye SK, Bogardus ST, Charpentier PA et al. A multicomponent intervention to prevent delirium in hospitalized older patients. *N Engl J Med.* 1999;340(9):669–676. doi:10.1056/NEJM199903043400901.

Inouye SK, Westendorp RG, Saczynski JS. Delirium in elderly people. *Lancet.* 2014;383(9920):911–22. doi:10.1016/S0140-6736(13)60688-1.

Kiely DK, Marcantonio ER, Inouye SK et al. Persistent delirium predicts greater mortality. *J Am Geriatr Soc.* 2009;57(1):55–61. doi:10.1111/j.1532-5415.2008.02092.x.

Mangusan RF, Hooper V, Denslow SA, Travis L. Outcomes associated with postoperative delirium after cardiac surgery. *Am J Crit Care.* 2015;24(2):156–163. doi:10.4037/ajcc2015137.

Marcantonio ER. Delirium. In: Medina-Walpole A, Pacala JT, Potter JF, eds. *Geriatrics Review Syllabus: A Core Curriculum in Geriatric Medicine.* 9th ed. New York, NY: American Geriatrics Society; 2016.

McKeith IG, Perry RH, Fairbairn AF, Jabeen S, Perry EK. Operational criteria for senile dementia of Lewy body type (SDLT). *Psychol Med.* 1992;22(4):911–922.

Pandharipande PP, Girard TD, Jackson JC et al. Long-term cognitive impairment after critical illness. *N Engl J Med.* 2013;369(14):1306–1316. doi:10.1056/NEJMoa1301372.

Siddiqi N, House AO, Holmes JD. Occurrence and outcome of delirium in medical in-patients: a systematic literature review. *Age Ageing.* 2006;35(4):350–364. doi:10.1093/ageing/afl005.

Vanderbilt Medical University. 2013. Delirium in the ICU: An Overview. Accessed August 17, 2015. http://www.icudelirium.org/delirium.html.

Wei LA, Fearing MA, Sternberg EJ, Inouye SK. The Confusion Assessment Method: a systematic review of current usage. *J Am Geriatr Soc.* 2008;56(5):823–830. doi:10.1111/j.1532-5415.2008.01674.x.

Weintraub D, Hurtig HI. Presentation and management of psychosis in Parkinson's disease and dementia with Lewy bodies. *Am J Psychiatry.* 2007;164(10):1491–1498. doi:10.1176/appi.ajp.2007.07040715.

Witlox J, Eurelings LS, de Jonghe JF, Kalisvaart KJ, Eikelenboom P, van Gool WA. Delirium in elderly patients and the risk of postdischarge mortality, institutionalization, and dementia: a meta-analysis. *JAMA.* 2010;304(4):443–451. doi:10.1001/jama.2010.1013.

Yang M, Marcantonio ER, Inouye SK, et al. Phenomenological subtypes of delirium in older persons: patterns, prevalence, and prognosis. *Psychosomatics.* 2009;50(3):248–254. doi:10.1176/appi.psy.50.3.248.

63

MENINGITIS

Nancy E. Villanueva

Case vignette

A 43-year-old man presents to the emergency room with a 4-day history of headaches, fever, nausea, and neck stiffness. His family reports a recent upper respiratory infection. On examination: febrile 101.8 F, blood pressure 108/70, heart rate 110/minute, respiratory rate 24/minute. Neurologic examination: lethargic, GCS 14 (disoriented to place and year), nuchal rigidity, motor strength symmetrical, cranial nerves II-XII intact. Based upon these findings, orders are placed for a metabolic panel, complete blood count (CBC) with differential and platelets, blood cultures, and a brain computed tomography (CT) scan. Intravenous fluids are started. A brain CT scan without contrast is obtained prior to performing a lumbar puncture (LP) due to the potential herniation risk. This concern is due to the altered level of consciousness, which could be from a space-occupying lesion or cerebral edema. The CT scan is negative, and an LP is performed. Opening pressure is elevated (200 mm H_2O). He is started on broad-spectrum antibiotic coverage pending results of cerebrospinal fluid (CSF) Gram stain and culture. Antibiotics are selected to cover Gram-positive and Gram-negative organisms. Additionally, he is placed on dexamethasone. Further management after admission includes follow-up of lab results, adjustment of antibiotic coverage, and close hemodynamic and neurologic monitoring.

Epidemiology

Bacterial meningitis is one of the most common central nervous system (CNS) infections (Heth, 2012). Despite advances in antimicrobial therapy, it continues to be a significant cause of morbidity and mortality. The incidence, demographics, and distribution of pathogens of meningeal infections vary by age and geographic regions. In the United States, the Centers for Disease Control and Prevention (CDC) estimate the rate of bacterial meningitis to be between 0.66 and 1.92 cases per 100,000 people (UpToDate, 2015). The development and utilization of vaccines that target the three most common agents of bacterial infection (*Streptococcus pneumonia, Haemophilus influenza,* and *Neisseria meningitidis*) have had significant impact on the incidence of the disease. This finding is in stark contrast to the undeveloped regions of the world (particularly sub-Saharan Africa) where epidemics of meningitis due to *N meningitidis* occur with incidence rates documented as high as 100 cases per 100,000 people (Manika and Joseph, 2014; Karen et al., 2014).

Other causative agents for the development of meningitis include both viral and fungal etiologies. Viral and fungal etiologies create an aseptic meningitis. The majority of cases of viral meningitis will be secondary to a primary infection at a different anatomic site. The route of exposure may be by inhalation, ingestion, or inoculation. The virus causes an associated viremia and CNS infection. Incidence of viral meningitis is higher in the summer months. Enteroviruses are the most common cause of aseptic meningitis (Russell, 2012).

A fungal causative agent must be considered in patients who have a compromised immune system. The most common causes of fungal meningitis are *Crytococcus neoformans* and *Cryptococcus gatti. Candida* meningitis is rare except for in patients who are immunosuppressed, have undergone a neurosurgical procedure, or have cancer (Manika and Joseph, 2014).

Societal significance

A population-based observational study examining the incidence and inpatient mortality for the most important causes of community and nosocomial bacterial meningitis between 1997 and 2010 in the United States was conducted by Castelblanco et al. (2014). In this study the incidence of hospital admissions due to bacterial meningitis in the National Inpatient Sample database was 50,822 cases for the five most commonly identified pathogens. The most frequent pathogen was *S pneumonia* followed by *N meningitides*, *H influenza*, *Staphylococcus* species and Gram-negative bacteria.

The cost associated with severe cases of meningococcal meningitis resulting in long-term sequelae was examined in a United Kingdom study by Wright et al. (2013). In this study the costs to the National Health Service were estimated to be between £160,000–£200,000 in the first year alone. Clearly this study illustrates the enormous potential impact of this disease.

Enteroviruses (primarily echoviruses and coxsackieviruses) are estimated to cause approximately 75,000 cases of aseptic meningitis yearly in the United States. It is the most common cause of viral meningitis (Russell, 2012; Jose, 2014). The incidence is higher in summer and early fall with increased time spent outside and increased potential for fecal-oral spread. Likewise with lighter clothing the opportunity for vector-borne causes of aseptic meningitis increases (e.g., arbovirus).

Meningitis caused by a fungal infection presents generally as a chronic meningitis picture. The rising incidence is related to the increasing number of individuals who are receiving immunosuppressive agents as part of their medical therapy. Conditions include cancer, AIDS, and inflammatory conditions such as rheumatoid arthritis (Hall and Kim, 2014).

Basic biologic and physiologic processes

Bacterial meningitis

Entry of the infectious agent into the CNS may occur in a variety of ways. The most common route is by hematogenous dissemination from a distant infectious focus seeding the meninges. Another route is by direct extension such as sinusitis, orbital cellulitis, mastoiditis, otitis media, and odontogenic source. Nosocomial infection may occur following a neurosurgical procedure, such as a craniotomy (Sarrazin et al., 2012; Manika and Joseph, 2014; Kourbeti et al., 2015; Mohran et al., 2012).

For community-acquired infections, the most likely organisms will vary depending on the age of the patient. Group B streptococci, *Escherichia coli*, and *Listeria monocytogenes* are seen in the neonate and infants up to 3 months. In the older infants, children, and adults less than 50 years of age streptococcus pneumonia and *N. meningitidis* are common pathogens. For adults older than 50 years of age, streptococcus pneumonia, *N. meningitidis*, *L. monocytogenes*, and Gram-negative bacilli are the most common agents (Manika and Joseph, 2014).

Staphylococcus aureus is the organism frequently associated with a nosocomial infection. Enteric Gram-negative bacteria (*E. coli*, *Klebsiella* species, *Acinetobacter baumannii*, and *Pseudomonas aeruginosa*) are also organisms associated with nosocomial infections (Manika and Joseph, 2014).

Viral meningitis

After the virus has been inhaled, ingested, or inoculated (infected arthropod vector such as a mosquito, tick, sand flies, and midges), it enters the lymphatic system and subsequently seeds the bloodstream. The viremia associated with this is when the CNS becomes infected.

Fungal meningitis

Because fungal meningitis is generally a chronic infection, the presentation differs from a bacterial or viral etiology. The patient generally has had symptoms for at least several weeks duration, and these symptoms can fluctuate in intensity. Risk factors include those individuals with an impaired or suppressed immune system (e.g., alcoholism, diabetes mellitus, asplenia, or cancer). In addition, individuals who are on immunosuppressive therapies (e.g., transplant, immune-modulating medications) are at a heightened risk (Hall and Kim, 2014; Jennifer John, 2014).

Common physical findings

Fever, neck stiffness, and altered mental status are often presented as the classic triad of symptoms for a patient presenting with acute meningitis (bacterial and viral). However, studies have shown that in only 44% of patients are these three symptoms actually present. When you query the symptoms (headache, fever, stiff neck, or altered mental status), at least two of the four symptoms will be present in 95% of the patients with bacterial meningitis. The absence of a stiff neck or a negative Kernig or Brudzinki sign does not eliminate the possibility of bacterial meningitis (Russell, 2012; Jose, 2014).

Central nervous system symptoms in viral meningitis are preceded with common complaints associated with a viral illness (fever and myalgias). The individual may also experience gastrointestinal symptoms with both enteroviruses and arboviruses. Altered level of consciousness is seen in an estimated two-thirds of patients with bacterial meningitis. In contrast, individuals with a viral etiology generally do not experience a change in consciousness. However, these patients can appear very ill. Seizures may also occur with bacterial meningitis. The incidence is estimated to be approximately 20%. The occurrence of seizures has also been associated with a poorer clinical prognosis. In addition, the physical examination should include a thorough inspection of the skin for the presence of a rash. This information can be utilized to aid in the determination of the etiology of the suspected meningitis. A rash is often seen with a viral etiology such as an enterovirus (Russell, 2012; Noto and Marcolini, 2014; Mohan et al., 2012; Manika and Joseph, 2014; Karen et al., 2014).

Relevant diagnostic tests

Laboratory

For definitive diagnosis, a lumbar puncture is required to obtain CSF for biochemical, cellular, and microbiological evaluation (Table 63.1). It is estimated that only 50% of patients with meningitis will show enhancement in the subarachnoid space. However, if the neurologic examination is abnormal, or the patent is immunocompromised, imaging of the brain must be obtained before performing a lumbar puncture. A CT scan of the brain is the preferred examination—this can be done quickly and will provide the practitioner with the information needed to determine if the lumbar puncture is safe to perform. The concern is for herniation if a supratentorial mass lesion (e.g., tumor, abscess) and/or cerebral edema is present. In addition, the CT scan will provide information regarding the possible presence of hydrocephalus. CSF studies include cell count and differential, glucose and protein concentrations, stains (gram, India ink, and acid-fast bacillus), cultures (aerobic, anaerobic, acid-fast bacillus, and fungal), antibody testing (arboviral), and polymerase chain reaction (PCR) testing for enteroviral, West Nile virus, and herpesvirus types 1 and 2 (Russell, 2012; Noto and Marcolini, 2014; Yuriko and Byers, 2014).

Cerebral spinal fluid analysis (adults)

1. Glucose—CSF glucose is normally two-thirds of the serum glucose. Bacterial infections alter the glucose transport across the blood-brain barrier, which results in a low CSF glucose.

2. Protein—ranges from 15 to 50 mg/dL. Elevated protein levels are seen due to the disruption of the junctions between the endothelial cells of the venules.
3. White blood cells (WBC) and differential—should have no WBCs in CSF. In bacterial meningitis the WBC differential shows a majority of neutrophils.
4. Gram stain—In 60%–90% the Gram stain is reported to be positive and is proportional to the concentration of the organisms in the CSF. If the patient has received antibiotics before CSF has been obtained, the yield of a positive Gram stain decreases by approximately 20%.
5. Culture—Identifies the organism(s) present and the sensitivities to antibiotic therapy.
6. Where suspicion is for a viral etiology, antibody testing and PCRs are indicated (Rodrigo, 2014).

In addition to the CSF studies, baseline laboratory studies (CBC with differential, basic metabolic panel, prothrombin time/international normalized ratio (PT/INR), erythrocyte sedimentation rate (ESR), C-reactive protein (CRP), and blood cultures should be obtained.

Table 63.1 Cerebrospinal Fluid Analysis

Value	Normal	Bacterial meningitis	Viral meningitis	Fungal meningitis
Opening pressure (mm H_2O)	<180	↑ 200–500	N/A	<250
WBC (mm³)	0–5	↑ 1000–5000	↑ 50–1000	↑ 20–2000
WBC differential	None	Predominance of neutrophils	Predominance of lymphocytes	Predominance of lymphocytes
Protein (mg/dL)	<50	↑ 100–500	<200	<50
Glucose (mg/dL)	Two-thirds of serum	↓ 40	<45	30–70

Sources: Rodrigo H. In Scheld WM, Whitley RJ, Marra CM [eds], *Infections of the Central Nervous System,* Philadelphia, Wolters Kluwer, 2014, 4–23; Russell B. *Continuum Lifelong Learning Neurol.,* 18(6), 2012; Noto A, Marcolini E. *Emerg Med Clin N Am.,* 32, 2014; Manika S, Joseph BD. In Hall WA, Kim PD [eds], *Neurosurgical Infectious Disease: Surgical and Nonsurgical Management.* New York, Thieme, 2014, 107–124.

Radiologic studies

Definitive diagnosis of meningitis is made based on the results of a lumbar puncture and CSF analysis. Neuroimaging studies should be obtained; however, when to obtain the studies is dependent on the clinical examination. A CT scan of the brain must be obtained prior to performing a lumbar puncture in the event of an abnormal examination or immunocompromised patient. This can be done quickly and will provide the practitioner with the information needed to determine if the lumbar puncture is safe to perform. The concern is for herniation if a supratentorial mass lesion (e.g., tumor, abscess) is present (Mohan et al., 2012)

In bacterial meningitis with a contrasted CT scan, enhancement is seen in about 50% of the patients. Magnetic resonance imaging (MRI) provides better visualization of the abnormalities seen in bacterial meningitis. These include inflammatory exudate and leptomeningeal enhancement. This is in contrast to a patient with a viral etiology where imaging studies are usually normal (Mohan et al., 2012).

Treatment

Until proven otherwise, the patient is treated with the presumptive diagnosis of bacterial meningitis. If there exists sufficient concern for an antiviral or fungal etiology, medications to address these concerns should be added to the patient's medication regimen. Once the causative etiology has been confirmed, the therapy can be tailored to that entity.

Supportive therapies include close neurologic assessments for changes in mental status, treatment for fever, and maintenance of fluid volume status.

Bacterial meningitis

Rapid diagnosis and initiation of broad-spectrum antibiotics are essential for improving patient outcome. Koster-Rasmussen reported a finding that a 1-hour delay in initiating antibiotics equated to a 30% increase in the odds of an unfavorable outcome (Heth, 2012). Clearly every effort should be made to obtain a CSF specimen prior to antibiotic administration, but this should not delay antibiotic administration. Selection of empiric antibiotics is based on the patient's age, immune status, risk factors, and resistance rates in the community. The antibiotics must possess good ability to penetrate the CNS and cover common Gram-positive and Gram-negative organisms. Once the culture results have been finalized, the antibiotics can be tailored (Manika and Joseph, 2014).

The use of adjunctive dexamethasone is widely discussed in the literature. There have been a number of meta-analyses and studies investigating the effect of dexamethasone on morbidity and mortality. Currently, dexamethasone is utilized when bacterial meningitis is suspected and discontinued if another etiology is found to be the causative agent (Russell, 2012; Karen et al., 2014).

Fungal meningitis

Antifungal agents will be utilized according to the culture and sensitivity results (Heth, 2012; Jennifer and John, 2014).

Viral meningitis

Once the etiology of the meningitis has been identified, the next step is to determine if there is a specific antiviral therapy available to treat the causative agent. Specific antiviral therapies are limited. Known antiviral therapies are available for meningitis caused by herpes simplex virus (HSV), cytomegalovirus (CMV), and herpes B virus. Acyclovir is utilized for HSV and also herpes B virus. Ganciclovir is recommended for CMV (Heth, 2012).

Prognosis

An efficient and expedient approach to evaluation and treatment is essential to ensure the most favorable outcomes for the patient. Potential complications associated with bacterial meningitis include hydrocephalus, ventriculitis, extraaxial fluid collections, cerebritis, abscess, cerebral edema, cranial nerve involvement, thrombosis/infarction, and vasculopathy. As a result, bacterial meningitis continues to carry significant morbidity and mortality. Sequelae of meningitis include seizure disorders, focal neurologic deficits, vision and hearing impairment, and cognitive dysfunction. It is estimated that one in four individuals will experience a consequence of bacterial meningitis. Viral etiologies as compared to bacterial etiologies have been found to be less associated with morbidity (Mohan et al., 2012).

Common questions

The practitioner is often asked for information on the illness and resources that are available to help them understand and cope with the illness. Being able to provide information and resources to family members and significant others is an integral part of providing care. The National Meningitis Association (NMA) and Meningitis Foundation of America (MFA) are two organizations that can provide information and support to families and those affected by meningitis.

Online resources

- Confederation of Meningitis Organisations (CoMO)—http://www.comomenigitis.org
- National Meningitis Association (NMA)—http://www.nmaus.org
- Meningitis Foundation of America—http://www.musa.org

References

Castelblanco RL, Lee M, Hasbun R. Epidemiology of bacterial meningitis in the USA from 1977 to 2010: A population-based observational study. *Lancet.* 2014;14:813–819.

Hall WA, Kim PD. Fungal infections of the central nervous system. In: Hall WA, Kim PD, eds. *Neurosurgical Infectious Disease: Surgical and Nonsurgical Management.* New York, NY: Thieme; 2014:68–80.

Heth JA. Neurosurgical aspects of central nervous system infections. *Neuroimag Clin N Am.* 2012;22:791–799.

Jennifer LH, John RP. Fungal meningitis. In: Scheld WM, Whitley RJ, Marra CM, eds. *Infections of the Central Nervous System.* 4th ed. Philadelphia, PA: Wolters Kluwer; 2014:687–710.

Jose RR. Viral meningitis and aseptic meningitis syndrome. In: Scheld WM, Whitley RJ, Marra CM, eds. *Infections of the Central Nervous System,* 4th ed. Philadelphia, PA: Wolters Kluwer; 2014:65–83.

Karen LR, Allan RT, van de B Diederik, Scheld WM. Acute bacterial meningitis. In: Scheld WM, Whitley RJ, Marra CM, eds. *Infections of the Central Nervous System,* 4th ed. Philadelphia, PA: Wolters Kluwer; 2014:365–419.

Kourbeti IS, Vakis AF, Ziakas P et al. Infections in patients undergoing craniotomy: Risk factors associated with post-operative meningitis. *J Neurosurg.* 2014;122(5):1113–1119.

Manika S, Joseph BD. Meningeal infections. In: Hall WA, Kim PD, eds. *Neurosurgical Infectious Disease: Surgical and Nonsurgical Management.* New York, NY: Thieme; 2014:107–124.

Mohan S, Jain KK, Arabi M, Shah GV. Imaging of meningitis and ventriculitis. *Neuroimag Clin N Am.* 2012;22:557–583.

Noto A, Marcolini E. Select topics in neurocritical care. *Emerg Med Clin N Am.* 2014;32:927–938.

Rodrigo H. Cerebrospinal fluid in central nervous system infections. In: Scheld WM, Whitley RJ, Marra CM, eds. *Infections of the Central Nervous System.* 4th ed. Philadelphia, PA: Wolters Kluwer; 2014:4–23.

Russell B. Acute bacterial and viral meningitis. *Continuum Lifelong Learning Neurol.* 2012;18(6):1255–1270.

Sarrazin JL, Bonneville F, Martin-Blondel G. Brain infections. *Diagnostic and Interventional Imaging.* 2012;93:473–490.

UpToDate. 2015 Epidemiology of bacterial meningitis in adults. http://www.uptodate.com/contents/epidemiology-of-bacterail meningitis-in-adults. Accessed February 24, 2015.

Wright C, Wardsworth R, Glennie L. Counting the cost of meningococcal disease: Scenerios of severe meningitis and septicemia. *Paediatr Drugs.* 2013;15(1):49–58.

Yuriko F, Byers K. Microbiological diagnosis of central nervous system infections. In: Hall WA, Kim PD, eds. *Neurosurgical Infectious Disease: Surgical and Nonsurgical Management.* New York, NY: Thieme; 2014:16–29.

64

ALZHEIMER'S DEMENTIA

LeAnn DeRungs

Dementia is the loss of cognitive function, a chronic, persistent, and progressively degenerative decline in brain function that negatively affects mental processes causing functional impairment. The *Diagnostic and Statistical Manual of Mental Disorders* (*DSM-5*) classifies dementia as a neurocognitive disorder (American Psychiatric Association, 2013). The diagnostic criteria for all-cause dementia must include functional impairment in two or more of the following areas: memory, executive thinking (reasoning and judgment), language, visuospatial ability, and attention (McKhann et al., 2011). Personality and behavior changes may also occur (Alzheimer's Foundation of America, 2015). Functional impairment in at least two areas is evident in the early stages; by the end stages of the disease, people have functional impairment in all areas. It is at the end stages of the dementing disease, and often earlier, when people with dementia will require full-time care (National Institute on Aging, 2015a).

Epidemiology

Alzheimer disease (AD) is the sixth leading cause of death in the United States and the fifth leading cause of death in people 65 years of age and older. A recent study reports the incidence of death due to AD is underreported, and it may be as high as the third leading cause of death in the United States after heart disease and cancer (James et al., 2014). Alzheimer's is not often listed on death certificates as cause of death because a more immediate cause of death is listed instead (James et al., 2014). Aspiration pneumonia is the most common reason for death in people with AD (Leonard, 2014). Prior to death, AD is one of the leading causes of disability and morbidity.

Age is the biggest risk factor for the onset of AD (National Institute of Neurological Disorders and Stroke, 2015).

In the United States, the number of people age 65 and older is expected to more than double from 40 million in 2010 to 88.5 million in 2050, leading to an increase in the incidence of AD (Grayson and Velkoff, 2010). By 2050, 13.5 million Americans are expected to have the disease, affecting families, caregivers, and the health-care system (Alzheimer's Association, 2015). In 2015, 18% of Medicare dollars ($113 billion) will be spent on caring for people with AD. Medicare costs are expected to increase to $589 billion in 2050. These figures do not include Medicaid dollars or out-of-pocket cost for individuals with the disease or the families affected (Alzheimer's Association, 2015).

Ages of people with Alzheimer disease in the United States, 2015

85+ years: 38%
75–84 years: 43%
65–74 years: 15%
<65 years: 4%

(Hebert et al., 2013)

Types of nonreversibile dementia

Alzheimer's is the most common form of dementia (Centers for Disease Control and Prevention, 2015). Some other forms of irreversible dementia include vascular dementia, Lewy body dementia, Parkinson dementia, frontal temporal lobe dementia (FTLD), and Huntington dementia. People can simultaneously have more than one type of dementia, referred to as mixed dementia. Mixed dementia is more common than previously recognized. In one study, 54% of people diagnosed with AD on autopsy showed pathology for another type of dementia (Alzheimer's Association, 2015). On autopsy, vascular dementia has been the most common coexisting type of dementia in mixed dementia, with Lewy body being the second most common type of coexisting dementia diagnosed. Dementia is confirmed only by autopsy. Until death occurs, the diagnosis is at best "probable Alzheimer disease." Neuropathologic confirmation is required to validate the clinical diagnosis of AD (Tierney et al.,1988).

Pathophysiology and stages of Alzheimer disease

Most people diagnosed with dementia who are over the age of 65 have Alzheimer dementia (National Institute of Neurological Disorders and Stroke, 2015). People whose onset of the disease occurs at age 65 or older are said to have late-onset AD. However, people diagnosed prior to age 65, who do not have an amyloid precursor protein (APP), presenilin 1, or presenilin 2 genetic mutation for the disease, are also said to have the late-onset type of Alzheimer dementia. People who develop Alzheimer dementia before age 65 and have an inherited genetic mutation for AD are diagnosed with early onset familial Alzheimer disease (FAD) (National Institute on Aging, 2015).

The cause of AD is not yet fully understood, and the disease most likely has more than one pathway. The pathophysiologic process of AD is thought to begin decades before the first symptoms of the disease are noted and before clinical diagnosis, known as the "preclinical phase" (Sperling et al., 2011; Morris, 2004). Not all people with preclinical biomarker evidence will develop AD, and not all older people who show pathology of the disease become symptomatic.

Between the preclinical phase and before criteria are met for a clinical diagnosis is the predementia phase of AD, referred to as mild cognitive impairment (MCI). In this phase of the disease, people will note a change in their cognition and have evidence of lower performance in one or more cognitive domains (memory, reasoning and judgment, language attention, and/or visuospatial ability) but are able to maintain independence in their daily functions (Albert et al., 2011). Not all people with MCI will go on to develop AD.

As stated previously, the definitive diagnosis of AD occurs by autopsy. The hallmark pathology of AD noted on autopsy is the accumulation of two types of protein: beta amyloid protein plaques outside the neurons in the brain and tau protein tangles inside the neurons of the brain. The beta amyloid plaques interfere with the communication between neurons leading to cell death. Tau tangles contribute to neuronal death by blocking essential molecules inside the neuron (Ballard et al., 2011). The number of neurofibrillary tangles is a pathologic marker of the severity of AD (Querfurth and Laferla, 2010).

Beta amyloid protein and tau protein are two important biomarkers used in Alzheimer research. The cerebral spinal fluid (CSF) that bathes the brain also bathes the spinal cord and can be found in the spinal sac and obtained by lumbar puncture. The CSF will be low in beta amyloid if the amyloid protein is being laid down and forming plaques in the brain, while tau will be high in the CSF if there is cell death in the neuron. Both a low amyloid level and a high tau level are indicators that Alzheimer pathology is occurring in the brain. However, at this time it is not known to what degree the pathology correlates with the onset of symptoms, or if any symptoms will occur.

Cell loss causes atrophy (shrinkage) of the brain. The smaller brain is noted on autopsy but can also be seen on magnetic resonance imaging (MRI) while people with AD are alive. MRIs are not used for the definitive diagnosis of AD; however, with improved diagnostic techniques and criteria, an earlier diagnosis may be possible (Ballard et al., 2011).

The hippocampus is vulnerable to damage in the early stages of AD (Mu and Gage, 2011). The hippocampus is the region of the brain most responsible for memory and forming new memories. In AD, the plaque buildup in this region makes it difficult for new memories to form. This loss in short-term memory, is demonstrated when people with AD are not able to remember a recent event (what they had for breakfast) but are able remember an event from their distant past (long-term memory). As the disease progresses, a person's long-term memories will also be lost.

Symptoms/Seven stages of Alzheimer disease

Dr. Barry Reisberg, clinical director of the New York University School of Medicine, developed a framework from which the following seven stages of Alzheimer's were gleaned (Alzheimer's Association, 2015). Memory loss is often the first symptom recognized in people with AD; however, other symptoms like poor judgment or difficulty finding words may occur first.

1. *No impairment*
2. *Very mild cognitive decline*—A person may notice and report word-finding difficulties, misplacing items, or memory lapses. However, family members, friends, or coworkers have not seen the change and it is not appreciated on exam.
3. *Mild cognitive decline*—Friends, family, or coworkers begin to notice difficulties, and a medical interview detects changes in memory or concentration. Word-finding difficulties, forgetting material that has just been read, losing or misplacing valuable objects, or increasing trouble planning or organizing are demonstrated or reported.
4. *Moderate cognitive decline*—Medical interview clearly detects symptoms. Patient forgets recent events, has difficulty managing finances and paying bills, shows impaired performance with mental arithmetic, forgets personal history, or becomes withdrawn or moody in social settings or when mentally challenged.
5. *Moderately severe cognitive decline*—People begin to need help with daily activities. They may not know the date or day of the week, forget where they are, be unable to recall personal data such as phone number and address, or need help choosing appropriate seasonal clothing to wear. They can still feed and toilet themselves and still know significant details about themselves and family members.
6. *Severe cognitive decline*—Personality changes may occur, memory worsens, and the patients require more help with daily activities such as personal hygiene, and dressing (may put clothes on over pajamas or wear things inside out). Patients may also have changes in sleep patterns (nap more or awake at night) and some incontinence of bladder or bowel. Behavioral changes include delusions or suspiciousness, and they may wander.
7. *Very severe cognitive decline*—Patients need help eating and toileting, and swallowing becomes impaired. Patients may also become less verbal, have difficulty holding up their head, lose the ability to smile, and muscles may become rigid.

Risk factors

According to the Alzheimer's Association, the late-onset form of AD is marked by a gene called apolipo-protein E (APOE). There are several forms of the gene, but the APOE alle 4 increases the risk of developing the disease. However, some people with the APOE alle 4 gene will not develop AD.

A small percentage of AD is caused by a mutation in the amyloid precursor protein (APP) and the presenilin 1 and presenilin 2 proteins. Mutations in these genes cause early onset AD, which starts before the age of 65 and as early as age 30. If the mutation is in the APP or the presenilin 1 gene, the chance of developing the disease is 100%, while having a mutation in the presenilin 2 gene offers a 95% chance of developing AD (Alzheimer's Association, 2015).

While age is the greatest risk factor for AD, cardiovascular risk factors such as smoking, diabetes, and obesity in midlife are also associated with dementia. Impaired glucose processing is a precursor to diabetes, and having the impairment alone without diabetes may increase the risk for dementia. New research shows high cholesterol and hypertension in midlife may be risk factors for dementia (Bendlin et al., 2010).

People with fewer years of education are at greater risk for AD. People with higher education are thought to have more "cognitive reserve" (Almeida et al., 2015). Cognitive reserve is the brain's ability to compensate for early brain changes due to disease. The hypothesis is that the more education (experience) a person has, the more compensatory mechanisms (alternate routes of neuron-to-neuron communication) the brain has to compensate for brain changes. However, less education may be associated with lower economic status, which can mean poorer nutrition, less health care, and more exposure to known environmental hazards.

Traumatic brain injuries (TBIs) may contribute to AD by disrupting normal brain function. People with repeated TBIs are at greater risk for dementia (Alzheimer's Association, 2015).

Prevention and treatment

There is no cure and no known prevention for AD. The class of medications used to slow the progression of the disease includes acetylcholinesterase inhibitor medications and NMDA receptor antagonists; both offer only a temporary slowdown to the progression of AD. Eliminating cardiovascular risk factors may reduce the risks for developing AD (Bendlin et al., 2010), and increasing cardiorespiratory fitness, through aerobic exercise, may help prevent the disease or delay its onset in older adults at risk for developing AD (Boots et al., 2015). Staying mentally challenged and socially engaged throughout life may also reduce the risk of developing AD (Alzheimer's Association, 2015).

Tips for caring for people with Alzheimer disease

- Speak slowly and repeat statements exactly the same way each time.
- Use concrete language and be specific, naming the person or object instead of using the words "this," "that," "him," "her," "he," or "she."
- Ask "yes" and "no" questions, and allow plenty of time for a response.
- Give a patient your full attention, showing that you are listening and are not in a hurry.
- Provide simple directions, one at a time.
- Always let the patient know what you are doing in the simplest of terms and apologize for any discomfort you caused.
- Watch for nonverbal communication, especially when assessing for pain.
- Remind the patient who you are.
- Reassure the patient knows that you will provide care.
- Provide the patient with a routine, and utilize the same nursing staff as much as possible.
- Avoid a busy room or too many caregivers in the room at one time.
- Once the patient's level of comprehension is established, discontinue asking orientation questions.
- Avoid asking, "do you remember?"

- An acute increase in memory difficulties or confusion may indicate delirium and be a sign of illness or metabolic distress (National Institute on Aging, 2015).

Remember the caregivers

AD places an enormous emotional, physical, and financial stress on informal caregivers, including family members and friends. Informal caregivers provide the majority of care for people with AD in the community and often do not identify themselves as caregivers, seeing themselves as only a wife, a daughter, a husband, a son, or a friend helping a person whom they care about. However, the intensive support required for a person with AD can negatively impact the caregiver's emotional and physical health and well-being. Informal caregivers often report symptoms of depression and anxiety (Cooper, 2010). For these reasons, it is important to introduce supportive services to patients and their families as early as possible.

Health-care services may include having a social worker present at clinic appointments to help arrange for professional home health visits, arranging for a meal service or transportation, and helping the caregiver to identify family members or friends who can help routinely. Depending on the patient's geographic location, there may be several agencies to assist the patient in remaining at home. There are local and state government agencies as well as private companies and/or volunteers to help with everything from meal preparation to transportation. Local Alzheimer's Association chapters have the most current information for their community agencies.

Alzheimer's Association 24/7 Helpline—800-272-3900; http://www.alz.org/

Alzheimer's Foundation of America Programs and Services—866-232-8484; http://www.alzfdn.org/AFAServices/tollfreehotline.html

Eldercare Locator—800-677-1116; http://www.eldercare.gov/Eldercare.NET/Public/Index.aspx

National Institute on Aging—https://www.nia.nih.gov/

National Institutes of Health, Alzheimer's Disease—http://search.nih.gov/search?utf8=%E2%9C%93&affiliate=nih&query=alzheimer+disease

National Institutes of Health, Alzheimer's Disease Research—https://www.nia.nih.gov/alzheimers/alzheimers-disease-research-centers

References

Albert MS, DeKosky ST, Dickson D et al. The diagnosis of mild cognitive impairment due to Alzheimer's disease: recommendations from the National Institute on Aging-Alzheimer's Association workgroups on diagnostic guidelines for Alzheimer's disease. *Alzheimers Dement.* 2011;7(3):270–279.

Almeida RP, Schultz SA, Austin BP et al. Effect of cognitive reserve on age-related changes in cerebrospinal fluid biomarkers of Alzheimer disease. *JAMA Neurol.* 2015;72(6):699–706.

Alzheimer's Association. Changing the trajectory of Alzheimer's disease: how a treatment by 2025 saves lives and dollars. 2015a. Available at www.alz.org/trajectory. Accessed June 22, 2015.

Alzheimer's Association. 2015 Alzheimer's disease facts and figures. *Alzheimers Dement.* 2015b;11(3):332–384.

Alzheimer's Association. Mixed dementia signs, symptoms, & diagnosis. 2015c Available at www.alz.org/dementia/mixed-dementia-symptoms.asp. Accessed June 26, 2015.

Alzheimer's Association. *Seven stages of Alzheimer's.* 2015d. Available at http://www.alz.org/nyc/in_my_community_63259.asp. Accessed June 22, 2015.

Alzheimer's Foundation of America. Symptoms. Available at www.alz.org/professionls _and_ researchers_behavoiral _symptoms_pr.asp. Accessed June 24, 2015.

American Psychiatric Association. *Diagnostic and Statistical Manual of Mental Disorders.* 5th ed. Washington, DC: American Psychiatric Association; 2013.

Ballard C, Gauthier S, Corbett A, Brayne C, Aarsland D, Jones E. Alzheimer's disease. *Lancet.* 2011;377(9770):1019–1031.

Bendlin BB, Carlsson CM, Gleason CE et al. Midlife predictors of Alzheimer's disease. *Maturitas*. 2010;65(2):131–137.

Boots EA, Schultz SA, Oh JM et al. Cardiorespiratory fitness is associated with brain structure, cognition, and mood in a middle-aged cohort at risk for Alzheimer's disease. *Brain Imaging Behav*. 2015;9(3):639–649.

Center for Disease Control & Prevention. Alzheimer's disease. Available at http://www.cdc.gov/aging/aginginfo/alzheimers.htm. Last updated March 5, 2015. Accessed June 26, 2015.

Cooper C, Katona C, Orrell M, Livingston G. Coping strategies, anxiety and depression in caregivers of people with Alzheimer's disease. *Int J Geriatr Psychiatry*. 2008;23(9):929–936.

Grayson VK, Velkoff VA. *The Next Four Decades: The Older Population in the United States: 2010 to 2050. No. 1138*. US Department of Commerce, Economics and Statistics Administration: US Census Bureau; 2010.

Hebert LE, Weuve J, Scherr PA, Evans DA. Alzheimer disease in the United States (2010–2050) estimated using the 2010 census. *Neurology*. 2013;80(19):1778–1783.

James BD, Leurgans SE, Hebert LE, Scherr PA, Yaffe K, Bennett DA. Contribution of Alzheimer disease to mortality in the United States. *Neurology*. 2014;82(12):1045–1050.

Leonard, WMPH. Alzheimer's disease complications. Available at.. www.healthline.com/health/alzheimers-disease-complications Accessed June.24, 2015. Published Aug. 29, 2014.

McKhann GM, Knopman DS, Chertkow H et al. The diagnosis of dementia due to Alzheimer's disease: recommendations from the National Institute on Aging-Alzheimer's Association workgroups on diagnostic guidelines for Alzheimer's disease. *Alzheimers Dement*. 2011;7(3):263–269.

Morris JC. Early-stage and preclinical Alzheimer disease. *Alzheimer Dis Assoc Disord*. 2004;19(3):163–165.

Mu Y, Gage FH. Adult hippocampal neurogenesis and its role in Alzheimer's disease. *Mol Neurodegener*. 2011;6(1):85.

National Institute on Aging. Acute hospitalization and Alzheimer's disease: a special kind of care. Available at www.Nia.nih.gov/Alzheimer's/publication/acute-hospitalization-and Alzheimer's disease. Published February 2009. Page Last Updated May 1, 2015. Accessed June 26, 2015.

National Institute on Aging. Alzheimer's disease fact sheet. Available at www.nia.nih.gov/alzheimers/publication/alzheimers-disease-fact-sheet. Accessed June 26,2015. Published May 2015. Updated June 9, 2015.

National Institute of Neurological Disorders and Stroke. Dementia hope through research. Available at www.ninds.nih.gov/disorders/dementia/detail_dementia.htm. Accessed June 24, 2015. Last updated February 23, 2015.

Querfurth HW, Laferla FM. Mechanisms of disease: Alzheimer's disease. *N Engl J Med*. 2010;362:329–344.

Sperling RA, Aisen PS, Beckett LA et al. Toward defining the preclinical stages of Alzheimer's disease: recommendations from the National Institute on Aging-Alzheimer's Association workgroups on diagnostic guidelines for Alzheimer's disease. *Alzheimers Dement*. 2011;7(3):280–292.

Tanzi RE, Bertram L. New frontiers in Alzheimer's disease genetics. *Neuron*. 2001;32(2):181–184.

Tierney MC, Fisher RH, Lewis AJ et al. The NINCDS-ADRDA work group criteria for the clinical diagnosis of probable Alzheimer's disease: a clinicopathologic study of 57 cases. *Neurology*. 1988;38(3):359–364.

65

PARKINSON'S DISEASE

Bruno V. Gallo and Alisabeth C. Hearron

Case vignette

A 66-year-old right-handed, recently retired man presents complaining of a resting tremor in his right hand that has been present for many months, but is not impairing his activities of daily living. His wife notes that more recently he walks while holding his right arm flexed, has a tendency to shuffle down their long hallways, seems to bend forward at the trunk, and takes longer and longer to complete many of his routine ADLs.

Overview

This example illustrates the classic Parkinson disease diagnosis triad: resting tremor, rigidity, and bradykinesia (slow movements). Postural stability and falls are often a late complication of the disorder. Generally, Parkinson disease presents asymmetrically, one side more affected, although, on careful neurologic examination, bilateral involvement is demonstrated.

Almost 200 years since Dr. James Parkinson first described the entity that would eventually bear his name, we know more; however, so much more needs to be learned to effectively approach every patient.

The natural history of the disorder stems from an unexplained loss of neurons, and the largest risk factor appears to be age. With the aging population, the impact is evident. Men have a slightly greater prevalence than women. Approximately 1.5 million in the United States carry the Parkinson disease diagnosis, thus affecting 0.3% of the general population but 3% of those older than 65 years of age (Lang and Lozano, 1998). With an average age of onset of 60, the prevalence in the population that is 80 years old or older is 10% (Lang and Lozano, 1998). Additionally, 5%–10% of PD patients have symptoms before the age of 40 (young-onset Parkinson disease [YOPD]). A major epidemiologic study suggests that genetic factors play a larger role in patients with YOPD, while environment insult plays a larger role in patients with PD onset after the age of 50 (Olanow et al., 2001).

As neuronal loss progresses, the development of motor symptoms leads patients to visit physicians. The diagnosis continues, to this day, to be made clinically. There are, in the spectrum of loss of neurons, premotor symptoms that appear and become clear in hindsight. These nonmotor presymptomatic signs would be a valuable place to begin to make the diagnosis, but that is an area of much research. In the "pathologic staging model," Braak and colleagues have described a degeneration of neurons in the brainstem (Braak et al., 2004).

This neurodegeneration then progresses to ultimately involve the loss of dopaminergic neurons. At this point, the motor manifestations make the clinical diagnosis an easier task.

Top:

Positron emission tomography (PET) scan showing striatal fluorodopa uptake of a normal brain (top left) versus PD (top right).

Bottom:

Gross pathology of the midbrain showing a normal brain (bottom left) versus PD (bottom right) (Marsden, 1994; Lang and Lozano, 1998).

Cardinal symptoms in making the diagnosis include the following:

- Tremor (usually resting)
- Rigidity
- Bradykinesia/akinesia
- Postural instability
  - Autonomic dysfunction
  - Neuropsychiatric dysfunction
  - Motor complications

Identifying patients in the premotor phases of the disease would be very advantageous for the patient. Imaging technologies have emerged, but these require the patient to already have a motor symptom (i.e., tremors) for a dopamine active transport (DAT) scan to be useful. There is active research underway in an effort to develop a synuclein scan, with the goal to diagnose patients without motor symptoms.

Physical examination findings

The patient is awake, alert, and oriented with no language deficits. His face is masked, and he has a decreased eye blink rate. He has a resting tremor of his right hand that appears pill rolling. The amplitude of the tremor is not marked, and the frequency is about 3–4 hertz. There is bradykinesia with testing of rapid alternating movements seen clearly on the right side compared to the left. It affects the right lower extremity as well. Cogwheeling and rigidity are elicited with a distraction maneuver on the left hand at the elbow and wrist of the right upper extremity. His sensation is normal throughout, and reflexes are intact and symmetric. No pathologic reflexes are noted. When walking he has no arm swing on the right upper extremity and has a tendency to turn "en bloc," using multiple steps to turn 180°. He is stable with no postural instability. Romberg sign is negative, and there is no retropulsion or anteropulsion.

Once the diagnosis is made, it is critical to assure the patient and family members and ensure that they are given the proper education to understand the road ahead. Literature and resources about the disorder are shared with everyone, and patients are encouraged to either maintain a healthy and active lifestyle including exercise and nutrition or begin one.

Symptomatic treatment

Literature regarding neuroprotective agents and medications that may help "slow down" the disease progression have been widely published. Once the diagnosis is made, in some cases, months to years may have passed before effective therapy is begun.

A complementary and multidisciplinary approach to the treatment of Parkinson disease must be adopted. Patients, caregivers, health-care professionals including movement disorder neurologists, neurology nurse practitioners, neurosurgeons, neuropsychologists, and therapists as well as support groups and families all become involved in the successful treatment of patients.

The management of early onset disease is very different from advanced therapy and beyond the scope of our discussion. In 2015 the mainstay of therapy for Parkinson disease remains medications. Available are oral, transdermal, continuous infusions of gels through an implanted jejunostomy pump, and in indicated cases subcutaneous injections. For those individuals with advanced disease, the implantation of electrodes in the brain using deep brain stimulation (DBS) has been a wonderful addition to therapy options.

Traditionally, therapy was initiated when motor symptoms interfered with the patient's ADLs. However, there is recent evidence by Shapira and Obeso that early therapy may have some long-term benefits (Shapira and Obeso, 2006).

In the author's opinion, the evidence is inconclusive but appears promising.

Physical therapy is another treatment that is essential. Therapy can be either formal, with a licensed therapist, or encouraged by support groups. Informal therapy may include Tai Chi, pool/swim therapy, carefully supervised weight lifting, and aerobic exercise and walking.

Pharmacologic treatment options

With the advent of levodopa in the late 1960s and early 1970s, the gold standard for therapy of Parkinson disease has remained carbidopa/levodopa. As a result of the treatment, long-term complications of the motor symptoms were reported for the therapy aimed at helping those motor symptoms. Even so, great strides have been made to develop medication choices that reduce the long-term motor complications of medical therapies. Additionally, advances have led many movement disorder neurologists to treat their patients using multiple medical therapies in a sophisticated fashion, reducing the untoward adverse sequela of long-term use. Physicians now also have the ability to provide medications that address the nonmotor symptoms of Parkinson disease (i.e., hallucinations, dementia, and dysautonomias). The prevention of deterioration and possible reversal of neurodegeneration remains a lofty goal in neuroscience to this day.

Amantadine has been available since the 1970s and in early disease, it may help with tremor and some of the slowness (bradykinesia). In advanced disease, it has a place in the treatment of dyskinesias that appear. This benefit may be a short-lived 6–12 months; nevertheless, it is a useful agent.

Another useful group of drugs are the MAO-B inhibitors. Although selegiline was the first of these to appear in the early 1990s, a newer agent rasagiline (Azilect) has shown some promise. Neither medication is approved as a "neuroprotectant," but is rather adjunctive therapy for the former and initial therapy and add-on therapy for advanced symptoms in the case of rasagiline (Olanow et al., 2009).

The dopamine agonists have been around for some time. They act on dopamine receptors in the striatum. They can be used as monotherapy or as adjunctive therapy to levodopa. Today we exclusively use the non-ergot alkaloids under the name Requip (ropinirole) and Mirapex (pramipexole). In 2007, a patch became available named Neupro (rotigotine). When launched, crystals formed in the patch and it was temporarily taken off the market. It took another 4 years to solve this issue before its reappearance in the United States in 2011. In our opinion it offers superior therapy when used in new-onset disease as a once daily therapy. And like most therapies, it reduces "off" time in a 24-hour period. This was proven in three studies when it was compared to placebo (Bigland et al., 2006).

Oral medications may be delivered in a pulsatile fashion, but the current theory is that this pulsatility results in the appearance of untoward long-term side effects such as dyskinesias and dystonias. Dyskinesias are uncontrollable wild asymmetric flailing movements of the arms, legs, trunk, and at times the face. They make the patient writhe and family members uncomfortable. It should be noted that patients prefer to be dyskinetic rather than "off" and unable to move, becuase patients can accomplish daily tasks with nontroublesome dyskinesias. Dystonias are slow, painful prolonged muscular contractions that can deform an articulation or joint and are referred to by patients as the "worst Charlie horses ever."

A common thread in the treatment of patients with Parkinson disease in recent years has been the continuous dopaminergic stimulation theory in an effort to avoid these adverse effects. An advanced therapy is the levodopa-carbidopa intestinal gel (Duopa) approved in the United States in February 2015. The gel holds the medication in suspension and is infused into the jejunum with a pump over 16–18 hours. This potentially avoids the peaks and troughs and pulsatile delivery of oral medications taken three, four, or more times each day.

Surgical treatment options

When DBS was first approved in the United States in 1997, it had indications for only essential tremors and unilateral tremors in PD patients with the target being the ventral intermediate nucleus of the thalamus (ViM). In 2002 an indication for PD was given with the targets of the subthalamic nucleus (STN) and the globus pallidus pars interna (Gpi). In 2003 another indication for dystonia was approved with the Gpi target. The indications for DBS in Parkinson disease patients are in those individuals when symptoms are no longer adequately controlled by medications. The best responders to this therapy are patients who responded to levodopa in the past and who present with increased "off" times, "on/off" motor fluctuations, tremors, disabling peak dose "on" dyskinesias, and painful dystonias. Selection of patients is stringent with detailed pre- and postoperative measurements using the Unified Parkinson Disease Rating Scale Questionnaire (UPDRS) usually administered by the neurologist or qualified nurse practitioner and a comprehensive neuropsychological battery. The UPDRS uses a four-point scoring system and measures a standardized core of 42 different assessments in four categories that include mood and behavior, activities of daily living, motor responses, and complications from therapy. With proper lead placement and in the hands of expert neurologists and nurse practitioners who have carefully selected the patients and postoperatively program their generators, DBS therapy can drastically improve quality of life and "on" time.

A typical DBS case requires the patient to be relatively awake and able to interact with the neurologist. The entire team has participated in getting the patient to this point with screening, qualification measurements such as motor testing and neuropsychological testing including intensive physical, occupational, and speech therapies.

Prognosis

Today the prognosis of patients with the diagnosis is excellent. With many therapies available to the practitioner, the quality of life we offer our patients is much improved over what was able to be provided 20 years ago. There are therapies that produce symptomatic benefit and can delay the need to start levodopa in some patients. When the gold standard of levodopa therapy produces untoward side effects, alternative options such as intestinal gels and DBS are available. Patients and caregivers have never been more educated and knowledgeable as to the many alternatives to augment standard medical care, and this helps provide a real team approach to treatment.

Common questions

Patients frequently ask about new therapies and cures

Patients get relief from motor complaints but continue to suffer from nonmotor complications. They ask about problems with disrupted sleep patterns, hallucinations, orthostatic hypotension, postural instability, depression, excessive sweating and drooling, and hypophonia (low voice volume). These produce for the practitioner a challenge that requires careful treatment options and often referrals to movement disorders specialists at centers for continued care.

Common pitfalls

Common pitfalls are patients asking to delay available new therapies today because they wish to "wait for the stem cell cure" which is not on the horizon. Other patients wish to hold out for gene therapy which, cannot be predicted despite researchers working diligently.

Common phone calls, pages, and requests with answers

Q: I have missed my doses of meds and never seem to take them on time. What should I do?

A: It is imperative that you take your medications when instructed and not miss doses. If you do miss a dose, it is acceptable to take it as soon as possible, but if close to the next dosing time, wait if you can.

Q: Are there any foods I should be eating or avoiding with my pills?

A: There has been a lot written about food and PD. To date there are no reasons to avoid certain foods or eat other foods. Eating a healthy balanced diet is best. Your Parkinson medications, particularly levodopa, are best taken on an empty stomach so as not to compete with mechanisms that absorb protein.

Q: What is the goal of treatment?

A: Knowing that there is no cure, the best thing is to establish a great working relationship with your medical team and understand that the therapies are there to provide the patient with the best quality of life. These include medical and surgical options.

Q: My Sinemet (carbidopa/levodopa) no longer works or lasts as long. What's happening?

A: All is not lost, this could be a sign of disease progression and results from the pulsatile fashion in which we administer the medication. Your physician will probably add another agent or change the interval between doses. Ultimately your doctor may consider advanced therapies to treat you and will carefully screen you as a candidate.

Q: I'm starting to fall and am having more difficulty walking. What gives?

A: Staying mobile and exercising as much as possible is your best option. When balance is affected, physical therapists can evaluate you for balance, gait training, and strengthening. The difficulty is from shorter steps or freezing of your gait, and may require a cane, a laser light cane, or a walker with or without a laser light. Your neurologists will help you through this. There are no "walking or balance" pills or surgeries.

Conclusion

The relevance of this integral approach to the diagnosis and treatment of Parkinson disease involves the entire medical team, including physician, nurse practitioner, and other allied health-care professionals to maximize patient quality of life and independence. It is the clear role of the nurse practitioner to look at the entire patient and to facilitate patient care outside the medical and surgical roles. Without such a dovetailed therapeutic approach, some patients may not be offered every available modality, and this we believe would not be optimal.

References

Bigland KM, Schwid S, Eberly S et al. Rasagiline improves quality of life in patients with early Parkinson's disease. *Mov Disord.* 2006;21(5):616–623.

Braak H, Ghebremedhin E, Rub U, Bratzke H, Del Tredici K. Stages in the development of Parkinson's disease-related pathology. *Cell Tissue Res.* 2004;318(1):121–134.

Lang AE, Lozano AM. Parkinson's disease. First of two parts. *N Engl J Med.* 1998;339(15):1044, 1049–1050.

Merritt's Textbook of Neurology. Pietro Mazzoni; Lewis P. Rowland Ed. 2001:362–373.

Olanow CW, Rascol O, Hauser R et al. A double-blind, delayed-start trial of rasagiline in Parkinson's disease. *N Eng J Med.* September 24, 2009;361:1268–1278.

Olanow CW, Watts RL, Koller WC. An algorithm (decision tree) for the management of Parkinson's disease (2001): treatment guidelines. *Neurology.* 2001;56(11 suppl 5):S1–S88.

Schapira AH, Olanow CW. Neuroprotection in Parkinson disease, mysteries myths and misconceptions. *JAMA.* 2004;291:356–364.

Shapira AH, Obeso J. Timing of treatment initiation in Parkinson's disease: a need for reappraisal? *Ann Neurol.* 2006;59(3):559–562.

Shults CW, Oakes D, Kieburtz K et al. Effects of coenzyme Q10 in early Parkinson disease evidence of slowing of the functional decline. *Arch Neurol.* 2002;59(10):1541–1550.

Siderwof A, Stern M. Pre-clinical diagnosis of Parkinson's disease, are we there yet? *Curr Neurol Neurosci Rep.* 2006;6(4):295–301.

Tanner CM, Ottman R, Goldman SM et al. Parkinson disease in twins: an etiologic study. *JAMA.* 1999;281:341, 345.

Watts RL, Koller WC, eds. *Movement Disorders: Neurologic Principles and Practice.* New York, NY: McGraw-Hill Professional Publishing; 1997.

66

STATUS EPILEPTICUS

Candice Osuga Lin, Simon Buttrick, and Odette A. Harris

Overview

Epidemiology and societal significance

- Status epilepticus (SE) affects 65,000–150,000 people in the United States each year (Treiman et al., 1998; Manno, 2011).
- One-third of patients with SE may develop refractory SE.
- Patients with refractory SE have almost 50% associated mortality (Kalviainen et al., 2005).

Basic biologic and physiologic processes

- SE is a seizure that lasts longer than 5 minutes (Mazurkiewicz-Beldzinska et al., 2014; Manno, 2011).
- SE is unlikely to stop without intervention (Mazurkiewicz-Beldzinska et al., 2014).
- SE could be a manifestation of other serious, treatable processes including brain tumors, infection, or hydrocephalus.
- SE in a patient with epilepsy could be due to decreased anticonvulsant serum levels due to recent medication changes, new medications in the regimen that may lower seizure threshold, infection, noncompliance, or alcohol abuse.
- Management of SE is to reduce morbidity and mortality.

SE is a seizure event that lasts for more than 5 minutes

- Patients often appear initially confused or in a twilight state.
- The tonic phase occurs, with mental status impairment and prolonged loss of consciousness.
- Body stiffening often with a piercing cry.
- Teeth clenching and tongue biting.
- The tonic phase is followed by a clonic phase with rhythmical muscle contractions with the entire body.
- May include urinary incontinence.
- Subtle tonic eye deviation, nystagmus, or other fine motor twitches.
- Postictal phase with confusion and lethargy.

Patients who are acutely ill may not have the above physical findings; rather their diagnosis of SE may be determined by an electroencephalogram (EEG).

Case vignette

MT is a 52-year-old right-handed female in the emergency room (ER) with severe headache, nausea, and vomiting. Upon admission she arched her body making a screeching noise. Her head deviated to the right and her jaws clenched as her arms and legs rhythmically shook. Immediately the ER staff assisted her to a side-lying position for airway protection as she was given supplemental oxygen and an intravenous (IV) line was started. She had a bedside fingerstick test for blood glucose while the vital signs were obtained: Glucose: 110, HR 102, BP 110/60, SaO$_2$ 96%. She was given 5 mg of IV lorazepam, and labs were obtained for STAT complete blood count (CBC)/erythrocyte sedimentation rate (ESR), basic metabolic panel (BMP), drug/toxicology screen, and pregnancy test. With no known risk factors for seizures (no recent trauma, surgery, or habits), a thorough workup ensued. She continued to convulse and was given fosphenytoin intravenously along with a fluid bolus of normal saline. After 10 minutes of continued tonic-clonic seizure activity, her body seemed to relax, repeated neurology exam found nystagmus with persistent eye deviation, and continued video EEG was started to assess for continued SE (Figure 66.1).

Common clinical examination findings

An accurate/thorough patient history is necessary (look for causes of SE).

- Note history of childhood febrile event, head injury, and dental work (risk for abscess)
- Establish onset of event
- Clarify patient medications (type, dose, and last time taken)

Relevant diagnostic tests

Table 66.1 presents tests for SE. Tests to establish potential underlying causes of SE include those for metabolic disturbances, electrolyte imbalance, hypoglycemia, drug toxicity/withdrawal (opioids, benzodiazepine, barbiturates, or alcohol), infection, tumors, stroke, hemorrhage, trauma, and hypoxia. SE can also occur due to inadequate antiepileptic drugs (AEDs).

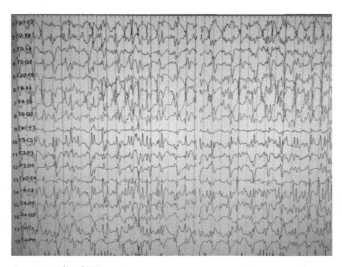

Figure 66.1 EEG showing generalized SE.

Table 66.1 Diagnostic Tests for SE

Test	Purpose	Abnormal findings
Electrolytes Sodium Calcium Magnesium Glucose	Assess for possible causes of SE	Hyponatremia, hypocalcemia, hypoglycemia
Complete blood count (CBC)	Assess for infection	Infection may be a precipitant for SE
Serum drug screen	Assess for drug and/or alcohol intoxication	May be a precipitant for SE
Antiepilepsy drug (AED) levels	Determine amount of drugs in the system	Low levels may be cause of SE
Arterial blood gases (ABGs)	Obtain baseline levels and determine oxygen saturation	Decreased oxygen saturation due to convulsive SE and medication administration
Continuous electrocardiogram (ECG) monitoring	Evaluate cardiovascular status, especially during medication administration	Phenytoin and other AEDs can cause dysrhythmias and hypotension
Electroencephalogram (EEG)	Evaluate the brain's electrical activity for ongoing seizures even if there are no clinical signs of seizures	Epileptiform discharges and seizure activity
Computed tomography (CT) brain scan	Evaluate for any brain abnormalities responsible for the SE	Abnormal scan with infarct, hemorrhage, tumor, or arteriovenous malformation
Pregnancy test	Evaluate for potential fetal concerns	
Magnetic resonance imaging (MRI) brain	Evaluate for any brain abnormalities responsible for the SE	Abnormal lesion like stroke, infection, tumor
Lumbar puncture	Assess for infection	Infection may be a precipitant for SE
Intracranial pressure monitor	Assess, measure, control intracranial pressure	Elevated intracranial pressure may be a precipitant for SE

Source: Modified from Baird M, Elsevier SB. *Manual of Critical Care Nursing.* 6th ed. St. Louis, MO: Mosby; 2011.

In children, SE is most commonly seen with prolonged febrile seizures. Children may have unique toxic exposure (ingestion).

Laboratory

- Fingerstick glucose
- CBC/ESR
- Basic metabolic panel
- Calcium (total and ionized)
- Magnesium
- Drug and toxicology screen—urine and blood
- AED levels
- Pregnancy test
- Arterial blood gas

Based on patient history, consideration may also be given to ordering a comprehensive toxicology panel for medications that frequently cause seizures (isoniazid, tricyclic antidepressants, theophylline, cocaine, sympathomimetics, alcohol, organophosphates, and cyclosporine).

Other laboratory tests may be ordered (liver function tests, serial troponins, type and hold, and coagulation studies [prothrombin time, partial thromboplastin time]), and an evaluation for inborn errors of metabolism may be conducted.

Electrophysiologic

Video/continuous EEG may be used to evaluate for nonconvulsive seizures if the patient is not waking up after convulsive events stop.

Radiologic

Scans may be normal and are not first priority in the treatment of SE; they are to evaluate potential causes for SE.

Computed tomography (CT)—Contrast-enhanced head CT scan to evaluate acute intracranial structural abnormalities (infarct, hemorrhage, tumor, or arteriovenous malformation)

Magnetic resonance imaging (MRI)—Gadolinium-enhanced MRI brain scan (stroke, infection, or tumor)

Review of relevant interventional procedures and surgeries

The management of SE involves swift intervention with clinician assessment, maintenance of patient safety, and minimization of sequelae. Treating the cause, if possible, will prevent recurrence as well as maximize patient outcome. Simultaneous assessment and management are crucial to emergently stop both clinical and electrographic seizure activity. Core vital sign evaluation with airway, breathing, and circulation is ongoing and interventions made as appropriate. Medication management is the first line of treatment.

- Airway
  - Position head to prevent aspiration
  - Suction prn
  - Consider bag valve mask/intubation
- Breathing
  - Ensure sufficient oxygenation
  - Consider nasal cannula, face mask, or ventilator support
- Circulation
  - Provide IV fluid (normal saline) and bolus prn
  - Provide IV access to give medication, nutrient resuscitation (reverse thiamine deficiency or treat hypoglycemia)
  - Consider all means of resuscitation including pressors if systolic blood pressure (SBP <90) or mean arterial pressure (MAP <70) low

Urinary catheter may also be placed to help evaluate systemic circulation.

Medication management is the key to treating SE, see the medication list in Table 66.2.

First-line medication:

- Lorazepam IV   0.15 mg/kg IV (can also be IM, PR, buccal, nasal)
- Midazolam IM   0.2 mg/kg IM (also available nasal/buccal)

or

- Diazepam Rectal 0.2 mg/kg PR adult

Table 66.2 Intermittent Drug Dosing in SE

Drug	Initial dose	Administrative rate and alternative dosing recommendations	Serious adverse effects	Considerations
Diazepam	0.15 mg/kg IV up to 10 mg per dose, may repeat in 5 minutes	Up to 5 mg/min (IVP)	Hypotension Respiratory depression	Rapid redistribution (short duration), active metabolite, IV contains propylene glycol
Lorazepam	0.1 mg/kg IV up to 3 mg per dose, may repeat in 5–10 min	Up to 2 mg/min (IVP)	Hypotension Respiratory depression	Dilute 1:1 with saline IV contains propylene glycol
Midazolam	0.2 mg/kg IM up to maximum of 10 mg	Peds: 10 mg IM (>40 kg); 0.2 mg/kg (intranasal)0.5 mg/kg (buccal)	Respiratory depression Hypotension	Active metabolite; renal elimination, rapid redistribution (short duration)
Fosphenytoin	20 mg PE/kg IV, may give additional 5 mg/kg	Up to 150 mg PE/min; may give additional dose 10 min after loading infusion Pediatrics: up to 3 mg/kg/min	Hypotension Arrhythmias	Compatible in saline, dextrose and lactated Ringer solution
Lacosamide	200–400 mg IV	200 mgIV over 15 minutes No pediatrics dosing established	PR prolongation Hypotension	Minimal drug interactions Limited experience in treatment of SE
Levetiracetam	1000–3000 mg IV Pediatrics: 20–60 mg/kg IV	2–5 mg/kg/min IV		Minimal drug interactions Not hepatically metabolized
Phenobarbital	20 mg/kg IV may give additional 5–10 mg/kg	Up to 50 mg/min IV; may give additional dose 10 min after loading infusion Pediatrics: up to 1 mg/kg/min	Hypotension Respiratory depression	IV contains propylene glycol
Phenytoin	20 mg/kg IV, may give an additional 5–10 mg/kg	Up to 50 mg/min IV; may give additional dose 10 min after loading infusion	Arrhythmias Hypotension Purple glove syndrome	Only compatible in saline IV contains propylene glycol
Topiramate	200–400 mg NG/PO	300–1600 mg/day PO divided 2–4 times daily No pediatric dosing established	Metabolic acidosis	No IV formulation available
Valproate sodium	20–40 mg/kg IV, may give an additional 20 mg/kg	3–6 mg/kg/in, may give additional dose 10 min after loading infusion Pediatrics: 1.5–3 mg/kg/min	Hyperammonemia Pancreatitis Thrombo cytopenia Hepatotoxicity	Use with caution in patients with traumatic head injury; may be a preferred agent in patients with glioblastoma multiforme

Source: Brophy GM et al., *Neurocrit Care,* 17, 3–23, 2012.

Table 66.3 RSE Dosing Recommendations

Drug	Initial dose	Continuous infusion dosing recommendations—titrated to electroencephalogram (EEG)	Serious adverse effects	Considerations
Midazolam	0.2 mg/kg; administer at an infusion rate of 2 mg/min	0.05 mg/kg/hr CI Breakthrough SE: 0.1–0.2 mg/g bolus, increase CI rate by 0.05 mg–0.1 mg/kg/hr every 3–4 hours	Respiratory depression Hypotension	Tachyphylaxis occurs after prolonged use Active metabolite, renally eliminated, rapid redistribution (short duration), does not contain propylene glycol
Pentobarbital	5–15 mg/kg, may give additional 5–10 mg/kg; administer at an infusion rate <50 mg/min	0.5–5 mg/kg/h CI Breakthrough SE: 5 mg/kg bolus, increase CI rate by 0.5–1 mg/kg/h every 12 hours	Hypotension Respiratory depression Cardiac depression Paralytic ileusAt high doses, complete loss of neurologic function	Requires mechanical ventilation IV contains propylene glycol
Propofol	Start at 20 mcg/kg/min, with 1–2 mg/kg loading dose		Hypotension (especially with loading dose in critically ill patients) Respiratory depressionCardiac failure Rhabdomyolysis Metabolic acidosisRenal failure (PRIS)	Requires mechanical ventilation Must adjust daily caloric intake (1.1 kcal/mL)
Thiopental	2–7 mg/kg, administer at an infusion rate <50 mg/min	0.5–5 mg/kg/h CI Breakthrough SE: 1–2 mg/kg bolus, increase CI rate by 0.5–1 mg/kg/h every 12 hours	Hypotension Respiratory depression Cardiac depression	Requires mechanical ventilation Metabolized to pentobarbital

Source: Brophy GM et al. *Neurocrit Care,* 17, 3–23, 2012.
Note: CI, continuous infusion; EEG, electroencephalogram; h, hour; IM, intramuscular; IV, intravenous; IVP, intravenous push, min; PRIS, propofol-related infusion syndrome.

Second-line medication:

- Fosphenytoin IV   20 mg PE/kg IV
- Valproate sodium   20–40 mg/kg IV
- Levetiracetam   1000–3000 mg IV

Refractory SE agents (Table 66.3):

- Midazolam   0.2 mg/kg bolus with IVF 0.1–0.04 mg/kg/hr
- Propofol   3–5 mg/kg bolus with IVF 5–10 mg/kg/hr
- Pentobarbital   2–3 mg/kg bolus with IVF 3–5 mg/kg/hr
- Ketamine   0.5 mg–4.5 mg/kg bolus with IVF 3–5 mg/kg/hr
- Thiopental

The initial AED administration is a benzodiazepine. When IV access is available, it is the preferred route and lorazepam is the preferred medication. However, medication can also be administered via intramuscular (IM), rectal, buccal, or nasal routes when IV access is not available. When giving IM, midazolam is preferred and is also available nasal or buccal. For rectal administration, diazepam is preferred.

If SE continues after adequate dosing, a second AED is introduced usually within 5–10 minutes. The second line of defense for medication management for SE with AE medication may include IV fosphenytoin/phenytoin, valproate sodium, levetiracetam, or continuous infusion of midazolam. The current preferred IV AED is fosphenytoin unless the patient has a history of primary generalized epilepsy, then valproate sodium is the drug of choice.

Despite these interventions, seizures may be refractory to medications. At this point, the initial intervention with the benzodiazepine may be repeated and a continuous infusion of AED is started or more frequent boluses of AED may be used. If seizures continue, a third medication may be considered.

- Therapeutic coma may be considered.
- Continuous infusion of midazolam, propofol, pentobarbital, or ketamine.
- Increased risks of complications including infection, prolonged hospitalization, and higher mortality (Marchi et al., 2015).

Note the use of ketamine is controversial. It has been shown to be effective in animal models but little clinical data are available (Brophy et al., 2012; Hocker et al., 2013; Manno, 2011).

Once the seizures stop and the patient is electrographically back to normal,

- Monitoring usually continues for 24–48 hours.
- Continuous infusion AED is titrated off.
- Upon withdrawal of the infusion, SE may recur, thus necessitating the return of the infusion or addition of another agent (Hocker et al., 2013).

Lumbar puncture may be performed as appropriate based on clinical presentation/history (to rule out meningitis and encephalitis).

Surgical decompression of hemorrhage/tumor/mass or repair of area traumatically injured may be necessary.

Common grading schemes

There are three types of SE: convulsive SE, nonconvulsive SE, and medically refractory SE:

Convulsive SE is the prototypical generalized convulsive seizure event with full-body rhythmical jerking that lasts for longer than 5 minutes. Patients may also experience recurrent seizure activity without recovery between events and thus be considered to be in status.

Nonconvulsive SE is sustained seizure activity seen on an EEG without the prototypical physical manifestations. These patients have mental status impairment with other physical findings such as agitation, automatisms, delirium, and/or eye deviation.

Medically refractory SE refers to those patients who continue to have clinical or electrographic SE after the initiation of two or more AEDs (Hocker et al., 2013).

Family counseling

- Supportive care for the patient and family is an ongoing intervention.
- Patient and family education regarding medication management and AED use is crucial. Consider creating a regular dosing schedule and list of potential medication interactions to help educate and reinforce regimen.

Prognosis

- Potential permanent neuronal injury with prolonged seizures
- Potential respiratory, cardiovascular, hematologic, renal, infectious, gastrointestinal, musculoskeletal, and epidermal complications (Hocker et al., 2013)
- 30-day mortality for patients with SE between 19% and 27% (Mazurkiewicz-Beldzinska et al., 2014)
- With refractory SE, 50% mortality (Malviainen, Eriksson, and Parviainen, 2005; Hocker et al., 2013)

Common questions

- *If I have SE will I have epilepsy?* Epilepsy can develop in 30% of the patients who have a single episode of SE (Manno, 2011).
- *Can I have children after having SE?* Patients should be provided with education regarding new medications and potential teratogenicity and risks with pregnancy and AED use.

Common pitfalls and medicolegal concerns

- Caution if patient has been given paralytics (i.e., intubation), as the muscle paralysis may stop but electrical brain seizure may continue (Greenberg, 2010).
- Seizures involve mandatory Department of Motor Vehicle (DMV) reporting. For patient and public safety, patients should not be allowed to drive and need to be monitored and stabilized on medications after having a seizure.
- Maximize each medication in the regimen to therapeutic dosing before going on to a second medication.
- Provide clear documentation of symptoms, assessment, and interventions.
- Ensure patient safety for adverse medication affects such as sedation, hypotension, arrhythmias, and/or potential allergic reactions and treat based on the patient.
- Consider pregnancy test as appropriate to ensure maternal/fetal safety.
- Serum AED levels may decrease with pregnancy.

Relevance to the advanced practice health professional

- The incidence of seizures may be high during the first postoperative week following some intracranial procedures; thus the advance practice professional should consider preoperative loading does of antiepileptic medication and maintenance medication as needed. Prophylactic treatment is often discontinued 6 months after surgery if seizures do not occur.
- Counsel patients and family regarding medication titration and the risk of seizures with medication adjustments. Some patients may elect to continue the AED as the sequelae of seizures could affect employment as well as driving.
- Approximately 30%–50% of patients with a brain tumor present with a seizure. There is an inverse relationship between the grade of malignancy of a glioma and a risk of seizure. In the patients with SE, 7% are caused by a brain tumor (Arik et al., 2014).
- Communication with the patient's primary care provider is imperative to facilitate ongoing patient care after an acute event is over and to prevent recurrence if there is a known cause.

Common phone calls, pages, and requests

How do you treat a patient already on AED with SE? For patients who have been on an AED and are in SE, prior to adding a second agent, give an IV bolus of that AED or half the loading dose, if available. Then titrate the AED to supratherapeutic levels once the AED levels are available to ensure proper dosing (Manno, 2011). These patients should be evaluated for any changes in their history, PE, and or medication patterns. Often their usual AED is subtherapeutic and thus benefits from bolus dosing.

References

Arik Y, Leijten FSS, Seute T, Robe PA, Snijders TJ. Prognosis and therapy of tumor-relatede vers non-tumor-related status epilepticus: a systemic review and meta analysis. *BMC Neurol.* 2014;14:152.

Baehr M, Frotscher M. *Duus' Topical Diagnosis in Neurology.* 5th ed. Stuttgart, New York: Theime; 2012.

Baird M, Elsevier SB. *Manual of Critical Care Nursing.* 6th ed. St Louis, Missouri: Mosby; 2011.

Bleck TP. Management approaches to prolonged seizures and status epilepticus. *Epilepsia.* 1999;40(suppl 1):S59–63.

Brophy GM, Bell R, Classen J et al. Guidelines for the evaluation and management of status epilepticus. *Neurocrit Care.* 2012;17:3–23.

Fujikawa DG. Neuroprotective effect of Ketamine administered after status epilepticus onset. *Epilepsia.* 1995; 36(2):186–195.

Gaspard N, Foreman B, Judd LM et al. Intravenous ketamine for the treatment of refractory status epilepticus: a restrospective multi-center study. *Epilepsia.* 2013;54(8):1498–1503.

Greenberg M. *Handbook of Neurosurgery.* 7th ed. New York, NY: Theime; 2010.

Hocker S, Wijdicks EFM, Rabinstein AA. Refractory status epilepticus: new insights in presentation, treatment and outcome. *Neurol Res.* 2013;35(2):163–168.

Kalviainen R, Eriksson K, Parviainen I. Refractory generalized convulsive status epilepticus: a guide to treatment. *CNS Drugs.* 2005;19(9):759–768.

Kilpatrick C. Epilepsy and its neurosurgical aspects. In: Kaye AH, ed. *Essential Neurosurgery.* 3rd ed. Hoboken, NJ: Blackwell Publishing; 2005: chap 21.

Marchi NA, Novy J, Faouzi M, Stahli C, Burnand B, Rossetti AO. Status epilepticus: impact of therapeutic coma on outcome. *Crit Care Med.* 2015;43(5):1003–1009.

Manno EM. Status epilepticus current treatment strategies. *Neurohospitalist.* 2011;1(1):23–31.

Mazurkiewicz-Beldzinska M, Szmuda M, Zawadzka M, Matheisel A. Current treatment of convulsize status epilepticus-a therapeutic protocol and review. *Anaesthesiol Intensive Ther.* 2014;46(4):293–300.

Silbergleit R, Lowenstein D, Durkalski V, Conwit R, Neurological Emergency Treatment Trials Investigators. RAMPART (Rapid anticonvulsant medication prior to arrival trial): a double-blind randomized clinical trial of the efficacy of intramuscular midazolam versus intravenous lorazepam in the prehospital treatment of status epilepticus by paramedics. *Epilepsia.* 52(suppl 8):45–47.

Synowiec AS, Singh DS, Yenugadhati V, Valeriano JP, Schramke CJ, Kelly KM. Ketamine use in the treatment of refractory status epilepticus. *Epilepsy Res.* 2013;105(1–2):183–188.

Treiman DM, Meyers PD, Walton NY et al. A comparison of four treatments for generalized convulsive status epilepticus. Veterans affairs status epilepticus cooperative study group. *N Engl J Med.* 1998;339(12):792–798.

67

DEMYELINATING SYNDROME
Multiple Sclerosis

Jeffrey Hernandez, Leticia Tornes, and Janice Y. Maldonado

Multiple sclerosis

Ms. D is a 36-year-old left-handed Caucasian woman born and raised in Michigan until age 30, when she moved to Miami, Florida. She was diagnosed in 2005 with a pituitary microadenoma (prolactin). Since diagnosis, annual magnetic resonance imaging (MRI) of her brain remained unchanged. However, in 2007 a demyelinating lesion perpendicular to the ventricle was seen that was typical of multiple sclerosis (MS). In hindsight, she could have been diagnosed with radiologically isolated syndrome (RIS) at that time. She was asymptomatic and was evaluated by a neurologist who repeated an MRI that showed "resolution" of the lesions. She was told not to worry about this and did not follow up.

In late fall of 2011, she had acute onset of paresthesias in the torso, below her breast, and of bilateral hands and feet. She reports the sensation began acutely without migration of symptoms. She then traveled home (Michigan) for the holidays and after about 10 days her symptoms resolved, except for hand paresthesias. She denied any new symptoms.

When she returned home, she was seen by another neurologist who ordered MRIs of the brain and cervical and thoracic spinal cord. She then presented to our office for evaluation. At the time she reported residual paresthesias with "stiffness" in her fingertips. She denied any current or previous fatigue, visual, bladder, bowel, memory, or gait abnormalities.

On physical exam she had a Hoffmann on the right and decreased vibration on the right toe, otherwise her exam was unremarkable. MRIs of the brain and cervical spine were reviewed (Figures 67.1 through 67.4). MRI of the brain revealed periventricular lesions (Dawson fingers), subcortical and juxtacortical lesions. The cervical cord revealed a dorsal lesion at C2.

At that point the patient was diagnosed with a resolving transverse myelitis and in conjunction with the brain MRI findings with clinically isolated syndrome (CIS). Acute therapy with steroids was not given as the patient was almost at baseline. Labs for other potential causes of central nervous system (CNS) demyelination were obtained that were all normal (Table 67.1). At that time she was started on a disease-modifying treatment with glatiramer acetate.

Ms. D did well; she was seen every 6 months in the clinic and had yearly MRIs without clinical or radiologic progression. However, in early 2015 she presented with pain with eye movement and blurred central vision. She was found to have optic disc swelling consistent with an acute optic neuritis. At this point she met criteria for Clinically Definite MS (CDMS) per the 2010 Revised McDonald Criteria, as there was a second attack disseminated in both space and time. She was given steroids for the acute exacerbation and transitioned to fingolimod for immunomodulation.

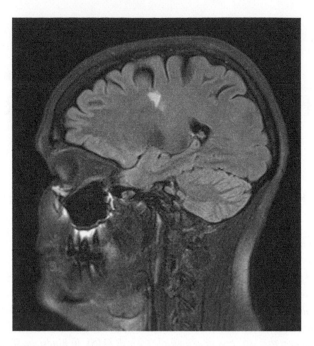

Figure 67.1 Brain MRI sagittal fluid–attenuated inversion recovery (FLAIR): Periventricular ovoid lesion (Dawson finger-like).

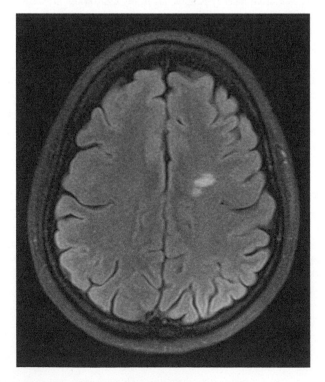

Figure 67.2 Brain MRI axial FLAIR: Periventricular ovoid lesion.

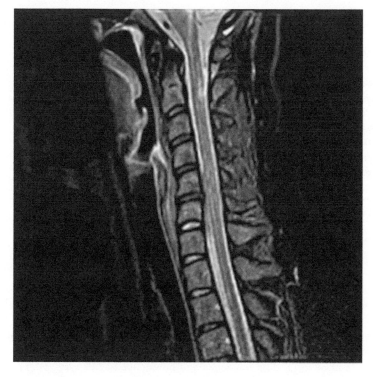

Figure 67.3   Cervical spine MRI sagittal T2: Dorsal lesion at C2 level.

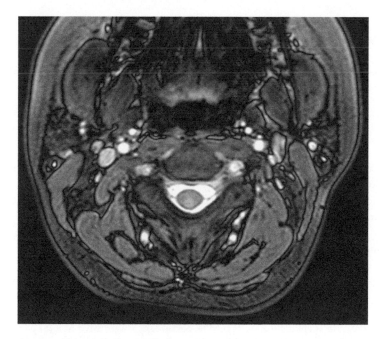

Figure 67.4   Cervical spine MRI axial T2: Dorsal lesion at C2 level.

Table 67.1 EDSS Table

0	Normal
1	No disability, minimal signs
2	Minimal disability in one area
3	Moderate disability in one area
4	Fully ambulatory without aid and severe disability in one area
5	Ambulatory without aid or rest for about 200 meters, disability severe enough to impair full daily activities
6	Unilateral assistance (cane or crutch)
7	Unable to walk more than 5 meters even with aid, wheelchair most of day, transfers alone
8	Essentially restricted to bed or chair, retains many self-care functions
9	Helpless bed patient; can communicate and eat
10	Death due to MS

Source: Kurtzke JF. *Neurology.* 1983, 33(11), 1444–1452.

Overview of multiple sclerosis

Epidemiology

MS is an autoimmune, inflammatory, demyelinating, and degenerative disorder of the CNS and one of the most common causes of disability in young adults. It is estimated that there are about 2.5 million people living with MS worldwide, with the onset typically occurring between the ages of 20 and 40 with a mean age of 30 (Milo and Kahana, 2010). The disease is at least four times more common in women than in men (Harbo, Gold, and Tintore, 2013). The incidence and prevalence of MS vary geographically, with higher frequency in Western Europe and North America (Koch-Henriksen and Sorensen, 2010).

Etiology and pathophysiology

MS was initially described as a disease of white matter, but we now know that it is characterized by inflammation, demyelination of white and gray matter, as well as axonal injury (Trapp et al., 1998). The etiology of MS is unknown but is likely the result of multiple factors including genetic and environmental (vitamin D, smoking, Epstein-Barr virus [EPV]) that trigger an immune response and leads to CNS injury (Wingerchuk, 2011).

Diagnosis

To establish a diagnosis of MS, lesions in the CNS must be separated both in time and space. The 2010 Revised McDonald Criteria include a simplified iteration of MRI requirements to establish the diagnosis of MS or CIS, allowing identification of MS with high probability at its first clinical manifestation (Polman et al., 2011). Lesions in MS will most commonly be in the periventricular white matter, brainstem, cerebellum, and spinal cord with highly specific lesions found in the corpus callosum and ovoid lesions perpendicular to the ventricles, named Dawson fingers (Figure 67.1). Importantly, the diagnosis of MS rests on ruling out other disorders that may have similar clinical presentations.

Clinical course

The clinical course of the disease varies greatly and is completely unpredictable. There are four defined MS disease courses: Relapsing Remitting MS (RRMS), Secondary Progressive MS (SPMS), Primary Progressive MS (PPMS), and Progressive Relapsing MS (PRMS) (Table 67.2).

Table 67.2 MS Disease Courses

Course	Percent at presentation	Characteristics and definitions
Relapsing remitting	85%	Relapse with recovery or recovery with some residual deficits, periods between "attacks," no progression (most common course)
Secondary progressive		Follows RRMS course, continuous progression (in about 50% of RRMS patients)
Primary progressive	10%–15%	Progression from onset, occasionally plateaus
Progressive-relapsing		Progressive from onset with superimposed relapses (most rare course)

Source: Compston A. et al., *McAlpine's Multiple Sclerosis*. 4th ed. London, Elsevier, 2006.

Two other disease courses have been described that were both present in our clinical case. These are disease courses seen prior to the diagnosis of CDMS.

- *Clinically Isolated Syndrome (CIS)*: CIS is the first clinical presentation of RRMS and usually presents as a syndrome: unilateral optic neuritis, transverse myelitis, or a brainstem attack (Miller et al., 2005). Patients with CIS and an abnormal brain MRI are likely to develop clinically definite MS (CDMS) (Fisniku et al., 2008).
- *Radiologically Isolated Syndrome (RIS)*: May be considered a presymptomatic phase of MS, usually an incidental image finding highly suggestive of an inflammatory demyelinating disease, in the absence of clinical signs and symptoms of MS. Patients should be closely monitored (Lublin et al., 2014).

Common signs and symptoms in MS

- *Central*: Fatigue, short-term memory loss, poor attention, word-finding difficulties, slow information processing, depression, Uhthoff phenomenon
- *Visual*: Optic neuritis, pale optic disc, poor visual acuity, blurred vision, visual field cut, scotoma
- *Cranial nerves*: Diplopia, internuclear ophthalmoplegia (INO), nystagmus, facial numbness, facial palsy, hearing loss, decreased palate elevation, dysarthria, dysphagia
- *Pyramidal dysfunction*: Hemiparesis, spasticity, hyperreflexia, Babinski sign, clonus, spasms, foot drop, spastic gait
- *Cerebellar*: Endpoint dysmetria, ataxia
- *Sensory*: Numbness/tingling (paresthesia), decreased sensation (hypoesthesia), neuropathic pain, "MS hug," loss of vibration, loss of position sense, Lhermitte phenomenon (cervical sensory changes, e.g., electric-like sensation down the upper back)
- Gastrointestinal (GI)/genitourinary (GU): Urinary urgency, frequency, retention, incontinence; constipation, bowel incontinence, sexual dysfunction

Diagnostic tests used in the evaluation of MS

Common serology that is sent during diagnostic testing for an MS patient includes: vitamin B_{12}, Sjogren panel, lupus panel, angiotensin-converting enzyme (ACE) level, thyroid studies, and other depending on individual case. If sending cerebrospinal fluid (CSF), both CSF and serum oligoclonal bands are sent to compare the two.

Common grading schemes

The Kurtzke Extended Disability Status Scale (EDSS) is used universally in assessing the MS patient's impairment and disability (Kurtzke, 1983).

Treatment

The pharmacologic treatment of MS is threefold and involves treatment of acute attacks, disease-modifying drugs, and symptomatic therapies. MS exacerbations will typically abate spontaneously without intervention; nonetheless, one can abbreviate the more severe MS flares with intravenous steroids, high-dose oral steroids, or adrenocorticotrophic hormone (ACTH). In cases when the attack is severe and refractory to steroid and/or ACTH therapy, plasma exchange statistically improved outcomes when compared to placebo (42.1% versus 5.9%) (Weinshenker et al., 1999).

In the last two decades, a number of drugs have been approved for the management of MS (Table 67.3). The injectable medications have a long-term safety profile and have been studied in CIS and found to delay both a second attack and MRI lesion activity (Coyle, 2008).

In addition to the injectable therapies, there are three oral medications and three infusions that are approved by the U.S. Food and Drug Administration (FDA) in the treatment of MS.

Natalizumab (Tysabri) is a monoclonal antibody infusion with a 67% reduction in relapse rates over 2 years compared to placebo (Polman et al., 2006). It is associated with the development of progressive multifocal leukoencephalopathy (PML), and the patient must be counseled on this risk.

Table 67.3 FDA-Approved Immunomodulating Medications for MS

Generic name	Brand name	Route and frequency	Adverse effects
Interferon beta–1a	Avonex Rebif	30 mcg intramuscularly (IM) weekly 44 mcg subcutaneously (SQ) three times weekly	Flu-like symptoms, injection site reactions (SQ injections)
Interferon beta–1b	Betaseron Extavia	0.25 mg SQ every other day	
Glatiramer acetate	Copaxone	20 mg SQ daily 40 mg SQ three times weekly	Idiosyncratic chest pain, injection site reaction
Natalizumab	Tysabri	Infusions: 300 mg intravenously (IV) every 28 days	Progressive multifocal leukoencephalopathy (PML)
Fingolimod	Gilenya	0.5 mg oral once daily	Bradycardia, atrioventricular (AV) block, macular edema, reductions in lymphocyte counts
Teriflunomide	Aubagio	7 mg oral once daily 14 mg oral once daily	Hair loss, black box: hepatotoxicity and teratogenesis, must chelate prior to pregnancy
Dimethyl fumarate	Tecfidera	240 mg oral twice daily	Nausea, abdominal pain, diarrhea, flushing
Peginterferon beta–1a	Plegridy	125 mcg SQ every 2 weeks	Flu-like symptoms, injection site reactions
Alemtuzumab	Lemtrada	Infusions: 12 mg for 5 days year one then 12 mg for 3 days year 2	Autoimmunity reactions, infusion reactions, and malignancies
Ocrelizumab	Ocrevus	Infusion: 300 mg IV on day 1 and day 15, then 600 mg IV every 6 months	Infusion reactions, upper and lower respiratory tract infections, and skin infections

Alemtuzumab (Lemtrada) is a CD-52 directed cytolytic antibody infusion with risk for autoimmune reactions, infusion reactions, and malignancy. More than 85% of patients remained free of MRI lesion activity 3 years later (Cohen et al., 2012). Ocrelizumab (Ocrevus) is a monoclonal antibody that depletes CD-20+ B cells approved for RRMS and PPMS. This is the first medication that has been FDA approved for the treatment of progressive MS, showing reduction in disability progression by 25% at 24 weeks when compared to placebo (Montalban et al., 2016, p. 212–216). In the RRMS clinical trials, ocrelizumab reduced relapse rates by 46% over 2 years when compared to the active comparator (Rebif 44 mcg TIW), and reduced disability progression by 40% at 24 weeks (Hauser et al. 2016, p. 224–228).

Patient and family counseling

Prognosis

The life span of a patient with MS is slightly less than the general population (Cook, 2012). In general, those with late onset of disease and those with a progressive course have a shorter survival (Ragonese et al., 2008). MS is the main cause of death in about 50% of patients. Results of disease-modifying treatments have shown a significant reduction of mortality among treated patients (Cook, 2012). Rapidly progressive and aggressive MS, severe complications from infections, and severe untreated depression can also lead to early death in MS patients. Males and those with late disease onset tend to progress more rapidly.

Common questions

Q: For how long will I need to use this medication?

A: MS is a chronic disease with no cure. We use medications as long as they are showing benefit in the hope of stabilizing the disease, slowing the progression, and preventing relapses.

Q: Should I continue to work?

A: Yes. Many patients do not develop significant disability and are gainfully employed. Some employment challenges may be resolved with work accommodations.

Q: What can make my MS worse?

A: At times MS symptoms may worsen due to excessive heat exposure, physical or emotional stress, dehydration, sleep deprivation, and any infection, especially if associated with fever.

Q: What should I do differently?

A. Limit time spent exposed to heat. Stay well hydrated, get adequate sleep, diet, and exercise. Have prompt evaluation and treatment of potential infections.

Q: Can I get pregnant? Can I breastfeed?

A: MS does not affect pregnancy, childbirth, or breast-feeding, in fact, the hormones of pregnancy may offer some protection. However, there is a higher risk of relapse for the 6 months postpartum (Vukusic et al., 2004).

Q: Will my child have MS?

A: Genetic factors play a role in susceptibility to MS and in disease progression. The child of a person with MS has an approximately 3%–5% risk of having the condition, compared to 0.2% in the general population (Sadovnick, Dircks, and Ebers, 1999).

Q: How can I combat my fatigue?

A: Address other *potential* causes for fatigue including poor sleep, sleep apnea, and depression. Next perform exercise in a cool area (pool is optimal). If fatigue continues the provider may be able to prescribe medication.

Common pitfalls and medicolegal concerns

- **It is not safe to get vaccinated if you have MS.**

    Vaccinations for the flu, hepatitis B, tetanus, measles, and rubella are usually safe, live virus vaccines are not. Always consult the treating physician before vaccination.
- **I don't want to know about MS, most patients end up in a wheelchair.**

    More than two-thirds of patients with MS do not ever need a wheelchair on a full-time basis. Although the course of MS is unpredictable, it is imperative that patients take the time to learn about the disease and how it can change over time in order to plan for the future.

Common phone calls, pages, and requests with answers

- **How to distinguish between a relapse and a pseudo-exacerbation.**

    A MS relapse is a new neurologic symptom lasting greater than 24 hours or a previously stable symptom, progressively worsening over 48 hours. A pseudo-exacerbation is a neurologic symptom that reappears or worsens in severity in the setting of an infection, physical/emotional stress, sleep deprivation, excessive heat exposure, or recent overexertion. One of the most commonly associated triggers for pseudo-exacerbations is a urinary tract infection.
- What resources are available for MS patients?

    The National MS Society—http://www.nmss.org

    The Multiple Sclerosis Foundation—https://www.msfocus.org

    The Multiple Sclerosis Association of America—https://mymsaa.org

Relevance to the advanced practice health professional

MS requires a multidisciplinary approach to promote positive patient outcomes. It is important to provide counseling and education during each encounter with the patient whether in the office or over the phone. This helps the patient and their family better cope with the diagnosis, symptoms, and possible adjustment to new roles in the household, and prepare to identify strategies to mitigate potential side effects. Education also is important in establishing reasonable expectations.

The advanced practice health professional may often perform many roles (e.g., social worker, case manager, etc.) and coordinate care with the multidisciplinary team on behalf of the MS patient and his or her family. They will also collaborate with the provider in evaluating the physical and psychosocial needs of the patient to make appropriate recommendations and interventions to improve and maintain the best possible quality of life.

References

Cohen J A, Coles AJ, Arnold DL et al. Alemtuzumab versus Interferon Beta 1a as first-line treatment for patients with relapsing-remitting multiple sclerosis: a randomised controlled phase 3 trial. *Lancet.* 2012;380(9856):1819–1828.

Compston A, Confavreux C, Lassmann H et al. *McAlpine's Multiple Sclerosis.* 4th ed. Elsevier London, UK: 2006.

Cook S. Life expectancy in multiple sclerosis: implications for clinicians. *Int J MS Care.* 2012;14(4):3–4.

Coyle PK. Early treatment of multiple sclerosis to prevent neurologic damage. *Neurology.* 2008;71(24 suppl 3):S3–S7.

Fisniku L K, Brex PA, Altmann DR et al. Disability and T2 MRI lesions: a 20-year follow-up of patients with relapse onset of multiple sclerosis. *Brain.* 2008;131(pt 3):808–817.

Hauser SL, Bar-Or A, Comi G et al. Ocrelizumab versus Interferon Beta-1a in relapsing multiple sclerosis. *N Engl J Med.* 2016;376:221–234.

Harbo HF, Gold R, Tintore M. Sex and gender issues in multiple sclerosis. *Ther Adv Neurol Disord.* 2013;6:237–248.

Kappos L, Radue EW, O'Connor P et al. A placebo-controlled trial of oral fingolimod in relapsing multiple sclerosis. *N Engl J Med.* 2010;362(5):387–401.

Koch-Henriksen N, Sorensen PS. The changing demographic pattern of multiple sclerosis epidemiology. *Lancet Neurol.* 2010;9(5):520–532.

Kurtzke JF. Rating neurologic impairment in multiple sclerosis: an expanded disability status scale (EDSS). *Neurology.* 1983;33(11):1444–1452.

Lublin FD, Reingold SC, Cohen JA et al. Defining the clinical course of multiple sclerosis: the 2013 revisions. *Neurology.* 2014;83(3):278–286.

Miller D, Barkhof F, Montalban X, Thompson A, Filippi M. Clinically isolated syndromes suggestive of multiple sclerosis, Part I: natural history, pathogenesis, diagnosis, and prognosis. *Lancet Neurol.* 2005;4(5):281–288.

Milo R, Kahana E. Multiple sclerosis: geoepidemiology, genetics and the environment. *Autoimmun Rev.* 2010;9(5):A387–394.

Montalban X, Hauser SL, Kappos L et al. Ocrelizumab versus placebo in primary progressive multiple sclerosis. *N Engl J Med.* 2016;376:209–220.

Noseworthy JH, Lucchinetti C, Rodriguez M, Weinshenker BG. Multiple sclerosis. *N Engl J Med.* 2000;343(13):938–952.

Polman CH, O'Connor PW, Havrdova E et al. A randomized, placebo-controlled trial of natalizumab for relapsing multiple sclerosis. *N Engl J Med.* 2006;354(9):899–910.

Polman CH, Reingold SC, Banwell B et al. Diagnostic criteria for multiple sclerosis: 2010 revisions to the McDonald criteria. *Ann Neurol.* 2011;69(2):292–302.

Ragonese P, Aridon P, Salemi G, D'Amelio M, Savettieri G. Mortality in multiple sclerosis: a review. *Eur J Neurol.* 2008;15(2):123–127.

Sadovnick AD, Dircks A, Ebers GC. Genetic counselling in multiple sclerosis: risks to sibs and children of affected individuals. *Clin Genet.* 1999;56(2):118–122.

Trapp BD, Peterson J, Ransohoff RM et al. Axonal transection in the lesions of multiple sclerosis. *N Engl J Med.* 1998;338(5):278–285.

Vukusic S, Hutchinson M, Hours M et al. Pregnancy and multiple sclerosis (the PRIMS study): clinical predictors of post-partum relapse. *Brain.* 2004;127(pt 6):1353–1360.

Weinshenker BG, Issa M, Baskerville J. Long-term and short-term outcome of multiple sclerosis: a 3-year follow-up study. *Arch Neurol.* 1996;53(4):353–358.

Weinshenker BG, O'Brien PC, Petterson TM et al. A randomized trial of plasma exchange in acute central nervous system inflammatory demyelinating disease. *Ann Neurol.* 1999;46(6):878–886.

Wingerchuk DM. Environmental factors in multiple sclerosis: Epstein-Barr virus, vitamin D, and cigarette smoking. *Mt Sinai J Med.* 2011;78(2):221–230.

68

INTOXICANTS

Timur M. Urakov and Rachel Hart

Case vignette

A 25-year-old man was brought to the emergency room (ER) from a nightclub where a fight broke out and he was later found unresponsive. The patient's blood pressure was 122/79, his pulse was 105, and his respirations were 9 breaths per minute and shallow. His Glasgow Coma Scale score was 3. He had a laceration to the scalp with blood over his head and face. The patient's pupils were constricted and nonreactive. His skin was cool and cyanotic. Glucose level was 55. Multiple track marks were visible on his forearms.

The patient was intubated and taken to computed tomography (CT) scanner immediately. A CT of the brain revealed no intracranial pathology. The patient was given naloxone and soon started to move spontaneously and followed simple commands. Laboratory analysis confirmed the presence of opioids and benzodiazepines in his bloodstream. The patient was extubated and admitted for observation to the intensive care unit (ICU). Low-dose clonazepam was started to prevent seizures associated with benzodiazepine withdrawal. Vitamins B$_{12}$ and folic acid were also administered intravenously.

Overview

Drug abuse is underrecognized in most patient populations. Approximately 5% of the adult population in the world uses an illicit drug, and 1% of adults use prescription opioids (Sauer, 2015). Whether it is a prescription medicine or illegal street drug like cocaine or heroin, neurologic implications can be detrimental if not identified in a timely manner (Wurcel, 2015). Exacerbating matters, substance use is typically denied or underreported by the patient and family/friends. Patients may also present for a reason not related to drug abuse; however, their care may be compromised by confounding factors in their diagnosis and treatment due to drug effects such as withdrawal during a hospitalization (Johnson, 1999).

Drugs causing intoxications can in general be divided into three groups: depressants, stimulants, and hallucinogens. Symptoms of withdrawal are usually the opposite of the effects of intoxication, and withdrawal from a depressant may be more life threatening than from a stimulant (Lago and Kosten, 1994). Care providers should also be cautious of their own safety as drug abuse may be associated with transmittable diseases like HIV, hepatitis, or tuberculosis especially in injection drug users (Haverkos, 1991).

Depressants

This class of drugs includes opioids, barbiturates, benzodiazepines, and alcohol. They all reduce brain activity resulting in altered consciousness, drowsiness, and respiratory depression. Patients may also be unable to protect their airway due to altered mental status.

Opioids act through a mu receptor present in the central nervous system. Drugs like dilaudid, morphine, methadone, and heroin all belong to the opioid family. Common presentation of overdose includes "pinpoint pupils" and decreased respiratory drive due to reduced sympathetic activity. Seizures are also possible but are more common with withdrawal (Bates et al.,2004). In less severe cases, patients may complain of constipation. Overdose treatment includes naloxone as well as symptomatic support. Caution should be applied when using naloxone, as effects may be immediate and patients may arise highly agitated (Barker and Hunjadi, 2008).

Withdrawal from opioids may present with flu-like symptoms including fever, rhinorrhea, nausea, stomach cramps, and diarrhea. In more severe cases, patients may experience anxiety, insomnia, anorexia, sweating, dilated pupils, and piloerection. Treatment of withdrawal is with clonidine, an α2 agonist that decreases sympathetic output making autonomic symptoms less intense (Cheskin, 1994). Buprenorphine with naloxone can also be used; however, it can also precipitate withdrawal if given too soon due to partial mu receptor agonism (Fudala et al.,1990). Methadone is used in long-term treatment.

Barbiturates act by keeping the α-aminobutyric acid (GABA) channel in open state and include phenobarbital, sodium thiopental, and pentobarbital. Overdose presents with depression of respiratory and central nervous system (CNS) functions. There is no ceiling effect on the drug actions, making them lethal at high doses (Hadden et al.,1969). There is no antidote for barbiturate overdose, and treatment is supportive with the goals of blood pressure maintenance and adequate oxygenation.

Withdrawal from barbiturates presents with anxiety, seizure, delirium, and cardiovascular collapse. Treatment includes long-acting benzodiazepines or barbiturate with taper.

Benzodiazepines increase frequency of GABA channel opening and at high doses result in amnesia, somnolence, ataxia, and respiratory depression to a lesser extent than barbiturates. Flumazenil competitively binds to GABA receptors in antagonistic fashion and can be used in severe cases of benzodiazepine overdose (Mordel et al.,1992). However, its use is not recommended since it can precipitate seizures.

Benzodiazepine withdrawal also leads to anxiety, insomnia, as well as tremor and life-threatening seizures. Treatment is with a long-acting benzodiazepine, like clonazepam.

Stimulants

Stimulants include cocaine, amphetamine, 3,4 methylenedioxymethamphetamine (MDMA), caffeine, and nicotine. They act by either increasing the activity of "stimulating" hormones like dopamine, norepinephrine, and serotonin, or reducing the activity of "inhibiting" GABA effects. Overall the effects lead to overburdened cardiovascular system and psychotic behaviors. Restraining of patients is contraindicated due to the high chance of rhabdomyolysis (Questel 1995).

Cocaine blocks reuptake of dopamine, norepinephrine, and serotonin from the synaptic cleft, therefore prolonging their activity on the postsynaptic membrane. Patients under cocaine intoxication present with euphoria, psychomotor agitation, grandiosity, hallucinations (tactile type is formication), and paranoid ideation (Lukas and Renshaw, 1998). The sympathetic system is overstimulated, and as a result pupils dilate, appetite decreases, and heart rate with blood pressure rises. Systemic vasospasm may have end-organ effect causing myocardial infarction, stroke, or placental infarction. Chronic cocaine users may present with nasal septum perforation (Kiesselbach plexus vasospasm) (Businco et al., 2008). Treatment of cocaine overdose is symptomatic with antipsychotics, benzodiazepines, and antihypertensives. Vitamin C promotes excretion of the drug.

Cocaine withdrawal presents with hyperphagia, hypersomnolence, fatigue, malaise, depression, and suicidality. Treatment is symptomatic plus with bupropion, bromocriptine, and selective serotonin reuptake inhibitors (SSRIs) for depression (Castells et al., 2016).

Amphetamines stimulate the release of dopamine, norepinephrine, and serotonin and at high doses decrease reuptake, like cocaine. Intoxicated patients present similarly to cocaine intoxication with mental status changes and sympathetic activation including fever and cardiac arrhythmias (Jones and Simpson, 1999). Treatment is with antipsychotics, benzodiazepines, antihypertensives (propranolol), and vitamin C. Withdrawal may include anxiety, irritability, somnolence, nightmares, and violent behavior.

Ecstasy (MDMA), as the name implies, has similar actions to amphetamines with more effect on serotonin than dopamine, and chronic use causes damage to serotonergic neurons. Intoxication presents with hyperthermia and social closeness (Jones and Simpson, 1999). It is treated symptomatically. In withdrawal, mood changes and depression are present.

Caffeine decreases GABA activity and thus improves wakefulness. At high doses it may lead to restlessness, insomnia, diuresis, muscle twitching, and cardiac arrhythmias. In withdrawal, it may contribute to headache, lethargy, depression, and even weight gain. Symptomatic treatment only is provided. Providing caffeine may alleviate some of the symptoms (Sawynok, 1995).

Nicotine acts on its receptors in the central, peripheral, and autonomic nervous systems. Intoxication may present with restlessness, insomnia, anxiety, and cardiac arrhythmias. Withdrawal results in irritability, headaches, anxiety, craving, and also weight gain. Addiction treatment includes bupropion, which can also lower threshold for seizures (Jorenby et al., 1999). Varenicline, used with nicotine patches, has the highest success rate as an antismoking drug (Tonstad et al.,2006).

Hallucinogens

Phencyclidine (PCP, aka Angel Dust) is an N-methyl-D-aspartate (NMDA) receptor antagonist, similar to an anesthetic ketamine. Intoxicated patients present with aggressive, impulsive behavior, and may exhibit fear and homicidality. Delirium, seizures, psychomotor agitation, vertical and horizontal nystagmus, tachycardia, and ataxia are also common. Treatment is with antipsychotics (haloperidol) and benzodiazepines. The patient should be placed in a low-stimulus environment and restraints considered to prevent injury to self or others. PCP withdrawal presents with depression, anxiety, irritability, restlessness, anergia, and disturbances of thought and sleep (McCarron et al.,1981).

Lysergic acid diethylamide (LSD, aka "acid") acts on serotonin receptors and presents with visual hallucinations and synesthesias, marked anxiety or depression, panic attacks, delusions, and pupillary dilation. Treatment is with antipsychotics and benzodiazepines. There are no withdrawal symptoms, though some patients may experience flashbacks (Ungerleider and Frank, 1976).

Cannabis (marijuana) binds to cannabinoid receptors located throughout the brain and body. Intoxication leads to euphoria, anxiety, disinhibition, paranoid delusions, perception of slowed time, conjunctival injection, impaired judgment, social withdrawal, increased appetite, dry mouth, and hallucinations. Use may precipitate schizophrenic episodes in a susceptible population (Vadhan et al., 2013).

Withdrawal from marijuana presents with mild symptoms or irritability, depression, insomnia, nausea, and anorexia. Most symptoms peak in 48 hours and last for 5–7 days. In chronic use, individuals can experience severe emesis due to downregulation of CNS cannabinoid receptors and upregulation of gut cannabinoid receptors (Batke et al., 2010). Treatment is with antiemetics.

The inhalants group is composed of volatile solvents, gases, aerosols, and nitrites—chemicals found around the household. Intoxication presents with unspecific symptoms of belligerence, assaultiveness, apathy, impaired judgement, blurred vision, altered mental status, and coma (Young et al., 1999). Treatment is symptomatic. Long-term effects may include permanent damage to the nervous system.

Alcohol

Alcohol is the most commonly abused substance. Intoxication presentation may vary and include talkative, flirtatious, aggressive, moody, or disinhibited behaviors. Treatment is with intravenous fluids including thiamine, dextrose, magnesium, and multivitamins ("banana bag"). Chronic cases may present with confabulation (memory deficits in Wernicke-Korsakoff syndrome) related to nutritional deficiencies such as thiamine (Nishimoto et al., 2017).

Patients suffering from chronic alcoholism present with several specific physical findings. Palpation of the abdomen reveals hepatomegaly and splenomegaly. Chronic damage to the liver contributes to portal hypertension evidenced by ascites, jaundice, and spider angiomas. Liver damage also reduces clearance of the body's toxic substances, which affects the nervous system resulting in hepatic encephalopathy and asterixis. In late stages of liver cirrhosis, lab values for liver markers may be falsely normal (Rausch et al., 2016).

Withdrawal can progress in stages. Early signs include trembling, irritability, anxiety, headache, tachycardia, and insomnia, treated with the "banana bag." Chronic alcohol abusers can experience visual, auditory, and tactile hallucinations in 12–24 hours after last consumption. At 48 hours, patients in withdrawal can experience tonic-clonic seizures. After 48–96 hours, patients may still present with autonomic instability, disorientation, hallucinations, and agitation, treated with benzodiazepines (Mayo-Smith, 1997). Addiction is treated with disulfiram, which inhibits acetaldehyde dehydrogenase and works by aversive conditioning (Larson et al., 1992). Naltrexone and gabapentin are used to decrease desire (Krystal et al., 2001).

Medicolegal concerns

Intoxicated patients may not be competent enough to make reasonable decisions in terms of their medical care as well as pose a potential danger to self and others. Inattention to key legal concepts when caring for an agitated patient may lead to significant liability. First, a care provider must determine a patient's ability to give or refuse consent for treatment. Second, if restraints are applied, it is the care provider's responsibility to ensure the patient's health and safety. By default, no one should touch or hold a patient against his or her will except in the case of an emergency, in which case the proper paperwork has to be established (Thomas and Moore, 2013).

Common phone calls, pages, and requests with answers

Q: A 55-year-old woman status post lumbar laminectomy and fusion 2 days prior has been on an extensive pain regimen including patient-controlled analgesia (PCA) pump with Dilaudid, breakthrough IV Dilaudid, and oral Percocet. Currently she is unresponsive, saturating 94% oxygen on 2 L nasal cannula, and pupils are small and nonreactive.

A: Opioid overdose is likely. Administer Narcan 0.4 mg IV.

Q: A 40-year-old man who was admitted 2 days ago with a concussion after a bar fight just had a seizure.

A: In view of head trauma, first rule out intracranial hemorrhage with a CT. Once negative, consider alcohol dependence.

Q: A 32-year-old businesswoman who had a Chiari decompression 2 days ago is complaining of severe headache. She has tried multiple medications, and imaging ruled out surgical complications.

A: Inquire about coffee consumption in her daily routine.

Q: A 22-year-old man, cocaine addict, who was admitted 3 days ago through the ER in an extremely agitated state and required restraints is now complaining of severe muscle pain and weakness. His urine has also been dark brown lately.

A: Evaluate for rhabdomyolysis associated with a restraint. Consider hydration, and rule out compartment syndrome in extremities.

Alcohol use disorders

Alcohol use disorders (AUDs) are prevalent in the United States, with 16.6 million adults over the age of 18 being diagnosed as having an AUD in 2013, while only 1.3 million adults received treatment for such at a specialized facility (National Institute on Alcohol Abuse and Alcoholism, 2015a). Alcohol-related deaths are the third leading preventable cause of death in the United States, with nearly 88,000 people dying from alcohol-related causes every year (NIAAA, 2015a). In 2010, the economic costs of excessive alcohol consumption were estimated to be $249 billion (Centers for Disease Control and Prevention, 2016). The health conditions related to alcohol dependence include liver cirrhosis, cancers, cardiovascular disease, and injuries. It is estimated that in 2012, 5.1% of the burden of disease and injuries globally were attributable to alcohol consumption (NIAAA, 2015a). Worldwide, among people ages 15–49, the leading risk factor for premature death and disability is alcohol misuse (NIAAA, 2015a). The long-term effects of alcohol misuse are unavoidable within the critical care patient population and require conscientious management to avoid serious and potentially fatal outcomes.

Alcohol withdrawal, alcoholic hallucinosis, and delirium tremens

A diagnosis of "alcohol withdrawal" as defined by the *Diagnostic and Statistical Manual of Mental Disorders–5* (APA, 2013) must include the criteria listed in Table 68.1 with clinical symptoms appearing anywhere from hours to days after a decrease or cessation in alcohol intake. Sudden abstinence in the setting of chronic alcohol consumption increases the possibility of developing withdrawal seizures, alcoholic hallucinosis, and delirium tremens. Withdrawal seizures occur in approximately 10% of patients and generally appear within 12–48 hours after decreased alcohol intake (Sarff and Gold, 2010, p. S495). Typically, seizures are not sustained status epilepticus, but rather brief tonic-clonic seizures. However, up to 60% of patients have multiple seizures with a previous history of withdrawal-related seizures being a significant risk factor for the development of seizures in future withdrawal episodes (Sarff and Gold, 2010, p. S495). Not all seizures occurring during an episode of alcohol withdrawal are related to the withdrawal itself; approximately 50% of seizures are a result of a separate physiologic cause such as repetitive brain trauma (Sarff and Gold, 2010, p. S495). Therefore, alcohol withdrawal seizures should remain a diagnosis of exclusion.

Alcoholic hallucinosis occurs in approximately 30% of patients experiencing alcohol withdrawal (Sarff and Gold, 2010, p. S495). Delirium tremens generally occur within 48–72 hours after the last drink in about 5% of alcoholics, but carry a mortality rate of 5%–15%, with early identification being key to

Table 68.1 Criteria for Alcohol Withdrawal as Defined by *DSM-V* (APA, 2013)

1. Cessation of (or reduction in) alcohol use that has been heavy and prolonged.
2. Two or more of the following symptoms that develop within several hours to a few days after the cessation of (or reduction in) alcohol use:
• Autonomic hyperactivity (sweating, pulse >100 bpm)
• Increased hand tremor
• Insomnia
• Nausea or vomiting
• Transient hallucinations (visual, tactile, or auditory)
• Psychomotor agitation
• Anxiety
• Generalized tonic-clonic seizures
3. The signs or symptoms discussed above cause clinically significant distress or impairment in social, occupational, or other areas of functioning.
4. The signs or symptoms are not attributable to another medical condition and are not better explained by another mental disorder.

Table 68.2 Substances and Their Effects

	Substance	Mechanism	Intoxication	Withdrawal
Depressants	Opioids	Mu receptor agonist	Respiratory depression Myosis Seizures	Anxiety Insomnia Diarrhea
	Barbiturates	Increases GABA R opening	Respiratory depression; CNS depression	Anxiety Seizures Delirium Cardiovascular collapse
	Benzodiazepines	Increases GABA R frequency	Amnesia Ataxia Stupor Somnolence	Anxiety Insomnia Seizures
Stimulants	Amphetamines	Stimulates DA, NE, 5HT release	Euphoria Impaired judgment Fever; Tachycardia	Anxiety Irritability Somnolence
	MDMA		Friendliness; Hyperthermia	Mood changes
	Cocaine	Blocks DA, NE, 5HT reuptake	Psychomotor agitation Grandiosity; Hallucinations Vasospasm	Depression Suicidal ideation
	Caffeine	Adenosine antagonist	Restlessness Diuresis Cardiac arrhythmias	Headache Lethargy Depression
	Nicotine	Nicotinic Ach R Agonist	Restlessness Anxiety Cardiac arrhythmias	Irritability Headache Weight gain
Hallucinogens	PCP	NMDA R Antagonist	Belligerence Psychosis Seizures Nystagmus Tachycardia Ataxia	Depression Anxiety Irritability
	LSD	5HT R Agonist	Mydriasis Visual hallucinations Synesthesia	Flashbacks
	Marijuana	Cannabinoid Receptor agonist	Euphoria Disinhibition Paranoid delusions Hallucinations	Irritability Depression Insomnia Nausea
	Inhalants	Unknown	Belligerence Impaired judgment	N/A Coma
Alcohol		Increases GABA channel opening	Aggression Mood swings; Disinhibition	Irritability Hallucinations Seizures

increasing the effectiveness of therapies (Mehta, 2016, p. 29). Delirium tremens are characterized by fluctuating levels of consciousness, attention and cognitive deficits, confusion, hallucinations, and hypertension. If not managed effectively, delirium tremens can lead to cardiovascular and respiratory collapse, electrolyte imbalances, arrhythmias, dehydration, and multiorgan dysfunction (Sutton and Jutel, 2016, p. 30).

Repeated withdrawal episodes can lead to a phenomenon known as the "kindling effect." The kindling effect is theorized to be a result of the increase in CNS hyperexcitability that occurs with each successive withdrawal episode and, in particular, plays a role in the development of withdrawal seizures (Sarff and Gold, 2010, p. S495). This increasing severity of alcohol withdrawal with each episode is thought to in part explain the development of benzodiazepine-resistant alcohol withdrawal.

Pathophysiology

Alcohol inhibits excitatory NMDA receptors, which results in a reduction of the neurotransmitter gluta-mate. Alcohol also activates the inhibitory GABA-A receptors. The cumulative result is that of anxiolytic and sedative effects as well as motor coordination impairment. Chronic alcohol use leads to decreased GABA-A receptor function and upregulated NMDA receptor function, creating a new adaptive physio-logic equilibrium that relies on alcohol for regulation. In the absence of alcohol, NMDA receptor function is increased/more sensitive to glutamate, and GABA-A receptors are reduced, resulting in an autonomic excitation that lacks inhibitory regulation (Mirijello et al., 2015, p. 353). Dysregulation of dopamine is also thought to play a role in alcohol withdrawal, potentially impacting the presence of hallucinations (Sarff and Gold, 2010, p. S494).

Common physical exam findings

Common symptoms associated with alcohol withdrawal are listed in Table 68.1. Other common exam findings are associated with chronic inflammatory liver disease or cirrhosis due to the toxic nature of alcohol metabolism in the liver. Exam findings consistent with cirrhosis include the following (Doig and Huether, 2014, p. 1460; Karnath, 2003):

- Hepatomegaly, splenomegaly
- Portal hypertension
- Esophageal varices
- Ascites
- Hepatic encephalopathy
- Jaundice
- Gynecomastia
- Spider angiomas
- Palmar erythema
- Asterixis

Relevant diagnostic tests

Laboratory tests

- *Complete blood count*: Thrombocytopenia is common, and anemia from nutritional deficiencies and/ or blood loss from the GI tract are common. (Dehydration is common in alcohol withdrawal and may mask anemias until rehydration can be achieved.) Macrocytic anemia may indicate a dietary deficiency of vitamin B_{12} and folate; thus, these levels may be checked as well.
- *Complete metabolic panel*: Assess for concurrent renal disease (possibly indicative of hepatorenal syn-drome), hypoglycemia (due to reduced glycogen stores and impaired gluconeogenesis), and elec-trolyte abnormalities including hypokalemia, hypomagnesemia, hyponatremia, hypophosphatemia,

and hypocalcemia. Hypomagnesemia is common due to dietary deficiencies and can lead to fatal arrhythmias including torsade de pointes. An ammonia level may also be helpful in cases of hepatic encephalopathy. Alcoholic pancreatitis is also common and can lead to hypocalcemia. Liver function tests including aspartate aminotransferase (AST) and alanine transaminase (ALT) elevations are useful in assessing for cirrhosis.

- *Coagulation studies*: As patients with cirrhosis at are risk for coagulopathies, prothrombin (PT) and international normalized ratio (INR) are useful, especially in the setting of active bleeding.
- *Urine analysis*: Include toxicology to assess for coingestion of other medications/recreational drugs, and assess for ketones to rule out associated alcoholic ketoacidosis. As alcoholism is an important risk factor for pneumonias, testing for *Streptococcus pneumoniae* urine antigen should be considered (Mehta, 2016, p. 29).
- *Ethanol*: An ethanol level may be useful to provide a point of reference. An ethanol level does not have to be zero before signs of alcohol withdrawal are apparent; chronic alcoholics may begin to exhibit withdrawal symptoms with a reduced ethanol level relative to their functioning baseline.
- If clinically indicated, other lab tests to consider include cardiac biomarkers, lipase/amylase if there are concerns for pancreatitis, and creatine kinase (CK) if there are concerns for rhabdomyolysis (e.g., the patient was found down for an unknown amount of time) (McKeown et al., 2015).

Imaging and other tests

- *Chest radiograph*: Alcoholism has been identified as a risk factor for the development of "typical" and atypical pneumonias, and aspiration pneumonia. A combination of altered oropharyngeal flora, blunted upper airway reflexes during inebriation, impaired normal defense mechanisms such as mucociliary clearance, and impaired innate immune responses such as the alveolar macrophage activation in the lower airways predispose alcoholics to the development of pneumonias. Additionally, alcoholics are also at an increased risk of sepsis and acute respiratory distress syndrome (Mehta, 2016, p. 30).
- *Electrocardiogram*: Increased autonomic hyperactivity found in alcohol withdrawal leads to tachycardia and hypertension. Electrolyte disturbances in addition to catecholamine release and reduced baroreflex sensitivity can lead to variable conduction patterns such as QT interval prolongation and reentry excitation, which has the potential to trigger ventricular tachycardia (Bar et al., 2007, p. 264). Hypomagnesemia can also predispose those in alcohol withdrawal to torsade de pointes.
- *Computed tomography*: CT specifically of the head is used to rule out intracranial bleeding as well as any other organic source of seizures. Cortical and cerebellar atrophy have been associated with chronic alcoholism (Garcia-Valdecasas-Campelo et al., 2007, p. 536). Additionally, coagulopathies may exist with chronic liver disease, which predispose the chronic alcoholic to intracranial bleeding. A head CT should be considered in patients with multiple seizures, with signs of head trauma, with an inappropriate level of consciousness, and with an unexpected failure to respond to treatment.

Interventional procedures that are frequently associated with alcohol withdrawal include the following:

- *Intubation*: Respiratory status can become a concern in alcohol withdrawal for many reasons: oversedation with benzodiazepines, withdrawal refractory to benzodiazepines requiring sedation, or other related physiologic processes (aspiration pneumonia, or significant GI bleed).

- *Esophagogastroduodenoscopy*: Gastrointestinal bleeding is commonly associated with alcoholism in the form of peptic ulcer disease and mucosal erosions. Esophageal varices are frequently found in alcoholic cirrhosis due to portopulmonary hypertension (Mehta, 2016, p. 31).
- *Other procedures*: Paracentesis may be necessary due to ascites (McKeown et al., 2015). Lumbar puncture should be considered to rule out meningitis.

Common grading schemes

The Clinical Institute Withdrawal Assessment—Revised (CIWA-Ar) is a 10-item scale used to grade the symptoms of withdrawal. It is the most commonly used tool to assess severity of withdrawal as well as response to treatment (Sullivan et al., 1989; p. 1353). This tool assigns points based on the presence and progression of symptoms; thus, a higher score indicates more acute and advanced withdrawal. Generally, a score of 10 or less is considered mild withdrawal, not requiring medication; 10–15 is considered moderate withdrawal, requiring medication; and greater than 20 is severe withdrawal (Awissi et al., 2013, p. S59). Of note, the CIWA-Ar does not include vital signs in the scoring system.

The CIWA-Ar requires patient participation to assess withdrawal severity. As intubated patients are frequently unable to participate in the assessment, the CIWA-Ar is not validated in the mechanically ventilated patient. While not directly correlated, the Richmond Agitation-Sedation Scale (RASS) is commonly used to assess withdrawal symptoms in the intubated patient (Awissi et al., 2013, p. S59).

Medication management

Benzodiazepines. Benzodiazepines such as lorazepam remain the first-line treatment of alcohol withdrawal. Through binding directly to GABA receptors, benzodiazepines exhibit anticonvulsant and sedation activity (Schmidt et al., 2016, p. 3). Current literature supports utilizing a symptom-triggered bolus benzodiazepine dosing strategy as opposed to a fixed-dose schedule for withdrawal management; a symptom-triggered approach has been found to prevent oversedation while maintaining effectiveness and to decrease total benzodiazepine requirements (Skinner, 2014, p. 314). Close monitoring of respiratory status is absolutely necessary as the large doses of benzodiazepines sometimes required to manage alcohol withdrawal can quickly lead to oversedation.

Dexmedetomidine. Dexmedetomidine is an α-2 adrenergic receptor agonist, centrally activating, which results in decreased norepinephrine synthesis and therefore less sympathetic nervous system stimulation. A key advantage of dexmedetomidine is the anxiolytic and sympatholysis effects achieved without respiratory depression, making dexmedetomidine appropriate for nonintubated patients. However, dexmedetomidine lacks GABA receptor activity and therefore has no anticonvulsant properties. Dexmedetomidine is appropriate as adjunctive therapy and has been proven to reduce overall benzodiazepine requirements (Schmidt et al., 2016, p. 6). Dexmedetomidine can cause marked bradycardia and hypotension, which are indications for discontinuation of the drug (Ferreira et al., 2015, p. 8).

Antipsychotics. As a dopamine antagonist, IV haloperidol has been used in alcohol withdrawal in the management of acute delirium and psychosis in conjunction with benzodiazepines. However, IV haloperidol is associated with an increased risk of cardiac dysrhythmias, particularly lengthening the corrected QT interval (or QTc) to >450 msec, predisposing the patient to torsade de pointes and sudden cardiac death (Meyer-Massetti et al., 2010, p. E14). In addition, IV haloperidol may lower the seizure threshold and has been linked with the development of pneumonias (hospital acquired and aspiration) (Ferreira et al., 2015, p. 9).

Anticonvulsants. Various anticonvulsants have been shown to be effective in reducing the probability of progression to seizures in alcohol withdrawal. These include carbamazepine, valproic acid, and gabapentin (Sachdeva et al., 2015, p. 5). Anticonvulsants may provide an additional benefit in treating withdrawal through "anti-kindling" properties, blocking progressive neuronal sensitization with repeat withdrawal episodes (Perry, 2014, p. 408). These medications may reduce the need for benzodiazepines but currently are not recommended to replace benzodiazepines (Hammond et al., 2015, p. 305). The use of anticonvulsants may be limited by medical comorbidities, side effects, and their limited usefulness in treating severe withdrawal symptoms or delirium tremens (Sachdeva et al., 2015, p. 5).

Propofol. Used primarily in severe and refractory withdrawal, propofol functions as a sedative and anxiolytic through GABA agonist receptor activity in addition to inhibiting glutamate at the NMDA receptors (Schmidt et al., 2016, p. 6). Propofol has a rapid onset of action as well as a short half-life (Perry, 2014 p. 407). Due to substantive respiratory depression, propofol requires intubation and mechanical ventilation. In addition, propofol may cause bradycardia and hypotension (Perry, 2014, p. 407).

Barbiturates. Barbiturates such as phenobarbital interact with GABA receptors in a method that is distinctly different from benzodiazepines. Phenobarbital creates a synergistic effect with benzodiazepines and may be used in refractory withdrawal (Schmidt et al., 2016, p. 5). While concerns for respiratory depression exist, preliminary research in utilizing barbiturates for alcohol withdrawal shows potential decreased rates of mechanical ventilation and decreased ICU as well as hospital length of stay (Ferreira et al., 2015, p. 7).

Supportive care. To prevent the development of Wernicke encephalopathy, thiamine supplementation is necessary. As thiamine assists with carbohydrate metabolism, it is imperative to address thiamine deficiency prior to any glucose administration. Due to frequent nutritional deficiencies found with chronic alcoholism, folate and multivitamin supplementation is also recommended. Additionally, it should be a priority to address electrolyte imbalances and hypovolemia (Schmidt et al., 2016, p. 3).

Common medicolegal concerns

*   Due to the stigma associated with the fields of substance abuse and mental health, confidentiality concerns abound. Substance abuse is identified as sensitive personal health information, and extreme care should be taken to protect privacy. Accidental disclosure of protected health information in social situations such as family dynamics and employment concerns are very real, and a heightened sense of awareness and caution is required. Under the Health Insurance Portability and Accountability Act (HIPAA) of 1996, health information cannot be disclosed without the patient's consent (Substance Abuse and Mental Health Services Administration, 2004, p. 2).

References

American Psychiatric Association. 2013. Substance related and addictive disorders. *In Diagnostic and Statistical Manual of Mental Disorders*, 5th ed. http://dsm.psychiatryonline.org.ezproxy.library.wisc.edu/doi/abs/10.1176/appi.books.9780890425596.dsm16.

Awissi DK, Lebrun G, Fagnan M et al. Alcohol, nicotine, and iatrogenic withdrawals in the ICU. *Critical Care Medicine.* 2013;41:S57–S68.

Bar KJ, Boettger MK, Koschke M et al. Increased QT interval variability index in acute alcohol withdrawal. *Drug and Alcohol DependenceI.* 2007;89:259–266.

Barker K, Hunjadi D. Meet Narcan: The amazing drug that helps save overdose patients. *JEMS.* 2008;33:72–76.

Bates JJ, Foss JF, Murphy DB. Are peripheral opioid antagonists the solution to opioid side effects? *Anesth Analg.* 2004;98:116–22, table of contents.

Batke M, Cappell MS, Others. The cannabis hyperemesis syndrome characterized by persistent nausea and vomiting, abdominal pain, and compulsive bathing associated with chronic marijuana use: A report of eight cases in the United States. *Dig Dis Sci.* 2010;55:3113–3119.

Businco LDR, Lauriello M, Marsico C, Corbisiero A, Cipriani O, Tirelli GC. Psychological aspects and treatment of patients with nasal septal perforation due to cocaine inhalation. *Acta Otorhinolaryngol Ital*. 2008;28:247–251.

Castells X, Cunill R, Pérez-Mañá C, Vidal X, Capellà D. Psychostimulant drugs for cocaine dependence. *Cochrane Database Syst Rev*. 2016;9:CD007380.

Centers for Disease Control and Prevention. 2016. Fact sheets – Alcohol use and your health. http://www.cdc.gov/alcohol/fact-sheets/alcohol-use.htm.

Cheskin LJ, Fudala PJ, Johnson RE. A controlled comparison of buprenorphine and clonidine for acute detoxification from opioids. *Drug Alcohol Depend*. 1994;36:115–121.

Doig A, Huether SE. Alterations of digestive function. In Kathryn L. McCance, Sue E. Huether, Valentina L. Brashers, Neal S. Rote, eds. Pathophysiology: The Biologic Basis for Disease in Adults and Children. 7th ed.. St. Louis, Missouri: Elsevier Mosby; 2014:1423–1485.

Ferreira J, Wieruszewski P, Cunningham D, Davidson K, Weisberg S. Approach to the complicated alcohol withdrawal patient. *Journal of Intensive Care Medicine*. 2015;1–12.

File:Myosis due to opiate use.jpg - Wikimedia Commons [Internet]. [cited 11 Jan 2017]. Available: https://commons.wikimedia.org/wiki/File:Myosis_due_to_opiate_use.jpg.

Fudala PJ, Jaffe JH, Dax EM, Johnson RE. Use of buprenorphine in the treatment of opioid addiction. II. Physiologic and behavioral effects of daily and alternate-day administration and abrupt withdrawal. Clinical Pharmacology & Therapeutics. *Wiley Online Library*; 1990;47:525–534.

Garcia-Valdecasas-Campelo E, Gonzalez-Reimers E, Santolaria-Fernandez F et al. Brain atrophy in alcoholics: Relationship with alcohol intake; liver disease; nutritional status, and inflammation. *Alcohol & Alcoholism*. 2007;42:533–538.

Hadden J, Johnson K, Smith S, Price L, Giardina E. Acute barbiturate intoxication. Concepts of management. *JAMA*. 1969;209:893–900.

Hammond, C, Niciu MJ, Drew S, Arias AJ. Anticonvulsants for the treatment of alcohol withdrawal syndrome and alcohol use disorders. *CNS Drugs*. 2015;29:293–311.

Haverkos HW. Infectious diseases and drug abuse. Prevention and treatment in the drug abuse treatment system. *J Subst Abuse Treat*. 1991;8:269–275.

Johnson MD, Heriza TJ, St Dennis C. How to spot illicit drug abuse in your patients. *Postgrad Med*. 1999;106:199–200, 203–6, 211–4 passim.

Jones AL, Simpson KJ. Ecstasy (MDMA) and amphetamine intoxications. Aliment Pharmacol Ther. *Wiley Online Library*. 1999;13:129–133.

Jorenby DE, Leischow SJ, Nides MA et al. A controlled trial of sustained-release bupropion, a nicotine patch, or both for smoking cessation. *N Engl J Med*. 1999;340:685–691.

Karnath B. Stigmata of chronic liver disease. *Hospital Physician*. 2003;14–16, 28.

Krystal JH, Cramer JA, Krol WF, Kirk GF, Rosenheck RA, Veterans Affairs Naltrexone Cooperative Study 425 Group. Naltrexone in the treatment of alcohol dependence. *N Engl J Med*. 2001;345:1734–1739.

Lago JA, Kosten TR. Stimulant withdrawal. *Addiction*. 1994;89:1477–1481.

Larson EW, Olincy A, Rummans TA, Morse RM. Disulfiram treatment of patients with both alcohol dependence and other psychiatric disorders: A review. *Alcohol Clin Exp Res*. 1992;16:125–130.

Lukas SE, Renshaw PF. Cocaine effects on brain function. *Cocaine Abuse*. Elsevier; 1998;265–287.

Mayo-Smith MF. Pharmacological management of alcohol withdrawal: A meta-analysis and evidence-based practice guideline. *JAMA*. American Medical Association; 1997;278:144–151.

McCarron MM, Schulze BW, Thompson GA, Conder MC, Goetz WA. Acute phencyclidine intoxication: Clinical patterns, complications, and treatment. *Ann Emerg Med*. 1981;10:290–297.

McKewon N, West P, VanDeVoort J et al., 2015. Withdrawal syndrome workup. *Medscape*. http://emedicine.medscape.com/article/819502-workup.

Mehta, Ashish J. Alcoholism and critical illness: A review. *World Journal of Critical Care Medicine*. 2016;5:27–35.

Meyer-Massetti C, Cheng CM, Sharpe BA, Meier CR, Guglielmo BJ. The FDA extended warning for intravenous haloperidol and torsades de pointes: How should institutions respond?" Journal of Hospital Medicine. 2010;5:E8–E16.

Mirijello, A, D'Angelo C, Ferrulli A et al., Identification and Management of Alcohol Withdrawal Syndrome. *Drugs*. 2015;75:353–365.

Mordel A, Winkler E, Almog S, Tirosh M, Ezra D. Seizures after flumazenil administration in a case of combined benzodiazepine and tricyclic antidepressant overdose. *Crit Care Med*. 1992;20:1733–1734.

National Institute on Alcohol Abuse and Alcoholism. 2015a. Alcohol facts and statistics. *National Institutes of Health*. http://www.niaaa.nih.gov/alcohol-health/overview-alcohol-consumption/alcohol-facts-and-statistics.

National Institute on Alcohol Abuse and Alcoholism. 2015b. Alcohol use disorder: A comparison between DSM-IV and DSM-5. *National Institutes of Health*. http://pubs.niaaa.nih.gov/publications/dsmfactsheet/dsmfact.pdf.

Nishimoto A, Usery J, Winton JC, Twilla J. High-dose parenteral thiamine in treatment of Wernicke's encephalopathy: Case series and review of the literature. *In Vivo.* 2017;31:121–124.

Perry, Elizabeth. Inpatient management of acute alcohol withdrawal syndrome." *CNS Drugs.* 2014;28:401–410.

Questel F, Dally S, Bismuth C. Rhabdomyolysis in cocaine abusers. *J Clin Forensic Med.* 1995/3;2, Supplement 1: 30.

Rausch V, Peccerella T, Lackner C, Yagmur E et al. Primary liver injury and delayed resolution of liver stiffness after alcohol detoxification in heavy drinkers with the PNPLA3 variant I148M. *World J Hepatol.* 2016;8:1547–1556.

Sachdeva A, Choudhary M, Chandra M. Alcohol withdrawal syndrome: Benzodiazepines and beyond. *Journal of Clinical and Diagnostic Research.* 2015;9:VE01–VE07.

Sarff MC, Gold J. Alcohol withdrawal syndromes in the intensive care unit. *Critical Care Medicine.* 2010;38:S494–S501.

Sauer A. 2015 World Drug Report finds drug use stable, access to drug & HIV treatment still low [Internet]. [cited 10 Jan 2017]. Available: https://www.unodc.org/unodc/en/frontpage/2015/June/2015-world-drug-report-finds-drug-use-stable--access-to-drug-and-hiv-treatment-still-low.html.

Sawynok J. Pharmacological rationale for the clinical use of caffeine. *Drugs.* 1995;49:37–50.

Schmidt, K, Doshi M, Holzhausen J, Natavio A, Cadiz M, Winegardner J. A review of the treatment of severe alcohol withdrawal. *Annals of Pharmacotherapy.* 2016;1–13.

Skinner R. Symptom-triggered vs. fixed-dosing management of alcohol withdrawal syndrome. *MedSurg Nursing.* 2014;23:307–329.

Substance Abuse and Mental Health Services Administration. The Confidentiality of Alcohol and Drug Abuse Patient Records Regulation and the HIPAA Privacy Rule: Implications for Alcohol and Substance Abuse Programs. *U.S. Department of Health and Human Services.* 2004 http://www.samhsa.gov/sites/default/files/part2-hipaa-comparison2004.pdf.

Sullivan J, Sykora C, Schneiderman J, Naranjo C, Sellers E. Assessment of alcohol Withdrawal: the revised clinical institute withdrawal assessment for alcohol scale (CIWA-Ar). *British Journal of Addiction.* 1989;84:1353–1357.

Sutton LJ, Jutel A. Alcohol withdrawal syndrome in critically ill patients: Identification, assessment, and management. *Critical Care Nurse.* 2016;36:28–39.

Thomas J, Moore G. Medical-legal issues in the agitated patient: Cases and caveats. *West J Emerg Med.* 2013;14:559–565.

Tonstad S, Tønnesen P, Hajek P et al. Effect of maintenance therapy with varenicline on smoking cessation: A randomized controlled trial. JAMA. *American Medical Association;* 2006;296:64–71.

Ungerleider JT, Frank IM. Management of acute panic reactions and flashbacks resulting from LSD ingestion. *Acute Drug Abuse Emergencies.* Elsevier; 1976:133–138.

Vadhan NP, Corcoran CM, Bedi GI, Lieberman JG, Haney M. Marijuana smokers at clinical high-risk for schizophrenia exhibit an enhanced subjective, behavioral and physiological response to smoked marijuana. *Compr Psychiatry.* 2013;54:e37.

Wurcel AG, Merchant EA, Clark RP, Stone DR. Emerging and underrecognized complications of illicit drug use. *Clin Infect Dis.* 2015;61:1840–1849.

Young SJ, Longstaffe S, Tenenbein M. Inhalant abuse and the abuse of other drugs. *Am J Drug Alcohol Abuse.* 1999;25:371–375.

69

HEADACHE

Jaclyn Baloga

One of the most common complaints in a neurology/neurosurgery patient setting is complaint of a headache. As medical providers, we must be able to recognize common causes, establish a differential diagnosis, and identify concerning signs and presentations.

There are a few categories of benign headaches, including migraine, tension-type, and cluster headache. More concerning pathologic headaches include headache due to a tumor or vascular lesion, hemorrhage, or infection (Bajwa and Wootton, 2014). This chapter addresses the most common and the most concerning causes of a headache.

Migraine

A typical presentation for a migraine headache is a progression that begins with a prodrome (symptoms of euphoria, depression, irritability, food craving, or constipation most commonly reported), then an aura (visual, auditory, somatosensory, or motor symptoms including photophobia, phonophobia, tinnitus, paresthesias, or jerking movements), then the headache that tends to be throbbing or pulsatile in nature and may be associated with nausea and vomiting, and last the postdrome once the headache resolves and symptoms of exhaustion can occur (Cutrer et al., 2014).

Tension type

A tension-type headache usually presents as mild to moderate, is usually bilateral, and is commonly described as "pressure-like," "band-like," or "heavy weight on my head." There is usually associated scalp muscle and trapezius muscle tenderness. No nausea or vomiting is usually reported, and it is not aggravated by activity (Taylor, 2014).

Cluster

Another benign headache is a cluster headache. These are unilateral, usually severe orbital or temporal attacks associated with autonomic symptoms such as lacrimation, rhinorrhea, diaphoresis, ptosis, or miosis on the same side as the headache. Cluster headache typically presents with patient agitation or restlessness (May, 2014).

Serious causes

More critical types of headaches include a subarachnoid hemorrhage, subdural hematoma, vascular malformations, brain tumors, cerebral spinal fluid (CSF) leak, or central nervous system (CNS) infection (Bajwa and Wootton, 2014). Serious causes need to be recognized quickly.

"Red flags"

There are signs and symptoms that are designated to be "red flags" for urgent causes of a headache. These warrant urgent evaluation.

- Sudden onset of severe headache
- Absence of similar headache in the past
- "Worst headache of my life"
- Focal neurologic deficits
- Associated seizures
- Mental status changes or fluctuation in consciousness
- Associated nuchal rigidity/meningismus
- Associated fever
- Papilledema
- Refractory or worsening pattern of headaches nonresponsive to treatment
- Onset or worsening of headache with exertion or Valsalva (Bajwa and Wootton, 2014)

Hemorrhage

A subarachnoid hemorrhage or subdural hematoma typically present with a sudden onset of a severe headache usually described as the "worst headache of my life." There may or may not be neurologic deficits, vomiting, or mental status changes (Singer et al., 2013). Headache associated with fever and meningismus is more concerning for an infectious etiology such as meningitis or intracranial abscess (Bajwa and Wootton, 2014).

Tumors/Lesions

Brain tumors or vascular abnormalities do not always present acutely. Both benign and malignant tumors can manifest similarly and need to be addressed urgently. Malignant tumors can be either primary (arising from cells within the CNS) or systemic from metastasis to the CNS. Headache is the biggest complaint in about half of patients with brain tumors. Pain is usually dull and constant. There can be associated nausea and vomiting. Typically, position changes such as forward flexion or Valsalva can exacerbate the pain due to an increase in intracranial pressure during these activities (Wong and Wu, 2014).

The classic triad of increased intracranial pressure includes:

- Headache
- Papilledema
- Nausea (Wong and Wu, 2014)

Cerebral spinal fluid leak

Positional or postural headache, with an onset or worsening of the headache in the upright position and alleviation of the headache when lying flat, is more indicative of a CSF leak. The headache is attributed to spontaneous intracranial hypotension (Sun-Edelstein and Lay, 2015). This should be strongly considered in a patient who recently underwent spinal or cranial surgery.

Nocturnal headache that awakens a patient from sleep is typical for a tumor-related headache due to vasodilation from an increase in carbon dioxide in the blood that regularly occurs during sleep. Seizures are more common with malignant lesions. Cognitive dysfunction, focal muscle weakness, and syncope are associated with brain tumors. Focal neurologic deficits can vary depending on the tumor location (Wong and Wu, 2014).

History and physical

Any patient who presents with a headache needs a full history and neurologic exam. A thorough history should include:

- Onset
- Intensity, frequency, and duration
- Change in headache pattern
- Number of days a month
- Known aura/prodrome?
- Quality and location
- Associated symptoms
- Family history of headaches or brain tumors
- Aggravating/alleviating factors, including effect of activity
- Response to treatment in the past
- Recent trauma, even minor especially if on anticoagulants
- Vision changes
- Effect of menstrual cycle in women
- Changes in weight, sleep, or lifestyle (Bajwa and Wootton, 2014)

A complete neurologic exam should be performed to include:

- Vital signs, especially blood pressure
- Neck and head auscultation for bruits
- Head, neck, and shoulder palpation including temporal arteries
- Examination of the spine and neck, including checking for resistance to passive neck flexion
- Gait and balance testing, including toe walk, heel walk, tandem walk, and Romberg test
- Cranial nerve examination
- Sensory, motor, and reflex examination
- Funduscopic exam to check for papilledema
- Cerebellar testing (Bajwa and Wootton, 2014)

Diagnostic tests

There is insufficient data for recommendations for neuroimaging in patients who present with a headache (Bajwa and Wootton, 2014). Any patient who presents with a "red flag" should get urgent neuroimaging with either brain computed tomography (CT) scan (better for evaluation of a hemorrhage) or brain magnetic resonance imaging (MRI) (better for evaluation of a tumor or CSF leak). Lumbar puncture is indicated with suspicion of subarachnoid hemorrhage with normal brain CT or with suspicion of infectious or inflammatory etiology (Bajwa and Wootton, 2014).

The following situations should consider neuroimaging:

- Abnormal neurologic finding on exam
- Change in pattern, severity, or frequency of the headache
- Worsening or no relief with appropriate therapy
- Onset with exertional activity or Valsalva
- Bruit finding on exam
- New onset of headache after 40 years old (Bajwa and Wootton, 2014)

Other relevant diagnostic tests may be indicated, such as laboratory studies including a complete blood count (CBC), complete metabolic panel (CMP), erythrocyte sedimentation rate (ESR), and noncardiac C-reactive protein (CRP) if there is clinical suspicion for an infectious, inflammatory, or metabolic cause of the headache. Elevation in white blood cell count on the CBC, elevation in ESR, and elevation in noncardiac CRP can be present in an infectious or inflammatory etiology. Metabolic abnormalities on the CMP can present from metabolic etiology for the headache.

Treatment

Treatment for headache varies based on the cause. Benign headaches can be treated conservatively as an outpatient. Medications including "triptans" (sumatriptan, rizatriptan), nonsteroidal anti-inflammatory drugs (NSAIDs) (ibuprofen, naproxen), acetaminophen, antiemetics (ondansetron, metoclopramide), and muscle relaxants (cyclobenzaprine, tizanidine) can be used to treat the symptoms. Oxygen therapy and octreotide are effective in treating cluster headaches (May, 2014). Preventative treatment is important. Verapamil is the agent of choice to prevent cluster headaches (May, 2014). Avoidance of triggers is important in migraine prevention. The more serious causes of headache usually require prompt referral to neurosurgery and may likely require inpatient care.

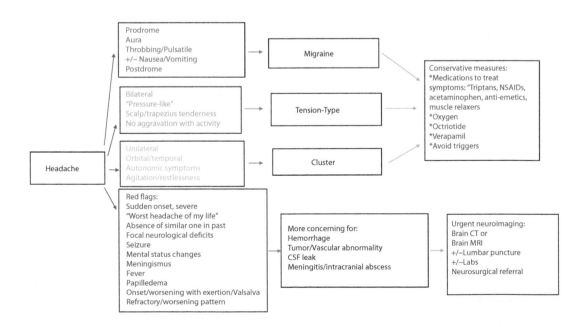

Patient counseling is important in the management and treatment of headaches. The patient should be taught to recognize and avoid potential triggers that can cause the headache. They need to be made aware of the "red flags" and when they should seek immediate medical attention.

Prognosis is determined based on the etiology of the headache. Benign causes such as migraine, cluster, and tension-type headaches have better prognoses as compared to serious causes such as hemorrhage, tumor, or infection (meningitis or abscess) understandably.

As an advanced practice health professional, it is our responsibility to evaluate and treat a patient complaining of a headache appropriately. We need to recognize when prompt imaging and neurosurgical evaluation is warranted and when conservative treatment is appropriate. Our management impacts patient health care and can prevent morbidity and mortality as well as limit unnecessary imaging.

References

Bajwa ZH, Wootton RJ. Evaluation of headache in adults. *UpToDate*. 2014. https://www.uptodate.com/contents/evaluation-of-headache-in-adults.

Cutrer FM, Bajwa ZH, Sabahat A. Pathophysiology, clinical manifestations, and diagnosis of migraine in adults. *UpToDate*. 2014. http://www.uptodate.com/contents/pathophysiology-clinical-manifestations-and-diagnosis-of-migraine-in-adults.

May A. Cluster headache: Epidemiology, clinical features, and diagnosis. *UpToDate*. 2014a. https://www.uptodate.com/contents/cluster-headache-epidemiology-clinical-features-and-diagnosis.

May A. Cluster headache: Treatment and prognosis. *UpToDate*. 2014b. https://www.uptodate.com/contents/cluster-headache-treatment-and-prognosis.

Singer RJ, Ogilvy CS, Rordorf G. 2013. Clinical manifestations and diagnosis of aneurysmal subarachnoid hemorrhage. *UpToDate*. https://www.uptodate.com/contents/clinical-manifestations-and-diagnosis-of-aneurysmal-subarachnoid-hemorrhage.

Sun-Edelstein C, Lay C. Headache attributed to spontaneous intracranial hypotension: Pathophysiology, clinical features, and diagnosis. *UpToDate*. 2015. http://www.uptodate.com/contents/spontaneous-intracranial-hypotension-pathophysiology-clinical-features-and-diagnosis.

Taylor FR. Tension-type headache in adults: Pathophysiology, clinical features, and diagnosis. *UpToDate*. 2014. http://www.uptodate.com/contents/tension-type-headache-in-adults-pathophysiology-clinical-features-and-diagnosis.

Wong ET, Wu JK. Clinical presentation and diagnosis of brain tumors. *UpToDate*. 2014. https://www.uptodate.com/contents/clinical-presentation-and-diagnosis-of-brain-tumors.

70

PERIPHERAL NERVE DISORDERS

Marine Dididze and Allan D. Levi

Case vignette

A 68-year-old female presented with 5 years of progressive pain and paresthesias involving the medial surface of her left foot. She underwent several negative lumbar magnetic resonance imaging (MRI) scans and resection of her navicular bone in an attempt to treat her pain. A mass was discovered along the medial aspect of her lower leg, and a MRI revealed a homogenously enhancing lesion involving the tibial nerve (Figure 70.1a). There was no history of medical problems and no family history of tumors or cutaneous lesions. Physical exam reveals a small, mildly tender mass located on the posteromedial surface of the left lower leg. She had full strength and normal sensation. Tinel sign is positive over the lesion and reproduced her symptoms.

Case summary

Based on the findings, the most likely preoperative diagnosis is a sporadic schwannoma. She was offered surgery for definitive diagnosis and symptom relief with the goal of gross total resection and preservation of neurologic function (Figure 70.1b, c). Intraoperatively, the tumor capsule was incised, the tumor was

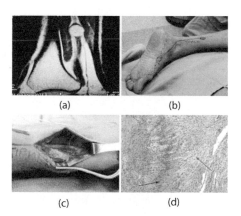

(a) (b)

(c) (d)

Figure 70.1 (a) Coronal T1 MRI with gadolinium showing a homogenously enhancing lesion involving the tibial nerve. (b) Preoperative image displaying the course of the tibial nerve and associated mass. (c) Intraoperative image of the tibial nerve following tumor resection. (d) Histologic stain showing Antoni A (*black arrow*) and Antoni B (*blue arrow*) configurations.

enucleated, and the parent fascicle sectioned under magnification following the absence of motor response with 1 mA of electrical stimulation. Final pathology confirmed the diagnosis with characteristic Antoni A and B configuration (Figure 70.1d). Postoperatively her pain and paresthesias resolved with preservation of motor function.

Overview

Schwannomas are classified as benign peripheral nerve sheath tumors. They arise from a single nerve fascicle, displacing other fascicles with tumor expansion. Histologically, these tumors are characterized by cellular areas with palisading configurations (Antoni A) and adjacent less cellular areas (Antoni B) (Figure 70.1d). S100 and Leu-7 are pathologic immunostains utilized to identify the neoplastic spindle cells present in schwannomas. In addition, microhemorrhages, cysts, hyalinization, and mineralization may be present. Ancient schwannomas, cellular schwannomas, and melanotic schwannomas are described variants. Although peripheral nerve sheath schwannomas (PNSSs) are often sporadic, multiple schwannomas occur in patients with neurofibromatosis type 2 (NF-2), schwannomatosis, Carney complex, and an unnamed syndrome including multiple nevi and leiomyomas. Sporadic schwannomas may present at any age (peak incidence third to sixth decades), and occur most commonly in the head, neck, and flexor surfaces of the extremities. Sensory roots most commonly give rise to spinal schwannomas. Schwannomatosis is a more recently described third form of neurofibromatosis. It is characterized by the development of multiple nonvestibular schwannomas. Although phenotypic overlap exists between schwannomatosis and NF-2, the absence of bilateral vestibular schwannomas, an NF-2 mutation, and classic ocular lesions on neuroophthalmologic exam can help to distinguish between the two clinically and molecularly distinct conditions. One-third of cases are anatomically confined to a single limb or spinal segment. While familial occurrence appears to be much less common than with NF-2, autosomal dominant inheritance has been described. Definitive diagnostic criteria include two or more nonintradermal schwannomas (one with histologic confirmation), absence of vestibular tumor on high-quality MRI, and lack of a constitutional NF-2 mutation in an adult over the age of 30. If a patient has a first-degree relative meeting criteria, they need only a single histologically diagnosed nonvestibular schwannoma.

A perineurioma is a distinct benign peripheral nerve sheath tumor that should be differentiated from a PNSS. They are classified according to anatomical location as intraneural and extraneural, with extraneural perineuriomas occurring in the skin and soft tissue as painless nodules. Clinically, this tumor tends to present as a slowly progressive mononeuropathy with marked motor loss in addition to sensory abnormalities in the appropriate distribution. Characteristic MRI findings include a homogenously enhancing, fusiform mass tracking along the length of the nerve (Figure 70.1a and b). Histologically, intraneural perineuriomas display features of hypercellularity in a whorl-like configuration ("onion bulbing-like") with a low mitotic index.

Evaluation of a peripheral nerve sheath tumor consists of a thorough history, including family history, general and neurologic physical examination, and advanced imaging (MRI or MR neurography). Neurologic signs and symptoms, as well as absent clinical stigmata of NF-1, can help direct a preoperative working diagnosis. Schwannomas typically present in middle-age adults as a painful mass. Less common presenting features include paresthesias, numbness, weakness, or a painless mass. Up to one-third of patients can have a positive Tinel sign on physical examination, which appears to be more common in schwannomas when compared to other peripheral nerve sheath tumors. MRI features of a schwannoma include gadolinium enhancement of a unilobular or fusiform lesion associated with a nerve, a "string sign" (string-like structure leaving or entering mass), or single or multiple "target signs" (Figure 70.1b).

Gross total resection with preservation of neurologic function is the ultimate goal of surgery, while utilizing established surgical principles for the resection of benign peripheral nerve tumors. The technique for schwannoma resection includes capsular incision, tumor enucleation, and sectioning of the parent fascicle under magnification. The capsule may be left behind if it is densely adherent to the parent fascicle. Direct stimulation and observation of a motor response may be utilized for identification of a functional fascicle tracking along the capsule, tumor, or its attachments. Schwannomas can typically be enucleated with preservation of the associated nerve; however, this may not be possible in some large tumors. When this is encountered, tumor debulking may be necessary. In a review of two large series of the surgical resection of peripheral nerve sheath tumors (LSUHSC and the University of Miami), postoperative function was preserved or improved in 89%–94% of patients. It is important to note that the risk of neurologic injury significantly increases if a diagnostic biopsy has been performed prior to definitive resection.

Pearls

- Peripheral nerve sheath schwannomas are benign tumors that may occur sporadically or as multiple tumors associated with the specific syndromes described.
- Schwannomatosis is a newly described syndrome characterized by multiple nonvestibular schwannomas.
- Perineuriomas are benign tumors that track along a nerve segment and more commonly present with slowly progressive mononeuropathies or plexopathies with a predisposition to loss of motor function.
- When operating on symptomatic schwannomas, the surgical goal is gross total resection with preservation of neurologic function. Direct low-amplitude electrical stimulation of the parent nerve and tumor can be utilized to help achieve this goal.

Other benign lesions

Intrinsic mass—Intraneural ganglion cyst (cyst within the epineurium). Typically, this is found at the peroneal nerve near the fibular neck. It produces predominantly deep peroneal nerve palsy (foot drop and strong eversion). Electromyography (EMG) helps to localize the lesion. Imaging reveals a cystic lesion. A cyst is derived from a neighboring joint. (For the peroneal nerve, its origin is from the superior tibiofibular joint.) An intraneural ganglion cyst is formed by propagation along the articular branch with extension into the parent nerve (common peroneal nerve). Surgery is to disconnect the articular branch connection and decompress the cyst.

Extrinsic masses—May compress the neighboring nerve by mass effect. First, protect the nerve(s) and then remove the tumor. Examples include [extraneural] ganglion cysts and lipomas.

Malignant—Malignant peripheral nerve sheath tumor (MPNST). This may form spontaneously, occur following radiation, or occur in patients with neurofibromas and NF-1. Suspect malignancy in patients with increasing pain, neurologic deficit, and rapid tumor growth. After definitive diagnosis, wide resection is preferred by many surgeons, often combined with radiation to produce a 5-year survival of about 50%. Do not perform aggressive resection based on intraoperative histology.

Nerve imaging

Image nerves at unusual sites of compression (localized clinically, such as with percussion tenderness) to rule out undiagnosed mass lesion with high-resolution ultrasound (US) or MRI.

541

Options/Techniques in nerve injury

Neurolysis—Circumferential dissection of the nerve. Done as the first part of a procedure. If an nerve action potential (NAP) is obtained across a neuroma in continuity, neurolysis alone is performed. Ninety percent of patients obtain favorable outcome at long-term follow-up.

Nerve repair—Direct repair performed to approximate nerve ends after transection or after a focal neuroma is resected (in the setting of an absent NAP). Mobilize stumps to obtain end-to-end repair if possible without tension. Techniques to shorten the nerve gap include mobilization of nerve ends by freeing up proximally and distally; transposition of the nerve to make a straighter line (such as for ulnar or radial nerves); and flexion of the joint gently and immobilization postoperatively in that position if necessary for several weeks. Early repair facilitates direct repair. Align fascicles as best as possible. Several fascicular or epineurial sutures using microsurgical technique may be placed with 8-0 to 10-0 suture. Immobilize for 3 weeks postoperatively to protect the suture line. Results with nerve repair (one suture line) are better than with nerve grafting (two suture lines).

Nerve grafting—If a gap exists: after stump retraction (following delay in treatment of transection/rupture) or after resection of a more lengthy neuroma in continuity (absent NAP). Resect neuroma back to normal nerve ends and good fascicular structure. Estimate the gap between stumps. Estimate the number of cable grafts needed to fill the face of the nerve(s). Harvest an appropriate estimation of sural nerve from the leg. Be generous with the nerve harvest. Err on taking more. Nerve shrinks. Avoid tension in the repair. Sometimes you may need or want an extra cable graft. Make an incision in the posterolateral leg obliquely from ankle to popliteal fossa as necessary. The nerve is identified midway between the lateral malleolus and the lateral edge of the Achilles tendon next to the lesser saphenous vein. If necessary, 30–40 cm of sural nerve from each leg may be obtained. Donor morbidity: expected sensory loss in dorsolateral foot and possibility for neuropathic pain following harvest.

Techniques:
Option 1: Suture in each graft individually, proximally and distally.
Option 2: Use fibrin glue to form a cable of grouped grafts. Freshen up ends with a sharp knife, and suture cabled grafts as one unit. Immobilize for 3 weeks.

Nerve transfer—Transfer of an expendable or redundant nerve, nerve branch, or fascicle-to-nerve transfers. May be used in preganglionic (avulsion) injury where standard nerve grafting techniques cannot be performed. An example in a patient with a severe brachial plexus injury would include intercostal nerve transfers used to obtain elbow flexion in brachial plexus reconstruction (usually three intercostal nerves T3-T5 are transferred from the chest to the musculocutaneous nerve in the axilla) to try to regain elbow flexion. Because of encouraging results with nerve transfers, these techniques are being employed in patients with postganglionic injury as a substitute for nerve grafts (which could also be done). A new approach to an upper trunk (C5-C6) brachial plexus injury would be to transfer the distal portion of the spinal accessory nerve to the suprascapular nerve to try to regain some shoulder stability (abduction and external rotation) and transfer a fascicle of the ulnar nerve in the proximal arm directly to the biceps branch of the musculocutaneous nerve to try to regain elbow flexion. These types of nerve transfers done closer to the muscle end-organs speed and perhaps improve recovery.

INDEX